THE AUTOIMMUNE DISEASES II

THE AUTOIMMUNE DISEASES II

Edited by

NOEL R. ROSE

Department of Immunology and Infectious Diseases
The Johns Hopkins University
School of Hygiene and Public Health
Baltimore, Maryland

IAN R. MACKAY

Centre for Molecular Biology and Medicine
Monash University
Clayton, Victoria, Australia

ACADEMIC PRESS, INC.

Harcourt Brace Jovanovich, Publishers

San Diego New York Boston London Sydney Tokyo Toronto

This book is printed on acid-free paper. ♾

Academic Press, Inc.
1250 Sixth Avenue, San Diego, California 92101

United Kingdom Edition published by
Academic Press Limited
24–28 Oval Road, London NW1 7DX

Library of Congress Cataloging-in-Publication Data

The Autoimmune Diseases II / [editors], Noel R. Rose, Ian R. Mackay
p. cm.
Includes bibliographical references and index.
ISBN 0-12-596922-8
1. Autoimmune diseases. I. Rose, Noel R. II. Mackay, Ian R. III. Title: Autoimmune diseases 2. IV. Title: Autoimmune diseases two.
[DNLM: 1. Autoimmune Diseases. WD 305 A9377]
RC600.A832 1991
616.97'8--dc20
DNLM/DLC
for Library of Congress 91-31705
CIP

PRINTED IN THE UNITED STATES OF AMERICA
92 93 94 95 96 97 BB 9 8 7 6 5 4 3 2 1

Contents

6
Molecular Mimicry
Robert S. Fujinami

7
B-Cell Epitopes in Natural and Induced Autoimmunity
Robert L. Rubin and Eng M. Tan

8
Disease-Specific Autoantibodies in the Systemic Rheumatic Diseases
Morris Reichlin

9
Molecular Analysis of Cytoplasmic Autoantigens in Liver Disease
M. Eric Gershwin, Michael P. Manns, and Ian R. Mackay

10
Autoimmune Diabetes Mellitus
William Hagopian and Åke Lernmark

11
Autoimmune Vasculitis
J. Charles Jennette, Drew A. Jones, and Ronald J. Falk

14

Autoimmune Aspects of Ocular Disease

Barbara Detrick and John J. Hooks

15

Autoimmune Arthropathy: Rheumatoid Synovitis

Gary S. Firestein and Nathan J. Zvaifler

16
Principles of Therapeutic Approaches to Autoimmunity
Hartmut Wekerle and Reinhard Hohlfeld

17
Autoimmunity: Horizons
Ian R. Mackay and Noel R. Rose

Contributors

Numbers in parentheses indicate the pages on which the authors' contributions begin.

Claude C. A. Bernard (47), Neuroimmunology Laboratory, Brain-Behavior Research Institute, La Trobe University, Bundoora, Victoria 3083, Australia

C. Lynne Burek (303), Department of Immunology and Infectious Diseases, Johns Hopkins University School of Hygiene and Public Health, Baltimore, Maryland 21205

Patrick Concannon (127), Immunology and Diabetes Research Programs, Virginia Mason Research Center, Department of Immunology, University of Washington School of Medicine, Seattle, Washington 98101

Roger L. Dawkins (317), Department of Clinical Immunology, Royal Perth Hospital, Perth, Western Australia 6001, Australia

Barbara Detrick (345), Division of AIDS, Vaccine Research and Development Branch, National Institute of Allergy and Infectious Diseases, National Institutes of Health, Rockville, Maryland 20892

Ronald J. Falk (279), Division of Nephrology, Department of Medicine, University of North Carolina School of Medicine, Chapel Hill, North Carolina 27599

Gary S. Firestein (363), Division of Rheumatology, University of California, San Diego Medical Center, San Diego, California 92103

Robert S. Fujinami (153), Department of Neurology, University of Utah School of Medicine, Salt Lake City, Utah 84132

M. Eric Gershwin (213), Allergy and Clinical Immunology, Division of Rheumatology, School of Medicine, University of California at Davis, TB 192, Davis, California 95616

William Hagopian (235), Robert H. Williams Laboratory, Department of Medicine, University of Washington, Seattle, Washington 98195

Ahvie Herskowitz (303), Department of Medicine, Johns Hopkins University School of Medicine, Baltimore, Maryland 21205

Reinhard Hohlfeld (387), Max-Planck-Institut für Psychiatrie, Abteilung für Neuroimmunologie, Deutsche Forschungsanstalt für Psychiatrie, Am Klopferspitz 18A, D-8033 Planegg-Martinsried, Germany

Peter N. Hollingsworth (317), Department of Clinical Immunology, Royal Perth Hospital, Perth, Western Australia 6001, Australia

John J. Hooks (345), Immunology and Virology Section, National Eye Institute, National Institutes of Health, Bethesda, Maryland 20892

J. Charles Jennette (279), Department of Pathology, University of North Carolina School of Medicine, Chapel Hill, North Carolina 27599

Drew A. Jones (279), Department of Medicine, University of Iowa, Iowa City, Iowa 52242

Åke Lernmark (235), Robert H. Williams Laboratory, Department of Medicine, University of Washington, Seattle, Washington 98195

Ian R. Mackay (1, 47, 213, 409), Centre for Molecular Biology and Medicine, Monash University, Clayton, Victoria 3168, Australia

Tom E. Mandel (47), The Walter and Eliza Hall Institute, Parkville, Victoria 3050, Australia

Michael P. Manns (213), Department of Gastroenterology and Hepatology, Zentrum Innere Medizin und Dermatologie, Medizinische Hochschule Hannover, D-3000 Hannover 61, Germany

Gerald T. Nepom (127), Immunology and Diabetes Research Programs, Virginia Mason Research Center, Department of Immunology, University of Washington School of Medicine, Seattle, Washington 98101

David A. Neumann (303), Department of Immunology and Infectious Diseases, Johns Hopkins University School of Hygiene and Public Health, Baltimore, Maryland 21205

Gustav J. V. Nossal (27), The Walter and Eliza Hall Institute of Medical Research, Post Office, Royal Melbourne Hospital, Melbourne, Victoria 3050, Australia

Clara M. Pelfrey (107), Cellular Immunology Section, Arthritis and Rheumatism Branch, National Institute of Arthritis and Musculoskeletal and Skin Diseases, National Institutes of Health, Bethesda, Maryland 20892

Morris Reichlin (195), Arthritis/Immunology Program, Oklahoma Medical Research Foundation, Department of Medicine, Oklahoma University Health Sciences Center, Oklahoma City, Oklahoma 73104

Noel R. Rose (1, 303, 409), Department of Immunology and Infectious Diseases, The Johns Hopkins University, School of Hygiene and Public Health, Baltimore, Maryland 21205

Robert L. Rubin (173), W. M. Keck Autoimmune Disease Center, Department of Molecular & Experimental Medicine, The Scripps Research Institute, La Jolla, California 92037

Alfred D. Steinberg (107), Cellular Immunology Section, Arthritis and Rheumatism Branch, National Institute of Arthritis and Musculoskeletal and Skin Diseases, National Institutes of Health, Bethesda, Maryland 20892

Eng M. Tan (173), W. M. Keck Autoimmune Disease Center, Department of Molecular & Experimental Medicine, The Scripps Research Institute, La Jolla, California 92037

Ranjeny Thomas (317), Department of Rheumatology, University of Texas, Southwestern Medical Center, Dallas, Texas

Hartmut Wekerle (387), Max-Planck-Institut für Psychiatrie, Abteilung für Neuroimmunologie, Deutsche Forschungsanstalt für Psychiatrie, Am Klopferspitz 18A, D-8033 Planegg-Martinsried, Germany

Nathan J. Zvaifler (363), Division of Rheumatology, University of California, San Diego Medical Center, San Diego, California 92103

Preface

The cordial reception accorded *The Autoimmune Diseases* indicated the need that existed for a book concentrating on the basic principles of self/nonself discrimination and the practical problems encountered in the diagnosis and treatment of an important group of human diseases. Since the first edition was published in 1985, further great strides have been made in the understanding of fundamental mechanisms and in the treatment of autoimmune diseases.

When the time was ripe for a second edition, we faced a dilemma. If all of the information in the first edition were to be combined with the pertinent newer knowledge, the resulting book would have become very unwieldy. For this reason, we decided to follow a different approach. Most of the original chapters were still valid, with some perhaps in need of updating, whereas the information in certain other areas had virtually exploded with new data and insights. Hence the decision was made to advise the readers of the new book to consult the first edition for information that had remained relatively unchanged, and to refer to this new volume, *The Autoimmune Diseases II,* for knowledge gained in the past six years.

The introductory chapter by the editors gives an account merging the historical and the contemporary study of autoimmunity and autoimmune disease. Gustav Nossal then reports on the current understanding of mechanisms of tolerance, and Claude Bernard and co-workers as well as Clara Pelfrey and Alfred Steinberg describe the newer lessons learned from experimental models. Two topics, molecular genetics and molecular mimicry as related to autoimmunity, have progressed greatly since the first volume was published. Gerald Nepom and Patrick Concannon, and Robert Fujinami discuss these advances. The introduction of new and more refined methods derived from molecular biology allows for the analyses of disease-specific antigenic determinants, with promise for great improvements in the diagnosis of autoimmune diseases. Chapters by Morris Reichlin, by Eric Gershwin and associates, and by Robert Rubin and Eng Tan describe these important developments in diagnostic methodology.

Subsequent chapters review in detail those autoimmune diseases in which quite significant progress has been made. They include diabetes mellitus by

William Hagopian and Åke Lernmark, vasculitis by Charles Jennette and colleagues, myocarditis by Noel Rose and colleagues, myositis by Peter Hollingsworth and colleagues, ocular disease by Barbara Detrick and John Hooks, and rheumatoid arthritis by Gary Firestein and Nathan Zvaifler.

Nothing has created more excitement in the realm of autoimmune diseases than the possibility that antigen-specific therapy may become feasible. Expectations of this sort are discussed in the chapter by Hartmut Wekerle and Reinhard Hohlfeld.

A new feature for *The Autoimmune Diseases II* is a brief and friendly comment by the editors on the subject matter of various of the chapters.

Finally, in "Horizons," the editors have presented some viewpoints of their own, looked in some dark corners for glimmers of light, and have even permitted themselves to make a few daring predictions. They have no doubt that the stage is set for a new and even more dramatic period of growth in the study of the autoimmune diseases.

The editors are deeply grateful to Hermine Bongers for her expert editorial assistance, and to Charles Arthur and Gayle Early of Academic Press for overseeing the publication process.

CHAPTER 1

The Immune Response in Autoimmunity and Autoimmune Disease

NOEL R. ROSE
Department of Immunology and Infectious Diseases
The Johns Hopkins University
School of Hygiene and Public Health
Baltimore, Maryland

IAN R. MACKAY
Centre for Molecular Biology and Medicine
Monash University
Clayton, Victoria, Australia

I. IMMUNOLOGIC RECOGNITION

The immune system of the host responds to foreign molecules while avoiding reactions against molecules (self-antigens) of the host itself. This ability to discriminate self from nonself, otherwise expressed as self-tolerance, is a fundamental property of the immune system. The intrinsic immunogenicity of self-antigens is obvious from the fact that they readily elicit an immune response when injected into a foreign species. It was known from Ehrlich's experiments at the turn of the century that the injection of foreign or allogeneic erythrocytes into goats would elicit an immune response, whereas the goat's own erythrocytes never did so (Mackay and Burnet, 1963). However, self/nonself discrimination is not absolute, nor would this be expected, given the molecular similarities between self and foreign molecules. Indeed, background or "natural" autoantibodies are well recognized and have even been assigned a physiologic role (Grabar, 1975); hence, regulatory mechanisms must exist to prevent "natural" autoimmunity from assuming pathogenic potential.

In this introductory chapter, we shall review some basic issues on the modes of emergence of autoimmunity, notwithstanding the various mechanisms designed to discourage it, and reasons that autoimmunity occasionally does have pathogenic consequences resulting in autoimmune disease.

The immune system recognizes molecules invading the host by availing itself of three different types of recognition structures: immunoglobulin (Ig) receptors, T-lymphocyte cell receptors (TcRs), and cell-surface products of class I or class II major histocompatibility complex (MHC) genes (Paul, 1989). The first two types of recognition structures are expressed only on B or T lymphocytes, while the class I MHC products are present on the surface of all nucleated cells of the body. Furthermore, Igs and TcRs are clonally distributed (i.e., each mature lymphocyte expresses a unique Ig molecule or TcR), whereas all cells of the body express the same class I MHC gene products. Class II MHC gene products are prominently expressed on cells that take up, process, and present antigen.

The generation of an immune response requires a sufficiently large repertoire of lymphocyte recognition structures so that any foreign antigenic epitope will find a complementary receptor. According to Burnet's clonal selection theory, an antigenic determinant selects its corresponding lymphocyte by binding to its Ig or TcR recognition structure and, in so doing, provides a proliferative stimulus resulting in a clone of cells, each bearing the same receptor (Burnet, 1959).

Lymphocytes bearing the Ig receptor are members of the B-cell lineage (Kincade and Gimble, 1989) and originate from a bone marrow stem cell under the direction of a particular mixture of the various colony-stimulating factors (CSFs) and interleukins (ILs) (Kincade *et al.*, 1989). The development from a precursor into a mature functional B cell is accompanied by programmed rearrangement and random assortment of the Ig-controlling genes (Perlmutter, 1989). Mature B cells secrete Ig molecules as antibodies of the corresponding specificity. A different diversity of Ig specificities derives from the N-terminal variable (V) portion of the molecule, especially the hypervariable or complementarity-determining regions (CDRs). The specificity as well as affinity of antibody binding depends on the amino acid sequences of these particular regions. The antibody molecule contains two types of polypeptide chains, light chains and heavy chains, which associate to form the functional molecule. The combining site (which relates to the unique idiotype) is derived from the V regions of the light and heavy chains. One constant (C) domain of the light chain and three or four C domains (of about 100 amino acids each) of the heavy chain make up the Fc region. This portion of the Ig molecule determines the isotype or class (M, G, A, E, or D) and subclass (G_1, G_2, G_3, G_4; S_1, S_2), on which depend many of its biological properties. The heavy and light chains of the Igs are each encoded by multiple genes that are physically separated on the chromosomes but are brought together to form a single compound gene. The V portions of the light chain are constructed from a V gene (encoding 95 amino acids) and a J gene (12 amino acids). The V domain of the heavy chain is created by combination of a V gene, J gene, and D gene. Since any one of several hundred V genes can combine with any of 4 to 6 J genes (and any of several D genes), the number of possible V regions is quite large. Diversity is further augmented by the association of different light chains and heavy chains.

Additional diversity is subsequently acquired because the V genes are themselves highly mutable and, in undergoing frequent somatic mutations, give rise to new specificities. These are generally beneficial, but some somatic mutations among V genes appear relevant to the acquisition of autoimmune specificities that may not be represented as such in the germ-line genes, perhaps as a result of evolutionary elimination (Mamula *et al.,* 1990). There is then no problem in envisioning a sufficient number of Ig receptors, $>10^6$, required to recognize any possible antigenic determinant, whether as a linear peptide sequence or a three-dimensional conformational configuration. The stages of development of B cells at which distinctions are made between antigenic determinants of self and non-self, and how this is effected, is discussed later in this chapter and by Nossal in Chapter 2 of this volume. However, we can note that even in health, a proportion of mature B cells is capable of binding self-antigens, albeit perhaps by a low-affinity IgM receptor (Roberts *et al.,* 1973).

The binding of its complementary antigenic determinant is an essential step for the B cell in the process of proliferation and differentiation. This process usually requires hormonelike factors, the ILs, supplied by accessory cells and cooperating (helper) T cells (Kincade *et al.,* 1989). Thc affinity of Ig for its antigenic determinant increases during the response, probably because somatically mutated B cells with a higher degree of affinity for antigen are favored.

T cells develop from the bone marrow stem cells as do B cells, probably under the direction of a slightly different mixture of CSFs (Sprent, 1989). However, T cells need to undergo an additional stage of maturation in the thymus, where products of the thymic stromal cells induce expression of TcR genes as well as CD4 or CD8 auxiliary surface markers. The TcR is a disulfide-linked heterodimer composed of α and β polypeptide chains. A minority of the T-cell population express TcRs consisting of γ and δ chains. The genes that encode the TcR chain show a striking homology to the V and C genes of the Ig molecule and so belong to the Ig supergene family. The genetic mechanisms that provide the necessary diversity of antigen-binding recognition structures are similar for T and B cells.

Although phylogenetically related to Ig molecules, the TcR gene products have quite distinctive recognition properties. T cells, unlike B cells, do not recognize antigenic determinants by their spatial configurations but actually "see" only short peptide sequences of the antigen, up to 10 or 12 amino acid residues. However, these must be recognized by the TcR in a dimensional pattern of which the antigenic peptide is just one component; TcR recognition requires joint presentation of the peptide sequence in the context of the cell-surface product of an MHC gene, class I or class II (Marrack and Kappler, 1987; Sinha *et al.*, 1990).

As stated above, TcR diversity is generated by processes of genetic rearrangement and reassortment similar to those regulating the formation of the Ig receptor. The complex processes that shape the T-cell repertoire are referred to in Chapters 2, 3, and 4 and discussed in the final Chapter 17. Somatic mutation does not seem to occur in mature lymphocytes of the T-cell lineage. After the T cells leave the thymus, therefore, they are incapable of changing the specificity of their antigen recognition. Hence if TcRs directed to self-antigens were to be totally eliminated in the thymus, they would not be regenerated in peripheral sites by somatic mutation of T-cell receptor genes.

When confronted by a congruent class II MHC product on an antigen-presenting cell, together with the appropriate antigenic fragment, the CD4+ T cell enters a reproductive cycle. Its reproduction is supported by the elaboration of growth factors, also members of the interleukin family, and the concurrent expression by the activated T cell of receptors for the ILs, particularly IL-2.

Class I MHC gene products are expressed on virtually all cells of the body and are the primary targets of CD8+ T cell-mediated cytotoxicity, such as seen in responses to viral, transplantation, or tumor antigens. Class II MHC products, on the other hand, are expressed mainly on antigen-presenting cells, including macrophages, dendritic cells, and B lymphocytes. Since the MHC locus is highly polymorphic, each individual is likely to differ in MHC phenotype. The MHC constitution of the antigen-presenting cell determines the ability of the CD4+ T cell to recognize a particular antigenic determinant; therefore, MHC class II genes act as immunoregulatory genes.

One function of the antigen-presenting cell is to prepare an antigenic molecule for T-cell recognition. The process involves hydrolytic cleavage of the antigenic protein into small peptide fragments, which then bind to the class II MHC receptor and are transported on the surface of the antigen-presenting cell. Antigen-presenting cells also secrete ILs that provide a "second" signal in concert with the antigenic signal to initiate T-cell proliferation (Weaver and Unanue, 1990; Dighiero *et al.*, 1986). The antigenic signal in the absence of the second signal is thought to be tolerogenic rather than immunogenic.

II. NORMAL SELF/NONSELF DISCRIMINATION AND TOLERANCE

A. B-Lymphocyte Tolerance

In general, B cells are capable of recognizing many self-antigens, as judged by the frequency of "natural" autoantibodies among the immunoglobulin molecules of normal individuals. On stimulation with a polyclonal activator like bacterial lipopolysaccharide, a high proportion of B cells produce autoantibodies to particular structures. These include cytoskeletal elements including laminin, vimentin, actin, and myosin; nuclear elements including single-stranded DNA; and even circulating proteins, e.g., thyroglobulin (Underwood *et al.*, 1985). Furthermore, B-cell hybridomas formed by fusion of B cells of normal mice (or normal humans) with plasmacytoma cells frequently produce monoclonal antibodies to self-antigens (Underwood *et al.*, 1985; Notkins and Prabhakar, 1986). The demonstration of naturally occurring autoantibodies in the sera of normal individuals indicates that B cells responsive to many self-antigens can persist under certain physiological conditions of the body. The fact that a pathological autoantibody response by self-reactive B cells does not occur under normal conditions could be because of the lack of appropriate T-cell help, or to regulatory effects that include antiidiotypic responses and suppressor influences (see Chapter 2 in this volume.

B. T-Lymphocyte Tolerance

The classic experiments of Billingham *et al.* in 1953 showed that tolerance is an acquired, not an innate property. The first suggestion by Burnet (1959) was that tolerance depended on clonal deletion of self-reactive cells, possibly in the thymus: exposure of immature cells to their corresponding antigen would result in their complete elimination. Direct evidence supporting this concept has become available only recently. The thymus receives from the bone marrow immigrant T-cell precursors with the genetic capacity for expressing TcRs for any antigenic determinant; the thymus exports only those T cells capable of responding to nonself-determinants. Therefore, positive and negative selective processes must take place in the thymus during T-cell maturation. T cells capable of recognizing MHC class II molecules in conjunction with a foreign antigenic determinant are favored, whereas T cells recognizing self-determinants are effectively eliminated. In fact, only a small proportion of precursor cells entering the thymus leave as mature T cells (Scollay and Shortman, 1985). The remainder of the precursor proportion is probably "programmed" for death by cell-suicide, referred to as apoptosis.

C. Selection Processes in the Thymus

An initial stage of positive selection, favoring T cells recognizing self-MHC molecules, probably only with low or intermediate affinities, occurs in the thymic cortex. Encountering thymic epidermal stromal cells that present the host's MHC molecule, such immature T cells remain viable and even proliferate, whereas all other T cells undergo apoptosis (Sha *et al.*, 1988). Thus only T cells that can recognize self-MHC continue the process of differentiation. In the thymic medulla, the maturing T cells may encounter self-antigens presented by bone-marrow-derived dendritic cells in conjunction with autologous MHC class II molecules. If a *positively selected* T cell reacts to high affinity with self-MHC, or with self-peptide/self-MHC complexes, it is eliminated (Adorini, 1990). This negative selection process can of course apply only to self-peptides that are represented in the medulla of the thymus. This would include self-MHC and other prominent cell-surface molecules, as well as autologous constituents transported by the blood to the thymic medulla. Many organ-specific and intracellular molecules would not get the opportunity to act as "deletogens."

D. Superantigens

The result of positive and negative selective processes is that only T cells that recognize foreign peptides in conjunction with self-MHC determinants survive. It has been difficult to document these dual processes because the number of T cells responsive to any particular peptide fragment is very small. However, a high proportion of T cells from nonimmunized mice respond to a few exceptional molecules referred to as superantigens. The minor lymphocyte-stimulating (Mls) alloantigen of the mouse, in conjunction with the appropriate MHC molecule, stimulates a significant portion of T cells. Moreover, most T cells recognizing the Mls determinant utilize a particular family of V genes, that is, genes coding for the variable combining portion of the TcR. Monoclonal antibodies specific for this V-gene family ($V_\beta 8.1$) provide a means for enumerating T cells with this particular specificity without depending on stimulation by the respective Mls antigen. Direct examination using labeled antibodies in mice has shown that many T cells with $V_\beta 8.1$ enter the thymic cortex, but most are eliminated when the T cells migrate to the medulla; consequently, they are not found in peripheral blood or lymphoid organs (Kappler *et al.*, 1988). Similar experiments have shown deletion of T cells specific for the class II MHC molecule I-E, for the MHC-like determinant on male cells, H-Y, and for superantigens, such as staphylococcal enterotoxin, which stimulate a large proportion of T cells (Kappler *et al.*, 1987; Kappler *et al.*, 1989). The effect of superantigens on the T-cell repertoire is discussed in Chapter 17.

E. Thymic Deletion—Lack of Interleukins?

The question arises why contact between a committed T cell and self-peptide/self-MHC in the thymus should result in clonal deletion, whereas a similar encounter in peripheral sites produces clonal proliferation. Evidence suggests that auxiliary growth factors, ILs, are required for the clonal proliferation in peripheral sites. The requisite ILs may not be available in the thymus and cannot save the self-reactive T cells from antigen-induced suicide.

F. Escape from Deletion

The central process of clonal deletion probably operates for potent and accessible self-antigens. Central (thymic) clonal deletion would not occur with antigens that are absent from the thymus or present only in small amounts. Organ-specific antigens, thyroglobulin for example, are probably not available in the thymus in significant amounts at any time during embryonic or later life. One can expect, therefore, that negative selection of T cells responsive with such self-antigens is either ineffective or lacking. The demonstration of T cells responsive to autologous thyroglobuiin, described above, accords with this prediction. Therefore, a search for risk factors for autoimmunity may have to go back to the processes that dictate repertoire generation in the thymus.

As described above, T cells reactive with certain major self-antigens are generally deleted during their maturation in the thymus by lethal contact with antigen plus MHC, but there is cogent evidence that all autoreactive T cells are not eliminated. As one line of evidence, there are the many examples of experimentally induced autoimmunity in which an organ-specific antigen, administered with a potent adjuvant, induces an experimental autoimmune disease. These examples include experimental autoimmune encephalomyelitis (EAE), thyroiditis (EAT), myasthenia gravis (EAMG), orchitis (EAO), each of which results from immunization with autologous or cross-reactive allogeneic or xenogeneic antigen (Rose, 1979) (and see Chapter 3 in this volume). In each case the autoimmune disease is T-cell dependent, since removal of T cells by neonatal thymectomy or treatment with specific monoclonal antibody to helper CD4+ T cells prevents their development (Vladutiu and Rose, 1975). The inducibility of these diseases means that a responsive autoimmune T-cell population must preexist, and can be called into action by an appropriate immunization procedure.

G. Checks on Breaking of Tolerance

We may well ask why self-destructive T-cell responses do not occur more often. The reasons may be that (1) the requisite antigen is sequestered and, therefore, not available in sufficient amounts to activate T cells; (2) antigen-presenting cells are unable to process and present self-antigens in an immunogenic form; (3) T cells are made unresponsive by particular concentrations of self-antigens; (4) T-cell responses become actively suppressed, nonspecifically or specifically; and (5) after antigenic contact, T cells do not receive a required second signal from a factor released by the antigen-presenting cell (Weaver and Unanue, 1990) and are thereby rendered anergic. As a further explanation, we suggest that T-cell tolerance is a quantitative phenomenon and that under normal circumstances only high-avidity T cells to self-antigens are likely to be eliminated during thymic maturation (Ada and Rose, 1988; Gammon and Sercarz, 1990). The low-avidity

T cells remaining at peripheral sites would be capable of reacting with a self-antigen only if it were presented in a sufficiently potent form, for example with an adjuvant.

H. Tolerance and Antigen-Presenting Cells

Does self-tolerance reside in the antigen-presenting cell? The ability of antigen-presenting cells to handle a number of self-antigens has been investigated. Some autologous antigens, including lysozyme and cytochrome c, bind to class II MHC products as effectively as do equivalent foreign molecules (Babbitt *et al.*, 1986; Lakey *et al.*, 1986), and would presumably be recognized by the corresponding T cells, if they were present. An even more convincing experiment has been reported in mice genetically lacking the circulating complement component C5. Transgenic mice given the gene for this complement component are able to process and to present the antigen to competent T cells in conjunction with syngeneic class II molecules (Liu and Stockinger, 1989). Therefore, all of the machinery necessary for antigen processing and presentation of many self-antigens is intact.

I. Peripheral Tolerance and Clonal Anergy

In view of experimental evidence that the cell populations required to generate an immune response to many self-antigens are normally not deleted, other mechanisms of self-tolerance must be considered. A critical requirement for the development of autoimmune disease is the proliferation of helper CD4+ T cells. These cells are capable of responding to fragments of antigen only when presented in conjunction with syngeneic class II MHC determinants. Helper T cells then induce the production of high-affinity autoantibodies by B cells, and facilitate the generation of cytotoxic CD8 T cells.

Given that not all self-reactive cells will be deleted intrathymically, additional peripheral mechanisms must operate to effect functional inactivation of self-reactive T and B cells. Among the several mechanisms suggested for peripheral immunoregulation are clonal anergy and active suppression.

The concept of anergy, developed by Nossal and Pike (1980) (see Chapter 2 in this volume) and initially applied to B cells, also applies to T cells (Adelstein *et al.*, 1991; Qin *et al.*, 1989; Rammensee *et al.*, 1989). The implication is that lymphocytes reactive with tolerated antigens are not physically deleted from the lymphocyte repertoire *in vivo*. In other words, lymphocytes capable of binding self-antigen are present, but incapable of proliferation in response to that antigen. The most striking evidence for the importance of anergy of peripheral lymphocytes has come from experiments using transgenic mice (Adelstein *et al.*, 1991).

When genes coding for an exogenous antigen, such as hen egg lysozyme, are inserted into the murine genome, the transgenic mice are incapable of responding to this otherwise exogenous antigen, because the antigen is present during embryogenesis and therefore is regarded as self. B cells capable of binding lysozyme can still be demonstrated in the peripheral lymphocyte population, but fail to proliferate. However, these B cells can undergo at least limited proliferation, if large quantities of ILs are added to the culture medium. These findings suggest that clonal anergy is not attributable to a failure of antigen recognition by the B cell; the anergic B cells recognize antigen but respond feebly or not at all, perhaps because they require supernormal amounts of auxiliary growth factors (Adams *et al.*, 1990). The question of peripheral T-cell anergy is readdressed later in this chapter, in Chapter 2, and in Chapter 17.

J. Suppression

When stimulated by their appropriate antigen, T lymphocytes undergo a process of repeated cell division that, if unchecked, could be disastrous. There must be means, therefore, of regulating immune responses, just as other physiological reactions of the body are controlled. These regulatory mechanisms can be grouped under the general heading of active suppression. A number of non-antigen-specific factors are capable of arresting the proliferation of T-cell clones (Peavy and Pierce, 1974). Certain mitogens, including concanavalin A, appear capable of initiating the production of suppressor factors by T lymphocytes (Dutton, 1972). In addition, specialized populations of T cells produce peptides that actively suppress T-cell proliferation. In general, these suppressor factors are produced by CD8+ T cells, and they act directly on CD4+ helper T cells (Jensen and Kapp, 1985). Some investigators suggest that antigen-specific CD4+ T cells serve as inducers of the CD8+ suppressor/effector cells. One idea is that elaborate suppressor circuits develop in which antigen-specific inducer T cells produce a factor that acts on suppressor-effector T cells to generate nonspecific suppressor factors that act, in turn, on the inducer (Eardley *et al.*, 1978). The concept remains controversial because the critical suppressor/effector T cell cannot be unequivocally identified.

Various types of suppressor T cells have been described. One type of suppressor T cell, which is antigen-specific at the effector level, is stimulated by the corresponding antigenic determinant (Green *et al.*, 1983); whether these are MHC-restricted, secrete cytokines, or display memory is uncertain. Another type of antigen-specific suppressor T cell is referred to as antiidiotypic; this type reacts with the variable portion of a particular TcR and thus can inactivate a specific population of T cells. Does this type of suppressor T cell see a T-cell receptor peptide in the context of MHC class II, and react with it in that context? Are there two types of suppressor factors, idiotypic and antiidiotypic, that bind, respectively, antigen or the antigen-specific T cell? Then there are types of suppressor T cells that are non-antigen-specific at the effector level; these appear to be activated after virus infections, e.g., measles, ultraviolet irradiation, and other stimuli. There is also the claimed existence of suppressor-inducer cells that have the naive phenotype, CD4,CD45RA (Sleasman *et al.*, 1991). Until answers are available on phenotype-functional relationships of putative suppressor T cells, the concept of immune suppression will remain controversial.

It is our view, in light of the evidence that all self-reactive T cells are not centrally deleted in the thymus, that peripheral immunoregulation must be important for maintaining self-tolerance under normal conditions. Several years ago, we proposed the concept of clonal balance (Rose *et al.*, 1981). It suggests that the totality of factors that stimulate the proliferation of helper T cells is closely balanced by other factors, specific and nonspecific, that impede T-cell proliferation. A small shift in this balance in one direction or the other is responsible for positive or negative responses to administration of antigen. The clonal-balance concept suggests that T cells reactive with self-antigens are normally held in a slight or pronounced negative balance. We are impressed by studies over the past 10 years that neonatal thymectomy can induce autoimmunity by removal of a suppressor population (see Chapter 3 in this volume), presumably because putative suppressor T cells generally receive a small *headstart* in thymic development. However, thymic development may be genetically abnormal, and animals with such genetic defects become deficient in their immunoregulation and might be expected to develop a number of autoimmune responses, similar to those seen in obese strain (OS) chickens or New Zealand mice. There is a reduction with aging in T cells that, by shifting the balance in favor of helper T cells, increases the prevalence of autoimmune responses in the aged (Calkins and Stutman, 1978). Postnatal thymectomy and cyclosporine treatment preferentially reduce the suppressor population at the expense of the previously peripheralized helper population and, therefore, a variety of autoimmune responses follow (Sakaguchi and Rose, 1988), as discussed in Chapter 3 in this volume. Limited doses of irradiation and cyclophosphamide have similar effects (Spellman and Daynes, 1978). The clonal-balance concept suggests that even a small shift in the helper : suppressor ratio may lead to autoimmunity, given other facilitating conditions. We must re-emphasize the limitation of this concept: so far, an identifiable population of antigen-specific suppressor T cells with distinctive phenotypic markers has not been identified in humans or in any other species.

III. AUTOIMMUNITY: FAILURE OF SELF-TOLERANCE

In spite of the elaborate strategies adopted by the body to maintain tolerance to self, autoimmunity is an ever-present hazard. We see no reason that an autoimmune response should not follow the same rules as a response to an extrinsic agent and, if this were the case, we should consider inductive and effector processes, acknowledging that in the established response, these will be occurring concurrently.

A. Inductive Mechanisms: Antigen-Related

These are listed in Table I, and the number suggests that no single mechanism will account for all instances of autoimmunity. Three general requirements, however, prevail: (1) self-reactive T cells and B cells remain in the immunological repertoire; (2) the cognate self-antigen is accessible; and (3) the antigen is processed and presented to helper T cells in conjunction with an MHC class II molecule by a competent antigen-presenting cell.

1. Sequestered Antigen

The most straightforward method of initiating autoimmunity occurs after the introduction of a constituent of the body that is normally sequestered from the immune system so that self-tolerance cannot develop. Such isolated components may be antigenic without any special manipulation, and do not require admixture with an adjuvant. The two most likely examples are antigens of sperm and lens. Injection of sperm induces the production of sperm-specific autoantibodies, even in the same species (Rose, 1974). Interestingly, these antibodies are generally not associated with any discernible disease, unless the original injection is given with an adjuvant (Freund *et al.*, 1953). The adjuvant may dictate the antibody class, favoring a complement-fixing isotype, to permit antibody and complement to penetrate the testis more readily, or may induce a persisting (unregulated) cell-

TABLE I
Inductive Mechanisms in Autoimmunity

Antigen-Related
Sequestered antigen
Molecular mimicry
Altered self-antigen
Self-antigen plus foreign determinant
Surrogate self-antigens—antiidotypic antibodies
Tumor autoantigens
APC-related
Self-antigen plus increased MHC class II expression
Tolerance—regulation-related
Nondeletion of anti-self specificities
Decreased suppression
Polyclonal activation
Failure of antiidiotypic control
Failure of peripheral tolerance

mediated immunity. These considerations emphasize the dichotomy between the autoimmune response itself (frequently harmless) and the occurrence of autoimmune disease.

In humans, vasectomy increases the levels of naturally occurring sperm antibody in 50 to 80% of subjects (Rose *et al.*, 1980). Vasectomy does not impair spermatogenesis, but blocks the exodus of mature spermatozoa through the vas deferens (Samuel and Rose, 1980). Sperm antigens, therefore, are continuously absorbed by the body. Following vasectomy, there is a striking accumulation of macrophages around the vas, sometimes accompanied by granuloma formation. This inflammatory infiltrate suggests that antigen is being taken up and processed. The spermatic antigen (or antigens) responsible for postvasectomy autoantibody production has not yet been characterized, but it is clear that native antigen is capable of inducing autoimmunity. Men who develop high titers of sperm antibody after vasectomy do not suffer from orchitis or aspermatogenesis, showing that the antibodies have no effect *in situ*. On the other hand, the relatively low fertility rate of men who have undergone surgical reversal of their vasectomy in order to restore fertility indicates that the antibodies to sperm are able to interfere with the competence of sperm exposed to antibody during its passage through the spermatic ducts (Thomas *et al.*, 1981).

2. Molecular Mimicry

The second mechanism for induction of autoimmunity is molecular mimicry, meaning the sharing of antigenic determinants between the host and some exogenous agent, usually an infecting microorganism. This concept is described in detail in Chapter 6 of this volume. A classic instance of molecular mimicry is poststreptococcal rheumatic fever. Epidemiologic and clinical evidence associates infection with β-hemolytic streptococci with the development of acute rheumatic fever, and repeated streptococcal infections are clearly associated with chronic carditis and rheumatic valvular disease (Stollerman, 1975). Experimentally, injection of rabbits with streptococcal suspensions induces antibodies that react with heart muscle (Zabriskie and Freimer, 1966). The antigen responsible for this cross-reaction has been identified with cardiac myosin, but it is not known whether the responsible antigen is present on all β-hemolytic streptococci or only certain rheumatogenic strains (Dale and Beachey, 1985). As a discordant note, it has not been possible to induce the characteristic pathological changes of rheumatic fever by immunization of animals with streptococci.

In recent years, there have been many other instances cited of possible molecular mimicry. Much of the evidence is based on the demonstration of closely similar but usually rather short amino acid sequences in polypeptides of microorganisms and bodily constituents. In only very few instances, however, has it been possible to induce an autoimmune response with the shared antigen. Hepatitis B virus polymerase has a 10-amino-acid sequence that is virtually identical with a peptide of myelin basic protein. Injection of this amino acid sequence into rabbits induces a disease resembling autoimmune encephalomyelitis (Fujinami and Oldstone, 1985). However, it is difficult to see the relevance of this to any spontaneous disease, since brain disease does not occur with hepatitis virus infection.

Heat-shock proteins (HSP) are highly conserved peptides found on prokaryotic as well as eukaryotic cells, and HSP from mycobacteria are capable of inducing antibody to mouse HSP (Kaufmann *et al.*, 1989). Great interest has been created by the observation that T cells from rats with adjuvant arthritis respond to a mycobacterial HSP of molecular mass 65 kDa, suggesting that rheumatoid arthritis may be the result of an autoimmune response instigated by the HSP from a microorganism (van Eden *et al.*, 1988) (see Chapter 3 in this volume). However, there is no evidence that patients with rheumatoid arthritis are abnormally responsive to the 65-kDa HSP. Despite the current enthusiasm for a role of HSP in the initiation of a range of autoimmune diseases (van Eden, 1990; Lamb and Young, 1990; Winfield, 1989; Kaufmann, 1990), we are uncommitted to this idea.

Molecular mimicry requires that presentation of an epitope differing only slightly from self is capable of initiating an immunologic response. That initial step depends on the *antigenic distance* between the exogenous and the endogenous antigenic determinants. A foreign determinant identical to self-antigens should not normally be immunogenic, whereas one that differs greatly from self would fail to give rise to an autoimmune (antiself) response. In order for the immune response to result in autoimmune disease, the antigenic distance should be slight, and the immune response should undergo *maturation* by somatic mutation, since a self-perpetuating cycle is probably required; that is, endogenous antigen must reinforce the initial response to the closely related foreign antigen. The absence of this second step may account for the difficulty experienced when an attempt is made experimentally to produce an autoimmune disease by the injection of a cross-reactive antigen. In addition, there is mounting evidence that autoimmune B cells see complex conformational epitopes rather than short linear epitopes (see Chapters 7 and 17 in this volume). Thus, molecular mimicry may have become *overstretched* as a general explanation of autoimmune responses. It will be noted that the discussions above have concerned antibody. It may be that molecular mimicry operates more effectively at the level of T-cell responses, a question requiring further investigation.

3. Altered Self-Antigens

An altered self-antigen may be misperceived by the body as a foreign entity. It is, for example, quite easy to show that heat-denatured albumin is antigenic in the host. Often antibodies to the denatured protein, however, do not react with the unaltered native albumin. Papain-treated red blood cells injected into the original donor mouse induce production of antibody directed only to the treated red blood cells, and fail to induce a hemolytic anemia by acting on the host's unaltered erythrocytes (Eyquem and Crepin, 1956). On the other hand, only minor changes in protein structure or amino acid sequence will permit antibodies or T cells reactive with denatured self-antigens to interact with the native counterpart. Papain-treated rabbit thyroglobulin injected without adjuvant into rabbits can induce both autoantibody production and transient thyroiditis, indicating that the immune response to the altered antigen can under some circumstances act effectively on native antigen *in situ* (Anderson and Rose, 1971).

Sometimes physiologic changes occurring in self-antigens are sufficient to induce an autoimmune response. When it reacts with its respective antigen, an antibody molecule undergoes a conformational change (Milgrom and Witebsky, 1960). Antibodies to changed Fc, called rheumatoid factors, can be shown to combine *in vitro* with immunoglobulin fixed to a solid surface. In rare cases, aggregates composed of rheumatoid factor and immunoglobulin occur in the body, suggesting that the rheumatoid factor is able to combine with unaltered immunoglobulin *in vivo* (Kunkel *et al.*, 1960).

Self-antigens may be altered through the action of exogenous chemicals and drugs. The hepatitis that follows the use of halothane anesthesia in some individuals, for example, has been attributed to an autoimmune reaction, although no convincingly objective evidence of autoimmunity has yet been published. Liver damage induced in mice by carbon tetrachloride has been studied to ascertain whether the chemical triggered an autoimmune response in genetically susceptible strains (Bhatal *et al.*, 1983; Beisel *et al.*, 1984). Mice differed greatly in their response to carbon tetrachloride injections, with some strains showing relatively little injury, whereas others developed active disease. Autoantibodies to liver antigens were sometimes present.

Certain infections are known to initiate autoimmune responses, which may contribute to the total picture of disease. Our investigations on myocarditis induced by Coxsackie B3 (CB3) exemplify autoimmunity due to infection (Rose *et al.*, 1987) (see Chapter 12 of this volume). After CB_3 infection, certain strains of mice developed an active myocarditis accompanied by heart-specific autoantibodies. The autoantigen involved was identified as the heavy chain of cardiac myosin (Neu *et al.*, 1987a). Using purified cardiac heavy chain as immunogen, the characteristic picture of myocarditis was produced in selected strains of mice. Since no antigenic cross-reaction between heart and Coxsackie virus could be detected, it was suggested (Neu *et al.*, 1987b) that the role of the virus is to alter and expose endogenous myosin as well as to provide local inflammation (Neu *et al.*, 1987b). These experiments are cited in more detail in Chapter 12 of this volume.

4. Self-Antigen Plus Foreign Determinant

There are several examples of self-constituents being rendered autoantigenic by addition of haptenic groups. In classic experiments by Weigle and his colleagues, rabbit thyroglobulin modified by sulfonilic and arsenilic substituents proved to be antigenic in rabbits (Weigle, 1965). Similar mechanisms may prevail in some of the human drug-induced autoimmune diseases. For example, some patients treated with α-methyldopa develop hemolytic anemia. The antibody involved is directed to determinants of the Rh series, showing that the autoimmune response is directed to a normal antigen of the red blood cell itself, and not to the drug (Worllege *et al.*, 1966). There are, as it happens, other explanations for drug-induced autoimmune reactions, such as an action of the drug in disturbing immune regulation. In any event, this type of drug-induced hemolytic anemia should be distinguished from the hemolytic anemia that follows penicillin administration, in which antibodies to penicillin combine with penicillin that previously attached to the surface of erythrocytes (Petz and Fudenberg, 1966). In such instances, the immune reaction is not directed to a self-antigen; the target cell is injured as an "innocent bystander" rather than being involved in an autoimmune response.

5. "Surrogate" Autoantigens

We use this term to describe an antiidiotype molecule that happens to mimic the configuration of a natural self-constituent. There are well-documented examples of the generation of an antibody response by antiidiotype, an "internal image" of an antigen, which is not as such encountered by the individual (Mackay, 1988). The concept of the antiidiotype mimicking the configuration of a host protein has been raised particularly in the context of antibody responses to viral infections (Plotz, 1983).

6. Tumor Autoantigens

Malignant tumors may be complicated by systemic diseases that are termed paraneoplastic. Among these are curious autoimmune syndromes that, until recently, have attracted little attention from immunologists. Among the early examples would be tumor-associated hemolytic anemia, particularly with ovarian cancers (Spira and Lynch, 1979). There is much interest in neurological syndromes, particularly cerebellar degeneration, that accompany ovarian cancers, with antibodies against Purkinje cells readily demonstrable by immunofluorescence (Lennon, 1989). Recently, examples of paraneoplastic pemphigus with acantholytic autoantibodies were described in association with various tumors (Anhalt *et al.*, 1990). Presumably the tumor expresses membrane antigens with epitopes that simulate those of natural self-constituents.

B. Inductive Mechanisms: Antigen Presentation

Since we maintain that self-reactive T cells are not entirely erased from the immunological repertoire (see earlier), then autoimmunity may be due to *hypereffective* antigen presentation. Hence the suggestion has been proffered that such aberrant MHC class II molecules on tissue cells may initiate an autoimmune response (Bottazzo *et al.*, 1983). Class II expression has been described in target organs in several autoimmune conditions. Examples include insulin-dependent diabetes, in which evidence was presented that class II molecules occur on islet cells (Bottazzo *et al.*, 1985); thyroiditis, in which class II molecules are newly expressed on follicular lining cells (Todd *et al.*, 1986); and primary biliary cirrhosis (Ballardini *et al.*, 1984), in which class II molecules are expressed on biliary ductular cells. Therefore, the proposal is that the tissue cell assumes the role of the *professional* antigen-presenting cell, and the expression of MHC class II together with an endogenous cell antigen stimulates self-reactive CD4+ helper T cells. It is known that gamma interferon can induce class II MHC expression on many epithelial and endothelial cells (Collins *et al.*, 1984). Since virus infection stimulates the production of gamma interferon, the concept suggests further that an initial virus infection could instigate the autoimmune process by evoking the secretion of gamma interferon by invading T cells that are combating the viral infection. In addition, if MHC class I antigens were similarly up-regulated, there would be the possibility for cytotoxic damage by CD8+ T cells. Unfortunately, it has been difficult to find direct evidence supporting this seductive hypothesis, and there is some evidence against it. For example, class II MHC expression in β cells of pancreatic islets has been induced in transgenic mice by inserting the class II MHC gene along with the insulin promotor: the effect was to damage the β islet cell but without any evidence at all of autoimmunity (Sarvetnick *et al.*, 1988). Perhaps the action of interleukins in addition to MHC class II expression on epithelial cells is required for autoimmune induction. Furthermore, self-peptides need to bind firmly to the class II molecule after endocytosis, rather than simply share expression at the cell membrane.

C. Inductive Mechanisms: Tolerance-Related

The winding down of an immune response is important physiologically. This may occur as the antigen is eliminated, but active immunoregulation participates as well. These regulatory processes are clearly relevant to those forms of autoimmunity in which there is persistence of the provoking antigen. Regulatory processes requiring discussion are suppression, antiidiotypic responses, and peripheral tolerance.

1. Nondeletion of Anti-Self

Despite the efficiency of intrathymic deletion of anti-self reactivity, this cannot be complete, as already noted. Hence some T cells with autoimmune potential, albeit weak, will be represented in the periphery.

2. Decreased Suppression

Operationally, suppression of autoimmunity can be demonstrated both in the body and in the test tube, even though the mechanisms involved in the process have not been determined. Injection of soluble syngeneic thyroglobulin without adjuvant, for example, fails to induce an immune response. In fact, animals thus treated do not respond to a later injection of thyroglobulin plus adjuvant (Kong *et al.*, 1982). This state of unresponsiveness lasts for at least a month and is antigen specific. It can be transferred to naive mice by injection of CD4+ spleen cells, operationally representing a population of antigen-specific suppressor cells. A similar state of unresponsiveness can be induced in mice in a more physiological manner by raising the normally low levels of circulating thyroglobulin after injection of thyroid-stimulating hormone or thyrotropin-releasing hormone. There is a very extensive and quite analogous literature on immune suppression in relation to EAE. Animals receiving central nervous system (CNS) preparations without adjuvants were rendered resistant to subsequent induction for EAE: this state was termed protection (Coates *et al.*, 1974). Protection was transferable adoptively with spleen cells, presumably of suppressor type (Bernard, 1977). These sets of experiments utilizing adoptive transfer protocols indicate that the presence of self-antigen in the absence of any adjuvantlike activity can play a role in maintaining unresponsiveness to self.

Recently there has been identified a population of cells in the thymus of mice capable of inhibiting production of thyroglobulin autoantibodies *in vitro* after injection with soluble thyroglobulin (Talor and Rose, 1989). These cells, which are antigen specific in their activity, migrate later to the spleen. They express the CD8 marker characteristic of cytotoxic T cells. The production of these cells in the thymus occurs primarily when thyroglobulin is injected without adjuvant. Their production is strain specific, since strains of mice known to be highly susceptible to the induction of autoimmunity, such as SJL, are deficient in the production of these antigen-specific suppressor cells. Moreover, the production of these cells declines with age, correlating with the increased propensity of older animals to develop autoimmunity. It has been difficult to identify antigen-specific suppressor cells in humans, but a decrease in the relative numbers or functional activity of nonspecific suppressor cells has been claimed in a number of autoimmune diseases, including rheumatoid arthritis and Hashimoto's thyroiditis (Goodwin, 1981; Volpé, 1987).

3. Polyclonal Activation

Since it is probable that B cells reactive with virtually all constituents of the body are present normally, nonspecific B-cell proliferation (polyclonal activation) can be expected to result in broad-scale autoantibody production. Under experimental conditions in the test tube, a general increase in the production of autoantibodies can be demonstrated after B-cell activation (Primi *et al.*, 1977). A striking feature of autoimmune disease, however, is the specificity of the autoantibodies produced (Rose, 1979). Thus, antibodies to actin are characteristic of chronic active hepatitis; antibodies to pyruvate dehydrogenase are diagnostic for primary biliary cirrhosis; and antibodies specific for glutamic acid decarboxylase of the β cells of the pancreatic islets are associated with insulin-dependent diabetes (see Chapter 10 of this volume). Even in systemic lupus erythematosus (SLE), a disease in which a large number of autoantibodies are produced, the spectrum of specificities is characteristic of lupus, in that antibodies to particular nuclear antigens can be demonstrated, but antibodies to organ-specific antigens are not usually found. Indeed it is slowly being appreciated that autoantibodies to particular nuclear, nucleolar, or cytoplasmic entities will define subsets of the lupus-related autoimmune diseases, even though we are still far from understanding why and how the subset-specific autoantibody relates to the disease in question (see Chapters 7 and 8 of this volume).

This marked disease-associated specificity of autoantibodies is seen even with respect to the portions of antigenic molecule recognized. We have recently found, for example, that patients with chronic thyroiditis consistently produce autoantibodies to a restricted portion of the thyroglobulin molecule—the most recently evolved part (Bresler *et al.*, 1990). The natural antibodies found in normal sera are directed to the more-primitive, shared portions of the thyroglobulin molecule.

Nonspecific B-cell proliferation can be induced in the body by graft-versus-host (GVH) reactions. Even in this instance, however, the autoantibodies produced are of predictable specificity. Autoantibodies to nuclear antigens and red-cell-surface antigens are produced, for example, whereas antibodies to thyroglobulin are not (van Rappard-van der Veen *et al.*, 1984); however, if thyroglobulin is given to the mouse at the time of induction of GVH disease, thyroglobulin antibodies are found subsequently (Kuppers *et al.*, 1988). These experiments show that the presence and concentration of antigen at the time of GVH-related lymphocyte proliferation may be critical in determining autoantibody specificity.

4. Idiotype Regulation

The concept of an internal regulation of immune responses by an idiotype network is based on the demonstrability of antibodies to idiotypic determinants on Fab regions of immunoglobulin molecules and B-cell antigen receptors, with the question of antiidiotypic responses to T-cell receptor molecules being more open. Antiidiotypic responses are demonstrable in various autoimmune diseases, and such responses probably do act to regulate autoimmunity, at least for B cells (Zanetti, 1985; Mackay, 1988). The success in treating autoimmune disease with plasma exchange or intravenous polyspecific IgG has been attributed, in part at least, to the presence in multiple donor IgG of antiidiotypes against pathogenic autoantibodies (Rossi *et al.*, 1989).

5. Peripheral T-Cell Tolerance

Since intrathymic deletion cannot (and for an effective repertoire should not) remove all degrees of antiself reactivity by T cells, regulatory processes must operate extrathymically. The explanations for nondeleted T cells failing to react with a cognate "self" peptide in the periphery could include (1) weak binding of that peptide to MHC molecules, (2) a receptor of low affinity on the T cell, (3) nondelivery of the putative second signal from the antigen-presenting cell, (4) lack of flux of facilitatory lymphokines, or (5) the process of clonal anergy in which the mature T cell becomes hyporesponsive to a peptide antigen. Peripherally induced T-cell anergy has been explicitly validated in transgenic mouse models (Adams, 1990). These show that transgenically derived polypeptides may elicit T responsiveness or, according to experimental conditions, induce nonresponsiveness to molecules that could not have had any representation in the thymus. One component of peripheral T-cell anergy could be a failure of T cells to undergo transition from the *naive* to the *activated-memory* phenotype.

D. Effector Mechanisms

When self-tolerance has been broken, by whatever means, the subsequent course of events depends largely on the activation of self-reactive T cells (Rose, 1989). They determine the selection of the various possible effector mechanisms that can lead to autoimmune disease. The CD4+ helper T cells induced by presentation of self-peptide plus MHC class II orchestrate the immune response by influencing the recruitment of additional CD4 helper cells, CD8 cytotoxic cells, and B cells. The CD4+ population probably contains subsets that differ in the mixture of facilitating ILs produced (Mosmann *et al.*, 1986), although the distinct Th1 and Th2 subsets identified in the mouse are not so evident in humans (Mosmann and Coffman, 1989). The various effector processes, listed in Table II, are discussed below.

1. B Cells and Autoantibodies

It is convenient to distinguish the multisystem from the organ-specific autoimmune diseases. In multisystem diseases, as illustrated by SLE, the major antigens

TABLE II
Effector Mechanisms in Autoimmunity

B cells—autoantibody	CD4 T cells—lymphokines	Cytotocix T cells
IgG antibody	Lymphokines	Specific cytolysis
Complement-mediated lysis	• Tumor necrosis factor	
	• Lymphotoxin	
Opsonization	• IFN-γ	
Antibody-dependent cell-mediated cytotoxicity	• Increased expression of MHC class I, class II)	
Anti-receptor antibodies	Granuloma formation	
• Blocking		
• Stimulating		
Immune complex formation		
• Local		
• Circulating		

are widely distributed in most tissues of the body, e.g., components of the nucleus. The formation of multiple antibodies is characteristic, but the particular mix of antibodies usually reflects the clinical characteristics of the patient: for example, antibodies to native DNA and histones in SLE, antibodies to tRNA synthetases in the polymyositic diseases, antibodies to centromere in the CREST variant (calcinosis, Raynaud's phenomenon, esophageal motility disturbances, sclerodactyly, and telangiectasia) of scleroderma, and antibodies to nuclear ribonucleoprotein (RNP) in mixed connective tissue disease (Burek and Rose, 1988). These expressions are described in Chapters 7 and 8 of this volume. The effectors of systemic disease are generally humoral, either antibody itself or deposited immune complexes.

In the case of the organ-specific autoimmune disease, the principal reactivity is specifically to the target organ (or a limited number of organs), and the antigen (or antigens) are unique to those organs. The principal antigens in chronic thyroiditis, for example, are thyroglobulin and thyroid peroxidase. Even if other autoantibodies are present, they are generally directed to analogous organ-specific antigens, such as those of stomach, adrenal cortex, pancreatic islet, or parathyroid. The effector mechanisms may be either, or both, humoral or cellular, depending primarily on the disposition of the antigen.

The B cell-stimulating interleukins, derived from CD4+ T cells, IL-4, IL-5, and IL-6, direct the proliferation of B cells and their differentiation into IgG secretors (Kishimoto and Hirano, 1989), whether they are responding to foreign or self molecules. In general, the development of autoimmune disease after autoimmunization corresponds to the appearance of IgG antibody. Natural autoantibodies are IgM and are usually innocuous. The class switch is T-cell dependent and is accompanied by somatic mutation, often resulting in greater antibody–antigen affinity (Shlomchik *et al.*, 1990). IgG antibody also penetrates tissues more readily than does IgM, and is able to cross the placenta. Most subclasses of IgG antibody are efficient activators of complement.

There are many instances in which autoantibody is clearly the pathogenic agent in autoimmune disease. For example, IgG autoantibodies to red-cell-surface antigens induce hemolytic anemia through cell-mediated lysis (Rose, 1979), or, more frequently, the antibodies sensitize (opsonize) the red cells for enhanced destruction by the mononuclear phagocytic system of the spleen, lymph nodes, and liver. Similar opsonization by cell-specific autoantibodies is responsible for the autoimmune leukopenias and thrombocytopenias. For that reason, removing the largest mass of mononuclear phagocytes by splenectomy alleviates the symptoms of some of these autoimmune blood diseases.

Antibody and complement are less likely to damage solid organs, because they are unable to attain at these loci the critical concentrations in tissue spaces. In some instances, local production of antibody may be important. The presence of germinal centers in the thyroid glands of patients with thyroiditis signifies the production of antibody within the gland, where it may contribute to the final pathological picture, by complement-dependent lysis or by cooperation with lymphocytes or monocytes, to produce antibody-dependent, cell-mediated cytotoxicity (Rose, 1989). This latter effect, which is more readily demonstrated in the test tube than in the body, depends on the capability of antibody to couple with a potential killer cell through its Fc receptor; the antibody directs the attachment of the killer cell to its target.

2. Antibodies to Cell Receptors

An important group of autoimmune diseases is attributable to autoantibody directed to physiological receptors on the cell surface. In myasthenia gravis, autoantibodies to the acetylcholine receptor block the transmission of impulses from the nerve to muscle at the myoneural junction (Lindstrom, 1979). A fascinating example of *receptor* interference is provided by the antibodies that block calcium channels in the Lambert–Eaton syndrome (Roberts *et al.*, 1985; Vincent *et al.*, 1989; Lennon and Lambert, 1989). In Graves' disease, antibodies to the thyroid-stimulating hormone (TSH) receptor on the thyroid epithelial cell act differently: these stimulate the cell and mimic the action of the TSH itself. Previously referred to as long-acting stimulators, these thyroid-stimulating antibodies are responsible for the hyperthyroidism characteristic of Graves' disease (Manley *et al.*, 1982). Antibodies to cell receptors were described in detail in *The Autoimmune Diseases I*.

3. Immune Complexes

In a number of autoimmune diseases, the primary pathology is the result of the production of antigen–antibody complexes. In SLE, as mentioned previously, the release of nuclear antigens into the bloodstream allows their combination with antinuclear antibody (Koffler *et al.*, 1974). These circulating complexes later localize in capillary beds of the kidney as well as of the skin, heart, brain, joints, and other organs. It is also shown that autoantigens, e.g., DNA, may circulate and become implanted in vulnerable tissues, e.g., the renal glomerulus. The complexes activate complement and attract leukocytes, which are directly responsible for the tissue damage (Theofilopoulos and Dixon, 1979). In the case of antigens that do not circulate in appreciable amounts, immune complexes may be formed locally. Visual evidence by immunofluorescence is available for immune complex deposition in the thyroid glands of patients with thyroiditis (Aichinger *et al.*, 1985).

4. CD4+ T Cells and Lymphokines—Cytokines

One subset of CD4+ cells releases lymphokines responsible for delayed hypersensitivity. Some cytokines, including the tumor necrosis factors (TNFs), can actually damage surrounding cells. Other lymphokines attract and activate inflammatory cells. Gamma interferon increases the activity of natural killer (NK) cells (Gillis, 1989), and also augments the expression of MHC class II by epithelial and endothelial cells, so enhancing the localization of CD4+ lymphocytes. MHC class I determinants are also increased on target cells through the action of gamma interferon, thereby augmenting the capacity of these cells to induce cytotoxic lymphocytes (CTL), and equally their susceptibility to lysis by activated antigen-specific CTL.

5. CD8+ Cytotoxic Lymphocytes

Cytotoxic T cells (CD8+) are said to require induction by CD4 helper cells. Because they have an antigen-specific receptor, the cytotoxic T cells are capable of a direct attack on antigen-bearing cells, with an activity restricted by the MHC class I products on the target cells. Such cells are able to reproduce the primary lesions in several experimental autoimmune diseases, including allergic encephalomyelitis and experimental autoimmune thyroiditis (Weigle, 1980). Acting in concert with CD4+ T cells, they are capable of also damaging the islet cells in mice with experimental diabetes (Bendelac *et al.*, 1977). There are indications from immunocytochemistry that CD8+ CTL are on the "front line" in autoimmune tissue injury involving cellular targets, but convincing evidence for their role as effectors is not available.

In reality, most autoimmune diseases are probably produced by a combination of several pathogenetic mechanisms. In chronic thyroiditis, for example, there is evidence of the simultaneous occurrence of complement-dependent cytotoxic antibody, antibody-dependent cell-mediated cytotoxicity, local immune-complex production, delayed hypersensitivity, and lymphokine production, as well as of the effects of cytotoxic T cells (Rose, 1989).

IV. NEW APPROACHES TO TREATMENT

In the past, treatment of autoimmune disease has relied mainly on global immunosuppression or on replacement of the functional deficit. However, specifically targeted immunotherapy is gradually coming closer to reality, as described in Chapter 16. In systemic autoimmune diseases, like SLE and rheumatoid arthritis, for example, it is still necessary to reduce the entire immunological response. Such treatment obviously leaves the patient vulnerable to infection as well as to the chronic side-effects of drug treatment. Organ-specific autoimmune diseases are more often treated by replacement, since insulin can replace some of the functions of the pancreatic islet cell, and thyroid hormone restores most of the functions of the thyroid gland. However, such replacement therapy is not ideal. It does not remedy the underlying autoimmune condition and, in the case of diabetes mellitus, there is the lifelong discomfort of daily injections.

In recent years, great effort has been expended in seeking more specific modes of preventing or arresting injurious autoimmune responses. Among the most promising approaches are the following: (1) reduction of the helper-inducer population (CD4+) of T cells; (2) reduction of activated T cells (anti-Ia or anti-IL-2 receptor); (3) antibody to particular MHC class II determinants; (4) antibody to particular TcR or to V region of TcR; and (5) surrogate peptide to block MHC class II binding. Details of these strategies are given in Chapter 16.

Methods of avoiding autoimmune responses are most effective if applied before the response is initiated. For that reason, increasing emphasis is placed on identifying individuals or populations at risk of developing autoimmune disease. They may be siblings of affected children, persons with particular HLA and other biomarkers, or individuals exposed to environmental agents. Identification of risk factors requires even greater insight into the fundamental causes of autoimmune disease.

REFERENCES

Ada, G. L., and Rose, N. R. (1988). *Clin. Immunol. Immunopathol.* **47,** 3–9.

Adams, T. E. (1990). *Mol. Biol. Med.* **7,** 341–357.

Adams, E., Basten, A., and Goodnow, C. C. (1990). *Proc. Natl. Acad. Sci. U.S.A.* **87,** 5687–5691.

Adelstein, S., Pritchard-Briscoe, H., Anderson, T. A., Crosbie, J., Gammon, G., Loblay, R. H., Basten, A., and Goodnow, C. C. (1991). *Science* **252,** 1223–1225.

Adorini, L. (1990). *Clin. Immunol. Immunopathol.* **55,** 327–336.

Aichinger, G., Fill, H., and Wick, G. (1985). *Lab. Invest.* **52,** 132–140.

Anderson, C. L., and Rose, N. R. (1971). *J. Immunol.* **107,** 1341–1348.
Anhalt, G. J., Kim, S. C., Stanley, J. R. *et al.* (1990). *N. Engl. J. Med.* **323,** 1729.
Babbitt, B. P., Matsueda, G., Haber, E., Unanue, E. R., and Allen, P. M. (1986). *Proc. Natl. Acad. Sci. U.S.A.* **83,** 4509–4513.
Ballardini, G., Bianchi, F. B., Mirakian, R., Pisi, E., Doniach, D., and Bottazzo, G. F. (1984). *Lancet* **ii,** 1009.
Beisel, K. W., Ehrinpreis, M. N., Bhathal, P. C., Mackay, I. R., and Rose, N. R. (1984). *Br. J. Exp. Pathol.* **65,** 125–131.
Bendelac, A., Carnaud, C., Boitard, C., and Bach, J. F. (1987). *J. Exp. Med.* **166,** 823–832.
Bernard, C. C. A. (1977). *Clin. Exp. Immunol.* **29,** 100–109.
Bhathal, P. S., Rose, N. R., Mackay, I. R., and Whittingham, S. (1983). *Br. J. Exp. Pathol.* **64,** 524–533.
Billingham, R. E., Brent, L., and Medawar, P. B. (1953). *Nature* **172,** 603–606.
Bottazzo, G. F., Pujol-Borrell, R., Hanafusa, T., and Feldmann, M. (1983). *Lancet* **2,** 1115–1119.
Bottazzo, G. F., Dean, B., McNally, J. M., MacKay, E. H., Swift, P. G., and Gamble, D. R. (1985). *N. Engl. J. Med.* **313,** 353–360.
Bresler, H. S., Burek, C. L., Hoffman, W. H., and Rose, N. R. (1990). *Clin. Immunol. Immunopathol.* **54,** 76–86.
Burek, C. L., and Rose, N. R. (1988). *In* "Diagnostic Immunopathology" (R. B. Colvin, A. K. Bhan, and R. T. McCluskey, eds.), pp. 87–119. Raven Press, New York.
Burnet, F. M. (1959). "The Clonal Selection Theory of Acquired Immunity." The University Press, Cambridge, England.
Calkins, C. E., and Stutman, O. (1978). *J. Exp. Med.* **147,** 87–97.
Coates, A. S., Mackay, I. R., and Crawford, M. (1974). *Cell Immunol.* **12,** 370–381.
Collins, T., Korman, A. J., Wake, C. T. *et al.* (1984). *Proc. Natl. Acad. Sci. U.S.A.* **81,** 4917–4921.
Dale, J. B., and Beachey, E. H. (1985). *J. Exp. Med.* **162,** 583–591.
Dighiero, G., Lymberi, P., Guilbert, B., Ternynck, T., and Avrameas, S. (1986). *Ann. N.Y. Acad. Sci.* **475,** 135–145.
Dutton, R. W. (1972). *J. Exp. Med.* **136,** 1445–1450.
Eardley, D. D., Hugenberger, J., McVay-Boudreau, L., Shen, F. W., Gershon, R. K., and Cantor, H. (1978). *J. Exp. Med.* **147,** 1106–1115.
Eyquem, A., and Crepin, Y. (1956). *Ann. Inst. Pasteur Paris* **90,** 364–367.
Freund, J., Lipton, M. M., and Thompson, G. E. (1953). *J. Exp. Med.* **97,** 711–726.
Fujinami, R. S., and Oldstone, M. B. A. (1985). *Science* **230,** 1043–1045.
Gammon, G., and Sercarz, E. (1990). *Clin. Immunol. Immunopathol.* **56,** 287–297.
Gillis, S. (1989). *In* "Fundamental Immunology" (W. E. Paul, ed.), 2nd Ed., pp. 621–638. Raven Press, New York.
Goodwin, J. S. (1981). "Suppressor Cells in Human Disease." Marcel Dekker, New York.
Grabar, P. (1975). *Clin. Immunol. Immunopathol.* **4,** 453.
Green, D. R., Chue, B., and Gershon, R. K. (1983). *J. Mol. Cell. Immunol.* **1,** 19–28.
Jensen, P. E., and Kapp, J. A. (1985). *J. Mol. Cell. Immunol.* **2,** 133–139.
Kappler, J., Roehm, N., and Marrack, P. (1987). *Cell* **49,** 273–280.
Kappler, J. W., Staerz, U., White, J., and Marrack, P. C. (1988). *Nature* **332,** 35–40.
Kappler, J., Kotzin, B., Herron, L. *et al.* (1989). *Science* **244,** 811–813.
Kaufmann, S. H. E. (1990). *Immunol. Today* **11,** 129–136.
Kaufmann, S. H. E., Munk, M. E., Koga, T. *et al.* (1989). *In* "Progress in Immunology" (F. Melchers *et al.*, eds.), Vol. VII, pp. 963–970. Springer-Verlag, Berlin.
Kincade, P. W., and Gimble, J. M. (1989). *In* "Fundamental Immunology" (W. E. Paul, ed.), 2nd Ed., pp. 41–67. Raven Press, New York.
Kincade, P. W., Lee, G., Pietrangeli, C. E., Hayashi, S. I., and Gimble, J. M. (1989). *Annu. Rev. Immunol.* **7,** 111–143.

Kishimoto, T., and Hirano, T. (1989). *In* "Fundamental Immunology" (W. E. Paul, ed.), 2nd Ed., pp. 385–411. Raven Press, New York.

Koffler, D., Agnello, V., and Kunkel, H. G. (1974). *Am. J. Pathol.* **74,** 109–124.

Kong, Y. M., Okayasu, I., Giraldo, A. A., Beisel, K. W., Sundick, R. S., Rose, N. R., David, C. S., Audibert, F., and Chedid, L. (1982). *Ann. N.Y. Acad. Sci.* **392,** 191–209.

Kunkel, H. G., Müller-Eberhard, H. J., Fudenberg, H. H., and Tomasi, T. B. (1960). *J. Clin. Invest.* **40,** 117–129.

Kuppers, R. C., Suiter, T., Gleichmann, E., and Rose, N. R. (1988). *Eur. J. Immunol.* **18,** 161–166.

Lakey, E. K., Margoliash, E., Flouret, G., and Pierce, S. K. (1986). *Eur. J. Immunol.* **16,** 721–727.

Lamb, J. R., and Young, D. B. (1990). *Mol. Biol. Med.* **7,** 311–321.

Lennon, V. A. (1989). *J. Neurol. Neurosurg. Psychiatry* **52,** 1438.

Lennon, V. A., and Lambert, E. H. (1989). *Mayo Clin. Proc.* **64,** 1498–1504.

Lindstrom, J. (1979). *Adv. Immunol.* **27,** 1–50.

Liu, R. H., and Stockinger, B. (1989). *Eur. J. Immunol.* **19,** 105–110.

Mackay, I. R. (1988). *In* "The Liver: Biology and Pathobiology" (I. M. Arias, W. B. Jakoby, and H. Popper, eds.), pp. 1259–1268. Raven Press, New York.

Mackay, I. R., and Burnet, F. M. (1963). "The Autoimmune Diseases." Charles C Thomas, Springfield, Illinois.

Mamula, M. J., Jemmerson, R., and Hardin, J. A. (1990). *J. Immunol.* **144,** 1835–1840.

Manley, S. W., Knight, A., and Adams, D. D. (1982). *Springer Semin. Immunopathol.* **5,** 413–431.

Marrack, P., and Kappler, J. (1987). *Science* **238,** 1073–1078.

Milgrom, F., and Witebsky, E. (1960). *J.A.M.A.* **174,** 56–63.

Mosmann, T. R., and Coffman, R. L. (1989). *Adv. Immunol.* **46,** 111–146.

Mosmann, T. R., Cherwinski, H., Bond, M. W., Giedlin, M. A., and Coffman, R. L. (1986). *J. Immunol.* **136,** 2348.

Neu, N., Rose, N. R., Beisel, K. W., Herskowitz, A., Gurri-Glass, G., and Craig, S. W. (1987a). *J. Immunol.* **139,** 3630–3636.

Neu, N., Craig, S. W., Rose, N. R., Alvarez, F., and Beisel, K. W. (1987b). *Clin. Exp. Immunol.* **69,** 566–574.

Nossal, G. J. V., and Pike, B. L. (1980). *Proc. Natl. Acad. Sci. U.S.A.* **77,** 1602–1606.

Notkins, A. L., and Prabhakar, B. S. (1986). *Ann. N.Y. Acad. Sci.* **475,** 123–134.

Paul, W. E. (1989). *In* "Fundamental Immunology" (W. E. Paul, ed.), 2nd Ed., pp. 3–38. Raven Press, New York.

Peavy, D. L., and Pierce, C. W. (1974). *J. Exp. Med.* **140,** 356–369.

Perlmutter, R. M. (1989). *In* "Progress in Immunology VII" (F. Melchers *et al.*, eds.), pp. 83–91. Springer-Verlag, Berlin.

Petz, C. D., and Fudenberg, H. H. (1966). *N. Engl. J. Med.* **274,** 171–178.

Plotz, P. H. (1983). *Lancet* **ii,** 224.

Primi, D., Hammerström, L., Smith, C. I., and Möller, G. (1977). *J. Exp. Med.* **145,** 21–30.

Qin, S., Cobbold, S., Benjamin, R., and Waldmann, H. (1989). *J. Exp. Med.* **169,** 779–794.

Rammensee, H. G., Kroschewski, R., and Frangoulis, B. (1989). *Nature* **339,** 541–544.

Roberts, A., Perera, S., Lang, B., Vincent, A., and Newsom-Davis, J. (1985). *Nature* **317,** 737–739.

Roberts, I. M., Whittingham, S., and Mackay, I. R. (1973). *Lancet* **ii,** 936–940.

Rose, N. R. (1974). *In* "The Inflammatory Process" (B. Zweifach, L. Grant, and R. McCluskey, eds.), Vol. 3, 2nd Ed., pp. 347–399. Academic Press, New York.

Rose, N. R. (1979). *In* "Principles of Immunology" (N. R. Rose, F. Milgrom, and C. J. van Oss, eds.), 2nd Ed., pp. 436–452. Macmillan Company, New York.

Rose, N. R. (1989). *Clin. Immunol. Immunopathol.* **53,** S7–S16.

Rose, N. R., Kong, Y. M., Okayasu, I., Giraldo, A. A., Beisel, K., and Sundick, R. S. (1981). *Immunol. Rev.* **55,** 299–314.

Rose, N. R., Beisel, K. W., Herskowitz, A., Neu, N., Wolfgram, L. J., Alvarez, F. L., Traystman, M. D., and Craig, S. W. (1987). *In* "Autoimmunity and Autoimmune Disease—Ciba Symposium No. 129" (D. Evered and J. Whelan, eds.), pp. 3–24. John Wiley & Sons, Chichester, U.K.

Rose, N. R., Lucas, P. L., Dilley, M., and Reed, A. H. (1980). *In* "Clinics in Andrology. V. Regulation of Male Fertility" (G. R. Cunningham, W.-B. Schill, and E. S. E. Hafez, eds.), pp. 197–204. Martinus Nijhoff Publishers, The Hague, The Netherlands.

Rossi, F., Dietrich, G., and Kazatchkins, D. (1989). *Immunol. Rev.* **110,** 135–149.

Sakaguchi, S., and Rose, N. R. (1988). *In* "Diagnosis and Pathology of Endocrine Diseases" (G. Mendelsohn, ed.), pp. 619–640. J. B. Lippincott, Philadelphia, Pennsylvania.

Samuel, T., and Rose, N. R. (1980). *J. Clin. Lab. Immunol.* **3,** 77–83.

Sarvetnick, N., Liggitt, D., Pitts, S. L., Hansen, S. E., and Stewart, T. A. (1988). *Cell* **52,** 773–782.

Scollay, R., and Shortman, K. (1985). *In* "Recognition and Regulation in Cell-Mediated Immunity" (J. D. Watson and J. Marbrook, eds.), pp. 3–30. Marcel Dekker, New York.

Sha, W. C., Nelson, C. A., Newberry, R. D., Kranz, D. M., Russell, J. H., and Loh, D. Y. (1988). *Nature* **336,** 73–76.

Shlomchik, M., Mascelli, M., Shan, H., Radic, M. Z., Pisetsky, D., Marshak-Rothstein, A., and Weigert, M. (1990). *J. Exp. Med.* **171,** 265–297.

Sinha, A. A., Lopez, M. T., and McDevitt, H. O. (1990). *Science* **248,** 1380–1388.

Sleasman, J. W., Henderson, M., and Barrett, D. J. (1991). *Cell. Immunol.* **133,** 367–378.

Spellman, C. W., and Daynes, R. A. (1978). *Cell. Immunol.* **38,** 25–34.

Spira, M. A., and Lynch, E. C. (1979). *Am. J. Med.* **67,** 753.

Sprent, J. (1989). *In* "Fundamental Immunology" (W. E. Paul, ed.), 2nd Ed., pp. 69–91. Raven Press, New York.

Stollerman, G. H. (1975). "Rheumatic Fever and Streptococcal Infection." Grune & Stratton, New York.

Talor, E., and Rose, N. R. (1989). *In* "Cellular Basis of Immune Modulation" (J. G. Kaplan, D. R. Green, and R. C. Bleackley, eds.), pp. 391–394. Alan R. Liss, New York.

Theofilopoulos, A. N., and Dixon, F. J. (1979). *Adv. Immunol.* **28,** 89–220.

Thomas, A. J., Pontes, J. E., Rose, N. R., Segal, S., and Pierce, J. M., Jr. (1981). *Fertil. Steril.* **35,** 447–450.

Todd, I., Londai, M., Pujol-Borrell, R., Mirakian, R., Feldmann, M., and Bottazzo, G. F. (1986). *Ann. N.Y. Acad. Sci.* **475,** 241–250.

Underwood, J. R., Pederson, J. S., Chalmers, P. J., and Toh, B. H. (1985). *Clin. Exp. Immunol.* **60,** 417–426.

van Eden, W. (1990). *Acta Pathol. Microbiol. Immunol. Scand.* **98,** 383–394.

van Eden, W., Thole, J. E. R., van der Zee, R. *et al.* (1988). *Nature* **331,** 171–173.

van Rappard-van der Veen, F. M., Kong, Y. M., Rose, N. R., Kimura, M., and Gleichmann, E. (1984). *Clin. Exp. Immunol.* **55,** 525–534.

Vincent, A., Lang, B., and Newsom-Davis, J. (1989). *Trends Neurol. Sci.* **12,** 496–502.

Vladutiu, A. O., and Rose, N. R. (1975). *Cell. Immunol.* **17,** 106–113.

Volpé, R. (1987). *N. Engl. J. Med.* **316,** 44–46.

Weaver, C. T., and Unanue, E. R. (1990). *Immunol. Today* **11,** 49–55.

Weigle, W. O. (1965). *J. Exp. Med.* **121,** 289–308.

Weigle, W. O. (1980). *Adv. Immunol.* **30,** 159–273.

Winfield, J. B. (1989). *Arthritis Rheum.* **32,** 1497–1504.

Worlledge, S. M., Carstairs, K. D., and Dacie, J. V. (1966). *Lancet* **2,** 135–139.

Zabriskie, J. B., and Freimer, E. H. (1966). *J. Exp. Med.* **124,** 661–678.

Zanetti, M. (1985). *Immunol. Today* **6,** 299–302.

CHAPTER **2**

Autoimmunity and Self-Tolerance

GUSTAV J. V. NOSSAL
The Walter and Eliza Hall Institute of Medical Research
Victoria, Australia

I. INTRODUCTION

When the nature of immunologic tolerance first came under scrutiny (Burnet and Fenner, 1949; Billingham *et al.*, 1953), the underlying assumptions about the immune response were rather simple. Antigen entered the body; it caused antibody formation and/or cellular immunity; tolerance induction meant putting a stop to all that by introducing the toleragen in fetal life. The challenge procedures used to test the tolerant state (skin graft rejection; antibody formation to an antigen administered in Freund's complete adjuvant) elicited strong and uniform responses in controls, so tolerance was seen as an all-or-none affair. There were no shades of grey. Little wonder then that, as the concept of autoimmunity in disease causation gradually gained acceptance (e.g., Mackay and Burnet, 1963), it too had a sharply etched quality. Autoimmunity was a breakdown of tolerance, a forbidden event, causing cataclysmic damage. It seemed entirely natural, therefore, to seek a single causative mechanism for tolerance, and a single etiology for autoimmunity. Uncomfortable facts such as low-titer antinuclear antibodies in healthy people, or skin grafts surviving for 20 days rather than 10, received only moderate attention.

The intervening years have seen an extraordinary increase in our knowledge of immune processes, which has highlighted the complexity of immunoregulation. No longer do we see the introduction of antigen into an adult animal as necessarily leading to immunity; we know that much depends on the route by which antigen enters and the form in which it is presented to the immune system, because the normal immune response depends on a cascade of intercellular interactions. This concept of the immune response as demanding a chain of events immediately raises the issue of multiple points at which the chain could be interrupted, and thus multiple causative mechanisms of tolerance. Given that possibility, it follows that autoimmunity could, in turn, have multiple causative mechanisms. It has become popular to regard the self-tolerance–autoimmunity problem as only one aspect of the wide field of immunoregulation. Yet simple examples of self-tolerance, such as the tolerance of one's own kidney versus the ferocity of the immune attack against an allogeneically transplanted one, are so dramatic as to create a yearning for an overriding paradigm. Three *single mechanism* theories of tolerance have had their ardent proponents down the decades, namely tolerance as due to repertoire purging (Burnet, 1957); tolerance resulting from antigenic signaling of a lymphocyte in the absence of a second signal due to associative antigenic recognition (Bretscher and Cohn, 1970); and tolerance arising from T cell-mediated suppression (McCullagh, 1970; Gershon and Kondo, 1971). In this chapter, the author will attempt to bring these into a modern perspective.

The biggest single operational obstacle to experimentation on the cellular mechanisms of tolerance induction has been the heterogeneity of lymphocytes. Only a small proportion of lymphocytes react with a given epitope, and then with varying avidities. If one wishes to examine in detail the cellular and biochemical processes occurring during tolerance induction, one must first, in some way, isolate this small subset. Two recent developments have been of extraordinary significance in breaking this logjam, namely the development of transgenic mice in which the majority of T or B lymphocytes express transgenes for a particular T-cell or immunoglobulin receptor; and the identification of certain *superantigens* that react with large sets of T lymphocytes. We shall review the great progress in tolerance research that has resulted from the exploitation of these models. Other aspects requiring attention include differential tolerance susceptibility of different lymphocyte subsets; the implications of immunoglobulin variable (V) gene hypermutation for tolerance and autoimmunity; and possible initiators of autoimmunity. From these considerations, a coherent if incomplete framework for thinking about tolerance and autoimmunity will emerge.

II. T-CELL TOLERANCE

A. Clonal Abortion of T Cells

The clonal-selection theory (Talmage, 1957; Burnet, 1957) was articulated before the distinction between T and B lymphocytes became clear, but it did lead to a logical way of thinking about tolerance. If immunity represented the selective activation of certain immunocytes, then tolerance could be seen as the selective destruction of such a set—in other words, the opposite of immunity. This thought was refined by Lederberg (1959), who saw lymphocytes as moving from a tolerance-sensitive, nonimmunizable stage of their ontogeny to an immunocompetent state in which they were no longer sensitive to tolerance induction but reacted to antigenic contact by immune activation. The first evidence consistent with clonal abortion as a mechanism of tolerance induction was provided by Nossal and Pike (1975) in relation to B cells, and it was not until several years later that clonal-frequency analysis for a parallel process in T cells came forward (Nossal and Pike, 1981). The relevant literature until 1983 has been summarized elsewhere (Nossal, 1983). One regrettable fact is that the enumeration of T cells competent to react with a given antigen is both complex and tedious, so the number of studies addressing the issue is not very large. Nevertheless, our early work made it quite clear that tolerance induction to foreign class I major histocompatability complex (MHC) antigens involved a functional clonal deletion of antiallogeneic cytotoxic T-lymphocyte precursors, which began in the thymus (Nossal and Pike, 1981).

1. Clonal Abortion by Superantigens

A peculiarity of T-cell recognition of certain self-antigens provided the next major step forward. It turns out, for example, that the murine class II MHC antigen I-E is recognized by T cells that express a T-cell receptor including the β chain coded for by the Vβ17a gene (Kappler *et al.*, 1987). A monoclonal antibody, KJ23a, has been prepared that can bind to all T cells expressing the Vβ17a gene product. Some normal mouse strains are characterized by a total absence of the I-E gene. In such strains, peripheral lymphoid tissues contain 4–14% of KJ23a-staining T cells. Mice that express I-E show only 0.1% of KJ23a-positive T cells. This suggested some active process of clonal deletion of Vβ17a-expressing T cells. When the thymus of I-E-possessing strains was examined, whereas the mature, medullary population showed an absence of Vβ17a-T cells, the immature thymocytes showed a persistence comparable to that in non-I-E-expressing strains. The results strongly suggested a clonal-abortion process occurring intrathymically during T-cell maturation.

Another interesting situation involves the polymorphic B-cell surface marker Mls. T lymphocytes from Mls-1^b mice respond strongly to stimulator cells from Mls-1^a strains even when there is no MHC difference between the strains. Kappler *et al.* (1988) found that virtually all T cells from Mls-1^b mice that expressed the Vβ8.1 gene could react to Mls-1^a, whereas McDonald *et al.* (1988) showed the same to be true for Vβ6-expressing T cells. Examination of peripheral versus thymic T lymphocytes with suitable clonotypic anti-T-cell-receptor monoclonal antibodies revealed essentially the same state of affairs as described for I-E, namely clonal abortion of anti-Mls cells within strains of the right Mls genotype.

There are about 20 Vβ genes and about 50 Vα genes in the mouse, and it is something of a puzzle to note that certain antigen–MHC combinations react with all cells bearing a particular β chain, regardless of which α chain is used. At the moment there is no known structural basis for this observation. The characteristic is not confined to self-antigens. Some bacterial toxins are very powerful T-cell mitogens, and it turns out that each toxin in this class stimulates T cells with defined Vβ expression (Janeway *et al.*, 1989; White *et al.*, 1989). In the case of these toxins, antigen processing destroys this property, so the association between T-cell receptor and antigen is different from the conventional one to self-MHC-bound peptide. The Kappler–Marrack group (e.g., Marrack *et al.*, 1989) have reasoned that such bacterial superantigens are of survival value to the pathogen, in that the vast flux of cytokines induced by massive T-cell activation is damaging to the host. This could provide a rationale for the evolution of self-superantigens. Those bacterial toxins that use a Vβ gene set that has been eliminated from the peripheral T-cell repertoire (because those V gene products also react with a self-antigen present in that host) are no longer toxic for the mouse strain concerned, so the mouse would survive that particular bacterial infection.

We are thus left with something of a dilemma concerning clonal abortion induced by superantigens. As it does not seem to depend on classical T-cell receptor and self-MHC-peptide interactions, is it really a good model for the processes guiding self-tolerance to the large array of self conventional antigens, against all of which we must become tolerant? Fortunately, the answer appears to be yes, as the following transgenic experiments demonstrate.

2. T-Cell Clonal Abortion in T-Cell-Receptor Transgenic Mice

Under suitable circumstances, transgenic mice can be produced in which the majority of the T- or B-cell population expresses receptors for antigen specified by the transgenes used. For example, Kisielow *et al.* (1988) used the αβ T-cell-receptor genes from a fully rearranged receptor of a cytolytic T-lymphocyte clone with activity against the male transplantation antigen, H-Y. In female mice lacking the H-Y antigen, at least 30% of the CD8+ T cells expressed the αβ receptor of the original clonal gene donor. In male mice, such cells were not found in the periphery, and within the thymus cortex, there was massive cell death of transgene-expressing cells due to clonal abortion. The only cells that escaped were those that either did not express the transgenes, or that possessed aberrantly low quantities of the accessory molecule CD8. Another interesting model is that of Pircher *et al.* (1989). An αβ T-cell receptor specific for a noncytopathic virus, to which mice can be rendered tolerant, was introduced as a pair of transgenes. In this case, drastic clonal abortion occurred within transgene-expressing CD4+ CD8+ cortical thymocytes in virus-positive mice. Finally, even γδ T cells can become victims of clonal abortion. When Dent *et al.* (1990)

introduced the genes for $\gamma\delta$ T-cell receptor specific for an allelic class I MHC gene product encoded by the Tla locus as a transgene, neither the peripheral lymphoid organs nor the thymus of mice possessing the relevant Tla allele had transgene-expressing T cells present.

From all of this work, it is quite clear that clonal abortion is a major mechanism of T-cell tolerance for those self-antigens that are expressed within the thymus.

3. The Pepton Hypothesis and Clonal Abortion

Many self-antigens are present only or chiefly as differentiation antigens in or on specific cells of various tissues or organs. How does the immune system become tolerant of such antigens? A novel hypothesis has been put forward by Boon and Van Pel (1989) termed the pepton hypothesis. This arose from the observation that, in essence, more or less any gene that mutates, including genes coding for cytosolic rather than plasma-membrane proteins, can create a new transplantation antigen evoking a T cell-mediated rejection response. When three such mutated genes were analyzed in detail, it was found that transfection of cloned gene fragments, comprising only the mutated exon and immediately adjacent intron regions, created cells that still acted as targets, i.e., effectively expressed the transplantation antigen of interest. This happened even though no expression vector was used.

Boon's hypothesis therefore embodies the suggestion that each self-protein contains at least one pepton, i.e., a T-cell epitope. Moreover, a new type of polymerase, not requiring a promoter, can lead to autonomous transcription of the pepton. The resultant peptide binds to class I MHC and the MHC–peptide complex makes its way to the cell surface. Active and efficient pepton transcription in the thymus could lead to thymic presentation of the whole self-pepton repertoire, in other words not just those antigens that have to be expressed on thymic cells, but indeed the whole universe of self-T-cell epitopes. As a result, clonal abortion might occur for *all* self-antigens, at least within the CD8+ population of T cells. As it now appears likely that intracellular association of peptides and class II MHC can also occur under certain circumstances, the Boon hypothesis might be expanded to comprise the whole universe of T-cell self-tolerance. If that were so, clonal abortion would be the complete Rosetta stone of self-tolerance within the T-cell compartment. However, it is clear that tolerance can also be induced extrathymically, as shown below. It remains to be determined how physiologically relevant these ancillary mechanisms are.

4. Mechanisms of Clonal Abortion

There is still controversy concerning the mechanisms of clonal abortion within the thymus. Some studies (e.g., Sprent and Webb, 1987; Matzinger and Guerder,

1989) imply that the toleragenic signal can be delivered only by a particular type of antigen-presenting cell, e.g., a dendritic cell. Other studies (e.g., Kisielow *et al.*, 1988; Pircher *et al.*, 1989) demonstrate that death can be widespread throughout the thymic cortex, where the density of accessory cells is rather sparse. In one interesting model (Smith *et al.*, 1989) anti-CD3 antibodies are added to fetal thymic organ cultures with the result that immature CD4+ CD8+ cortical thymocytes die in very large numbers by the process of apoptosis. The earliest events following ligand binding, e.g., phosphoinositol hydrolysis and calcium mobilization, resemble the earliest events in activation of mature T cells, but in these immature thymocytes, lead instead to cell death. These studies, superficially at least, suggest that ligation of the T-cell receptor alone, without a second signal from an accessory cell, can lead to clonal abortion. In that case, the requirement for accessory cells in some models might be attributable simply to limited tissue distribution of the toleragen under consideration.

B. Clonal Anergy of T Cells

Clonal anergy is a term introduced by our group (Nossal and Pike, 1980) to describe functional silencing of an immunocyte without its actual destruction. The concept was first proven for B cells, anergy induction being much more readily induced in immature than in mature cells. The experimental demonstration of clonal anergy was anticipated by the theory of Bretscher and Cohn (1970), who postulated that a union of antigen with a receptor on the lymphocyte surface (Signal 1 only) would lead to tolerance, unless accompanied by Signal 2, delivered by a helper T cell recognizing an associated epitope of the antigen. In the case of the T cell, the greater sensitivity of immature cells to anergy induction has not been so clearly established, perhaps because abortion is the main mechanism while the cells are in the thymus. However, some results are consistent with this possibility (Ramsdell and Fowlkes, 1990). The first direct evidence for T-cell anergy came from the work of Lamb *et al.* (1983). They showed that human CD4+ T-cell clones reactive to peptides of the influenza virus hemagglutinin could be rendered unresponsive by incubating them with peptide alone. The cells were not killed but rather rendered anergic and thus not able to proliferate in response to specific antigen and accessory cells. A similar conclusion in a murine system was reached by Jenkins and Schwartz (1987), who also showed that the anergic cells fail to produce interleukin (IL)-2. Costimulatory signals from accessory cells, probably requiring direct cell contact, are required if the cell is to be activated rather than rendered anergic. Interestingly, many of the early biochemical events during anergy induction resemble those of immune activation (Schwartz, 1989). Clearly, much remains to be done to elucidate the mechanisms that allow the cell to "decide" between anergy or activation.

Can clonal anergy of T cells be a reality *in vivo?* This question can now be answered definitively in the affirmative. Rammensee and Bevan (1987) noted that when substantial numbers of splenic lymphocytes are injected intravenously into class I MHC-incompatible recipients, donor-derived T cells persist in the recipients, and a mutual tolerance develops: host lymphocytes become non-responsive to the donor, and donor lymphocytes, to the host. This is perhaps a special case, as MHC antigens are expressed particularly strongly on lymphoid and hemopoietic cells. However, anergy toward class I or class II MHC antigens can also be induced when the toleragen is expressed only on particular parenchymal cells. Once again, the transgenic approach has been of great help here. The most interesting studies are those in which a transgene has been placed under the control of a promoter that targets expression precisely to a particular organ or tissue. In a sense, the transgene-coded protein becomes a surrogate for the multitude of tissue-specific cell-surface molecules, which could become targets of an immune attack. A good example is to place a foreign MHC gene under the control of the insulin promoter, which leads to expression of the transgene in the β cells of the pancreatic islets of Langerhans (Allison *et al.*, 1988; Morahan *et al.*, 1989a; Burkly *et al.*, 1990; reviewed in Miller *et al.*, 1989). Interestingly, class I transgene expression leads to some form of nonimmunologic damage to the β cells, whether the transgene is syngeneic or allogeneic to the host animal. When allogeneic class I is involved, the mice become tolerant of the class I antigen, as shown by skin grafting or by cell-mediated lympholysis experiments performed on splenocytes *in vitro*. Importantly, thymic lymphocytes do *not* show *in vitro* tolerance. The tolerance wanes as the β cells die and is thus clearly associated with the continued presence of the antigen. This is a powerful argument against the notion that tolerance is really induced within the thymus by conventional clonal abortion through "leakiness" of transgene expression. Also, the absence of *in vitro* tolerance within the thymic population at any time argues against transport of β cell-derived antigen to the thymus via accessory cells. It is difficult to escape the conclusion that tolerance is induced peripherally, probably through clonal anergy, possibly while the T cells recently emigrated from the thymus are still immature. The problem then remains how *all* the T cells get modified by such a small source of tissue. This point is rendered even more difficult by the recent finding that most of the T cells in different lymph (and thus cells patrolling the tissues) are of memory and not naive phenotype (Mackay *et al.*, 1990). Presumably shed MHC antigens from dying β cells could be processed by macrophages and other accessory cells in draining lymph nodes, a site through which naive T cells do traffic. In that regard, it is of interest that IL-2 can restore the *in vitro* reactivity of the tolerant splenocytes, suggesting that the tolerance lesion may lie in the CD4+ helper cell compartment rather than the CD8+ cytotoxic T-cell compartment. If so, tolerization by processed antigen could work. If not, processed antigen would be unlikely to be the toleragen, because only internal peptides associate with class I MHC, save for a few exceptional circumstances (Braciale *et al.*, 1987).

There is a second model thrusting in the same general direction, which involves the class I K^b transgene under the control of the metallothionein promoter (Morahan *et al.*, 1989b). This directs expression chiefly to the liver, kidney, and exocrine pancreas. In this model also, skin graft tolerance to the foreign class I is produced and lasts for life. It survives adult thymectomy, x-irradiation with marrow protection and grafting of nontransgenic syngeneic thymus. This indicates a peripheral mechanism as, even if transgene expression "leaks" to the thymus, the transplanted thymus or donor-derived nontransgenic cells would not express the foreign class I antigens.

C. T-Cell-Mediated Suppression

For most of the 1970s, it was fashionable to ascribe many tolerance phenomena, if not the whole of tolerance, to suppressor T cells. Now the pendulum has swung in the opposite direction, and the concept does not figure prominently in discussions on tolerance. Yet there is a wealth of experimental evidence, particularly in various transplantation models, to show that there are circumstances in which the adoptive transfer of T cells abrogates immune responses and confers tolerance at least at the operational level. It is also evident that large doses of antigen given intravenously or sometimes orally can powerfully inhibit later immune responses. A review of the vast literature on T cell-mediated suppression is outside the scope of the present chapter, but some subjective comments may be helpful. It is unlikely that a separate lineage of T cells, the sole duty of which is to suppress immune responses, exists. Both CD4+ and CD8+ T cells can secrete lymphokines, in combinatorial patterns and ratios that depend (*inter alia*) on the method of antigen presentation (Kelso, 1989). Some of these lymphokines can be powerfully inhibitory to immune responses. For example, interferon-γ can inhibit IL-4-dependent isotype switching and other aspects of antibody formation (Snapper and Paul, 1987) and tumor necrosis factor (TNF) can trigger cytotoxic phenomena. It is possible that antigen-specific suppression is attributable to the activation of T cell clones into the localized synthesis of lymphokines antagonistic to those made by helper T cells or accessory cells that are required for immune activation. It is also possible that suppression involves the inhibition of idiotype-bearing helper T cells by antiidiotypic CD8+ T cells. As regards suppressor phenomena noted exclusively *in vitro,* these could on occasion have quite a trivial explanation, such as addition of T cells that consume a lymphokinelike IL-2, required for the ongoing immune response and made in limiting amounts within the culture. I believe a majority of immunologists would now not see suppression as the dominant mechanism of self-recognition. This should not minimize its importance, however, as the true establishment or reestablishment of tolerance remains a dream in the two situations that confront us clinically, namely autoimmune diseases and organ transplantation. If suppressor phenomena are an important aspect of the regulation of immune responses, as I believe they are, then we should endeavor to learn enough about them to use them intelligently in therapy.

III. B-CELL TOLERANCE

A. Earlier Studies on Clonal Abortion and Clonal Anergy

The thought that B cells, too, could be rendered tolerant by antigen goes back at least 20 years. Weigle's group, working with adult mice, found that large doses of soluble antigen could silence B-cell populations as well as T cells (Chiller *et al.*, 1970). The first evidence of a special sensitivity of immature B cells to negative signaling came from Cooper's group using antiimmunoglobulin μ heavy chain antibodies (reviewed in Lawton and Cooper, 1974). We were the first to attack the problem at the clonal level by enumerating antibody-forming cell precursor (AFCP) numbers using microculture techniques (Nossal and Pike, 1975; 1978; 1980). This work clearly demonstrated three things. First, hapten-specific B cells were exquisitely sensitive to negative signaling by hapten–protein conjugates during the period when they moved from pre-B to B-cell status, that is, when the Ig receptors were first appearing on the cell membrane. Second, multivalency of the antigen was important; the more a conjugate crosslinked the receptor, the stronger the negative signal. These two points were independently made by Metcalf and Klinman (1976; 1977) at about the same time. Third, while large doses of toleragen led to a reduction in the number of hapten-specific B cells that appeared, smaller doses could still induce tolerance without affecting actual hapten-binding B-cell numbers. We thus argued that *strong* negative signaling involved *clonal abortion,* an actual removal of the B cell from the population; whereas weaker negative signaling induced *clonal anergy,* a tolerant state that did not lead to death of the B cell.

This capacity of one reagent to cause the two disparate effects could be amply confirmed by use of the *universal toleragen,* anti-μ chain antibody (Pike *et al.*, 1982). When either newborn splenic or adult bone marrow pre-B cells were asked to mature into B cells in the presence of various concentrations of a monoclonal anti-μ chain antibody, it took about 10 μg/ml to prevent B-cell appearance, i.e., to cause clonal abortion. A 100-fold lower concentration allowed B cells with a normal Ig receptor complement to emerge, but these cells were completely unable to proliferate or form antibody. Indeed, even 100 pg/ml still induced anergy in half the B cells. This is a striking example of the sensitivity of maturing B cells to anergy induction. This earlier body of work has been reviewed in more detail elsewhere (Nossal, 1983).

B. Transgenic Models for Study of Clonal Abortion and Clonal Anergy

The development of transgenic mouse models has been particularly revealing with respect to B-cell tolerance and has supported many of the earlier insights. It may be worthwhile to begin with some negative results. Models in which the transgene leads to the production of low concentrations of a *soluble* form of class I MHC antigen (Arnold *et al.*, 1988) or a xenogeneic insulin (Whiteley and Kapp, 1989) fail to lead to B-cell tolerance. This agrees with the experiments in which experimental tolerance was hard to induce in B cells with monovalent antigens. However, one elegant model (Goodnow *et al.*, 1988; 1989; 1990) shows that monovalent antigens can lead to tolerance in the B-cell compartment, at least for B cells displaying receptors of high affinity for the transgenic antigen. These experiments relied on doubly transgenic mice. One strain was rendered transgenic for the antigen, hen egg lysozyme (HEL), another for both the μ and δ heavy and κ light chain genes specifying a high-affinity anti-HEL. When the strains were crossed, some progeny were doubly transgenic. It was clear that these possessed a preponderant population of transgene-expressing B cells with an IgM^{dull} IgD^{bright} phenotype, which had *not* been deleted but which were unreactive to challenge with HEL in either T-independent or T-dependent form. Interestingly, adoptive transfer studies from antibody-alone transgenics to antigen-alone transgenics showed that anergy could be induced perfectly well in mature B cells, immature cells enjoying no special advantage. When B cells from doubly transgenic animals were adoptively transferred into syngeneic, HEL-free mice, the anergy could not be reversed, but the selective down-regulation of surface IgM was.

While it is naturally satisfying to the author to see the concept of clonal anergy validated also for the B cell, it is nevertheless important to focus on the apparent discrepancies. Why does HEL cause B-cell tolerance, but insulin does not? One reason may be affinity; the anti-HEL transgenes were chosen for high-affinity antibody. Molarity is also important; there are founder lines in the HEL system that yield lower HEL serum concentrations, which do not lead to anergy. And why does an apparently monomeric protein work when our model and others required epitopic multivalency? The most likely explanation is *in vivo* matrix-generating mechanisms; HEL is "sticky" and could adhere to cell surfaces and/or self-aggregate. However, it is not excluded that monomeric antigen can tolerize high-affinity B cells.

A transgenic model illustrating clonal abortion of B cells has also been presented (Nemazee and Bürki, 1989a,b). In this, mice were rendered transgenic for the IgM form of monoclonal antibody 3-83, which has a moderately high affinity for H-2K^k and a low affinity for H-2K^b. In the absence of H-2K^k or K^b in the transgenic mouse, abundant transgene-expressing B cells were found, constituting up to 90% of the B cells of the animal. In the presence of H-2K^k, the bone marrow contained significant numbers of B cells bearing small amounts of transgene product, but anti-H-2K^k B cells were absent from the spleen and lymph nodes. The results indicated that clonal deletion of transgene-bearing cells was occurring during the pre-B and B-cell transition in the marrow. Interestingly, the same was true when H-2K^b was expressed, either on all cells, or just on liver parenchymal cells, as in the metallothionein-K^b transgenic model. This indicates that an abundant cell-surface antigen, such as class I MHC, can cause deletion even when the affinity of the interaction is not particularly high. It also indicates that tolerance can be induced peripherally, perhaps in B cells that have recently emigrated from the bone marrow.

Why does this model show deletion, but the HEL model shows anergy? Perhaps the answer lies in the strength of the negative signal. A strongly crosslinking stimulus may cause clonal abortion, just as saturating concentrations of anti-μ antibodies do. A weakly crosslinking stimulus may cause anergy, just as low concentrations of anti-μ do. A noncrosslinking stimulus may have no effect or perhaps may cause anergy in only very high affinity B cells.

C. Negative Signaling Involving the Fc Receptor

There is a substantial literature documenting the fact that soluble immune complexes in the zone of antigen excess can deliver powerful negative signals to the relevant B cells (reviewed in Feldmann and Nossal, 1972; Sinclair, 1990). This has led some to speculate that all B-cell tolerance of self-antigens might be associated with that kind of end-product inhibition. Any activation of an anti-self B cell would be followed by rapid complexing of the secreted antibody with the ubiquitous self-antigen, perhaps in the vicinity of the B cell, before the antibody reaches the circulation. The resulting complex quickly shuts off the B cell in question and all others like it in nearby areas. Is any more required to ensure an absence of self-reactivity? Conceptually, this idea is not appealing, as it fails to discriminate between self-antigens and long-persisting foreign antigens, e.g., in parasitic infestations. Antibody-mediated negative feedback may well be a major factor in limiting the levels of antibody reached in the latter. Experimentally, the notion could conceivably explain the HEL anti-HEL model, though no immune complexes have been noted, which is difficult to explain given the large number of transgene-expressing immunocytes. However, it does not fit comfortably with the anti-H-2K^k transgene model, nor with the demonstration of clonal anergy in very young mice that could not yet have formed substantial quantities of antibody

(Nossal and Pike, 1980). We prefer to regard this very powerful and important end-product feedback control as exemplifying the subtlety of immunoregulation and ensuring that antibody formation does not become excessive under circumstances in which it proves impossible to eliminate an antigen from the body.

D. Tolerance Mechanisms and Affinity Maturation of Antibodies

When a foreign antigen persists for some time in the body, or when an antigen is injected repeatedly, it is a general rule that the affinity of antibody for the antigen increases with time. The reason for this affinity maturation is that the V genes of immunoglobulin heavy and light chains are subject to a very high rate of somatic mutation (hypermutation), and that those cells, the V genes of which code for antibody of higher affinity, are preferentially selected for further multiplication (Weigert *et al.*, 1970; Rajewsky *et al.*, 1987; Berek and Milstein, 1987). It is widely believed that B-cell hypermutation and antigenic selection take place in specialized structures, the germinal centers (MacLennan and Gray, 1986). The question then arises as to what happens when a B cell, appropriately dividing in response to some foreign antigen, fortuitously mutates to high-affinity recognition of a self-antigen. This must happen from time to time, given the number of self-antigens. As selection of mutant cells within the germinal center appears to be independent of T cells, such a B cell could easily continue to multiply. Obviously, its restimulation outside the germinal center would require T-cell help, which would be absent because of T-cell tolerance, but it might nevertheless be advantageous for this cell to be eliminated or silenced in some way. Linton *et al.* (1989) have obtained some evidence that those B cells responsible for immunologic memory go through a *second window* of tolerance susceptibility shortly after activation, that is, a period during which contact with soluble antigen in the absence of T-cell help renders them inactive or eliminates them. This is the circumstance that might apply within germinal centers. Our group has produced some evidence (Nossal and Karvelas, 1990) to demonstrate that the injection of soluble protein antigen before, or even shortly after, challenge immunization largely prevented the appearance of B cells able to produce specific antiprotein IgG_1 antibody in clonal microcultures. The normal-affinity maturation among B cells was also prevented. We now require adoptive transfer studies to elucidate whether this was owing to a direct effect of soluble antigen on B cells, or whether it was attributable (in whole or in part) to T cell-mediated effects, either tolerance or helper cells or some form of suppression.

E. The Basis of B-Cell Tolerance

The above results indicate that the concept of B-cell tolerance is now on a firm footing, but, as with T-cell tolerance, that more than one cellular mechanism is at work. Obviously the easiest target for tolerance induction is the B cell being formed in the bone marrow, where strongly crosslinking antigenic encounters lead to its death, and weaker signals, to anergy. B cells in the periphery can still be eliminated or rendered anergic, but now stronger signals are required. Antigen–antibody complexes, which crosslink the Ig receptor and also the Fc receptor, are very strongly down-regulatory for the B cell unless T-cell help is concurrently at hand. There may be a further phase of great sensitivity to tolerance induction shortly after the activation of B cells responsible for secondary responses. Given the fact that antibodies vary so greatly in their affinity, and also the large number of cross-reactions between antigens and antibodies, it is obvious that some B cells with anti-self reactivity must be permitted within the body. Their total elimination would require the total elimination of the B-cell repertoire. Thus what is required is that high-affinity anti-self B cells be eliminated by clonal abortion or silenced through clonal anergy; and furthermore, that low-affinity anti-self B cells not be permitted to survive and divide if they mutate toward high-affinity anti-self. This probably involves both T-cell regulatory circuits and direct B-cell tolerance effects. It is a failure of such censorship that permits autoantibody production. There is mounting evidence that this involves antigen-driven events and, in many cases, extensive somatic V gene mutation (Shlomchik *et al.*, 1987).

IV. TOLERANCE BREAKDOWN AND AUTOIMMUNITY

The immune system is based on selection rather than instruction and is composed of cells that carry only one specific kind of recognition structure, the Ig or T-cell receptor. As the system does not know beforehand what it must recognize, the set or repertoire of recognition units is degenerate and redundant. Immunity depends on clonal selection; tolerance, on clonal deletion or silencing. In each case, just beyond the population being activated or silenced, there are immunocytes that *might* have been activated or silenced had circumstances been slightly different, because the affinity of their receptors for the antigen in question was just below the required threshold. The immune system therefore contains cells with autoimmune potential, and it is, in a sense, not surprising that dysregulation sometimes occurs and leads to frank autoimmune disease.

The etiology of autoimmune diseases is undoubtedly multifactorial. The clearest evidence for this comes from genetic analysis of autoimmune diseases in inbred strains of laboratory animals, in which it is usual to find at least four genes segregating, all of which contribute to disease incidence. In the context of breakdown of tolerance, most theories of autoimmunity can be grouped under four headings, namely, failed self-censorship, abnormal presentation of autoantigens, hyporesponsiveness, or hyperresponsiveness (Table I).

TABLE I
Tolerance Breakdown and Autoimmunity

A. Failed self-censorship (nondeletion)
T cells: intrathymic escape from negative selection
escape from peripheral deletion/anergy
B cells: escape during pre-B to B-cell transition
B. Aberrant antigen presentation
Leakage of sequestered antigen
Tolerated autoantigen on nontolerated carrier
Molecular mimicry ± autoimmune cascade
"Ectopic" MHC molecules
C. Hyporesponsiveness
Predisposition to infection → autoimmunity (e.g., AIDS)
D. Hyperresponsiveness
Polyclonal activation of B cells (e.g., lupus mice)
E. Other mechamisms
Failure of T-cell suppression
Infections → lymphokines → B-cell activation
Structural defects in target organs
Vicious circle: damage → antigen release → damage, etc.

A. Failed Self-Censorship

Self-tolerance within the T-cell compartment depends on intrathymic elimination of those T cells potentially directed against self-peptide–MHC complexes expressed in the thymus and peripheral silencing of T cells directed against self-peptide–MHC complexes expressed extrathymically. If these negative selective mechanisms were to fail, the scene would be set for autoimmunity. One extensively studied model in which failed self-censorship may be at work is the insulin-dependent diabetes of nonobese diabetic (NOD) mice (e.g., Nishimoto *et al.*, 1987; Slattery *et al.*, 1990). These mice have a peculiar class II MHC genotype, lacking I-E altogether and possessing a unique I-A gene, I-A^{NOD}. If the mice are rendered transgenic for, e.g., I-A^k, diabetes is completely prevented. One interpretation of this is that the I-A^k but not the I-A^{NOD} MHC molecule can present a peptide intrathymically that is also a critical autoantigen on the pancreatic B cell. Clonal abortion would occur in the I-A^k transgenic but not the littermate NOD mice. The latter would permit peripheralization of the putatively autoimmune T cells. Of course, it is not excluded that the transgenic but not the littermate NOD mice can respond to some pathogen, which is responsible for autoimmunity. Given the fact that any one individual expresses only a small subset of the large array of MHC genes that a species possesses, it is probable that failure of self-censorship at the T-cell level contributes to at least some autoimmune diseases. Failed self-censorship at the B-cell level is likely to be at least a factor in those situations in which multiply mutated autoantibodies are recognized in a disease.

B. Aberrant Antigen Presentation

One of the earliest notions in autoimmunity was that it might be triggered by the release of sequestered antigens. While it is now clear that tolerance pertains to many antigens that do not exist in readily measurable concentrations in extracellular fluids, and thus that the sequestered-antigen idea is not tenable in its original form, there are still situations in which an unusual presentation of antigen may contribute to autoantibody formation. Presentation of a tolerated antigen on a nontolerated carrier is one example; molecular mimicry, in which an epitope that is shared between a self-antigen and a pathogen triggers autoantibody formation is a specialized example of altered presentation. The epitope concerned is obviously embedded in a highly foreign, nontolerated biochemical environment within the pathogen. Molecular mimicry can also work in reverse, where self-tolerance of an autoantigen impedes a response to a shared epitope on a pathogen.

Immunogenic mimicry could start an autoimmune cascade. Consider normal cellular turnover, in which cells die, and their constituent parts are dealt with by a mixture of proteolytic degradation and autophagocytes without significant autoantibody formation. Suppose mimicry permits antibody formation to some intracellular constituent, say an epitope on a small nuclear ribonucleoprotein. The existence of this antibody could alter the balance of disposition of the constituents of the dying cell, e.g., most of the small nuclear ribonucleoprotein particles displaying the epitope could be opsonized and enter professional antigen-presenting cells, thus making the *whole* particle more immunogenic than it would otherwise be. In that case, other and nonmimicked epitopes within that same particle could elicit autoantibody formation, and a cluster of autoantibodies to a variety of epitopes on the subcellular constituent concerned would appear.

The sudden appearance of class II MHC on a cell is another specialized example of abnormal presentation. If nontolerated T-cell epitopes are suddenly presented on a cell in association with class II MHC, it makes the cell a logical target for autoimmune attack versus that epitope, whereas a cell lacking class II MHC would not be susceptible. Admittedly, this form of abnormal presentation is not so attractive a concept as formerly, in view of the fact that class II association usually occurs not for endogenously synthesized peptides but for exogenous antigens, which need to be endocytosed and processed.

C. Hyporesponsiveness

The strong MHC association in many autoimmune diseases prompts the persisting claim that autoimmunity may have something to do with an inadequate immune response to some infectious agent, one that most people deal with adequately, but which is not removed by individuals of a particular MHC genotype because the T-cell epitopes of the pathogen concerned cannot be adequately presented by those MHC molecules. Attempts to find causative microorganisms for autoimmune diseases have been legion, and, most recently, a new interest in retroviruses has emerged. For example, Talal *et al.* (1989) invoke a retrovirus as a possible cause in 20 to 30% of patients with Sjögren's syndrome, and Ciampolillo *et al.* (1989) have suggested retroviral involvement in Graves' disease. Obviously, these important claims will have to be examined very seriously. However, there are theoretical reasons making it unlikely that hyporesponsiveness based on deficiencies in MHC genotype is the cause of autoimmunity. These reasons are similar to those that make MHC genotype-based susceptibility to infectious diseases an uncommon event. B- and T-cell responses to a single protein antigen are usually polyclonal, not only because a protein usually has more than one epitope but also because a selective immune system randomly assembles light- and heavy-chain V genes, thus finding many solutions for specificity toward a given epitope. Moreover, even a virus displays not just one but several antigenic proteins, and more complex pathogens, correspondingly more. Should a particular MHC genotype prejudice against response to one protein, it is unlikely to do so against a second. Therefore, on balance, the author is disinclined to regard specific hyporesponsiveness to a causative virus as a major cause of autoimmunity. If viruses are involved in disease initiation, it seems more likely that MHC genotype would influence the reaction to some critical autoantigen released from the damaged target organ.

D. Hyperresponsiveness

Polyclonal activation of B lymphocytes is a feature of many animal models of multisystem autoimmunity, and particularly the lupus erythematosuslike models. This manifests itself in hypergammaglobulinemia and an increase in the number of antibody-producing cells found in the spleen or other lymphoid tissue. A significant proportion of these activated cells display anti-self reactivity, e.g., make antinuclear antibody. However, as Edberg and Taylor (1986) have noted, there are significant differences between anti-DNA antibodies derived through immortalizing randomly stimulated B cells, and those found in systemic lupus erythematosus. The latter are, in general, of higher avidity, display fewer cross-reactions, react more frequently with double-stranded DNA, and display multiple somatic V-gene mutations (Shlomchik *et al.*, 1987). It is difficult to escape the conclusion that they have been shaped by antigenic stimulation and selection. Thus, hyperresponsiveness to any stimulus is not likely to be the cause of lupus, although it may represent one step in a dysregulation that later conspires with failed self-censorship and/or aberrant antigen presentation to produce the disease state.

E. Other Mechanisms

The above list of possible contributory factors to autoimmunity is by no means exhaustive. A failure of T cell-mediated suppression is less favored now than a decade ago, but must be considered, as the vast literature on suppressor T cells undoubtedly contains a selection of valuable findings. Polyclonal B-cell activation due to high lymphokine concentrations may contribute to those autoantibodies that accompany some severe infections. Structural defects in target organs probably contribute both to undue fluxes of autoantigens and to the amount of damage inflicted by a given quantum of autoaggression. The *vicious circle* hypothesis, first enunciated by Mackay and Burnet (1963), remains attractive. A *forbidden* clone of immunocytes, i.e., one that has escaped self-censorship, damages a target organ, thus causing autoantigen release, consequent stimulation and proliferation of the forbidden clone leading to further target organ damage, and so on.

The early literature on autoimmunity concentrates on autoantibodies because that is what could be easily measured. Now it is clear that in many situations, it is really autoaggressive T cells that are the initiators of damage, and uncovering the details of their specificity and regulation is a formidable task. Fortunately, the process of isolating and cloning T cells that infiltrate damaged tissue has begun, and, in animal models of spontaneous autoimmunity, has been achieved before frank disease is manifest. This should help in defining the most important T-cell epitopes that are the targets of autoimmunity.

Just like tolerance, autoimmunity is a quantitative concept, a matter of balance. Clearly, some level of autoantibody formation is quite normal, and autoimmune disease results only when the amount, duration, or affinity of autoantibody, or of autodirected T-cell activity, pass some normal limit. The mechanisms may differ for different autoimmune diseases, or even in different cases of one autoimmune disease.

V. CONCLUSIONS

The paradigm of regarding self-tolerance and autoimmunity as directly opposite concepts, both subject to a variety of cellular and molecular mechanisms, remains as valid as when it was first articulated. What has changed in our perceptions is that we no longer seek a single, simple cause of autoimmunity any more than a single, simple mechanism of tolerance induction. Clonal abortion and clonal anergy of T and B cells come close to the single, simple mechanism of tolerance; failure of those two mechanisms of repertoire purging comes close to the cause of autoimmunity. However, so many factors influence normal repertoire purging, and so many influence the activation of any cell that may have escaped purging, that this bald articulation does not do credit to the huge body of knowledge that has accumulated about immunoregulation. What is perhaps of greater importance is to examine each model of tolerance, and each clinically important example of tolerance breakdown, in considerable detail. In all probability, different models will highlight different facets of immunoregulation within the above broad framework. If so, different control strategies will emerge for the various situations, be these autoimmune diseases, organ transplants, or defects of immunoregulation such as allergies or immunodeficiencies. The students of tolerance and autoimmunity find themselves in much the same trouble as all immunologists; understanding of an immune phenomenon demands knowledge of the system as a whole. This being so, the search for underlying broad principles and the profound exploration of particular fragmentary models must continue to proceed in parallel.

ACKNOWLEDGMENTS

Original work summarized in this review was supported by the National Health and Medical Research Council, Canberra, Australia, by Grant AI-03958 from the National Institute of Allergy and Infectious Diseases, U.S. Public Health Service, and by the generosity of a number of private donors to The Walter and Eliza Hall Institute of Medical Research.

REFERENCES

Allison, J., Campbell, I. L., Morahan, G., Mandel, T. E., Harrison, L. C., and Miller, J. F. A. P. (1988). *Nature* **333,** 529–533.

Arnold, B., Dill, O., Kuhlbeck, G., Jatsch, L., Simon, M. M., Tucker, J., and Hämmerling, G. J. (1988). *Proc. Natl. Acad. Sci. U.S.A.* **85,** 2269–2273.

Berek, C., and Milstein, C. (1987). *Immunol. Rev.* **96,** 23–42.

Billingham, R. E., Brent, L., and Medawar, P. B. (1953). *Nature,* **172,** 603–606.

Boon, T., and Van Pel, A. (1989). *Immunogenetics* **29,** 75–79.

Braciale, T. C., Morrison, L. A., Sweetser, M. T., Sambrook, J., Gething, M.-J., and Braciale, V. L. (1987). *Immunol. Rev.* **98,** 95–114.

Bretscher, P., and Cohn, M. (1970). *Science* **169,** 1042–1049.

Burkly, L. C., Lo, D., and Flavell, R. A. (1990). *Science* **248,** 1364–1368.

Burnet, F. M., (1957). *Aust. J. Sci.* **20,** 67–69.

Burnet, F. M., and Fenner, F. (1949). "The Production of Antibodies," 2nd edn. pp. 142. Macmillan, London.

Chiller, J. M., Habicht, G. S., and Weigle, W. O. (1970). *Proc. Natl. Acad. Sci. U.S.A.* **65,** 551–56.

Ciampolillo, A., Marini, V., Mirakian, R., *et al.* (1989). *Lancet* May 20, 1096–1100.

Dent, A. L., Matis, L. A., Hooshmand, F., Widacki, S. M., Bluestone, J. A., and Hedrick, S. M. (1990). *Nature* **343,** 714–719.
Edberg, J. C., and Taylor, R. P. (1986). *J. Immunol.* **136,** 4581–4587.
Feldmann, M., and Nossal, G. J. V. (1972). *Transplant. Rev.* **13,** 3–34.
Gershon, R. K., and Kondo, K. (1971). *Immunol.* **21,** 903–914.
Goodnow, C. C., Crosbie, J., Adelstein, S., Lavoie, T. B., Smith-Gill, S. J., Brink, R. A., Pritchard-Biscoe, H., Wotherspoon, J. S., Loblay, R. H., Raphael, K., Trent, R. J., and Basten, A. (1988). *Nature* **334,** 676–682.
Goodnow, C. C., Crosbie, J., Jorgensen, H., Brink, R. A., and Basten, A. (1989). *Nature* **342,** 385–391.
Goodnow, C. C., Adelstein, S., and Basten, A. (1990). *Science* **248,** 1373–1379.
Janeway, C. A., Yagi, J., Conrad, P., Katz, M., Vroegop, S., and Buxser, S. (1989). *Immunol. Rev.* **107,** 61–88.
Jenkins, M. K., and Schwartz, R. H. (1987). *J. Exp. Med.* **165,** 302–319.
Kappler, J. W., Roehm, N., and Marrack, P. C. (1987). *Cell* **49,** 273–280.
Kappler, J. W., Staerz, U., White, J., and Marrack, P. C. (1988). *Nature* **332,** 35–40.
Kelso, A. (1989). *Curr. Opin. Immunol.* **2,** 215–225.
Kisielow, P., Blüthmann, H., Staerz, U. D., Steinmetz, M., and von Boehmer, H. (1988). *Nature* **333,** 742–746.
Lamb, J. R., Skidmore, B. J., Green, N., Chiller, J. M., and Feldmann, M. (1983). *J. Exp. Med.* **157,** 1434–1447.
Lawton, A. R., and Cooper, M. D. (1974). *Contemp. Top. Immunobiol.* **3,** 193–225.
Lederberg, J. (1959). *Science* **129,** 1649–1653.
Linton, P.-J., Decker, D. J., and Klinman, N. R. (1989). *Cell* **59,** 1049–1059.
MacDonald, H. R., Schneider, R., Lees, R. K., Howe, R. C., Acha-Orbea, H., Festenstein, H., Zinkernagel, R. M., and Hengartner, H. (1988). *Nature* **332,** 40–45.
Mackay, C. R., Marston, W. L., and Dudler, L. (1990). *J. Exp. Med.* **171,** 801–817.
Mackay, I. R., and Burnet, F. M. (1963). "Autoimmune Diseases." Charles C Thomas, Springfield, Illinois.
MacLennan, I. C. M., and Gray, D. (1986). *Immunol. Rev.* **91,** 61–85.
Marrack, P., Pullen, A. M., Herman, A., Callahan, J., Choi, Y., Potts, W., Wakeland, E., and Kappler, J. W. (1989). *In* "Progress in Immunology VII" (F. Melchers, ed.), pp. 3–12. Springer-Verlag, Berlin.
Matzinger, P., and Guerder, S. (1989). *Nature* **338,** 74–76.
McCullagh, P. J. (1970). *Aust. J. Exp. Biol. Med. Sci.* **48,** 369–379.
Metcalf, E. S., and Klinman, N. R. (1976). *J. Exp. Med.* **143,** 1327–1340.
Metcalf, E. S., and Klinman, N. R. (1977). *J. Immunol.* **118,** 2111–2116.
Miller, J. F. A. P., Morahan, G., Allison, J., Bhathal, P. S., and Cox, K. O. (1989). *Immunol. Rev.* **107,** 109–123.
Morahan, G., Allison, J., and Miller, J. F. A. P. (1989a). *Nature* **339,** 622–624.
Morahan, G., Brennan, F. E., Bhathal, P. S., Allison, J., Cox, K. O., and Miller, J. F. A. P. (1989b). *Proc. Natl. Acad. Sci. U.S.A.* **86,** 3782–3786.
Nemazee, D., and Buerki, K. (1989a). *Nature* **337,** 562–566.
Nemazee, D., and Buerki, K. (1989b). *Proc. Natl. Acad. Sci. U.S.A.* **86,** 8039–8043.
Nishimoto, H., Kikutani, H., Yamamura, K., and Kishimoto, T. (1987). *Nature* **328,** 432–434.
Nossal, G. J. V. (1983). *Annu. Rev. Immunol.* **1,** 33–62.
Nossal, G. J. V., and Karvelas, M. (1990). *Proc. Natl. Acad. Sci. U.S.A.* **87,** 1615–1619.
Nossal, G. J. V., and Pike, B. L. (1975). *J. Exp. Med.* **141,** 904–917.
Nossal, G. J. V., and Pike, B. L. (1978). *J. Exp. Med.* **148,** 1161–1170.
Nossal, G. J. V., and Pike, B. L. (1980). *Proc. Natl. Acad. Sci. U.S.A.* **77,** 1602–1606.

Nossal, G. J. V., and Pike, B. L. (1981). *Proc. Natl. Acad. Sci. U.S.A.* **78,** 3844–3847.
Pike, B. L., Boyd, A. W., and Nossal, G. J. V. (1982). *Proc. Natl. Acad. Sci. U.S.A.* **79,** 2013–2017.
Pircher, H., Bürki, K., Lang, R., Hengartner, H., and Zinkernagel, R. M. (1989). *Nature* **342,** 559–561.
Rajewsky, K., Förster, I., and Cumano, A. (1987). *Science* **238,** 1088–1094.
Rammensee, H.-G., and Bevan, M. J. (1987). *Eur. J. Immunol.* **17,** 893–895.
Ramsdell, F., and Fowlkes, B. J. (1990). *Science* **248,** 1342–1349.
Schwartz, R. H. (1989). *Cell* **57,** 1073–1081.
Shlomchik, M. J., Marshak-Rothstein, A., Wolfowitz, C. B., Rothstein, T. L., and Weigert, M. G. (1987). *Nature* **328,** 805–811.
Sinclair, N. R. St.C. (1990). *Autoimmunity* **6,** 131–142.
Slattery, R. M., Kjer-Nielson, L., Allison, J., Charlton, B., Mandel, T. E., and Miller, J. F. A. P. (1990). *Nature* **345,** 724–726.
Smith, C. A., Williams, G. T., Kingston, R., Jenkinson, E. J., and Owen, J. J. T. (1989). *Nature* **337,** 181–184.
Snapper, C. M., and Paul, W. E. (1987). *Science* **236,** 944–947.
Sprent, J., and Webb, S. R. (1987). *Adv. Immunol.* **41,** 39–133.
Talal, N., Dauphinee, M. J., Dang, H., Alexander, S., and Garry, R. (1989). *Prog. Immunol.* **7,** 837–841.
Talmage, D. W. (1957). *Annu. Rev. Med.* **8,** 239–256.
Weigert, M. G., Cesari, I. M., Yonkovich, S. J., and Cohn, M. (1970). *Nature* **228,** 1045–1047.
White, J., Herman, A., Pullen, A. M., Kubo, R., Kappler, J., and Marrack, P. (1989). *Cell* **56,** 27–35.
Whiteley, P. J., and Kapp, J. A. (1989). *Prog. Immunol.* **7,** 826–832.

CHAPTER **3**

Experimental Models of Human Autoimmune Disease: Overview and Prototypes

CLAUDE C. A. BERNARD
Neuroimmunology Laboratory
La Trobe University
Bundoora, Victoria, Australia

TOM E. MANDEL
The Walter and Eliza Hall Institute
Parkville, Victoria 3050, Australia

IAN R. MACKAY
Centre for Molecular Biology and Medicine
Monash University
Clayton, Victoria, Australia, and
Brain-Behaviour Research Institute
La Trobe University
Bundoora, Victoria, Australia

I. AN OVERVIEW OF MODELS

A. INTRODUCTION

The complexity of human autoimmune disease requires comparable models for a reductionist understanding of etiology and pathogenesis, and for devising optimal treatments. The earliest models, dating back to 1933, depended on the logical procedure of immunizing animals with emulsions of normal (neural) tissues (Rivers *et al.*, 1933). However, the regular induction of autoimmune disease by this means could not be achieved until the immunogenic potency of the tissue inocula could be enhanced by emulsification in complete Freund's adjuvant (CFA) of the tissue extract, brain, testis, thyroid gland, etc. The ensuing model autoimmune diseases replicated many of the features of the naturally occurring human counterparts, including comparable signs and histopathology and a strong genetic requirement, and allowed for an analysis of effector processes, which were shown to depend essentially on activated T lymphocytes.

In 1959, a new experimental model was recognized in New Zealand. This was a mouse strain derived by selective inbreeding, New Zealand Black (NZB), that spontaneously developed an "acquired" hemolytic anemia. Mating of these mice with another related inbred line, New Zealand White (NZW), produced an F_1 that developed an autoimmune disease simulating human systemic lupus erythematosus (SLE). Subsequently there were recognized other strains of mice with a similar disease expression; collectively these are known as *lupus mice.*

In more recent years, various other experimental models have been developed, each illustrating particular features relevant to the induction and/or expression of autoimmune disease, as shown in Fig. 1. The figure divides these experimental models into *spontaneous* and *induced.* We shall follow the schema in Fig. 1 for a brief commentary on models of autoimmunity as of 1992, with more detailed analysis of prototypic examples, spontaneous autoimmune diabetes mellitus in nonobese diabetic (NOD) mice, and induced experimental autoimmune encephalomyelitis (EAE) in inbred mice.

B. Spontaneous Models of Autoimmune Disease

Lupus mice have been the best studied of the spontaneous models of autoimmunity. It is only recently, however, with the introduction of molecular techniques, that real insights into the complex genetics of these mice have been possible. Murine lupus is described in Chapter 4 of this volume. The reader is directed also to the considerations on pathogenesis by Yoshida *et al.* (1990) in which B cells, T-cell dependency, the role of the major histocompatibility complex (MHC) and thymic perturbations are discussed. The origins of antibodies to DNA and their idiotypes are reviewed by Mackworth-Young and Schwartz (1988). The likelihood that anti-DNA arises by specific antigen-driven stimulation, and that somatic mutations among B cells confer specificity on the autoantibodies, is presented by Schlomchik *et al.* (1990).

Evidence for the important role of MHC class II molecules and antigen presentation has come from studies in which the I-A^{bm12} mutation is crossed onto NZB.H-2^b mice (Chiang *et al.*, 1990), resulting in a greatly augmented capacity of the mice to make anti-DNA. This change in these mutants replicates the *hot spot* at residue 71 of the I-Eβ chain of MHC class II. Analysis of the molecular genetics of murine lupus models appears to exclude disease-specific immu-

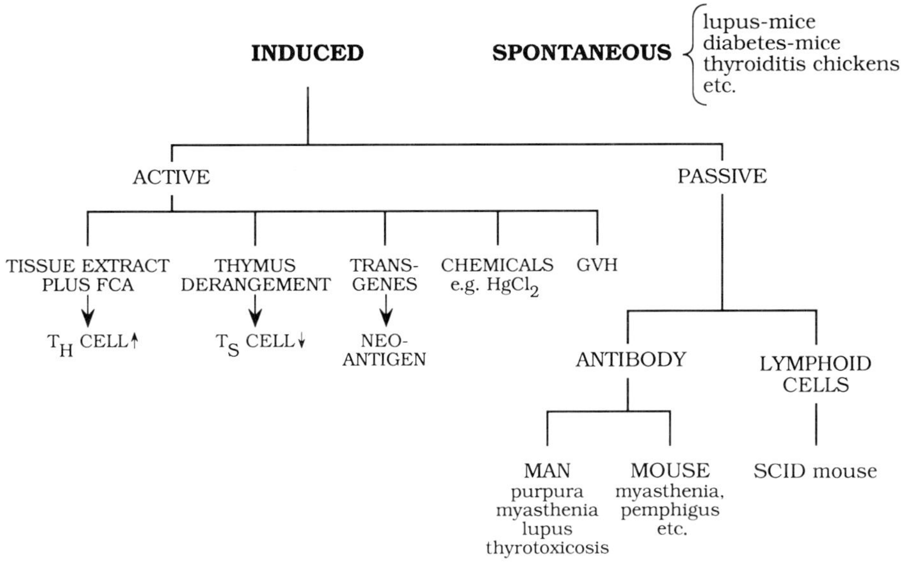

FIG. 1 A schematic outline of contemporary experimental models of autoimmune diseases, as described in the text. Reprinted with permission from *Gastroenterologia Japonica*. Mackay, I. R. (1991).

noglobulin (Ig) 1g genes or T-cell receptor (TcR) αβ genes and indicates that the B- and T-cell repertoires are normal (Theofilopoulos *et al.*, 1989). The role of an expanded population of double-negative autoreactive T cells (CD4−CD8−) that have escaped tolerogenesis and become subject to down-regulation of the CD4 and CD8 accessory molecule is a subject of discussion (Theofilopoulos *et al.*, 1989; Adams *et al.*, 1990).

There are also spontaneous models of organ-specific autoimmune disease in animals. One of these is the nonobese diabetic mouse, described in detail subsequently in this chapter. Another is autoimmune thyroiditis that can develop in various species (Bigazzi and Rose, 1975), and which closely resembles the features of human autoimmune thyroiditis, reviewed by Charreire (1989). The most striking predisposition to spontaneous autoimmune thyroiditis is shown by the obese chicken (Wick *et al.*, 1989).

C. Immunization with Autologous Tissues

Immunization of experimental animals with tissue extracts in Freund's adjuvant is the classical method for inducing an autoimmune disease model, beginning with encephalomyelitis (*vide supra*). We can note the convincing induction of autoimmune thyroiditis in 1956 when rabbits were thus immunized with autologous thyroid tissue (Witebsky and Rose, 1956). Other models induced by immunization with tissue and adjuvants include experimental autoimmune orchitis (Bernard *et al.*, 1978; Kohno *et al.*, 1983), experimental autoimmune neuritis (Geczy *et al.*, 1984; Shin *et al.*, 1989), experimental autoimmune myasthenia gravis (Berman and Patrick, 1980; Christadoss *et al.*, 1982), experimental autoimmune uveitis (Gery *et al.*, 1986; Caspi *et al.*, 1988, and this chapter, *vide infra*) and collagen-induced arthritis (Trentham *et al.*, 1977). Since EAE is so widely recognized and accepted as the prototype for antigen-specific T cell-mediated autoimmune diseases, we have elected to give detailed attention to the EAE model in this chapter.

Moreover, because certain forms of EAE can be induced, characterized by recurrent paralysis, histologic lymphocytic infiltrations, and demyelination, the chronic relapsing EAE model can be regarded as a valid facsimile of multiple sclerosis (MS) and the postinfectious encephalopathies (Raine, 1984; Wisniewski *et al.*, 1985; Waksman, 1989).

We shall emphasize how the application of modern cellular and molecular techniques to EAE has facilitated characterization of the subset of T cells involved, their T-cell receptor use, and the MHC restriction elements for the autoantigen myelin basic protein. This knowledge has kindled great interest in biotherapies that already have been successfully applied to EAE and some other experimentally induced autoimmune diseases with expectations of applicability to human autoimmune disease (Marx, 1990).

D. Thymus Perturbation: Cyclosporin, Thymectomy

1. Normal T-Cell Differentiation

T cells differentiate in the thymus from progenitors that enter the organ early in its development. These progenitors soon begin to express simultaneously CD4+ and CD8+, and low levels of CD3. These CD4+CD8+ T cells become *positively* or *negatively* selected. Positive selection depends on proliferation according to the capacity to react with MHC molecules displayed on thymic cortical epithelial cells, and negative selection depends on inhibition or deletion according to the capacity to react with MHC molecules coexpressing self-antigens displayed on bone marrow-derived dendritic cells in the thymic medulla or at the corticomedullary junction (Marrack and Kappler, 1987; von Boehmer, 1988; Benoist and Mathis, 1989). Actual clonal deletion is operative for certain self-antigens including Mls and I-E (Kappler *et al.*, 1987a; 1987b; Marrack *et al.*, 1988). However, our impression is that deletional tolerance operates only for an incomplete array of self-antigens to which autoimmune reactivity would have catastrophic results. In any event, the selection process is strongly biased in favor of those T cells that would react with MHC molecules that coexpress foreign peptides. The final differentiated phenotype, that expresses either CD4 or CD8 as well as high levels of the TcR, is exported to the periphery as the naive T cell that displays functional MHC-restriction in terms of antigen responsiveness, and is nonreactive with *major* self-antigens (Bevan 1977; Zinkernagel *et al.,* 1978; Kisielow *et al.,* 1988; Sha *et al.,* 1988; Nikolic-Zugic and Bevan, 1990).

The actual mechanisms of positive and negative selection are still unclear. Affinity or avidity may be relevant, so that cells reacting strongly with a self-peptide coexpressed with MHC, and thus potentially harmful, are deleted by apoptosis, whereas cells reacting less strongly become positively selected. Also, MHC molecules expressed in the thymus on cortical epithelial cells and on medullary bone-marrow-derived cells may be seen differently by T-cell receptors (Marrack *et al.,* 1988). Even more opaque are the processes in the thymus that govern the generation and export of T cells with suppressor properties, assuming that such cells do exist and have a thymic origin. Finally, selection must likewise operate on the newly recognized class of T cells with $\gamma\delta$ receptors. Whatever the processes might be, they are subject to error, resulting in export to the periphery of nondeleted autoreactive cells, and failure of export of cells with requisite suppressor properties. The thymus-perturbation models of autoimmune disease described in the following sections are based on interference with the normal orderly processes of T-cell differentiation and selection in the thymus.

2. Cyclosporin A

Cyclosporin A (CsA) in mice causes faulty T-cell development. Gao *et al.* (1988) showed that sublethally irradiated (600 R) mice given repeated injections of CsA had anomolous T-cell development, associated with blocking of the differentiation of the immature CD4+CD8+ *double positive* cells into single positive cells; this results in incomplete deletion of cells with autoreactive potential. Jenkins *et al.* (1988) similarly showed that differentiation of *single positive* T cells was inhibited by CsA, and autoreactive cells were not deleted. The site of action of CsA in the thymus is uncertain. It may be the thymic microenvironment, because the effects were seen primarily in the medulla with reduction in the number of epithelial cells, macrophages, and dendritic cells, whereas the cortex was spared (Kanariou *et al.,* 1989). We note the claim that transplanted thymus from CsA-treated mice into athymic recipients induced organ-specific autoimmunity in normally resistant strains (Sakaguchi and Sakaguchi, 1988); confirmation of these data is awaited. Siegel *et al.* (1990) tested the effect of CsA *in vitro* on the differentiation of 16-day gestation murine fetal thymus in organ culture and showed that after 8 days *in vitro* the development of mature TcR$\alpha\beta$-expressing cells was inhibited and, particularly, those cells expressing CD4 were selectively eliminated. The effects of CsA in interfering with development of CD4+ T cells are reproduced by treating neonatal mice with an anti-CD4 monoclonal antibody (MAb) (MacDonald *et al.*, 1988), which also abrogates deletion on self-reactive cells.

3. Neonatal Thymectomy

Post-thymectomy organ-specific autoimmune disease was first reported by Nishizuka and Sakakura (1969) who showed that thymectomy within a few days of birth resulted in ovarian but not testicular dysgenesis. Subsequently, perinatal thymectomy was shown to result in various organ-specific autoimmune diseases in strains of mice that rarely if ever develop such diseases spontaneously. The diseases induced have included thyroiditis (Kojima *et al.*, 1976), oophoritis (Taguchi *et al.*, 1980), gastritis and macrocytic anaemia (Kojima *et al.*, 1980), orchitis (Taguchi and Nishizuka, 1981; Tung *et al.*, 1987a, 1987b) and epididymoorchitis (Tung *et al.*, 1987a, 1987b). In regard to other species, Welch *et al.* (1973) showed that neonatal thymectomy increased the severity of spontaneous autoimmune thyroiditis in the obese chicken, and Silverman and Rose (1974) reported equivalent data for spontaneous thyroiditis in Buffalo rats. These data led Penhale *et al.* (1975) to demonstrate that thyroiditis could be induced in some strains of rats after adult thymectomy and repeated sublethal irradiation; presumably a neonate-like state was produced by these procedures in susceptible rat strains. These results on thymectomy in spontaneously autoimmune animals gave a perspective to the earlier observations in mice by Nishizuka and Sakakura (1969).

The obligatory requirement of T cells, both for the initiation of organ damage (Taguchi and Nishizuka, 1980; Sakaguchi *et al.*, 1982a; Sakaguchi *et al.*, 1985), as well as for its prevention (Penhale *et al.*, 1976; Sakaguchi *et al.*, 1982b), was repeatedly noted. Smith *et al.* (1989) showed that thymectomy performed in mice within 3 days of birth allowed the expansion and functional expression of potentially autoreactive cells that had been exported soon after birth, resulting in a range of organ-specific autoimmune diseases in mice that are otherwise resistant to these. Thymectomy in older mice failed to have this effect. Autoreactive T cells are apparently produced in the thymus and not deleted within this early postnatal period, and can apparently *leak out*. With increasing maturity, the export of potentially autoreactive cells is in some way regulated, perhaps by the later development and export of a subset of T cells with suppressor potential that inhibits the expression of anti-self activity. Thus there appears to be a finely tuned developmental process in the thymus that results in a balance of peripheral T cells tipped in favor of control of potential autoreactive cells, but experimentally modifiable so that autoimmunity predominates.

4. Gastritis as an Example of Post-Thymectomy Autoimmunity

The reality of post-thymectomy autoimmunity is strikingly illustrated by the induction of autoimmune gastritis in mice by this procedure. Until recently, experimental gastric autoimmunity has been relatively neglected, and the models described have not been particularly convincing (Whittingham *et al.*, 1990). However, neonatal thymectomy at 2 to 4 days in selected strains of mice produces a remarkable facsimile of human autoimmune gastritis. This is all the more interesting because of the recent molecular characterization of the autoantigen associated with the gastric parietal cell, and the observation that the reactivity of the human and murine parietal cell autoantibody is apparently identical.

In humans, autoimmune gastritis at its terminal stage results in malabsorption of vitamin B_{12} and pernicious anemia. Sera characteristically react by immunofluorescence with gastric parietal cells, and an autoantigen reactive with gastritis sera was identified as a 92-kDa polypeptide. This molecule corresponded with that of the H^+/K^+ adenosine triphosphatase (H^+/K^+ATPase) enzyme, also known as the proton pump, that delivers hydrogen ions into the gastric cavity (Karlsson *et al.*, 1988). Subsequently, there was identified a second reactive antigen of 60 to 90 kDa that co-localized with the 92-kDa autoantigen by immunogold electron microscopy, and was co-precipitated by autoantibodies to gastric parietal cells (Toh *et al.*, 1990). Various lines of evidence established that the two reactive antigens were the α and β subunits of the ATPase (Gleeson and Toh, 1991). Murine autoantibodies that develop after thymus perturbation have a reactivity identical with that of human gastric parietal cell autoantibodies, i.e., with the α and β subunits of the H^+/K^+ATPase of the gastric parietal cell (Mori *et al.*, 1989; Jones *et al.*, 1991). This reactivity is exhibited by whole mouse serum and by MAbs derived by fusion of splenocytes of the thymectomized mice. Moreover, the mice develop a gastritis histologically similar to that of the human counterpart. It is yet to be ascertained whether this progresses to the gastric atrophy that is the end stage of human autoimmune gastritis. The murine gastritis is T-cell related, to the extent that its initiation requires thymic perturbation, and its transfer to syngeneic mice among certain strains requires T cells rather than antibody (Fukuma *et al.*, 1988). It is of interest that transfer of disease by splenocytes in mice is particularly effective in nude mice with a T-cell deficient periphery (Gleeson and Toh, 1991). Whether the actual destruction of gastric parietal cells is mediated by cells or antibody is still unresolved for human and murine gastritis.

E. Transgenes

The injection of transgenes into fertilized ova of mice can result in the expression of a foreign protein that, in postnatal life, can interfere with the function of a particular tissue or elicit an immune response akin to autoimmunity. The examples cited here relate to pancreatic β islet cells, which have been intensively studied, and to liver.

1. Transgenic Diabetes

Hanahan (1985) introduced the gene for the simian virus 40 T-antigen (SV40Tag) with the rat insulin promoter so that the SV40Tag was expressed in pancreatic β islet cells. Some mice developed islet hyperplasia and β islet-cell tumors that eventually killed the animals, and others died of hypoglycemia resulting from islet hyperfunction; however, lines of transgenic mice were bred that expressed the transgene and survived to a moderate age. Adams *et al.* (1987) made the very interesting observation that mice that expressed SV40Tag in their β islet cells could either develop an autoimmune response within the islets, or become tolerant to this protein; if there was a delayed expression of the hybrid insulin-SV40 gene, there could be a failure of prenatal tolerance with a consequent production of *autoantibodies* to the nontolerated protein. What determines whether a transgenic gene product is expressed early, possibly during prenatal life, resulting in a failure of its immune recognition and functional tolerance, or late, with consequent autoantibody production and islet destruction, is still not understood. It would be of interest to treat the mice with presumed late expression of the transgene with anti-CD4 antibodies to prevent the development of an autoimmune response, since this type of treatment is effective in various situations in which it produces long-lasting tolerance to foreign proteins (Benjamin and Waldman, 1986; Benjamin *et al.*, 1986; Goronzy *et al.*, 1986; Gutstein *et al.*, 1986; Qin *et al.*, 1987, Carterton *et al.*, 1988; Charlton and Mandel 1989b).

Since hyperexpression of MHC gene products with immune activation is described in the target cells of endocrine autoimmune disease, several groups have used MHC-transgenic mice to study the involvement of these molecules in endocrine autoimmunity. Lo *et al.* (1988) and Sarvetnick *et al.* (1988) inserted an MHC class II transgene on a rat insulin promoter, and these transgenic mice expressed the MHC class II product and did indeed become diabetic; however, there was no inflammatory islet-directed response. In similar studies on transgenic mice that expressed either foreign or self-MHC class I proteins on their β islet cells, there was development of diabetes, regardless of whether the MHC gene was self or nonself (Allison *et al.*, 1989); these mice were tolerant to the foreign transgene product but only while it was still expressed, and tolerance rapidly waned when the target cells were destroyed (Morahan *et al.*, 1989a). Other foreign transgenic products that can result in diabetes include calmodulin (Epstein *et al.*, 1989) and the H-ras oncoprotein (Efran *et al.*, 1990), but in these instances, likewise, there is no evidence that the immune system is involved in the pathogenesis of the disease. Perhaps there is aberrant expression of a foreign protein that interferes with insulin secretion (Parham, 1988). Immune mechanisms seem excluded, since (1) insulin secretion *in vitro* by fetal islets from MHC class I transgenic mice is severely affected, even when the islets are removed well before functional immune cells reach the periphery; (2) there is defective function of fetal transgenic islets transplanted into athymic (nude) mice; and (3) similar insulin defects occur when the transgene is bred into nude mice (Mandel *et al.*, 1991).

When interferon-γ transgenic mice were produced (Sarvetnick *et al.*, 1988, 1990), these animals did show insulitis and diabetes. Recently a similar model of apparently immune-mediated diabetes was described in transgenic mice when the gene for influenza virus hemagglutinin (HA) was linked to an insulin promoter (Roman *et al.*, 1990).

Clearly those transgenic mouse models (SV40Tag, interferon γ, influenza virus HA) that show features indicative of immunopathological destruction of β islet cells do appear to be valid experimental models of the spontaneous autoimmune diabetes, whether seen in NOD mice, BB rats, or humans. It is less evident whether the transgenic models that do not display an apparent immune pathogenesis also have a human counterpart, since most humans with type I diabetes have evidence of immune involvement (Eisenbarth, 1986) including autoantibodies and, when tissue is available, evidence of insulitis (Gepts, 1965; Foulis *et al.*, 1986). There are, however, some instances in which these features are not present. Thus in the large survey by Foulis *et al.* (1986), most histological samples showed insulitis, albeit patchy in its distribution, but none of the few individuals who developed severe diabetes before the age of 18 months had any evidence of insulitis and indeed had what appeared to be well-granulated β islet cells despite clinically typical diabetes. Perhaps these unusual patients had a different form of diabetes in which insulin secretion by their β cells was abnormal, as in the MHC transgenic models. Also, conceivably, such patients could be expressing a "natural" transgenic product, e.g., viral proteins limited to β islet cell expression.

2. Transgenic Hepatitis

In experiments to assess pathogenic effects of the hepatitis B virus surface antigen (HBsAg), a construct containing genes for HBsAg and mouse albumin regulatory sequences was introduced into mice (Moriyama *et al.*, 1990). The injection of spleen cells from donor mice primed to respond to peptides of HBsAg induced immune-mediated liver cell destruction simulating chronic hepatitis in man.

Another model of chronic hepatitis was reported in mice in which a transgene for an allogeneic class I MHC molecule was linked to the β-metallothionein (βMT) promoter; this directed the expression of the transgene product to the liver when a heavy metal (zinc) was given (Morahan *et al.*, 1989b). When the transgenic mice were irradiated and then reconstituted with syngeneic spleen cells, there developed a chronic but self-limited hepatitis as a result of an attack by the transferred donor cells against liver cells expressing the transgene product.

A more direct model of autoimmune hepatitis was produced by introduction of an ovine growth hormone transgene linked to the βMT promoter since, in these mice, chronic hepatitis developed spontaneously when the transgene was activated by the feeding of zinc (Orian *et al.*, 1991). Thus a host response to an induced transgene product to which neonatal tolerance had not been established elicited immune-mediated tissue damage and simulated naturally occurring autoimmune hepatitis.

F. Mercuric Chloride and Analogs

Various drugs are known to induce autoimmune reactions. It is widely assumed that the drug attaches to a host protein, and the ensuing configuration suffices to initiate a response to the native protein. However, the likelihood that other mechanisms can operate is illustrated by the well-studied model of mercury-induced autoimmunity in the Brown Norway rat. The disease, induced by subcutaneous injection of mercuric chloride into rats, includes a T cell-dependent polyclonal activation of B lymphocytes expressed as lymphoproliferation, hypergammoglobulinemia, and production of autoantibodies to nuclei, and particularly to glomerular basement membrane with an ensuing glomerulonephritis. There is an initial proliferation of CD4+ cells that are subject to regulation by a suppressor population that limits the disease in the host, and can transfer resistance to syngeneic animals.

The mercuric chloride model is of interest from three standpoints. First, the target of the autoimmune attack is a class II MHC molecule (Ia). Second, the model vindicates the reality of autoregulatory processes in autoimmunity, as judged by studies on autoantiidiotypic antibodies (Neilson and Phillips, 1982) and regulatory (suppressor?) T cells that are evoked by the expanding autoreactive T-helper population (Rossert *et al.*, 1988). Third, mercuric chloride nephritis is a prototype for other drug-induced autoimmune models in animals [e.g., gold salts that induce disease in mice associated with nucleolar autoantibody (Robinson *et al.*, 1986)], and D-penicillamine that induces renal disease in Brown Norway rats (Tournade *et al.*, 1990a, 1990b). There is a good likelihood that at least some drug-induced autoimmune diseases in man have a similar basis.

G. Graft-versus-Host Disease (GVHD)

The occurrence of graft-versus-host reactions has long been known to elicit immunologic abnormalities in experimental animals and in humans after treatment with donor bone marrow. GVHD results from cytotoxic T cells in the donor tissue attacking host cells bearing foreign MHC antigens, in skin, intestine, liver, and other sites. GVHD may be acute or chronic; the latter resembles (to a degree) multisystem autoimmune disease and is ameliorated by immunosuppression (Storb, 1989). Gleichman and colleagues (1984) have reasoned that experimental GVHD is a valid model for human autoimmunity and that, as a model, GVHD has similarities with autoimmunity induced by drugs such as mercuric chloride, particularly the induction by anti-MHC class II T cells. This idea is supported by recent experiments of Tournade *et al.* (1990a; 1990b).

A point of interest is whether donor T cells must *directly* recognize foreign Ia on the host B cells that make the autoantibodies present in GVHD as a *cognate interaction,* or whether sufficient help is generated by lymphokines to stimulate all B cells as a *bystander interaction.* The conclusion of Morris *et al.* (1990), based on double-congenic chimeric mice, indicated that cognate interaction was necessary. In the very interesting report of Saitoh *et al.* (1990) on GVHD in a semiallogeneic host, the CD8+ (presumably regulatory) subset was depleted by MAb to the Ly2 molecule. This caused a striking histologic insulitis and cholangitis resembling the lesions of human primary biliary cirrhosis (PBC). Of particular interest, the affected mice produce the range of mitochondrial antibodies specifically seen in PBC (see Chapter 9 of this volume).

Although not strictly a graft-versus-host model, the wasting disease in athymic rats resulting from *asymmetrical* reconstitution with the OX-22^{high} vis-à-vis the OX-22^{low} subset of T cells is equivalent (Powrie and Mason, 1990). The OX-22^{high} subset appears to correspond with Th1 in mice, and the OX-22^{low}, with Th2; the data point to an important regulatory role of the Th2-like subset over CD4+ T cells that have autoaggressive potential.

H. Antiidiotypes as Surrogate Autoantigens

The heuristic concept of the *idiotypic network* (Jerne, 1974) has had a remarkably influential effect on immunologic theory and experimentation. As one corollary of the concept, the structure of the idiotype of an antibody can mimic that of another potential antigen, quite unrelated to that reactive with the antibody itself, and creates what is termed the internal image of that antigen. It also follows that a surrogate autoantigen may be generated by an antiidiotypic reaction to the idiotype of an autoantibody (Mackay 1988). One of the common cross-reactive idiotypes of anti-DNA antibodies is 16/6, the serum levels of which correlate with disease activity in human SLE. A human monoclonal IgM antibody carrying the 16/6 idiotype was used to immunize mice, and this created a model of SLE in which the full range of lupus antibodies was induced, together with glomerulonephritis of immune-complex type. Presumably the Ab2 (antiantibody) created an immunogenic surrogate DNA that was sufficient to initiate the disease, as discussed by Schoenfeld and Mozes (1990). As another example, an Ig light chain from a lupus-prone MRL-1pr/1pr mouse carried a sequence homologous to the 70-kDa U1-RNP polypeptide, and elicited antibodies to ribonucleoprotein (RNP) and DNA (Pucetti *et al.*, 1990). An experimental study with similar implications was reported by Iribe *et al.* (1989). An antiidiotypic MAb was raised against a MAb reactive with a species-specific epitope of mouse type II collagen; immunization with this Ab2 rendered the recipients susceptible to arthritis on challenge with human type II collagen.

I. Passive Transfer Models

The passive transfer of disease by serum or cells from individuals with an autoimmune disease establishes the pathogenic role of the transfer inoculum.

1. Human-to-Human Transfer by Serum

The first example is the heroic self-transfer by Harrington and colleagues of serum from cases of idiopathic (autoimmune) thrombocytopenic purpura, resulting in striking decreases in platelet levels (Harrington *et al.*, 1990). Later there were described "experiments of nature" in which maternally transmitted autoantibody from mothers caused autoimmune expression in the fetus; the several examples include myasthenia gravis, thyrotoxicosis, lupus erythematosus, and thrombocytopenia, with congenital heart block caused by the maternal Ro antibody attracting particular interest (Scott *et al.*, 1983).

2. Human-to-Mouse Transfer by Serum

Examples of autoimmune diseases that have been transferred to mice by inoculation of human serum include myasthenia gravis (Toyka *et al.*, 1977), the Lambert–Eaton myasthenic syndrome (Lambert and Lennon, 1988) and pemphigus vulgaris (Anhalt *et al.*, 1982). To facilitate transfer of autoimmune disease by serum, a neonatally tolerant mouse model was developed by repeated injections of human IgG into mice during pregnancy (Mundlos *et al.*, 1990). The *in utero* tolerized mice retained human autoantibodies in the circulation for periods of weeks. However, the prolonged circulation of autoantibodies to intracellular antigens did not induce any evidence of autoimmune disease, indicating that serum autoantibody is optimally reactive only with targets exposed on the cell surface.

3. Human-to-Mouse Transfer by Cells

Mice with congenital severe combined immune deficiency (SCID) will accept xenogeneic grafts and can in fact be immunologically reconstituted by transfer of human lymphoid cells (McCune *et al.*, 1988; Mosier *et al.*, 1988). Hence such mice could be a useful model for passive transfer of cell-mediated autoimmune lesions. One example is the transfer of disease by an inoculum of peripheral blood lymphocytes (PBL) from patients with PBC. The recipients developed mitochondrial antibody in serum and typical periductular biliary lesions (Krams *et al.*, 1989), but similar lesions occurred after inoculation of PBL from some normal individuals. Thus a confounding effect of a GVH reaction could complicate the interpretation of these experiments. There are reports of attempted transfer of other autoimmune diseases into SCID mice by lymphoid cells, either PBL or synovial cells, from patients with rheumatoid arthritis (Tighe *et al.*, 1990) or systemic lupus erythematosus (Duchosal *et al.*, 1990). The recipient mice were reconstituted to the degree that circulating IgG was of human type, and autoantibodies, rheumatoid factor, or antinuclear antibody were demonstrable, but a convincing counterpart of the corresponding human disease was not elicited.

II. THE NON-OBESE DIABETIC MOUSE

A. INTRODUCTION

Animal models of severe insulinopenic diabetes were, until recently, usually surgically or drug-induced and were thus not true etiologic models of the spontaneously occurring autoimmune disease of humans. Streptozotocin in multiple subdiabetogenic doses produced an indolent disease in a few strains of mice with mononuclear cell infiltrates in and around the islets of Langerhans—*insulitis* (Like *et al.*, 1976, 1978). To the extent that diabetes induced in this way was highly strain dependent and had histological appearances similar to those of human diabetic insulitis, it resembled human insulin-dependent diabetes mellitus (IDDM). However, at the same time, spontaneously occurring models of IDDM became identified. One such model in a Wistar/Furth rat colony at the BioBreeding Laboratory in Canada (Nakhooda *et al.*, 1977; Seemayer *et al.*, 1980), was named Bio-Breeding Wistar (BB/W). A large proportion of young adults developed severe insulinopenic diabetes, both sexes were equally affected, and the pancreas showed insulitis before overt diabetes developed. Thus, this model seemed to be a close homolog of human IDDM, but BB/W rats were severely lymphopenic and immunosuppressed (Jackson *et al.*, 1981; Jackson *et al.*, 1984; Colle *et al.*, 1981), particularly in their T-cell compartment, and thus differed from humans with IDDM.

In 1980 a murine model of spontaneous diabetes was described in Japan (Makino *et al.*, 1980; Tochino, 1986) and was referred to as the non-obese diabetic (NOD) mouse. The initial diabetic mouse was detected as part of a screening program of CTS mice that had cataracts and micro-ophthalmia; since cataracts occur in diabetes, CTS mice were screened, and a diabetic female was detected in 1974. By 1980 some 1500 mice had been studied (Makino *et al.*, 1980). Diabetes was initially detected in female mice aged around 200 days, but in later generations, the age of onset decreased markedly; males also developed diabetes but much less frequently. The disease was rapidly fatal without insulin treatment. Glycosuria was first detected at 90 days, and thereafter the number of affected female mice increased steadily to 50% by 130 days and 80% by 210 days. Males first developed diabetes about 60 days after the females, and their diabetes incidence peaked at less than 20% by 210 days. Histologic insulitis was present from an early age, and 90% of females and 60% of males had this by 5 weeks. Thus, insulitis preceded diabetes and was present in more animals than eventually developed diabetes. Makino *et al.* (1980) also noted that insulitis disappeared when all islet β cells had been destroyed. NOD mice do not have lymphopenia (Kataoka *et al.*, 1983) in contrast to BB rats, but rather a lymphocytosis (Prochazka *et al.*, 1987).

NOD mice are now widely available, and the many colonies have a differing incidence of IDDM, yet the disease still fulfills the initial Japanese description by Makino *et al.* (1980): an acute onset of severe diabetes mainly in young adult females but only ~20% in males, and insulitis virtually invariably present in both sexes from a very young age and persisting to old age or until β islet cells are totally destroyed.

B. Genetic Studies

Makino *et al.* (1985) crossed NOD and C57BL/6 (B/6) mice and found no insulitis in either B/6 mice or in F_1 animals; in $(F_1 \times F_1)F_2$ mice a low incidence (1–5%) was seen. In backcrosses of NOD to F_1 mice, the incidence of insulitis increased to around 25%. These data indicated an effect on insulitis development of two recessive genes on independent autosomal chromosomes, but there were no data on diabetes incidence in that study.

Hattori *et al.* (1986) showed that the NOD mouse has a unique MHC class II complex. When NOD mice were crossed with C3H, diabetes in the progeny depended on homozygosity for the NOD MHC. Serologic analysis showed that NOD mice were H-2K^d and H-2D^b at class I, but when the class II region was analyzed, the NOD I-A was evidently unique, since the mice failed to express I-E because they had no message for the Eα gene (Fushijima *et al.*, 1989). Hattori *et al.* (1986) further determined the linkage of diabetes to inheritance of Aβ, and showed that there was no diabetes in F_1 mice, but it appeared in backcrosses, in 16% of females and 2% of males. In F_2 intercrosses, 2.5% became diabetic, and all diabetic mice were homozygous for a unique NOD 9.5-kb band by restriction fragment length polymorphism (RFLP) analysis. Because of the relatively low incidence of diabetes in backcross females they postulated that there was at least one, and probably two or more, susceptibility genes in addition to the gene linked to the MHC. Polygenic effects are reported in the BB rat (Jackson *et al.*, 1984) in which a non-MHC-linked gene determines lymphopenia, and the other is MHC linked, with both necessary for development of diabetes. Also, in humans, there is only a 20% concordance for diabetes in patients sharing both histocompatibility regions, and 5% in those sharing only one with the affected first-degree relative (Gorsuch *et al.*, 1982).

Analysis of the fine structure of the I-Aβ and I-Aα chains revealed a five-nucleotide variation in the β chain that resulted in two amino acid substitutions, from proline-aspartic acid in I-A^d to histidine-serine in I-A^{NOD} (Acha-Orbea and McDevitt, 1987). This highly conserved region is also altered in a similar way in Caucasians with diabetes (Todd *et al.*, 1987; Morel *et al.*, 1988), but not in Japanese (Awata *et al.*, 1990) who have an asp residue at position 57, a feature that is highly protective for diabetes in non-Japanese. The NOD I-Aβ sequence is present in the related sister strains of NOD mice (ILI and CTS), but these mice do not develop diabetes (Koide and Yoshida, 1989). Thus, this MHC-linked gene alone does not determine diabetes, and some other gene(s) must be involved. The DNA-sequencing data support the results from breeding studies. Recently, it was shown by Slattery *et al.* (1990), Miyazaki *et al.* (1990), and Lund *et al.* (1990) that the expression of non-NOD I-A antigens in transgenic NOD mice can prevent diabetes, although insulitis may still be present, and when 57asp or 56pro is present in the I-Aβ molecule, diabetes is prevented. The absence of expression of I-E seems also to be important for the generation of diabetes susceptibility. When NOD mice were crossed with transgenic C57BL/6 mice that expressed I-E, the NOD progeny were also resistant to the development of insulitis and presumably also of diabetes (Nishimoto *et al.* 1987).

Wicker *et al.* (1987) analyzed the genetic predisposition of NOD mice to develop insulitis and diabetes in breeding studies using NOD crossed with C57BL/10 (B10), selected because B10 mice do not develop diabetes or insulitis, and fail to express I-E. Insulitis and diabetes proved to be under partially overlapping but distinct genetic control, with insulitis determined by a single gene not linked to the MHC, whereas diabetes was determined by at least three independent gene complexes, one linked to the MHC. The severity of insulitis, rather than its presence, was greatly influenced by MHC linkage. In contrast to other studies that implicated MHC homozygosity in NOD mice, three backcross MHC heterozygous females with diabetes were detected and were more intensively studied by Wicker *et al.* (1989). These authors postulated either a crossover event between the MHC and a putative MHC-linked diabetogenic gene, or a dominant MHC-linked diabetogenic gene with low penetrance in the heterozygous state. By pedigree analysis of their progeny, the latter hypothesis was favored.

C. The Insulitis Lesion

Insulitis in NOD mice is almost invariable, occurs early in life, and occurs even in mice that do not develop overt diabetes. By the age of 210 days, all females and almost all males have insulitis, and this incidence rapidly increases from 0% in both sexes at 21 days, to >80% in females and almost 60% in males by 5 to 6 weeks (Makino *et al.*, 1981). Insulitis appears to be a necessary but not sufficient event to produce β-cell destruction, and other factors apart from the homing of lymphoid cells to the islets seem necessary. The initiation of insulitis probably begins with macrophage infiltration into the islets. The infiltrating macrophages may present islet β antigens to T cells, and these activated T cells induce insulitis. Macrophages also may initiate insulitis in the BB/W rat (Lee *et al.*, 1988; Kolb-Bachofen and Kolb, 1989), and in mice made diabetic with multiple low doses of streptozotocin (Kolb-Bachofen *et al.*, 1988). The early presence of macrophages in islets was reported by Lee *et al.* (1988) and by Charlton *et al.* (1988), who showed that giving silica to NOD mice prevented diabetes. However, the initial damage that causes the release of β-cell antigens for presentation to the cells of the immune system remains unknown.

In the initial histopathologic study of the NOD pancreas, Fujita *et al.* (1982) reported that mononuclear cells first appeared at 4 weeks and were present in most mice by 5 weeks, and earlier in females. The severity of the infiltrate varied between islets in the same sample. Mononuclear cells were first seen in periductal regions opposite to but outside the islets. Fujita *et al.* (1982) noted that infiltrating cells were initially separated from the endocrine cells by a thin sheet of connective tissue, and there was a conspicuous filling of periductal lymphatics with small lymphoid cells. With increasing age the islets became surrounded by a thick ring of lymphoid cells that eroded into the islet, gradually destroying the β cells but leaving the other endocrine cells intact (see Fig. 2). As β cells were destroyed, the infiltrate disappeared, leaving small atrophic islets lacking β cells. Kanazawa *et al.* (1984) studied mice aged from 3 to 22 weeks and reported that insulitis began at 6 weeks with an initial preponderance of IgM+ lymphocytes that formed follicular structures surrounded by T cells. Both Lyt-1+ and Lyt-2+ cells were seen and were regarded as being CD4+ and CD8+, respectively, since Lyt-1 was then regarded as a CD4 marker; also detected were asialo-GM1+ (ASGM1) cells that were considered to be natural killer (NK) cells. Subsequently, however, it was shown that Lyt-1 is not a unique marker for CD4 cells, and ASGM1 is not specific for murine NK cells.

Miyazaki *et al.* (1985) used immunofluorescence microscopy to show that T cells predominated in the infiltrate and were located adjacent to the endocrine cells, whereas B lymphocytes were fewer and more peripherally located. Koike *et al.* (1987) used immunohistochemistry to identify the surface phenotypes of infiltrating cells; over 90% were Thy-1+ and Lyt-1+. The T cells were predominantly CD4+, with some CD8+ cells present. The age of the mice at the end of

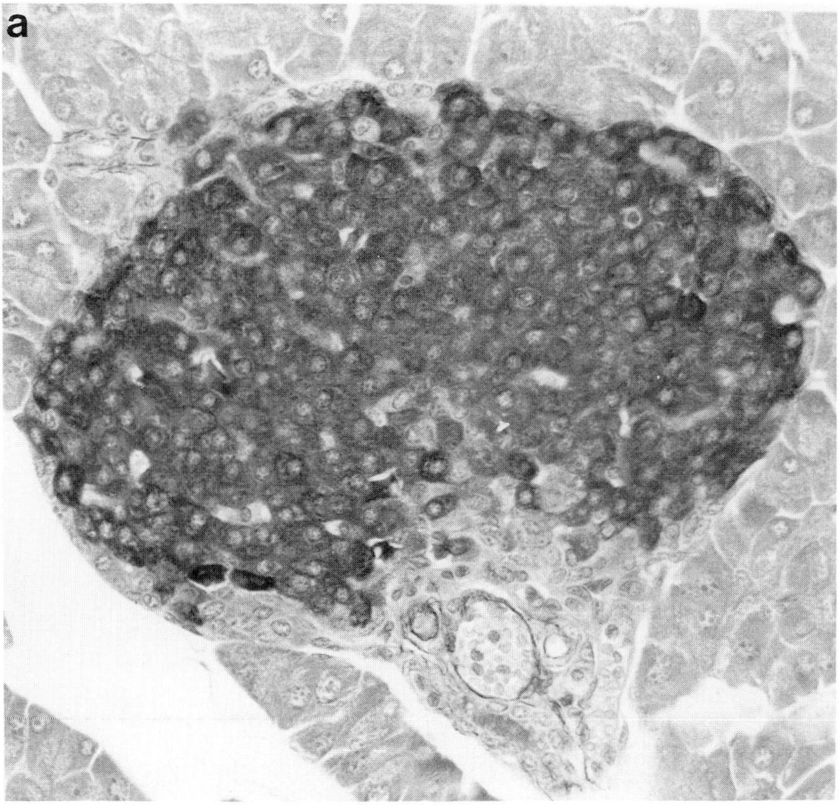

FIG. 2 Histologic evolution of spontaneous insulitis in the NOD mouse. A. A normal mouse islet with selective staining of insulin-containing β cells. The unstained cells, mainly at the islet periphery, are the glucagon-producing α cells, somatostatin-secreting δ cells and pancreatic polypeptide cells (aldehyde fuchsin ×400). B. Islet from a prediabetic NOD mouse with insulitis showing slight invasion by mononuclear cells with the endocrine cells still intact (aldehyde fuchsin ×400). C. An atrophic islet from a NOD mouse with established diabetes showing depletion of β cells and loss of insulitis, as seen when the target β cells are destroyed (aldehyde fuchsin ×400).

the experiment was only 15 weeks, and presumably, most were prediabetic. Similar results were obtained by Ikehara *et al.* (1985) in prediabetic mice aged around 5 months. However, phenotypic markers on mononuclear cells are not necessarily totally specific for a particular cellular subset since L3T4, the CD4 marker in mice, is present also on some macrophages/monocytes, and Lyt-1 is present on at least some CD8 T cells. Accordingly, Signore *et al.* (1989) used double staining to study the natural history of the infiltrate on cryostat sections. They detected insulitis at 5 weeks and, with age, the severity of the lesion increased, and more islets became affected; however, there was no significant variation in the proportions of mononuclear cell subsets with age, and they

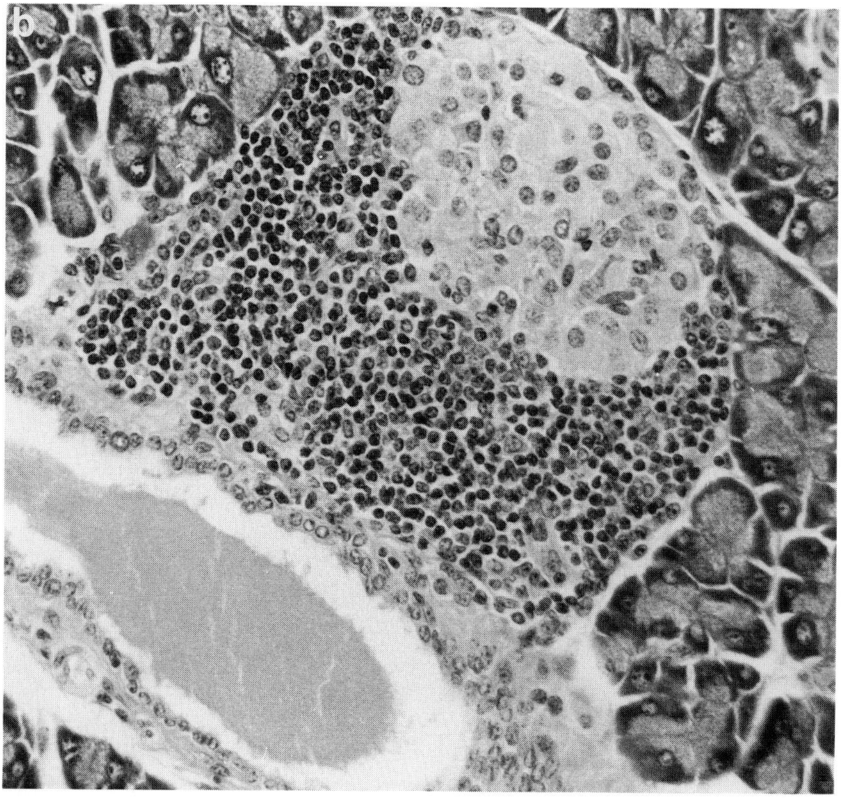

FIG. 2 (*Continued*)

reported a slight excess of B over T lymphocytes. Interestingly, with double staining, there were more L3T4+ cells than Thy-1+ cells, suggesting that some of the former were nonlymphoid, possibly macrophages. This conclusion was strengthened by many of the L3T4+ cells being stained with antibodies to MHC class II; T cells in the mouse are MHC class II (Flavell *et al.*, 1986; Araneo *et al.*, 1985). CD4+ cells predominated over CD8+ cells, with a constant small proportion of presumably activated IL-2R+ cells.

D. Immunologic Status of Non-Obese Diabetic Mice

1. Target Antigens and Autoantibodies

Reactive autoantigens in the NOD islets have been extensively investigated, notably cytoplasmic antigens, the 64-kDa antigen described in human IDDM,

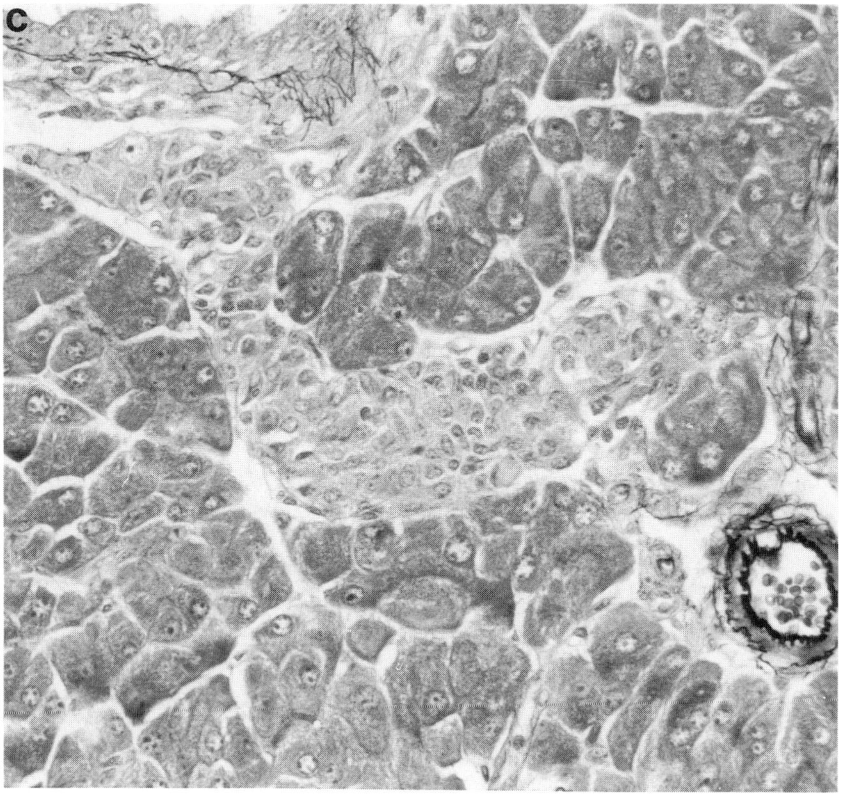

FIG. 2 *(Continued)*

the insulin molecule, and others. Viral antigens have been detected on the surface of β cells (Suenaga and Yoon, 1988), including the retrovirus p73 antigen that is cross-reactive with insulin (Serreze *et al.*, 1988a). An "occult" MHC class I-like antigen was recognized on the β cells of NOD mice after exposure to interferon γ (Leiter *et al.*, 1989).

The expression of MHC molecules on β cells has been controversial, i.e., whether or not class II antigens can ever be expressed, either constitutively or endogenously. Hanafusa *et al.* (1987) claimed that I-A antigens were present on islet endocrine cells, whether or not insulitis was present. Formby and Miller (1990) suggested that aberrant class II expression occurred on NOD islet cells from an early age, and Timsit *et al.* (1989) inferred that it was present, since they could prevent diabetes with antibodies to MHC class II. Conversely, Signore *et al.* (1987) failed to detect class II determinants on islet cells of NOD mice but could detect these on islet-infiltrating cells, of which some were also IL-2R+.

Insulin is a suggested target since insulin autoantibodies (IAb) are commonly present in NOD mice, and in humans with IDDM. Pontesilli *et al.* (1987) reported that IAb, detected by a solid-phase enzyme-linked immunosorbent assay (ELISA), were present in almost all NOD mice from the earliest age studied (75 days), but control non-NOD mice also had IAb, at lower titer. However, only one IAb+ female eventually developed diabetes. Anti-insulin-reactive T cells were not detected in NOD mice (Hurtenbach and Maurer, 1989). Recently a 65-kDa heat-shock protein was suggested as a target antigen (Elias *et al.*, 1990), adding to the long list of potentially pathogenic cross-reactions in which this heat-shock protein has been implicated.

MAb have been used in attempts to define islet cell antigens by Yokono *et al.* (1985) and Hari *et al.* (1986). An anti-islet cell MAb raised by fusing spleen cells from islet cell surface antigen (ICSA)+ NOD mice with lymphoma cells recognized two major polypeptides of 28 kDa and 64 kDa; the MAb did not lyse ^{111}In-labeled rat insulinoma (RIN) cells in a complement-mediated assay, but antibody-dependent cell-mediated cytotoxicity (ADCC) was detected when high antibody and effector-cell levels were used. The antibody also inhibited glucose-mediated insulin secretion by isolated rat islets. This work is unconfirmed. Pontesilli *et al.* (1989) described a cytotoxic antibody to an islet cell surface trypsin-sensitive antigen (ICSAb) generated by fusing spleen cells from recently diabetic NOD mice with P3X cells. The MAbs produced were screened against RIN cells, and one line produced a stable IgM MAb reactive against ICSAb. This antibody labeled 35% of isolated viable BALB/c islet cells but did not label fixed or frozen human or murine islets.

Islet cell cytoplasmic antibodies (ICAb), a feature of human autoimmune diabetes, and islet cell surface antibodies (ICSAb) have been well investigated in NOD mice. ICAb identified by immunofluorescence on Bouins' fixed pancreas sections were present in about 50% of NOD mice but not in controls. In contrast, ICSAb were absent in young NODs but developed later, and were present in a few older mice. ICAb and ICSAb were, however, not detected on frozen sections of mouse pancreas but only in Bouins' fixed tissue. Reddy *et al.* (1988) reported that IAb and ICAb were present in about 50% of the animals by 15 days of age; in a longitudinal study, both Abs were frequently present but did not necessarily predict the occurrence of diabetes. Whereas these Ab were not clearly predictive, no mouse developed diabetes without the prior presence of both. Michel *et al.* (1989) reported the early presence of IAb, long before diabetes occurred in IAb+ mice, and the antibodies were found mainly in the diabetes-prone females. In contrast, Zeigler *et al.* (1989) showed that IAb levels were predictive of later onset of diabetes, and higher levels were seen in those mice that became overtly diabetic; by 6 weeks, 37% of females but no males were IAb+. Our experience (Colman *et al.*, unpublished) on the appearance and titer of IAb in a large cohort of NOD mice of both sexes, from lines with a low and high incidence of diabetes (Baxter *et al.*, 1989), is that IAb are nonpredictive.

Other manifestations of abnormal humoral immunity in NOD mice include lymphocytotoxic IgM antibodies that appear several weeks after insulitis. These are not predictive of the occurrence of diabetes and appear in F_1 mice that do not usually develop insulitis (Lehuen *et al.*, 1990). Thus, in common with other mouse strains susceptible to development of autoimmune disease, NOD mice are prone to dysregulated B-lymphocyte function independent of T-cell malfunction.

Atkinson and Maclaren (1988) showed that NOD serum contained an autoantibody that immunoprecipitated the 64-kDa antigen from detergent lysates of biolabeled murine islet cells. This antibody occurred in newly diagnosed diabetes, was present at weaning, but quickly disappeared in diabetic mice and was absent in old nondiabetic NOD mice and in three control strains. This islet-cell antigen is presumably similar to the 64-kDa antigen described in patients and BB rats with IDDM (Baekkeskov *et al.*, 1982, 1984, 1987; Colman *et al.*, 1987; Atkinson *et al.*, 1988). This antigen is now identified as glutamic acid decarboxylase (Baekkeskov *et al.*, 1990).

2. Mononuclear Cell Populations

BB/W rats are profoundly lymphopenic, particularly in respect to T cells, and thus differ sharply from humans with IDDM, who lack immune deficits (Drell and Notkins, 1987). In NOD mice, lymphoid populations in the blood and spleen of 12-week-old adult NOD females showed moderate depletion, predominantly of T cells and Fc-receptor+ cells, but no differences in macrophage numbers; there was a slight increase in B lymphocytes (Kataoka *et al.*, 1983). The spleen contained far fewer T cells than did the spleen of age- and sex-matched ICR control mice. The methods used to enumerate cell numbers were not precise and, although there were differences between these two strains, even when adjusted for body weight, doubt exists on the accuracy of the data. Other studies generally show moderate lymphocytosis and increased T cells in spleen and lymph nodes (Ikehara *et al.*, 1985; Prochazka *et al.*, 1987). The slight peripheral lymphopenia in young prediabetic NOD mice is followed with increasing age by moderate lymphocytosis, particularly in females (Pontesilli *et al.*, 1987). Thus, T cells account for more than 50% of blood mononuclear cells compared with 30% in three unrelated control strains, and B lymphocytes are somewhat reduced in NOD mice, to around 40%. Wang *et al.* (1987) stated that in blood, CD4+ T cells composed 43% of the total mononuclear population.

3. Functional Studies

NOD mice generally have augmented immune responsiveness. Both antibody responses and delayed-type hypersensitivity (DTH) against sheep red blood cells were either increased or not different from those of ICR mice (Kataoka *et al.*, 1983). When challenged with herpes simplex virus, NOD mice had a high mortality, suggesting a strongly reduced capacity to respond to this challenge, although whether this was owing to defective cytotoxic T-cell responses or to an inability to generate an appropriate humoral response was not elucidated. Ikehara *et al.* (1985) reported increased responses both to T-cell (PHA and Con A) and a B-cell (LPS) mitogen. NOD mice are also responders to the H-Y antigen (Chandler *et al.*, 1988). The variable immune responses could be explicable by a defect in suppressor-cell activity (Kataoka *et al.*, 1983). Reduced suppressor activity was also indicated by data from Serreze and Leiter (1988), and from Bach's group, who have consistently maintained that a primary immune defect in NOD mice is a disorder of immunoregulation (Bendelac *et al.*, 1987, 1988; Timsit *et al.*, 1988; Boitard *et al.*, 1988, 1989; Bedossa *et al.*, 1989; Dardenne *et al.*, 1989).

NOD mice appear to be relatively resistant to the induction of classical neonatal tolerance and, despite the presence of lymphoid chimerism, they generally do not accept donor skin permanently and show a frequent reversion of *in vitro* tolerance, as measured by mixed lymphocyte responses and the generation of cytotoxic T cells (Bendelac *et al.*, 1989a). In contrast to other strains of mice that can accept immunomodified islet allografts, NOD mice destroy these, although this may be owing to recurrence of disease rather than rejection (Wang *et al.*, 1987).

4. Mechanism of β-Cell Destruction

The cells ultimately responsible for β-cell destruction are almost certainly T cells (Nagata *et al.*, 1989a; 1989b), either CD4+ or CD8+, and both subsets are required for transfer of disease (Wicker *et al.*, 1986; Bendelac *et al.*, 1987; Miller *et al.*, 1988); B cells are not involved (Bendelac *et al.*, 1988). The CD8+ subset is particularly implicated (Charlton *et al.*, 1988; Young *et al.*, 1989; Nagata *et al.*, 1989a; 1989b) Kay *et al.*, 1989), but CD4+ cells are also involved (Wang *et al.*, 1987; Hanafusa *et al.*, 1988; Charlton *et al.*, 1988), possibly by acting as helper cells. Whether the cells are antigen specific or nonspecific is still uncertain, and there are claims that the effector cells have features of NK cells (Kay *et al.*, 1989). The mode of destruction of islet grafts in NOD mice is also controversial, with claims that they are destroyed in an MHC-restricted manner (Terada *et al.*, 1988), or that there is nonrestricted β-cell killing (Wang *et al.*, 1987).

5. Cyclophosphamide

Cyclophosphamide (CP) is usually used to suppress immune reactivity, but it may also increase immune responses, perhaps by selectively depleting regulatory (suppressor?) cells and allowing effector cells to become dominant (Bach and Strom, 1985). In NOD mice given CP, about 70% developed overt diabetes within 1 to 2 weeks, equally in both sexes (Harada and Makino, 1984). Diabetes occurred even in mice aged 3 weeks at the time of the first injection, and the frequency of disease was sharply increased in older mice. In females the maximal prevalence was not increased, but the age of onset was sharply reduced. Three other strains given CP did not develop diabetes. Yasunami and Bach (1988) also found that CP accelerated disease in young females, again without increasing total frequency, but sharply increased the disease frequency in males to over 80%, from the usual 12–40%; spleen cells from CP-treated diabetic donors transferred disease to irradiated syngeneic recipients, thus excluding any toxic effect of CP on islet β cells. CP treatment of F_1 hybrids between NOD and a variety of other strains was nonpromoting, indicating that strong genetic predisposition in susceptible NOD mice was related to immune regulatory control.

A low-diabetes-incidence line of NOD/Wehi mice, with disease virtually absent in males (Baxter *et al.*, 1989), showed a high incidence of overt diabetes within 14 to 16 days after a single large dose of CP (Charlton *et al.*, 1989); diabetes was prevented if the treated mice were given syngeneic spleen and lymph node cells from young prediabetic donors soon after CP. When fetal pancreas isografts were transplanted some days after the recipients were treated with CP, when residual CP or its metabolites were absent from the circulation, these were also destroyed. CP had no diabetogenic effect in many other strains (Charlton *et al.*, 1989). The effect of CP was prevented with silica (Charlton *et al.*, 1988), and with Mab against CD4 cells (Charlton and Mandel, 1988), or CD8 cells (Charlton *et al.*, 1988); even elimination of a small subset of T cells bearing the Vβ8 TcR (Bacelj *et al.*, 1989) was effective, and data suggest that T cells with the Vβ8.3 receptor is the critical population (Bacelj *et al.*, 1990).

6. Thymectomy

Early perinatal thymectomy has immunomodulatory effects as described earlier. Dardenne *et al.* (1989) performed thymectomy in NOD mice at either 3 or 7 weeks of age and found that diabetes was sharply increased in females but not in males, but there was no effect of delayed thymectomy.

7. Adoptive Transfer

Insulitis and diabetes can be transferred with lymphoid cells from diabetic donors, and splenocytes transferred disease to young sublethally irradiated (775 R) recipients (e.g., Wicker, *et al.*, 1986). In suitably irradiated (>600 R) recipients, as few as 2×10^6 cells sufficed, although 5×10^6 cells were optimal. The irradiated recipients needed to be over 4 weeks old, although before 3 weeks of age, irradiation was not required for adoptive transfer (Bendelac *et al.*, 1987). Splenocytes from chronically diabetic NOD mice also transferred disease, suggesting the long persistence of immunologically active cells (Wicker *et al.*, 1986), equivalent to the situation in human recipients of a pancreas transplant from either an identical twin (Sibley *et al.*, 1985), or even an HLA-identical sibling (Sibley and Sutherland; 1988). With the identical twins, immunosuppression was not used initially, since the graft should have been retained, but with the MHC-identical donor–recipient combinations, this disease frequently recurred despite immunosuppression. Hanafusa *et al.* (1988) transferred spleen and lymph-node cells from CP-treated diabetic NOD mice to T cell-depleted syngeneic recipients; with unseparated T cells there was a high incidence of insulitis compared with mice not receiving cell transfers. Depletion of T cells from the transferred inoculum abrogated transfer of insulitis; but depletion only of the CD8+ cells did allow transfer of insulitis, suggesting that CD4+ cells were critical.

Adoptive transfer of diabetes is possible without experimental manipulation of the recipients (Bendelac *et al.*, 1987; Bedossa *et al.*, 1989). Insulitis and diabetes resulted when 2×10^7 spleen cells from diabetic mice were transferred into neonatal recipients, and diabetes developed by 3 weeks of age. Bendelac *et al.*, (1987) used purified (B-cell-free) T cells and demonstrated that both CD4+ and CD8+ T cells were required, and males were as susceptible as females. However, after the age of 3 weeks, NOD mice become resistant to adoptive transfer, presumably because immunoregulatory processes develop that override the capacity of transferred cells to cause disease. Bedossa *et al.* (1989) reported that diabetes in recipients was preceded by MHC class II expression on vascular cells in the islets, so there may have been augmented "homing" of T cells to the islets. After adoptive transfer, the time between insulitis and destruction of β islet cells is short compared with that in natural disease. Initially, the infiltrating cells were mostly CD4+, and about 30% of these were activated, being IL-2 receptor positive; however, when β islet cell damage was occurring, CD8+ cells were dominant and were presumably the effector cells. The requirement for both CD4 and CD8 cells from diabetic donors for successful adoptive transfer was confirmed by Miller *et al.* (1988).

Cloned cells from either infiltrated islets or lymphoid organs of diabetic mice are also effective under certain conditions. Haskins *et al.* (1988) produced an islet-reactive T-cell line from spleen and lymph-node cells by stimulating the cells with NOD islets. A line was cloned by limiting dilution and repeated stimulation with islet antigens, and 2 subclones derived. The original line and both clones were CD4+ but CD8-. One clone produced large amounts of IL-2, and when stimulated with antigen presenting cells (APC) and islet antigen, this clone also homed to a NOD islet graft in $(CBA \times NOD)F_1$ mice, suggesting that even *in vivo* it could recognize islet-specific antigens; a NOD pituitary graft was not infiltrated (Bradley *et al.*, 1990). Haskins *et al.* (1989) derived a panel of islet-specific T-cell clones and showed that they respond *in vitro* to islet antigens from a variety of mouse strains, but only when APCs bearing NOD class II MHC antigens were present. All clones were CD4+ and CD8-, and most caused damage to NOD islet grafts after adoptive transfer. This line would also produce diabetes in young NOD mice (Haskins and McDuffie, 1990). Some clones were also transferred to (CBA × NOD)F_1 hybrid mice that do not develop insulitis spontaneously, and marked insulitis resulted.

Whether the cells present in lymphoid organs are representative of the cells involved in islet damage is uncertain. Reich *et al.* (1989a) cloned and expanded T cells from the islets of recently diabetic NOD mice and showed that they were either CD4+ or CD8+, in contrast to data reported by Haskins *et al.* (1989). The CD4+ clones did not respond to BALB/c islets, but the CD8+ clones did. Since BALB/c and NOD mice share an MHC class I (H-$2K^d$) locus, the data were interpreted as indicating antigen specificity and MHC restriction. Neither CD4+ nor CD8+ clones alone caused insulitis after adoptive transfer, but when used together, produced an intense insulitis by 28 days in most islets with reduction of β cells and even diabetic symptoms in some mice. When TcR expression was analyzed, it was found that most islet-specific clones expressed the Vβ5 TCR. $V\beta_5$+ cells are normally deleted in I-E+ mice and, since NOD mice are I-E- (Hattori *et al.*, 1986), it was suggested that the absence of deletion of these TCR-bearing cells contributed to pathogenesis.

8. Diabetes in Diabetes-Resistant Recipients

Non-NOD mice do not develop diabetes, and hybrids between NOD and other strains do so rarely. However, diabetes can be adoptively transferred by NOD bone-marrow stem cells to (NOD × non-NOD) F_1 hybrids (Serreze *et al.*, 1988b), but the recipients need lethal irradiation (1000 R), and transfer has to be with NOD cells. Serreze *et al.* (1988b) concluded that the presence of the diabetogenic alleles in the putative effector cells was sufficient to produce diabetes, and the onset and frequency of disease was remarkably similar to that seen naturally in NOD mice. Also, destruction of β cells occurred in all donor-matched islet grafts. However, cells other than T cells and their precursors were also transferred and included precursors of nonlymphoid APCs that may eventually home to the thymus and become involved in T-cell education. Transfer of bone marrow cells from diabetes-prone BB/W rats is capable of transferring disease to diabetes-resistant (BB/W)F_1 rats when 2-deoxyguanosine-treated thymus from diabetes-resistant donors was also transplanted (Georgiou *et al.*, 1988). Adoptive transfer of NOD bone marrow cells into lethally irradiated C57BL/6 and B10.BR/cd recipients also resulted in insulitis, with 10% developing diabetes (LaFace and Peck, 1989). The low incidence of diabetes despite a high incidence of insulitis was attributed to the need for additional but unknown host susceptibility factor(s).

E. Prevention of Diabetes

1. Sex Hormones

Protective effects of male sex hormones are well established in NOD mice, as in other experimental autoimmune diseases. Castration at 5 weeks of age was protective in females, but in males, resulted in a female incidence of diabetes (Makino *et al.*, 1981). The mode of action of the sex hormones is presumably by effects on immunoregulation.

2. Thymectomy

Neonatal thymectomy reduces the severity and incidence of insulitis (Ogawa *et al.*, 1985; Ikehara *et al.*, 1985), but its effect on diabetes was not reported. Neonatally thymectomized mice were free of insulitis at 8 weeks, but after parabiosis to normal syngeneic partners, insulitis developed in the thymectomized partners within 2 weeks (Ikehara *et al.*, 1985). After neonatal thymectomy in the low-diabetes-incidence NOD/Wehi mice, diabetes was virtually abolished, and insulitis was also greatly reduced (Slattery and Mandel, 1988 unpublished). The mice were not followed to a sufficient age to establish the preventive effect with certainty.

3. Cyclosporine A and FK506

Cyclosporine A (CsA) acts specifically on T cells, in contrast to most other immunosuppressive agents that have a broader action (Bach and Strom, 1985). Mori *et al.* (1986) found that if CsA treatment was started before hyperglycemia developed, and was continued until 160 days, diabetes was prevented; as little as 2.5 mg/kg orally on alternate days completely prevented diabetes, and insulitis was greatly diminished; once glucose intolerance was present, CsA was ineffective. Wang *et al.* (1988) showed that disease recurrence in islet isografts was prevented in prediabetic, but not in diabetic NOD mice given CsA. Spleen cells from prediabetic NOD mice treated *in vitro* with both CsA and IL-2 for 72 hr and reinfused into the original donors greatly reduced the incidence of diabetes; mice given cells treated with either agent alone were not protected (Formby *et al.*, 1988). These findings point to a preferential activation of a suppressor population. The new immunosuppressant FK506, which also apparently is specific for T cells, can prevent diabetes in NOD mice (Miyagawa *et al.*, 1990).

4. Antibodies to T-Cell or MHC Molecules

In earlier studies, both conventional antithymocyte globulin, and an MAb against the pan-T cell marker Thy-1, reduced but did not abolish diabetes (Harada and Makino, 1986). MAbs against major subsets of T cells have been variably effective. Koike *et al.* (1987) treated 2-week-old females with large doses (2 mg/dose i.p.) of the cell-depleting rat IgG2b anti-CD4, GK1.5, twice weekly for 12 weeks. Insulitis was prevented, but studies beyond 12 weeks were not reported. Shizuru *et al.* (1988) treated NOD mice with GK1.5 and found that this not only prevented the progression of disease but even prevented diabetes. In contrast, Charlton and Mandel (1989a) treated NOD/Wehi mice weekly with the non-cell-depleting rat IgG2a anti-CD4, H129, from 25 to 100 days of age; this almost totally prevented insulitis during treatment but, after cessation of treatment, insulitis recurred. Its severity in mice at 180 days was similar to that of 100-day-old untreated mice. MAbs against potentially larger T-cell subsets (e.g., those expressing CD3, a universal component of the TcR) are effective even after a single dose given neonatally (Hayward and Shreiber, 1989). The incidence of insulitis in treated females was only 8% at 10 weeks and 25% at 32 weeks, with less than 10% of the mice being diabetic by 32 weeks. An MAb to the IL-2R, directed to activated T cells, proved effective in young mice when given before insulitis developed (Kelley *et al.*, 1988). As noted above, MAb treatment is effective in diabetes accelerated by CP (Charlton and Mandel, 1988; Charlton *et al.*, 1988; Bacelj *et al.*, 1989); notably when given peritransplant, the MAb to TcR anti-Vβ8 prevents disease recurrence in isografts of fetal pancreas in spontaneously diabetic mice (Bacelj *et al.*, 1990).

Diabetes in NOD mice is prevented also by Mab directed against MHC class II antigens, whether treatment is started neonatally or delayed until weaning (Boitard *et al.*, 1988).

5. Cytokines

Cytokines may mediate the action of many types of immunotherapy. In NOD mice, tumor necrosis factor-α (TNFα) reduced insulitis without causing upregulation of MHC class II expression, and suppressed the adoptive transfer of diabetes to young male mice (Jacob *et al.*, 1990). Satoh *et al.* (1989) tested mouse IFN-γ, human IL-1α, IL-2, TNFα, and mouse GM-CSF, but only TNFα suppressed insulitis and reduced the incidence of diabetes. Human recombinant interleukin-2 (rIL-2) given at 250 U twice weekly from 6 weeks also greatly reduced diabetes to 17 versus 75% in controls at 20 weeks (Serreze *et al.*, 1990). Treatment with poly[I:C], an inducer of IFN α/β, was even more effective and completely prevented diabetes at 20 weeks, but had to be given continuously. Serreze *et al.* (1990) suggested that, in the presence of these stimulators, the defective T-cell suppressor function, claimed to be the cause of autoreactivity (Serreze and Leiter, 1988), is increased to more normal levels.

6. Viruses

Lymphocytic choriomeningitis virus (LCMV), a virus that infects mainly CD4+ T cells, can prevent diabetes in NOD mice (Oldstone 1988). Infection with LCMV was preventive when neonatal mice were infected intracerebrally, and the incidence of diabetes was reduced when virus was injected at 6 weeks, from 95% in untreated females of 9 months to 6%. The ablation of T helper cells produced an immunologic regulatory imbalance, and adoptive transfer of bone marrow and spleen cells from infected mice was successful in preventing disease in lethally irradiated (850 R) recipients. The effect of the virus is limited to the Th-1.2+, CD4+, CD8-, lymphocytes and not bone marrow cells (Oldstone, 1990). Furthermore, and as indicated by the fact that several other CD4+-dependent immune responses were not affected by LCMV infection, the immunosuppressive effect on murine diabetes appears to be selective (Oldstone, 1990). In a further study aimed at determining whether the entire genome of LCMV or only part of it was needed to prevent diabetes in NOD mice, only the S RNA segment, encoding two of the major structural glycoproteins, was required for that immunosuppressive effect (Oldstone *et al.*, 1990). Oldstone (1990) suggested that viral genes or their expressed products could be used to attack or treat specific cells that may be causing disease. A similar protective effect of virus infection can be seen in BB/W rats (Dyrberg *et al.*, 1988).

7. Adoptive Transfer of Putative Suppressor Cells

In a model of adoptive transfer of diabetes in irradiated adult recipient mice, diabetes was prevented if lymphoid cells from young nondiabetic donors were transferred simultaneously with the cells from a diabetic donor (Boitard *et al.*, 1989). Thus the presence of a suppressor-cell population in the lymphoid pool of prediabetic mice may override the effect of effector cells present in the cell inoculum from diabetic donor. A similar explanation was invoked for the protective effect seen with transfer of normal prediabetic cells in the diabetes induced by CP (Charlton *et al.*, 1989). In a variant of the suppressor-cell transfer experiment, a line of autoreactive T cells, generated from newly diabetic mice and injected into nondiabetic NOD recipients, prevented diabetes and insulitis up to 1 year of age (Reich *et al.*, 1989b); these cells were CD3+, CD4+, CD8-, and stained homogeneously for the Vβ2 TcR. Formby *et al.* (1988) took spleen cells from prediabetic NOD mice, activated these *in vitro* for 72 hr with CsA and IL-2; retransferred back into the same animals, these cells conferred markedly protective effects. In all, these data are of interest in further validating adoptive transfer protocols as evidence for the reality of immune suppression.

8. Tolerance Induction

Tolerance to semiallogeneic spleen cells in neonatal NOD mice can be induced by injecting 10^6 cells i.v. (Bendelac *et al.*, 1989). In these experiments tolerance was demonstrated using donor skin grafts, proliferative and cytotoxic responses *in vitro* to donor cells, and by the presence of chimerism. Insulitis and diabetes were both markedly reduced but not fully prevented. Donor T cells were not required in the initial inoculum, since T-cell depletion of the transferred cells was also effective. Interestingly, whereas significant protection from disease was seen and chimerism was present, permanent skin allograft acceptance was not achieved. Viable cells were required to produce an effect since irradiation of the cells abrogated protection.

9. Bone Marrow Transfer

The role of T cells in disease production in NOD mice is now well established, but the precise mode of development of the autoreactive cells is still uncertain. A defect in bone marrow stem cells may be present since Ikehara *et al.* (1985) found that when 2×10^7 allogeneic bone marrow cells from young BALB/c athymic (nude) donors were transplanted into lethally irradiated NOD females aged 5 months, both insulitis and diabetes were absent when the recipients were examined 3 months later. LaFace and Peck (1989) showed that NOD mice could be protected totally from insulitis and diabetes with lethal irradiation followed by B10.BR/cd hemopoietic cells.

10. Other Treatments

a. Free Radical Scavengers. Killing of β cells may be mediated in many types of insulitis by free-O_2 radicals resulting from superoxide production at the site of inflammation; hence, free radical scavengers that can inactivate or destroy these radicals may prevent β-cell damage. Klandorf *et al.* (1989) found that dimethylsulfoxide (DMSO) or its derivatives, methyl-sulfonylmethane (MSM) or dimethylsulfide (DMS), added to drinking water of NOD mice at weaning, produced marked alterations in diabetes incidence. In contrast to the expected results, 2.5% DMSO *increased* the rate of appearance as well as the frequency of diabetes in females and also in males, in which the incidence was increased from 21 to 79%, whereas MSM had no effect, and DMS reduced the prevalence of diabetes. However, when a modified diet AIN-76, which had previously been shown to decrease the frequency of diabetes in BB rats (Scott *et al.*, 1985), was fed to the mice, the effect of DMSO was to reduce the incidence of diabetes to 36%. The conclusion was that DMSO augmented the uptake of potentially diabetogenic constituents in the food and, in the presence of genetic susceptibility, increased the rate of diabetes. Two enzymes that act on superoxide radicals, superoxide dismutase and catalase, will prevent β-cell destruction in allografts in diabetic NOD mice (Nomikos *et al.*, 1989). These grafts had been exposed before transplantation to 95% O_2, a procedure that often prevents allograft rejection in nondiabetic mice but not disease recurrence in spontaneously diabetic animals.

b. Nicotinamide. This prevents diabetes induced with large doses of streptozotocin (STZ) (Dulin *et al.*, 1969; Stauffacher *et al.*, 1970; Lazarow *et al.*,

1950; Lazarus and Shapiro, 1973), as well as insulitis induced by low-dose STZ (Rossini *et al.*, 1978). Also, nicotinamide prevented diabetes and reduced insulitis in prediabetic NOD mice and, in 4 of 6 mice treated from the first appearance of glycosuria, there was reversal of glycosuria; however, treatment of established diabetes with nicotinamide was generally ineffective (Yamada *et al.*, 1982). The action of nicotinamide may be immunological, and perhaps on ADCC; ADCC was found to increase when NOD mice developed diabetes, but when NOD spleen cells were tested for ADCC against human red blood cells *in vitro* in the presence of nicotinamide, lysis was markedly inhibited. Nicotinamide is thought to act in STZ diabetes by preventing the STZ-induced reduction of intracellular content of nicotinamide adenine dinucleotide (NAD) (Ho and Hashim, 1972; Anderson *et al.*, 1974; Yamamoto and Okamoto, 1980).

c. Immunomodulator OK-432. Toyota *et al.* (1986) tested a streptococcal preparation OK-432 as an immunomodulator in NOD female mice by giving weekly i.p. injections from 4 to 24 weeks; diabetes occurred in 0 of 17 mice compared with 14 of 17 controls. OK-432 apparently stimulates IFN-γ and IL-2 production, and reportedly activates macrophages, NK cells and cytotoxic T cells (Satoh *et al.*, 1980; Saito *et al.*, 1982; Wakasugi *et al.*, 1982; Ichimura *et al.*, 1985). The mode of action of OK-432 as an antiimmune drug is not yet clear.

d. Diet. Diet itself has been shown to modify diabetes in NOD mice (Elliott *et al.*, 1988) as well as in BB rats (Scott *et al.*, 1985; Elliott *et al.*, 1984). In NOD mice, only animals that had been fed meat meal or casein developed the expected incidence of diabetes (27%), and a diet of lactalbumin and gluten reduced the incidence to 2.4 and 4.6%, respectively (Elliott *et al.*, 1988).

e. 2 Acetyl-4-tetrahydroxybutylimidazole (THI). Recently we (Mandel T. E., Koulmanda M. & Mackay I. R., 1991, unpublished observations) have shown that THI given to NOD mice in drinking water can prevent spontaneous and CP-induced diabetes. THI is a contaminant in caramel color and is widely found in common foods and beverages. At the dose used (400 ppm), this drug produced T-lymphopenia, but in more recent studies we have data that suggests that the diabetic protective effect is not due to lymphopenia per se. The mode of action of THI is currently being investigated in more detail.

III. EXPERIMENTAL AUTOIMMUNE ENCEPHALOMYELITIS

A. Introduction

Experimental autoimmune encephalitis (EAE) remains the most widely studied and informative of the experimentally induced models of autoimmune disease, and is the prototype for an antigen-specific and T cell-mediated attack on the target organ. There are two types of EAE, acute or chronic relapsing, depending on species, the age of the animal, the nature of the encephalitogenic inoculum, etc. Acute EAE is induced by injection with purified myelin proteins (Bernard *et al.*, 1983a), peptides thereof (Hashim *et al.*, 1978; Bernard and Carnegie, 1975; Kono *et al.*, 1988) or T-cell lines or clones specific for these myelin antigens (Ben-Nun *et al.*, 1981a; Zamvil *et al.*, 1985a; Sakai *et al.*, 1988a; 1988b). Chronic relapsing EAE is marked by extensive demyelination and inflammation (Raine, 1984). It is induced in young animals, particularly guinea pigs, and requires neural components additional to myelin basic protein (Raine, 1984).

Acute and chronic relapsing EAE have been the subjects of numerous reviews (Paterson, 1979; Bernard *et al.*, 1983a; Raine, 1984; Wisniewski *et al.*, 1985; Lebar, 1987). Our purpose here is to discuss the recent developments in EAE that have contributed new knowledge on pathogenesis, expression of autoimmune lesions, and prevention. In particular, we shall describe new or alternative antigenic inocula that induce lesions identical to those seen in classical EAE, including the utilization of *Bordetella pertussis* to enhance antigenicity, the demyelinating effect of antibodies as opposed to cells, the role of vasogenic edema in the production of tissue lesions, the interplay between the MHC and T-cell receptor use in relation to genetic predisposition, and possibilities for immunotherapeutic modulation that could be applicable to human disease. We can emphasize that the routine production of various autoimmune diseases in mice has been an important development, particularly because of the possibility of using inbred strains for studies of cell transfer, congenic strains for immunogenetic studies, and cultured mouse lymphoid tissue for immune induction and other types of *in vitro* experimentation (Bernard, 1976; Bernard and Carnegie, 1975; Bernard *et al.*, 1976).

B. Enhancing Effect of Pertussis on Experimental Autoimmune Disease

Bordetella pertussis or derivatives are potent adjuvants and enhancers of experimentally induced autoimmune disease. Pertussis has been particularly exploited to induce EAE in mice as well as experimental autoimmune orchitis (EAO) (Bernard *et al.*, 1978; Kohno *et al.*, 1983) and experimental autoimmune uveitis (EAU) (Gery *et al.*, 1986; Caspi *et al.*, 1988).

1. Enhancement of EAE with Pertussigen

Levine and co-workers (Levine *et al.*, 1966) found that pertussis vaccine and extracts from *B. pertussis* rich in histamine-sensitizing factor facilitated the induction of EAE in rats and mice. Subsequently EAE was routinely induced in mice (SJL/J) provided that, in addition to the emulsion of mouse spinal cord or MBP with FCA, pertussis vaccine was given as a co-adjuvant (Bernard and

Carnegie, 1975; Bernard *et al.*, 1976). Pertussigen, one of the biologically active proteins from *B. pertussis,* was found to be a potent adjuvant in promoting EAE in mice receiving mouse spinal cord homogenate (MSCH) in CFA supplemented with *Mycobacterium tuberculosis* (MT) (Munoz *et al.*, 1984). An effective regimen consisted of an intravenous dose of 400 μg pertussigen within a few minutes of injection of the MSCH-CFA emulsion (Fig. 3). Pertussigen by other routes (e.g., i.m., s.c., i.p.) facilitated the induction of EAE but was less efficient. Within 11 to 13 days, a severe form of EAE regularly developed, although paralysis seldom extended to the forelimbs. Pertussigen given 5 days after the injection of MSCH-CFA resulted in milder EAE, but paralysis persisted for some 74 days, the duration of the experiment. Histologic studies on mice 15 to 20 days after the onset of paralysis revealed typical lesions of EAE (Raine 1984), whereas mice with residual evidence of EAE after 74 days showed no clear histologic evidence of EAE lesions in the brain and spinal cord (Munoz *et al.*, 1984). Whereas these findings differ from those obtained with protocols for chronic

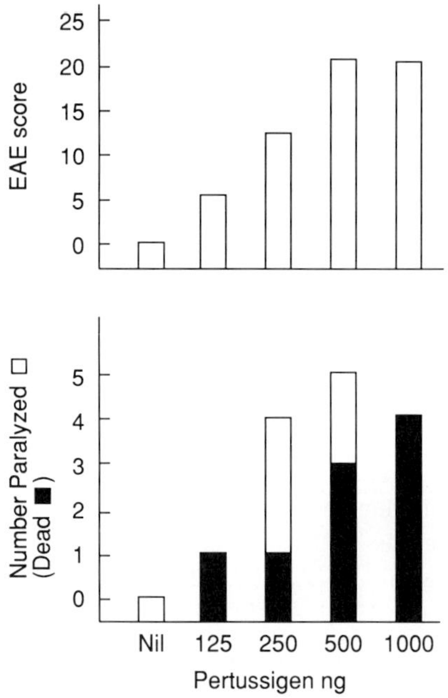

FIG. 3 Titration of pertussigen for its ability to promote EAE in susceptible (SJL × BALB/c) F_1 mice (5 per group) receiving 4 mg MSC emulsified in CFA-H37. Nil, pertussigen not given. Upper graph gives the EAE score and the lower graph, the number of mice with definite paralysis (score of 2 or greater) and the number of mice dying from EAE. Reprinted with permission from Munoz, J. J., Bernard, C. C. A. and Mackay, I. R., *Cellular Immunology,* (1984), **83,** 92–100.

relapsing EAE in SJL/J mice (Lublin *et al.*, 1981; Fritz *et al.*, 1983a), the chronic EAE induced in our experiments appeared early after immunization, was long lasting and had a high incidence (Munoz *et al.*, 1984).

2. Enhancement of EAO with Pertussis

EAO could be induced consistently in mice (BALB/c) by immunization with a homologous testicular homogenate emulsified in CFA together with at least 1 μg of an extract of *B. pertussis* rich in pertussigen (Bernard *et al.*, 1978; Kohno *et al.*, 1983). Serum antibody to testicular antigens appeared within 20 days after immunization. The lesions were located in testis (100%), rete testis (37%), cauda epididymis (21%), and vas deferens (37%), and were characterized by peritubular and/or intratubular accumulation of eosinophils, neutrophils, lymphocytes, and macrophages, and were followed by aspermatogenesis. Late lesions included massive necrosis and extensive fibrosis of the seminiferous tubules. Disruption of a blood–testis barrier on day 20 was evidenced by the detection of (1) perfused lanthanum deposits between Sertoli cells and surrounding inflammatory cells inside the seminiferous tubules; (2) deposits of endogenous mouse IgG in germinal epithelium; and (3) probably immune complexes (granular C3) surrounding seminiferous tubules. Murine EAO differed from that of the guinea pig in the lack of involvement of the ductus efferentes, the extensive necrosis, the abundant polymorphonuclear leukocytes in the lesion, and the absolute requirement for concomitant injection of *B. pertussis* extract.

3. Enhancement of EAU with Pertussis

EAU has been studied mainly in rats and a few other species, including primates, in which the disease is produced with one or the other of two antigens, interphotoreceptor-binding protein (IRBP) (Lai *et al.*, 1982) and the retinal soluble antigen, S-Ag (Pfister *et al.*, 1985). Both proteins are components of the retinal photoreceptor cell layer, the site of the autoimmune attack in autoimmune uveoretinitis (Gery *et al.*, 1986). However, with the exception of the mouse, inbred strains are not readily available and, further, the disease in the rat tends to be acute and severe with rapid destruction of the photoreceptor cells, thus differing from chronic posterior uveitis seen in humans. A murine model of EAU was developed by Caspi *et al.* (1988) in strains of mice that developed a chronic disease resembling human uveitis, and was produced with either of the two antigens, S-Ag and IRBP. Although all mouse strains tested showed immune responses to both antigens as measured by lymphocyte responsiveness and antibody production, actual ocular disease was restricted to only a few strains; these showed that the uveitogenic response to the two antigens was mutually exclusive.

Initially, EAU could be produced in mice only with an intensive immunization protocol that required the use of quite large amounts of antigen as well as CFA and *B. pertussis* organisms, and a preimmunization dose of CP. This treatment schedule produced a slow-onset disease that was chronic and largely confined to the posterior segment with focal retinal damage. The histopathological features included vasculitis, retinal granulomata, retinal folds, focal serous detachments, and loss of photoreceptors (Chan *et al.*, 1990). There was also some subretinal neovascularization in a few animals and mild vitritis. The predominant infiltrating cells in the granulomas were macrophages, while the major cells seen in the vitreous were CD4+ T cells. The disease was typically relapsing, showing two peaks of activity at 5 and 10 weeks after immunization. Later, Caspi *et al.* (1990) used pertussis toxin rather than the whole organism, and a single immunization with antigen sufficed without the requirement for CP. In addition, the severity of the disease could be modulated so that either a chronic or an acute disease could be produced.

C. Encephalitogenic Inocula Alternative to Myelin Basic Protein

1. Myelin Proteolipid Protein

There are constituents of myelin other than myelin basic protein (MBP) that clearly induce EAE. The myelin proteolipid protein (PLP) is a potent inducer of acute and chronic EAE (Williams *et al.*, 1982; Cambi *et al.*, 1983; Yoshimura *et al.*, 1985; Yamamura *et al.*, 1986; Tuohy *et al.*, 1989), and PLP-responsive cell lines, as well as PLP-specific T-cell clones, will transfer adoptively EAE into naive syngeneic recipients (Satoh *et al.*, 1987; van der Veen *et al.*, 1990). Both the T-cell lines and clones had the phenotypes of T helper/inducer cells (CD4+CD8-) and induced severe acute EAE within 2 weeks after injection (Satoh *et al.*, 1987; van der Veen *et al.*, 1990). Thus, and as for EAE induced by MBP, a PLP-sensitized T cell appears to be sufficient to induce inflammatory lesions with, in some cases, evidence of demyelination.

2. Endothelial Cell Membranes

Guinea pigs and rhesus monkeys immunized with an emulsion of cultured brain endothelial cell membrane components and FCA, supplemented with MT, develop a chronic or relapsing form of EAE (Tsukada *et al.*, 1987, 1988). The encephalitogenic component is uncharacterized, but neither MBP nor PLP could be detected in the brain endothelial cell samples used; in addition, no proliferative responses to these characteristic myelin antigens were observed either in guinea pigs or monkeys, and none of the immunized guinea pigs gave a positive delayed-type hypersensitivity (DTH) skin reaction to MBP or PLP

(Tsukada *et al.*, 1987, 1988), although there was a positive DTH reaction to the immunizing antigen.

The first signs of disease induced by endothelial cell membranes were loss of body weight and hair, followed by the development of ataxia, flaccid paralysis of the hind legs, and occasional myoclonus, occurring at days 14–21 and 21–30 for guinea pig and monkey, respectively (Tsukada *et al.*, 1987, 1988). In surviving animals, there was chronic progressive disease. Histologically, in the acute phase, there were infiltrates of mononuclear cells attached to cerebral endothelial cells, and small focal perivascular hemorrhages and edema; in the chronic phase, there was severe loss of myelin particularly in the cerebellum, cerebrum, pons, and midbrain (Tsukada *et al.*, 1987, 1988). In this respect the presence of diffuse demyelination is in keeping with the histopathologic features of MS (Prineas, 1985), and thus emphasizes the use of this model for immunologic and pathogenic studies of naturally occurring demyelinating diseases.

3. Myelin Oligodendrocyte Glycoprotein (MOG)

Molecules with epitopes exposed at the external side of the myelin membrane could be accessible targets for demyelinating immune responses. MOG is the molecule recognized by the MAb 8-18C5 raised against a rat cerebellar glycoprotein preparation (Linington *et al.*, 1984). MOG was demonstrated immunohistochemically on oligodendrocyte surfaces and in the outermost lamellae of myelin sheaths (Linington *et al.*, 1988; Lebar *et al.*, 1986; Brunner *et al.*, 1989). It is central nervous system (CNS) specific since antibodies to MOG do not react with peripheral nerves (Linington *et al.*, 1984; Lebar *et al.*, 1986). MOG is a surface marker of oligodendrocyte maturation (Scolding *et al.*, 1989) and, during CNS development, expression corresponds with myelination; MOG is not demonstrable in glial cells before myelin sheath formation (Linington *et al.*, 1988). The encephalitogenic capacity of MOG has not yet been studied, partly because of its low abundance in CNS tissue, but it is clearly a target for immune attack, as judged by the potent capacity of antibody to MOG to cause demyelination (*vide infra*).

D. Major Histocompatibility Complex and T-Cell Interaction

1. Class I and Class II MHC Molecules

The genes of the major histocompatibility complex (MHC) on chromosomes 6 (man) and 17 (mouse) are contained within three regions with distinct gene products, the class I, class II and complement molecules, reviewed by Moeller (1983) and Tait (1990), and described by Nepom and Concannon in Chapter 5 of this volume.

Class I molecules, HLA-A, B, and C in man and H2-K, D, L in mice, are composed of two polypeptide chains: a polymorphic 45-kDa protein non-covalently linked to β_2 microglobulin and a 12-kDa monomorphic molecule on the membrane of all nucleated cells. The α_1 and α_2 domains of an alpha helix of the 45-kDa molecule fold to form an antigen-binding groove, surrounded by most of the polymorphic residues (Bjorkman *et al.*, 1987a, 1987b; Townsend *et al.*, 1989). CD8+ (T-cytotoxic) cells recognize endogenously derived cellular peptide antigens bound to Class I molecules (Townsend *et al.*, 1986, 1989).

Class II molecules, expressed as heterodimers primarily on dendritic cells, macrophages, and B lymphocytes, are encoded by HLA-DR, DQ, and DP genes in man and by H2-I-A and I-E genes in mice (Kaufman *et al.*, 1984). They consist of two glycoprotein molecules, a 34-kDa α chain and a 28-kDa β chain. As with class I MHC molecules, there are sequences on the hypervariable region of the α_1 and β_1 chains of class II molecules that have binding affinity for a site, the agretope, on immunogenic structures (Babbit *et al.*, 1985; Guillet *et al.*, 1987; Sette *et al.*, 1987). Crosslinking of MHC class II molecules with radio-labeled peptides suggests that there is a single antigen-binding site on class II molecules (Luescher *et al.*, 1988). CD4+ (T-helper) cells recognize antigenic fragments after endocytosis and subsequent association with class II molecules on the cell surface. In exceptional circumstances, there can be recognition by CD4+ T cells of *self* peptides associated with class II molecules, with potential for autoimmune induction.

2. EAE Susceptibility and the MHC

The response to encephalitogenic challenge is strain dependent in mice, with only a few strains being highly susceptible to EAE, e.g., SJL/5 (H-2^s) (Bernard 1976), and BIOPL and PL/J (H2^u) (Fritz *et al.*, 1983b). Nonsusceptibility is not because of an absence of, or a defect in, the relevant antigen in the target tissue, because MBP purified from resistant strains will induce EAE in susceptible animals (Bernard 1976). Since equivalent findings are available for rats (Williams and Moore, 1973; Gaser *et al.*, 1973), guinea pigs (Lisak *et al.*, 1975; Kies *et al.*, 1975; Geczy *et al.*, 1984), and rabbits (Villarroya *et al.*, 1990), genetic predisposition based on MHC molecules is clearly a feature in all species. There is clear analogy here with the genetic risk for multiple sclerosis in Caucasians conferred by the HLA susceptibility alleles DR2 and Dw2 (Tiwari and Terasaki 1985; Olerup *et al.*, 1989).

3. T-Cell Recognition: The Bimolecular Complex

Fritz *et al.* (1983b) made the important observation that the *N*-terminal 1–34 amino acid peptic fragment of guinea pig or rat MBP caused EAE in PL/J (H-2^u) and (PL x SJL)F_1 mice, but not in the SJL/J (H-2^s) mice. Conversely SJL/J and

A.SW (H-2^s) mice developed EAE after injection with the *C*-terminal 89–169 fragment of MBP. Furthermore, the encephalitogenic response to MBP peptides in (PL × SJL)F_1 was not codominant, in that only MBP peptide 1–37 caused EAE (Fritz *et al.*, 1983b). It was postulated that I-A^s-restricted T cells that recognized the MBP peptide 89–169 could be either inactivated or suppressed, or that the level of I-A^s expression by (PL × SJL)F_1 antigen-presenting cells was insufficient for effective priming of MBP-reactive I-A^s-restricted T cells.

Further studies have fully confirmed that there is preferential binding of encephalitogenic peptides with I-A class II molecules, noting one exception in which the response to MBP peptide 35–47 is associated with the I-E molecule (HLA-DR in man) (Acha-Orbea *et al.*, 1988; Zamvil *et al.*, 1988b). In addition, an imbalance in the level of MHC class II gene expression may partly account for the hierarchy in the recognition of MBP epitopes (Urban *et al.*, 1988; Fritz *et al.*, 1985; Fritz and Skeen, 1987; Zamvil *et al.*, 1985b; Sobel and Colvin, 1985). However, not all MBP determinants are encephalitogenic, since, as shown by Zamvil *et al.* (1986), the acetylated *N*-terminus peptide AcN1-20 contains an I.A^u restricted dominant encephalitogenic epitope; when this peptide is deacetylated, it fails to induce EAE, yet retains immunogenicity (Zamvil *et al.*, 1986; Zamvil and Steinman, 1990).

The identification of multiple encephalitogenic epitopes on MBP illustrates the utility of EAE as a prototypic model for the genetically complex human autoimmune disorders, including demyelinating diseases. Zamvil *et al.* (1988a) and Urban *et al.* (1989) have shown that separate autoantigens, or multiple discrete T-cell epitopes of a single antigen, may at least partly account for the association of more than one class II MHC gene (i.e., DQ, DR) with autoimmune conditions.

There is a remarkable restriction in the use of the TcR chain molecules among autoreactive CD4+ lymphocytes in EAE. The TcR is a transmembrane heterodimer composed of a 45-kDa α-chain and 43-kDa β-chain. Each TcR α and β chain has two components, a variable domain that determines antigen recognition and a constant domain to which is attached a transmembrane portion. The gene encoding the α chain is located on chromosome 14 in man and mouse, and the gene encoding the β chain is located on chromosome 7 (man) and chromosome 6 (mouse). As for immunoglobulins, the structural diversity of the TcR is generated through the somatic recombination of different variable (V), diversity (D) (for β chain only), and joining (J) gene segments, as well as random insertion and/or deletion of nucleotides occurring during T-cell differentiation (Davis, 1988).

Studies in mice with EAE, using cell-surface staining with specific MAbs against the TcR Vβ chain, Southern transfer analysis, and direct TcR gene sequencing, have shown a striking restriction of the TcR utilization against the immunodominant epitope of MBP (Acha-Orbea *et al.*, 1988; Urban *et al.*, 1988; Burns *et al.*, 1989). Data indicate that this may also pertain to human diseases (Oksenberg *et al.*, 1989, 1990; Ota *et al.*, 1990; Wucherpfennig *et al.*, 1990). Thus, in the PL mouse strain, over 89% of the encephalitogenic T cells directed against MBP peptide 1–9 utilize Vβ8.2, and 100% utilize the Vα4 family. In B10PL mice, 70% utilize Vβ8.2; 58%, Vα2.3; and 42%, Vα4.3 (Urban *et al.*, 1988; Zamvil *et al.*, 1988b; Acha-Orbea *et al.*, 1988). Both Vα2.3- and Vα4.3-bearing T cells were shown to have the same J gene, $J\alpha_{39}$ (Urban *et al.*, 1988). In the Lewis rat 100% of the encephalitogenic T cells that recognize the MBP peptide 72–86 expressed the T-cell receptor β chain homologous to the mouse Vβ8.2, and 73% had the rat homolog of Vα2 (Burns *et al.*, 1989; Vanderbark *et al.*, 1989). It is of particular interest that in the two species, different epitopes of MBP are presented by different MHC class II molecules, yet both species use the same TcR V genes and possibly the same Jα region. Thus the same construction of the TcR recognizes particular antigen–MHC associations across different species. The V-region disease hypothesis enunciates that a specific ligand, the malatope, selects a given V region of the TcR to initiate pathogenic T-cell responses (Heber-Katz, 1990).

E. Specific Effector Processes in EAE

1. T Cells

Susceptibility to EAE in mice is a dominant trait in part controlled by MHC genes (Bernard, 1976). Resistance is associated with the inability of the CD4+ helper cells (Ly1.2+ Ly2.2-) to express a specific cell-mediated immune (CMI) response to the autoantigen, MBP. However, both susceptible and resistant strains can express CMI to the tuberculin derivative in adjuvant preparations. Since EAE in mice is dependent on T helper cells (Bernard, 1976; Bernard *et al.*, 1977; Pettinelli and McFarlin, 1981; Bernard and Mackay, 1983), resistance to EAE should be associated with a specific failure of T lymphocytes to recognize and/or respond to the encephalitogenic sequence of the MBP molecule (Bernard, 1976; Bernard *et al.*, 1977). In line with this, neonatal thymectomy results in conversion from susceptibility to resistance (Arnason *et al.*, 1962; Bernard *et al.*, 1976). As further evidence for the essential participation of T-helper cells in EAE, continuous lines of MBP-reactive T_H cells will adoptively transfer EAE (Ben-Nun *et al.*, 1981a; Ben-Nun and Lando, 1983), T_H cells are present in inflammatory EAE lesions (Traugott *et al.*, 1986), and inhibition and/or reversal of EAE can be effected in rats and in mice by MAb against CD4, the surface marker expressed by MHC class II-restricted T_H lymphocytes (Brostoff and Mason, 1984; Waldor *et al.*, 1985).

2. Antibody

EAE as a prototypic model could clarify the debate whether antibody can have damaging effects *in vivo* on neural tissues. We note here that it is now well established that MS is associated with an excessive production of immunoglobulins within the CNS, but the antigenic specificity of these remains unknown. Recently, evidence has accumulated in both EAE and MS that antibodies against defined myelin antigens can produce immune-mediated demyelination. We can note an important new model to identify demyelinating antibodies since, when specific antimyelin antibodies are injected into animals sensitized for acute EAE when the blood–brain barrier is known to be breached, extensive demyelination ensues (*vide infra*).

a. Antibody to MOG. In acute EAE produced in Lewis rats by injection of purified MBP or by passive transfer of monospecific MBP-reactive T lymphocytes, there is little or no demyelination despite widespread inflammation (Raine, 1984). However, extensive CNS demyelination can be induced in these animals by i.v. injection of a purified MAb to MOG, clone 8-18C5 (Linington *et al.*, 1984), at the time when the blood–brain barrier is breached (Schluesener *et al.*, 1987). Antibody to MOG alone in control animals had no effect, nor did injection of normal mouse IgG in animals with EAE. In other forms of EAE, antibody to MOG increased the severity of the disease and augmented demyelination (Lassmann *et al.*, 1988; Linington *et al.*, 1988). As further evidence that antibody to MOG within the CNS causes demyelination, intrathecal injection of the MAb 8-18C5 in normal rats induced demyelinating lesions on the surface of the spinal cord (Lassmann and Linington, 1987).

The likelihood that MOG is a target antigen in demyelinating diseases is better shown by the presence of antibodies to MOG in rats with chronic relapsing EAE (Linington and Lassmann, 1987), and the occurrence of cross-reactive idiotypes on these specific autoantibodies (Gunn *et al.*, 1989). Notably, the demyelinating activity of serum in chronic relapsing EAE, assayed *in vivo* by intralethal injection into normal rats, correlates with the titer of antibody to MOG (Linington and Lassmann, 1987). These studies suggest that although MOG is present in low amounts of myelin (Linington *et al.*, 1984), it must have a high immunogenic potential since immunization with homogenates of whole CNS generates detectable levels of antibodies to MOG (Linington and Lassmann, 1987).

There is additional *in vitro* evidence that antibody to MOG has demyelinating activity. Although antibodies against the major myelin proteins, MBP and PLP, are present in EAE sera with demyelinating activity (Lassmann and Linington, 1987), polyclonal antibodies raised against preparations of MBP, PLP, or myelin-associated glycoprotein (MAG) do not cause demyelination in cultured CNS tissue (Glynn and Linington, 1989). Antibodies against myelin glycolipids can cause demyelination in cultured CNS tissue (Raine, 1984), but such antibodies are not a prerequisite for demyelination, either *in vitro* (Lebar *et al.*, 1976) or *in vivo* (Schwerer *et al.*, 1984). Hence antibodies against other myelin antigens must participate in demyelination (Schwerer *et al.*, 1984). In this context, we note that EAE sera with no reactivity against MBP, PLP, or cerebrosides, but containing antibodies against the CNS myelin glycoprotein M2, will cause demyelination *in vitro* (Lebar *et al.*, 1976; Lebar *et al.*, 1979). It now appears that glycoprotein M2 described by Lebar *et al.* (1976; 1986) is actually identifiable as MOG (Glynn and Linington, 1989; Lebar *et al.*, 1986) as judged by immunologic cross-reactivity, tissue and cellular localization, and molecular weight. That *in vitro* demyelination by EAE sera may indeed be attributed to antibody to MOG is validated by the effects of purified MAb to MOG antibody on aggregating cell cultures from fetal rat brain (Kerlero de Rosbo *et al.*, 1990). In this culture system, the cellular differentiation and organization, as well as the chemical composition of the myelin membrane formed, closely resemble what is found *in vivo* (Honegger, 1985). In these cultures, the MAb 8-18C5 induced antibody-specific and dose-related demyelination (Kerlero de Rosbo *et al.*, 1990). Hence demyelination induced by antibody to MOG represents a specific immune-mediated lesion that could likewise participate in demyelinating diseases of man.

b. Demyelination by Other Myelin-Specific Antibodies. There is evidence for demyelinating effects of other myelin-specific antibodies, as judged by injection of the antibody into animals sensitized for acute EAE. The i.v. injection of a MAb raised against Theiler's murine encephalomyelitis virus, but cross-reacting with a determinant on myelin and oligodendrocytes, caused extensive demyelination *in vivo* in SJL mice with acute EAE (Yamada *et al.*, 1990). An antibody to galactocerebroside had the same effect (Lassmann and Linington, 1987). The question therefore arises whether immunoglobulins isolated from serum and/or brain of patients with MS (Bernard *et al.*, 1983b) would cause demyelination in an equivalent assay system.

F. Nonspecific Effector Processes in EAE: Vasogenic Edema

In both acute EAE and the first phase of chronic EAE, there are similar neurological deficits expressed in rodents by a typical ascending paralysis that progresses from a limp tail to severe paresis of the hindlimbs, usually followed by a full recovery (Simmons *et al.*, 1984). This characteristic neurologic lesion was originally attributed to neuronal damage at sites of focal lesions, but other explanations now seem likely.

1. Immune-Mediated Vasogenic Edema

Investigations of hindlimb motor function in adult female Lewis rats with MBP-induced acute EAE were conducted using an objective behavioral measure of motor ability (Simmons *et al.*, 1981). There was no apparent hindlimb motor deficit in the absence of overt signs of EAE, despite histologic evidence of severe inflammatory lesions that persisted in the CNS until the postrecovery test (Simmons *et al.*, 1981). Thus an explanation for motor dysfunction in rodents with acute EAE must account for the limited and qualitatively similar nature of the deficits, their transient nature, and their typical ascending progression, and there should also be a valid pathologic correlate.

In rodents, the arterial supply to the lower spinal cord is derived solely from the descending branch of a single radicular artery, *A. radicis magna* (Woolam and Millen, 1955; Tokioka, 1973). Since abnormalities of carbohydrate metabolism had been detected in spinal cord tissue slices from rats with EAE (Smith, 1966), we investigated the possibility that the characteristic progression of lesions resulted from ischemia due to obstructed flow in the long single-input arterial supply to the lower spinal cord. The progression of paralysis did in fact correlate with a progressive ascending accumulation of lactic acid in the spinal cord (Simmons *et al.*, 1982), but lactate accumulation was not attributable to focal ischemia, indicating that blood flow to the lower spinal cord regions was intact during EAE (Simmons *et al.*, 1982). Rather, metabolic disturbance appeared to be owing to neural tissue anoxia caused by vasogenic edema after breakdown of the blood–brain barrier during EAE (Barlow, 1956; Levine *et al.*, 1965; Paterson, 1972; Leibowitz and Kennedy, 1972; Oldendorf and Towner, 1974; Daniel *et al.*, 1981). As judged by the large amounts of specific plasma proteins extravasated into the neural tissue in rats with EAE, a caudo–rostral progression of vasogenic edema appeared to correlate with both ascending paralysis and lactate accumulation, in the absence of significant demyelination (Kerlero de Rosbo, *et al.*, 1985). These data indicate that the ascending paralysis is induced by edema during EAE, with nerve root endoneurium as the functionally vulnerable site. In other words, the signs of EAE in rodents are explained anatomically by progressive disturbance of the nodes of Ranvier in nerve root myelinated fibers (Simmons *et al.*, 1982; 1984). Finally, because vasogenic edema has been detected in the lesions of MS (Takeoka *et al.*, 1983; Newcombe *et al.*, 1982), its relevance to neurologic impairment in human disease needs careful assessment.

2. Non-Immune-Mediated Vasogenic Edema: Tunicamycin

The above concept of deficits due to vasogenic edema is supported by a newly described model of neurological impairment that is quite independent of immune mechanisms. This is produced by injection of the neurotoxin, tunicamycin. The signs depend on the age of the animals (Peterson and Jago, 1977). Thus in young adult rats, the neurologic signs are virtually identical to those of typical acute EAE; in baby rats there is a stiff-legged staggering gait, tremor of the body musculature and convulsions; and in old rats there are no neurologic signs except depression. Vasogenic edema, as indicated by an increase in extravasated plasma proteins into the CNS in tunicamycin-treated young adult rats, was shown to be located, as in EAE rats, mostly in the spinal cord, and coincided exactly with the onset of clinical paralysis, i.e., 48 hr after injection of the toxin (Kerlero de Rosbo *et al.*, 1987). Degradation of MBP, assessed throughout the CNS as an index of demyelination, was never observed (Kerlero de Rosbo *et al.*, 1987). Neurologic impairment in young adult rats given tunicamycin simulates that observed in adult rats with EAE and points to a localization of edema in the spinal cord, rather than in the brain as observed in baby rats. Indeed, the differences in neurologic symptoms of tunicamycin toxicity at different ages in rats is explicable by the different sites of vasogenic edema in the CNS. The relevance to MS may be in a possible pharmacologic control of vasogenic edema and alleviation of paralysis. In this context, we note that in experimental autoimmune neuritis, the putative experimental model for the polyneuropathies (Bernard *et al.*, 1983b; Geczy *et al.*, 1984, 1985; Milner *et al.*, 1987; Hartung and Toyka, 1990), the onset of the disease is delayed in rats treated with reserpine, which indirectly inhibits opening of the blood–nervous system barrier by depleting vasoactive amines (Brosnan and Tansey, 1984). As an explanation for the action of tunicamycin on the blood–CNS barrier, tunicamycin binds to membranes (Kuo and Lampen, 1976; Heifetz *et al.*, 1979). As focal damage to endothelial cells in the cerebral vasculature of baby rats treated with tunicamycin has been observed (Finnie and Mukherjee, 1986), the possibility exists that binding of tunicamycin to the endothelial cell membrane may directly affect vascular permeability. The detection of antiendothelial cell antibodies and immune complexes in sera of animals with acute and chronic relapsing EAE (Tsukada *et al.*, 1986), and in patients with MS (Tanaka *et al.*, 1987; Tsukada *et al.*, 1989a), neurologic-Behcet syndrome and myelopathies (Tsukada *et al.*, 1989b), supports the suggestion that damage to the CNS endothelium can cause increased vascular permeability and thus is an important factor in experimentally induced and naturally occurring demyelinating disorders.

G. Immunotherapy of EAE

EAE has proved to be a most applicable model disease for the analysis of immunotherapy for autoimmune disorders including MS (Bernard *et al.*, 1983a), rheumatoid arthritis (Mackay *et al.*, 1991), and others. Initially, inhibition or reversal of EAE depended on the use of nonspecific immunosuppressive and antiinflammatory drugs (Brandiss *et al.*, 1965; Paterson, 1972; Bernard *et al.*, 1977). Subsequently, immunologically specific procedures were used depending on protection-suppression induced by whole CNS tissue or purified proteins or peptides (Hashim, 1981; Driscoll *et al.*, 1976; Higgins and Weiner, 1988; Bernard *et al.*, 1975; Bernard, 1977) or analogs of these (Teitelbaum *et al.*, 1974). More recently, MAbs against T-cell surface markers have been successfully used to prevent or suppress EAE (Brostoff and Mason, 1984; Waldor *et al.*, 1985). Currently, the EAE model is being used to assess the effect of oral administration of purified autoantigens as well as the effect of interference with events at the inductive stage of the disease by blocking MHC molecules or components of the TcR.

1. Oral Administration of Myelin Basic Protein

The oral administration of soluble antigens has long been recognized as an effective method of producing immunological unresponsiveness to a variety of sensitizing antigens (Mattingly and Waksman, 1978; Titus and Chiller, 1981; Rubin *et al.*, 1981). In recent years, this method of tolerance induction has been successfully applied to the prevention and suppression of EAE in Lewis rats (Bitar and Whitacre, 1988; Higgins and Weiner, 1988; Lider *et al.*, 1989; Fuller *et al.*, 1990). Oral MBP before or after EAE induction dramatically suppresses signs of EAE with a significant decrease in histologic lesions and concurrently a decrease in lymphocytic proliferative response and antibody production to MBP. This suppression is specific, dose dependent, and still effective even 8 weeks after feeding of MBP (Bitar and Whitacre, 1988; Higgins and Weiner, 1988; Fuller *et al.*, 1990). It is interesting to note that such a suppression is inducible not only with the intact MBP molecule, but also with encephalitogenic and nonencephalitogenic fragments of MBP. Lider *et al.* (1989) report that the suppression of EAE by oral administration of MBP is mediated by antigen-specific CD8+ T lymphocytes. Simplicity and lack of adverse effects prompt consideration for the application of this method of tolerance in man.

The suppressive effects of orally administered autoantigen are not limited to EAE, but pertain also to other models including adjuvant arthritis (Zhang *et al.*, 1990), collagen-induced arthritis (Nagler-Anderson *et al.*, 1986; Thompson and Staines, 1986) and uveitis (Nussenblatt *et al.*, 1990).

2. Interference with MHC Class II Molecules

In the mouse (SJL), MAb to I-A injected before immunization prevents EAE (Steinman *et al.*, 1981) and, given after the appearance of lesions, or in mice with chronic relapsing EAE, greatly reduces the frequency of relapses and death (Sriram and Steinman, 1983). There are equivalent data for EAE in monkeys, although acute deaths are recorded in some monkeys given anti-I-A Mab (Jonkers *et al.*, 1988).

Another approach has been the prevention of EAE with nonimmunogenic peptides of MBP (mimotopes) that block the interaction of T cells with I-A molecules (Sakai *et al.*, 1989). In $H2^u$ strains of mice, the encephalitogenic *N*-terminal peptide 1–9 of MBP is immunodominant as a T-cell stimulus, provided that it is acetylated at the *N*-terminus (Zamvil *et al.*, 1986). Accordingly, Sakai *et al.* (1989) investigated the inhibitory effect *in vivo* of competitor nonpathogenic peptides (MBP peptide 1–20 and acetylated MBP peptide 9–20) on induction of EAE by the acetylated *N*-terminal MBP peptide 1–11. Coinjection of mimotopes prevented EAE if the competitor (mimotope) to inducer (encephalitogen) ratio was in excess (Sakai *et al.*, 1989).

There is a new approach to immunotherapy of EAE that involves MBP linked to cells, or cell-derived membranes, that express MHC class II molecules (Ben-Nun and Yossefi, 1990). Thus, when SJL/J mice were innoculated with MSCH intraperitoneally, together with MBP-pulsed or MSCH-pulsed syngeneic macrophages and/or B cells, EAE was dramatically reduced in frequency and severity. Moreover, glutaraldehyde fixation of the cells or membranes that presented MBP/MHC class II did not impair their ability to alleviate EAE (Ben-Nun and Yossefi, 1990).

3. *Vaccination* against Effector T Cells

Autoimmune T cell clones or lines, if used in suboptimal doses and/or *attenuated* by irradiation or hydrostatic pressure, prevent or suppress EAE in rats (Ben-Nun *et al.*, 1981b; Lider *et al.*, 1987; Lohse, 1989). The process(es) that underlie *T-cell vaccination* remain unclear, but presumably the immunogen is the configuration of the T-cell receptor on the cultured cell lines, and the responding protective T cell is antiidiotypic to this (Lider *et al.*, 1987); favoring this, T-cell clones with specific reactivity against EAE-inducing T cells have been isolated from rats recovering from EAE. Since the nucleotide and deduced amino acid sequences are known for the rearranged rat TcR α- and β-chain genes that recognize the MBP peptide, Vandenbark *et al.* (1989) vaccinated Lewis rats with synthetic peptides corresponding to the hypervariable region of the TcR Vβ8 molecule; T cells specific for the TcR Vβ8 peptide passively transferred protection to naive syngeneic recipients (Vandenbark *et al.*, 1989). Similarly, Howell *et al.* (1989) found that EAE in Lewis rats was prevented by vaccination with synthetic peptides corresponding to the idiotypic determinants of the TcR β-chain VDJ region and Jα regions that determined recognition of MBP peptide 72–86. Moreover, Hashim *et al.* (1990) reported that immunization with a synthetic peptide corresponding to residues 39–59 of the TcR Vβ8 generated peptide-specific antibodies that, when injected into Lewis rats, protected against EAE.

4. Monoclonal Antibodies to the T-Cell Receptor

The very limited heterogeneity of the TcR used by encephalitogenic T-cell clones allows for the prevention or treatment of EAE using MAb prepared against the TcR molecule (Acha-Orbea *et al.*, 1988; Urban *et al.*, 1988). Most of the T cells reactive against the MBP N-terminal peptide in H-2^u mice use Vβ8.2; hence, Mabs against this T-cell receptor component were injected into mice to prevent or suppress EAE. Such treatment with Vβ8-specific antibodies does lead to reduction of EAE in both the B10 PL and (PL × SJL)F_1 mice, whether treated before or after sensitization (Acha-Orbea *et al.*, 1988; Urban *et al.*, 1988). However, some anti-Vβ8 antibodies-treated mice developed just as severe a disease as did the untreated controls. Hence, to improve the efficacy of treatment with anti-TcR Mab, Zaller *et al.* (1990) used a combination of Vβ8 and Vβ13 specific antibodies and found in B10 PL mice that this combination led to a near-complete protection against EAE, and marked suppression of paralysis (Zaller *et al.*, 1990).

IV. CONCLUDING REMARKS

Macfarlane Burnet, in one of his rare indulgences in double entendre, wrote a paper entitled "Life's Complexities: Misgivings about Models" (Burnet, 1969 p. 364) containing the following quotation: "Appropriately applied they have given us most of our *understanding* of living systems. I am less confident about how far they have helped in the *control* of those systems for the purposes of human need or desire." We acknowledge that whereas models of human autoimmune diseases can be developed by various protocols, from selective inbreeding to high-technology experimentation (e.g., transgenic mice), none exactly simulates the spontaneous human counterpart; however, we emphasize in this chapter how models of autoimmunity are in fact bringing us much closer to the understanding and control of aberrant systems that result in human autoimmune disease.

A. Combination of Errors

Autoimmune disease is clearly multifactorial in cause, and our models clearly point to several levels of genetic anomaly, well illustrated in spontaneous disease (NOD mouse, lupus mice), and induced disease (EAE). Thus the susceptible phenotype is the product of a *combination of errors,* but there is still uncertainty on the *weighting* of the genetic component, since there always seems to be an element of randomness in either the actual occurrence, or the timing of autoimmune expression. The environmental contribution will clearly be greater in the outbred human than in the genetically tailored laboratory animal: models prove the need for deeper analyses of genetic elements in human autoimmunity.

B. Intrathymic Events

Experimental immunology has pointed to an orderly progression of intrathymic selection, positive and negative, of thymocytes destined for the peripheral repertoire. The importance of these events is illustrated by the outcome of experimental perturbation by cyclosporin or thymectomy. In either case, there is uncontrolled expansion of clones of cells with *forbidden* reactivity with self-antigens. We infer that since the main culprit in autoimmunity, the CD4 T cell, is not subject to postthymic somatic genetic changes (cf. B cells), autoimmunity must depend on forbidden emigrants from the thymus which, under appropriate circumstances, become expanded into a pathogenic clone.

C. Critical Importance of MHC

The models clearly illustrate the importance of MHC molecules in the genesis of autoimmunity. These may operate at two levels. The first is in repertoire generation in the thymus, since MHC molecules direct the expansion of T cells so as to provide for optimal reactivity with the *antigenic universe.* Deletion of anti-self-reactivity depends on the presentation of self-antigens by MHC molecules on bone marrow-derived medullary cells. Deletional tolerance depends on the efficiency of this process. MHC molecules are also critical in the activation of T cells for antigen reactivity, since the T cell sees peptide antigens only in the context of an MHC molecule. Certain molecular configurations in the hypervariable regions of MHC class II molecules seem capable of presenting self-antigens very efficiently and, if a responding CD4 T cell has escaped deletion, the stage is set for autoimmunity. The occurrence of anti-DNA antibodies in NZB/W lupus mice and the ablation of susceptibility to disease in NOD mice by the transgenic replacement of I-Aβ chain, are two pertinent illustrations.

D. Amplification of Responding Cells

Given that T cells with autoreactive potential can escape from the thymus, these still must be clonally expanded for disease to occur. This is modeled rather crudely in the experimentally-induced autoimmune diseases by adjuvant effects of various types (e.g., Freund's adjuvant or pertussis). We assume that the role of adjuvants is to facilitate the engagement of autoreactive cells with antigen, and perhaps allow the optimal generation of a memory population.

E. The Suppression Enigma

Immunosuppression remains the most opaque aspect of contemporary immunology, since the models argue very strongly for its existence (e.g., CP augmentation of NOD diabetes and T-cell vaccination against EAE), yet the effectors of suppression are still *veiled.* There has been interest in various marker molecules on the T-cell surface revealed by MAbs but, curiously, most of these putative suppressor markers turn out to be members of the integrin, selectin, or other families of adhesion or homing molecules. We leave the reader with the uncontested validity of the adoptive transfer of suppression in various of the models, and we await the resolution of this enigma.

F. Effectors

The ability of autoreactive CD4+ T-cell lines to adoptively transfer autoimmunity clearly points to a primordial role of T cells in the pathogenic events leading to autoimmune diseases. Since the activated CD4 T lymphocyte is a major source of most lymphokines, we suspect that many of these molecules potentiate the inflammatory processes involved in the destruction of the target tissues. The role of antibodies as effectors of autoimmunity is less defined. However, available data indicate that, at least in some models, humoral autoimmunity acts in synergism with specific or nonspecific T-cell responses. This is best exemplified by one of the adoptive transfer models of EAE, where extensive demyelination occurs following the injection of a reduced number of encephalitogenic T cells in the presence of anti-MOG antibody.

G. Treatment of Autoimmune Disease

More than anything else, the autoimmune models are pointing the way toward new and more gentle treatment of autoimmune diseasc in man. Among the successful strategies in animals are vaccination with autoantigen with both pathogenic and nonpathogenic potential, injection of blocking peptides analogous to MHC molecules, or components of the TcR (mimotopes), and immunosuppressive MAbs directed to MHC and TcR molecules. Certain technical aspects need to be considered including definition of T-cell use in each individual to be treated, the ablation of antimouse responses to injected Mab or deleterious anti-idiotypic response to the active site of the injected antibody. The models also point to the possibility of attacking the *downstream* effector processes, including the cytokine molecules and the integrin–selectin molecules that mediate the inflammatory components of the autoimmune response.

ACKNOWLEDGMENTS

We thank very warmly our laboratory colleagues Dr. Nicole Kerlero de Rosbo and Dr. Merrill Rowley for discussion and suggestions. Ms. Margaret Richards provided invaluable help in preparing this manuscript. We record our appreciation to Emeritus Professor G. Singer and Professor Kim Ng (CCAB) and Professor A. W. Linnane (IRM), for facilities. Investigations from the authors' laboratories were supported by grants from the National Health and Medical Research Council of Australia, the National Multiple Sclerosis Society of Australia, and donations from several benefactors.

REFERENCES

Acha-Orbea, H., and McDevitt, H. O. (1987). *Proc. Natl. Acad. Sci. U.S.A.* **84,** 2435–2439.

Acha-Orbea, H., Mitchell, D. J., Timmerman, L., Wraith, D. C., Tausch, G. S., Walder, M. K., Zamvil, S. S., McDevitt, H. O., and Steinman, L. (1988). *Cell* **54,** 263–273.

Acha-Orbea, H., Steinman, L., and McDervitt, H. O. (1989). *Annu. Rev. Immunol.* **7,** 371–405.

Adams, S., Zordan, T., Sainis, K., and Datta, S. K. (1990). *Eur. J. Immunol.* **20,** 1435–1443.

Adams, T. E., Alpert, S., and Hanahan, D. (1987). *Nature* **325,** 223–228.

Allison, J., Campbell, I. L., Morahan, G., Mandel, T. E., Harrison, L. C., and Miller, J. F. A. P. (1989). *Nature* **333,** 529–533.

Anderson, T., Schein, P. S., McMenamin, M. G., and Cooney, D. A. (1974). *J. Clin. Invest.* **54,** 672–677.

Anhalt, G. J., Labib, R. S., Voorhess, J. J., Beals, T. F., and Diaz, L. A. (1982). *N. Engl. J. Med.* **306,** 1189–1196.

Araneo, B. A., and Yowell, R. L. (1985). *J. Immunol.* **135,** 73–79.

Arnason, B. G., Jankovic, B. D., Waksman, B. H., and Wennerstein, L. (1962). *J. Exp. Med.* **116,** 177–186.

Atkinson, M. A., and Maclaren, N. K. (1988). *Diabetes* **37,** 1578–1590.

Atkinson, M. A., Maclaren, N. K., Riley, W. J., Scharp, D. W., and Holmes, L. (1988). *Diabetes* **37** (Suppl. 1), 98A.

Awata, T., Kuzuya, T., Matsuda, A., Iwamoto, Y., Kanazawa, Y., Okuyama, M., and Juji, T. (1990). *Diabetes* **39,** 266–269.

Babbit, B. P., Allen, P. M., Matsueda, G., Haber, E., and Unanue, E. R. (1985). *Nature* **317,** 359–361.

Bacelj, A., Charlton, B., and Mandel, T. E. (1989). *Diabetes* **38,** 1492–1495.

Bacelj, A., Charlton, B., and Mandel, T. E. (1990). *In* "Lessons from Animal Models of Diabetes, III" (E. Shafrir, ed.), pp. 121–125. Smith and Gordon, London.

Bach, J.-F., and Strom, T. B. (1985). *In* "The Mode of Action of Immunosuppressive Agents", 2nd Ed., pp. 175–239. Elsevier, Amsterdam.

Baekkeskov, S., Dryberg, T., and Lernmark, A. (1984). *Science* **224,** 1348–1350.

Baekkeskov, S., Kristensen, J. K., Srikanta, S., Bruining, G. J., Mandrup-Poulsen, T., DeBeaufort, C., Soeldner, J. S., Eisenbarth, G., Lindgren, F., and Lernmark, Å. (1987). *J. Clin. Invest.* **79,** 926–936.

Baekkeskov, S., Nielsen, J. H., Marner, B., Bilde, T., Ludvigsson, J., and Lernmark, Å. (1982). *Nature* **298,** 167–169.

Baekkesov, S., Aanstoot, H-J., Christgau, S., Reetz, A., Solimena, M., Cascalho, M., Folli, F., Richter-Olesen, H., and Camilli, P.-D. (1990). *Nature* **347,** 151–156.

Barlow, C. F. (1956). *J. Neuropathol. Exp. Neurol.* **15,** 196–207.

Baxter, A. G., Adams, M. A., and Mandel, T. E. (1989). *Diabetes* **38,** 1296–1300.

Bedossa, P., Bendelac, A., Bach, J.-F., and Carnaud, C. (1989). *Eur. J. Immunol.* **19,** 1947–1951.

Bendelac, A., Carnaud, C., Boitard, C., and Bach, J. F. (1987). *J. Exp. Med.* **166,** 823–832.

Bendelac, A., Boitard, C., Bendossa, P., Bazin, H., Bach, J.-F., and Carnaud, C., (1988). *J. Immunol.* **141,** 2625–2628.

Bendelac, A., Carnaud, C., Boitard, C., and Bach, J.-F. (1989a). *J. Exp. Med.* **166,** 823–832.

Bendelac, A., Boitard, C., Bach, J.-F., and Carnaud, C. (1989b). *Eur. J. Immunol.* **19,** 611–616.

Benjamin, R. J., and Waldmann, H. (1986). *Nature* **320,** 449–451.

Benjamin, R. J., Cobbold, S. P., Clark, M. R., and Waldman, H. (1986). *J. Exp. Med.* **163,** 1539–1552.

Ben-Nun, A., and Lando, A. (1983). *J. Immunol.* **130,** 1205–1209.

Ben-Nun, A., and Yossefi, S. (1990). *Eur. J. Immunol.* **20,** 357–361.

Ben-Nun, A., Wekerle, H., and Cohen, I. R. (1981a). *Eur. J. Immunol.* **11,** 195–199.
Ben-Nun, A., Wekerle, H., and Cohen, I. R. (1981b). *Nature* **293,** 60–61.
Benoist, C., and Mathis, D. (1989). *Cell* **58,** 1027–1033.
Berman, P. W., and Patrick, J. (1980). *J. Exp. Med.* **151,** 204–223.
Bernard, C. C. A. (1976). *J. Immunogenet.* **3,** 263–274.
Bernard, C. C. A. (1977). *Clin. Exp. Immunol.* **29,** 100–109.
Bernard, C. C. A., and Carnegie, P. R. (1975). *J. Immunol.* **114,** 1537–1540.
Bernard, C. C. A., and Mackay, I. R. (1983). *Clin. Exp. Immunol.* **55,** 211–216.
Bernard, C. C. A., Carnegie, P. R., and Mackay, I. R. (1983a). *In* "Multiple Sclerosis" (J. F. Hallpike, C. W. M. Adams, and W. W. Tourtellotte, eds.), pp. 477–503. Chapman and Hall, London.
Bernard, C. C. A., Leydon, J., and Mackay, I. R. (1977). *Int. Arch. Allergy* **53,** 555–559.
Bernard, C. C. A., Leydon, J., and Mackay, I. R. (1976). *Eur. J. Immunol.* **6,** 655–659.
Bernard, C. C. A., Mackay, I. R., Whittingham, S., and Brous, P. (1975). *Cell. Immunol.* **22,** 297–310.
Bernard, C. C. A., Mitchell, G. F., Leydon, J., and Bargebos, A. (1978). *Int. Arch. Allergy* **56,** 256–263.
Bernard, C. C. A., Roberts, I. M., and Townsend, E. (1983b). *In* "Molecular Aspects of Neurological Disorders" (L. Austin and P. L. Jeffrey, eds.), pp. 235–248. Academic Press, Sydney Australia.
Bevan, M. J. (1977) *Nature* **269,** 417–418.
Bigazzi, P. E., and Rose, N. R. (1975). *Prog. Allergy* **19,** 245–274.
Bitar, D. M., and Whitacre, C. C. (1988). *Cell Immunol.* **112,** 364–370.
Bjorkman, P. J., Saper, M. A., Samraoui, B., Bennett, W. S., Strominger, J. L., and Wiley, D. C. (1987a). *Nature* **329,** 506–512.
Bjorkman, P. J., Saper, M. A., Samraoui, B., Bennett, W. S., Strominger, J. L., and Wiley, D. C. (1987b). *Nature* **329,** 512–518.
Boitard, C., Bendelac, A., Richard, M. F., Carnaud, C., and Bach, J.-F. (1988). *Proc. Natl. Acad. Sci. U.S.A.* **85,** 9719–9723.
Boitard, C., Yasunami, R., Dardenne, M., and Bach, J.-F. (1989). *J. Exp. Med.* **169,** 1669–1680.
Bradley, B. J., Wang, Y., Lafferty, K. J., and Haskins, K. (1990). *J. Autoimmunity* **3,** 449–456.
Brandiss, M. W., Smith, J. W., and Friedman, R. M. (1965). *Ann. N.Y. Acad. Sci.* **122,** 356–368.
Brosnan, C. F., and Tansey, F. A. (1984). *J. Neuropathol. Exp. Neurol.* **43,** 84–93.
Brostoff, S. W., and Mason, D. W. (1984). *J. Immunol.* **133,** 1938–1942.
Brunner, C., Lassmann, H., Waehneldt, T. V., Matthieu, J.-M., and Linington, C. (1989). *J. Neurochem.* **52,** 296–304.
Burnet, F. M. (1969). *Aust. Ann. Med.* **4,** 363–367.
Burns, F. R., Li, X., Shen, N., Offner, H., Chou, Y. K., Vandenbark, A., and Heber-Katz, E. (1989). *J. Exp. Med.* **169,** 27–39.
Cambi, F., Lees, M. B., Williams, R. M., and Macklin, W. B. (1983). *Ann. Neurol.* **13,** 303–308.
Carterton, N. L., Wofsy, D., and Seaman, W. E. (1988). *J. Immunol.* **140,** 713–716.
Caspi, R. R., Chan, C.-C., Leake, W. C., Higuchi, M., Wiggert, B., and Chader, G. J. (1990). *J. Autoimmunity* **3,** 237–246.
Caspi, R. R., Roberge, F. G., Chan, C.-C., Wiggert, B., Chader, G. J., Rozenszajn, L. A., Lando, Z., and Nussenblatt, R. B. (1988). *J. Immunol.* **140,** 1490–1495.
Chan, C.-C., Caspi, R. R., Ni, M., Leake, W. C., Wiggert, B., Chader, G. J., and Nussenblatt, R. B. (1990). *J. Autoimmunity* **3,** 247–255.
Chandler, P., Fairchild, S., and Simpson, E. (1988). *J. Immunogenet.* **15,** 321–330.
Charlton, B., Bacelj, A., Slattery, R. M., and Mandel, T. E. (1989). *Diabetes* **38,** 441–447.
Charlton, B., and Mandel, T. E. (1988). *Diabetes* **37,** 1108–1112.

Charlton, B., Bacelj, A., and Mandel, T. E. (1988). *Diabetes* **37,** 930–935.
Charlton, B., and Mandel, T. E. (1989a). *Autoimmunity* **4,** 1–7.
Charlton, B., and Mandel, T. E. (1989b). *Immunol. Cell. Biol.* **67,** 1–7.
Charreire, J. (1989). *Adv. Immunol.* **46,** 263–334.
Chiang, B.-L., Bearer, E., Ansari, A., Dorshkind, K., and Gershwin, M. E. (1990). *J. Immunol.* **145,** 94–101.
Christadoss, P., Lennon, V. A., Krco, C. J., and David, C. S. (1982). *J. Immunol.* **128,** 1141–1144.
Colle, E., Guttman, R. D., and Seemayer, T. (1981). *J. Exp. Med.* **154,** 1237–1242.
Colman, P. C., Campbell, I. L., Kay, T. W. H., and Harrison, L. C. (1987). *Diabetes* **36,** 1432–1440.
Daniel, P. M., Lam, D. K. C., and Pratt, O. E. (1981). *J. Neurol. Sci.* **52,** 211–219.
Dardenne, M., Lepault, F., Bendelac, A., and Bach, J.-F. (1989). *Eur. J. Immunol.* **19,** 889–895.
Davis, M. M. (1988). *Hosp. Pract.* **23,** 115–128.
Drell, D. W., and Notkins, A. L. (1987). *Diabetologia* **30,** 132–143.
Driscoll, B. F., Kies, M. W., and Alvord, E. C., Jr. (1976). *J. Immunol.* **117,** 110–114.
Duchosal, M. A., McConahey, P. J., Robinson, C. A., and Dixon, F. J. (1990). *J. Exp. Med.* **172,** 985–988.
Dulin, W. E., Wyse, B. M., and Kalamazoo, M. S. (1969). *Diabetes* **18,** 459–466.
Dyrberg, T., Scwimmbeck, P. L., and Oldstone, M. B. A. (1988). *J. Clin. Invest.* **81,** 928–931.
Efran, S., Fleischer, N., and Hanahan, D. (1990). *Mol. Cell. Biol.* **10,** 1779–1783.
Eisenbarth, B. S. (1986). *N. Engl. J. Med.* **314,** 1360 1368.
Elias, D., Markovits, D., Reshef, T., van der Zee, R., and Cohen, I. R. (1990). *Proc. Natl. Acad. Sci. U.S.A.* **87,** 1576–1580.
Elliott, R. B., and Martin, J. M. (1984). *Diabetologia* **26,** 297–299.
Elliott, R. B., Reddy, S. N., Bibby, N. J., and Kida, K. (1988). *Diabetologia* **31,** 62–64.
Epstein, P. N., Overbeek, P. A., and Means, A. R. (1989). *Cell* **58,** 1067–1073.
Finnie, J. W., and Mukherjee, T. M. (1986). *J. Comp. Pathol.* **96,** 205–216.
Flavell, R. A., Allen, H., Burkly, L. C., Scherman, D. H., Waneck, G. L., and Widera, G. (1986). *Science* **233,** 437–443.
Formby, B., Miller, N., and Peterson, C. M. (1988). *Diabetes* **37,** 1305–1309.
Formby, B., and Miller, N. (1990). *Proc. Natl. Acad. Sci. U.S.A.* **87,** 2438–2442.
Foulis, A. K., Liddle, C. N., Farquharson, M. A., Richmond, J. A., and Weir, R. S. (1986). *Diabetologia* **29,** 267–274.
Fritz, R. B., Chou, C. H.-J., and McFarlin, D. (1983a). *J. Immunol.* **130,** 1024–1026.
Fritz, R. B., Chou, C. H.-J., and McFarlin, D. E. (1983b). *J. Immunol.* **130,** 191–194.
Fritz, R. B., and Skeen, M. J. (1987). *Immunogenetics* **25,** 161–166.
Fritz, R. B., Skeen, M. J., Jen-Chou, C. H., Garcia, M., and Egorov, I. K. (1985). *J. Immunol.* **134,** 2328–2332.
Fujita, T., Yui, R., Kusumoto, Y., Serizawa, Y., Makino, S., and Tochino, Y. (1982). *Biomed. Res.* **3,** 429–443.
Fukuma, K., Sakaguchi, S., Kuribayashi, K., Chen, W. L., Morishita, R., Sekita, K., Uchino, H., and Masuda, T. (1988). *Gastroenterology* **94,** 274–283.
Fuller, K. A., Pearl, D., and Whitacre, C. C. (1990). *J. Neuroimmunol.* **28,** 15–26.
Fushijima, Y., Koide, Y., Kaidoh, T., Nishimura, M., and Yoshida, T. O. (1989). *Diabetologia* **32,** 118–125.
Gao, E.-R., Lo, D., Cheney, R., Kanagawa, O., and Sprent, J. (1988). *Nature* **336,** 176–179.
Gasser, D. L., Newlin, C. M., Palm, J., and Gonatas, N. K. (1973). *Science* **181,** 872–873.
Geczy, C. L., Roberts, I. M., Meyer, P., and Bernard, C. C. A. (1984). *J. Immunol.* **133,** 3026–3036.
Geczy, C. L., Raper, R., Roberts, I. M., Meyer, P., and Bernard, C. C. A. (1985). *J. Neuroimmunol.* **9,** 179–191.

Georgiou, H. M., Lagarde, A. C., and Bellgrau, D. (1988). *J. Exp. Med.* **167,** 132–148.
Gepts, W. (1965). *Diabetes* **14,** 619–633.
Gery, I., Mochzuki, M., and Nussenblatt, R. B. (1986). *Prog. Retinal Res.* **5,** 75–109.
Gleeson, P. A., and Toh, B. H. (1991). *Immunol. Today* **12,** 233–238.
Gleichmann, E., Pals, S. T., Rolink, A. G., Radaszkiewicz, T., and Gleichmann, H. (1984). *Immunol. Today* **5,** 324–332.
Glynn, P., and Linington, C. (1989). *CRC Crit. Rev. Neurobiol.* **4,** 367–385.
Goronzy, J., Weyand, C. M., and Fathman, C. G. (1986). *J. Exp. Med.* **164,** 911–925.
Gorsuch, A. N., Spencer, K. M., Lister, J., Wolf, E., Bottazzo, G. F., and Cudworth, A. G. (1982). *Diabetes* **31,** 862–866.
Guillet, J.-G., Lai, M-Z., Briner, T. J., Buus, S., Sette, A., Grey, H. M., Smith, J. A., and Gefter, M. L. (1987). *Science* **235,** 865–870.
Gunn, C., Suckling, A. J., and Linington, C. (1989). *J. Neuroimmunol.* **23,** 101–108.
Gutstein, N. L., Seaman, W. E., Scott, J. H., and Wofsy, D. (1986). *J. Immunol.* **137,** 1127–1132.
Hanafusa, T., Sugihara, S., Fujino-Kurihara, H., Miyagawa, J.-I., Miyazaki, A., Yoshioka, T., Yamada, K., Nakajima, H., Asakawa, H., Kono, N., Fujiwara, H., Hamaoka, T., and Tarui, S. (1988). *Diabetes* **37,** 204–208.
Hanafusa, T., Fujino-Kurihara, H., Miyazaki, A., Yamada, K., Nakajima, H., Miyagawa, J., Kono, N., and Tarui, S. (1987). *Diabetologia* **30,** 104–108.
Hanahan, D. (1985). *Nature* **315,** 115–122.
Harada, M., and Makino, S. (1984). *Diabetologia* **27,** 604–606.
Harada, M., and Makino, S. (1986). *Exp. Anim.* **35,** 501–504.
Hari, J., Yokono, K., Yonezawa, K., Amano, K., Yaso, S., Shii, K., Imamura, Y., and Baba, S. (1986). *Diabetes* **35,** 517–522.
Harrington, W. J., Minnich, V., Hollingsworth, J. W., and Moore, C. V. (1990). *J. Lab. Clin. Med.* **115**(5), 636–645. (Reprinted from original 1951 version of the publication).
Hartung, H. P., and Toyka, K. V. (1990). *Ann. Neurol.* **27** (Suppl.), S57–S63.
Hashim, G. A. (1981). *J. Immunol.* **126,** 419–423.
Hashim, G. A., Carvalho, E. F., and Sharpe, R. D. (1978). *J. Immunol.* **121,** 665–670.
Hashim, G. A., Vandenbark, A. A., Galang, A. B., Diamanduros, T., Carvalho, E., Srinivasan, J., Jones, R., Vainiene, M., Morrison, W. J., and Offner, H. (1990). *J. Immunol.* **144,** 4621–4627.
Haskins, K., Portas, M., Bergman, B., Lafferty, K., and Bradley, B. (1989). *Proc. Natl. Acad. Sci. U.S.A.* **86,** 8000–8004.
Haskins, K., Portas, M., Bradley, B., Wegmann, D., and Lafferty, K. (1988). *Diabetes* **37,** 1444–1448.
Haskins, K., and McDuffie, M. (1990). *Science* **249,** 1433–1436.
Hattori, M., Buse, J. B., Jackson, R. A., Glimcher, L., Dorf, M. E., Minami, M., Makino, S., Moriwaki, K., Kuzuya, H., Imura, H., Strauss, W. M., Seidman, J. G., and Eisenbarth, G. S. (1986). *Science* **231,** 733–735.
Hayward, A. R., and Shreiber, M. (1989). *J. Immunol.* **143,** 1555–1559.
Heber-Katz, E. (1990). *Clin. Immunol. Immunopathol.* **55,** 1–8.
Heifetz, A., Kennan, R. W., and Elbein, A. D. (1979). *Biochemistry* **18,** 2186–2192.
Higgins, P. J., and Weiner, H. L. (1988). *J. Immunol.* **140,** 440–445.
Ho, C. K., and Hashim, S. A. (1972). *Diabetes* **21,** 789–793.
Honegger, P. (1985). *In* "Cell Culture in the Neurosciences" (J. E. Bottenstein and G. Sato, eds.), pp. 223–243. Plenum Press, New York.
Howell, M. D., Winters, S. T., Tsaiwei, O., Powell, H. C., Carlo, D. J., and Brostoff, S. W. (1989). *Science* **246,** 668–670.
Hurtenbach, U., and Maurer, C. (1989). *J. Autoimmunity* **2,** 151–161.
Ichimura, O., Suzuki, S., Saito, M., Sugawara, Y., and Ishida, N. (1985). *Int. J. Immunopharmacol.* **7,** 263–270.

Ikehara, S., Ohtsuki, H., Good, R. A., Asamoto, H., Nakamura, T., Sekita, K., Muso, E., Tochino, Y., Ida, T., Kuzuya, H., Imura, H., and Hamashima, Y. (1985). *Proc. Natl. Acad. Sci. U.S.A.* **82,** 7743–7747.

Iribe, H., Kabashima, H., and Koga, T. (1989). *J. Immunol.* **142,** 1487–1494.

Jackson, R. A., Buse, J. B., Rifai, R., Pelletier, D., Milford, E. L., Carpenter, C. B., Eisenbarth, G. S., and Williams, R. M. (1984). *J. Exp. Med.* **159,** 1629–1636.

Jackson, R. A., Rassi, T., Crump, T., Haynes, B., and Eisenbarth, G. S. (1981). *Diabetes* **30,** 887–889.

Jacob, C. O., Aiso, S., Michie, S. A., McDevitt, H. O., and Acha-Orbea, H. (1990). *Proc. Natl. Acad. Sci. U.S.A.* **87,** 968–972.

Jenkins, M. K., Schwartz, R. H., and Pardoll, D. M. (1988). *Science* **241,** 1655–1658.

Jerne, N. K. (1974). *Ann. Inst. Pasteur* **125c,** 373–389.

Jones, C. M., Callaghan, J. M., Gleeson, P. A., Mori, Y., Masuda, T., and Toh, B.-H. (1991). *Gastroenterology* **101,** 287–294.

Jonkers, M., van Lambalgen, R., Mitchell, D., Durham, S. K., and Steinman, L. (1988). *J. Autoimmunity* **1,** 399–414.

Kanariou, M., Huby, R., Ladyman, H., Colic, M., Sivolapenko, G., Lampert, I., and Ritter, M. (1989). *Clin. Exp. Immunol.* **78,** 263–270.

Kanazawa, Y., Komeda, K., Sato, S., Mori, S., Akanuma, K., and Takaku, F. (1984). *Diabetologia* **27,** 113–115.

Kappler, J. W., Roehm, N., and Marrack, P. (1987a). *Cell* **49,** 273–280.

Kappler, J. W., Wade, T., White, J., Kushnir, E., Blackman, M., Bill, J., Roehm, N., and Marrack, P. (1987b). *Cell* **49,** 263–271.

Karlsson, F. A., Burman, P., Loof, L., and Mardh, S. (1988). *J. Clin. Invest.* **81,** 475–479.

Kataoka, S., Satoh, J., Fujita, H., Toyota, T., Suzuki, R., Itoh, K., and Kumagai, K. (1983). *Diabetes* **32,** 247–253.

Kaufman, J. F., Auffray, L., Korman, A. J., Shackelford, D. A., and Strominger, J. (1984). *Cell* **36,** 1–13.

Kay, T. W. H., Campbell, I. L., Malcolm, L., and Harrison, L. C. (1989). *Cell. Immunol.* **120,** 341–350.

Kelley, V. E., Gaulton, G. N., Hattori, M., Ikegami, H., Eisenbarth, G., and Strom, T. B. (1988). *J. Immunol.* **140,** 59–61.

Kerlero de Rosbo, N., Honegger, P., Lassmann, H., and Matthieu, J.-M. (1990). *J. Neurochem.* **55,** 583–587.

Kerlero de Rosbo, N., Jago, M. W., Carnegie, P. R., and Bernard, C. C. A. (1987). *J. Neurol. Sci.* **78,** 281–294.

Kerlero de Rosbo, N., Bernard, C. C. A., Simmons, R. D., and Carnegie, P. R. (1985). *J. Neuroimmunol.* **9,** 349–361.

Kies, M. W., Driscoll, B. F., Lisak, R. P., and Alvord, E. C. Jr. (1975). *J. Immunol.* **115,** 75–79.

Kisielow, P., Teh, H. S., Bluthmann, H., and von Boehmer, H. (1988). *Nature* **335,** 730–733.

Klandorf, H., Chirra, A. R., DeGruccio, A., and Girman, D. J. (1989). *Diabetes* **38,** 194–197.

Kohno, S., Munoz, J. J., Williams, T., Teuscher, C., Bernard, C. C. A., and Tung, K. S. K. (1983). *J. Immunol.* **130,** 2675–2682.

Koide, Y., and Yoshida, T. O. (1989). *Int. Immunol.* **2,** 189–192.

Koike, T., Itoh, Y., Ishii, T., Ito, I., Takabayashi, K., Maruyama, N., Tomioka, H., and Yoshida, S. (1987). *Diabetes* **36,** 539–541.

Kojima, A., Taguchi, O., and Nishizuka, Y. (1980). *Lab. Invest.* **42,** 387–395.

Kojima, A., Tanaka-Kojima, Y., Sakakura, T., and Nishizuka, Y. (1976). *Lab. Invest.* **34,** 550–557.

Kolb-Bachofen, V., Epstein, S., Kiesel, U., and Kolb, H. (1988). *Diabetes* **37,** 21–27.

Kolb-Bachofen, V., and Kolb, H. (1989). *Autoimmunity* **3,** 145–155.

Kono, D. H., Urban, J. L., Horvath, S. J., Ando, D. G., Saavedra, R. A., and Hood, L. (1988). *J. Exp. Med.* **168,** 213–217.

Krams, S. M., Dorshkind, K., and Gershwin, M. E. (1989). *J. Exp. Med.* **170,** 1919–1930.

Kuo, S. C., and Lampen, J. O. (1976). *Arch. Biochem. Biophys.* **172,** 574–581.

LaFace, D. M., and Peck, A. B. (1989). *Diabetes* **38,** 894–901.

Lai, Y. L., Wiggert, B., Liu, Y. P., and Chader, G. J. (1982). *Nature* **298,** 848–849.

Lambert, E. H., and Lennon, V. A. (1988). *Muscle Nerve* **11,** 1133–1145.

Lassmann, H., and Linington, C. (1987). *In* "A Multidisciplinary Approach to Myelin Diseases" (G. S. Crescenzi, ed.), pp. 219–225. NATO-ASI Series. Plenum, New York.

Lassmann, H., Brunner, C., Bradl, M., and Linington, C. (1988). *Acta Neuropathol. (Berl)* **75,** 566–576.

Lazarow, A., Liambies, J., and Tausch, A. J. (1950). *J. Lab. Clin. Med.* **36,** 249–258.

Lazarus, S. S., and Shapiro, S. H. (1973). *Diabetes* **22,** 499–506.

Lebar, R. (1987). *Path. Biol.* **35,** 275–283.

Lebar, R., Boutry, J.-M., Vincent, C., Robineaux, R., and Voisin, G. A. (1976). *J. Immunol.* **116,** 1439–1446.

Lebar, R., Lubetzki, C., Vincent, C., Lombrail, P., and Boutry, J.-M. (1986). *Clin. Exp. Immunol.* **66,** 423–443.

Lebar, R., Vincent, C., and Fischer-Le Boubennec, E. (1979). *J. Neurochem.* **32,** 1451–1460.

Lee, K.-U., Kim, M. K., Amano, K., Pak, C. Y., Jaworski, M. A., Metha, J. G., and Yoon, J.-W. (1988). *Diabetes* **37,** 1035–1057.

Lehuen, A., Bendelac, A., Bach, J.-F., and Carnaud, C. (1990). *J. Immunol.* **144,** 2147–2151.

Leibowitz, S., and Kennedy, L. (1972). *Immunology* **22,** 859–869.

Leiter, E. H., Christianson, G. J., Serezze, D. V., Ting, A. T., and Worthen, S. M. (1989). *J. Exp. Med.* **170,** 1243–1262.

Levine, S., Hirano, A., and Zimmerman, H. M. (1965). *Am. J. Pathol.* **47,** 209–221.

Levine, S., Wenk, E. J., Devlin, H. B., Pieroni, R. E., and Levine, L. (1966). *J. Immunol.* **97,** 363–368.

Lider, O., Reshef, T., Beraud, E., Ben-Nun, A., and Cohen, I. R. (1987). *Science* **239,** 181–183.

Lider, O., Santos, L. M. B., Lee, C. S. Y., Higgins, P. J., and Weiner, H. L. (1989). *J. Immunol.* **142,** 748–752.

Like, A. A., Appel, M. C., Williams, R. M., and Rossini, A. A. *Lab. Invest.* (1978) **38,** 470–486.

Like, A. A., and Rossini, A. A. (1976). *Science* **193,** 415–417.

Linington, C., and Lassmann, H. (1987). *J. Neuroimmunol.* **17,** 61–69.

Linington, C., Bradl, M., Lassmann, H., Brunner, C., and Vass, K. (1988). *Am. J. Pathol.* **130,** 443–454.

Linington, C., Webb, M., and Woodhams, P. L. (1984). *J. Neuroimmunol.* **6,** 387–396.

Lisak, R. P., Zweiman, R., Kies, M. W., and Driscoll, B. (1975). *J. Immunol.* **114,** 546–549.

Lo, D., Burkley, L. C., Widera, G., Cowing, C., Flavell, R. A., Palmiter, R. D., and Brinster, R. L. (1988). *Cell* **53,** 159–168.

Lohse, A. W. (1989). *Curr. Opin. Immunol.* **1,** 718–726.

Lublin, F. D., Maurer, P. H., Berry, R. G., and Tippett, D. (1981). *J. Immunol.* **126,** 819–822.

Luescher, I. F., Allen, P. M., and Unanue, E. R. (1988). *Proc. Natl. Acad. Sci. U.S.A.* **85,** 871–874.

Lund, T., O'Reilly, L., Hutchings, P., Kanagawa, O., Simpson, E., Gravely, R., Chandler, P., Dyson, J., Picard, J. K., Edwards, A., Kioussis, D., and Cooke, A. (1990). *Nature* **345,** 727–729.

MacDonald, H. R., Hengartner, H., and Pedrazzini, T. (1988). *Nature* **335,** 174–176.

Mackay, I. R. (1988). *In* "The Liver: Biology and Pathology" (I. M. Arias, W. B. Jakoby, H. Popper, D. Schachter, and D. A. Shafritz, eds.), 2nd Ed., pp. 1259–1268. Raven Press, New York.

Mackay, I. R., Rowley, M. J., and Bernard, C. C. A. (1991). *In* "Monoclonal Antibodies and Immunotherapy in Arthritis: Clinical and Experimental Aspects" (T. F. Kresina, ed.), pp. 75–100. Marcel Dekker, New York.

Mackworth-Young, C., and Schwartz, R. S. (1988). *CRC Crit. Rev. Immunol.* **8,** 147–173.

Makino, S., Kunimoto, K., Muraoka, Y., Mizushima, Y., and Katagiri, K., and Tochino, Y. (1980). *Exp. Anim.* **29,** 1–13.

Makino, S., Kunimoto, K., Muraoka, Y., and Katagiri, K. (1981). *Exp. Anim.* **30,** 137–140.

Makino, S., Muraoko, Y., Kishimoto, Y., and Hayashi, Y. (1985). *Exp. Anim.* **34,** 425–432.

Mandel, T. E., Allison, J., Campbell, I. L., Koulmanda, M., Malcolm, L., Cutri, A., and Miller, J. F. A. P. (1991). *Autoimmunity* **9,** 47–54.

Marrack, P., and Kappler, J. (1987). *Science* **238,** 1073–1079.

Marrack, P., Lo, D., Brinster, R., Palmiter, R., Burkly, L., Flavell, R. H., and Kappler, J. (1988). *Cell* **53,** 627–634.

Marx, J. (1990). *Science* **249,** 246–249.

Mattingly, J., and Waksman, B. (1978). *J. Immunol.* **121,** 1878–1883.

McCune, J. M., Namikawa, R., Kaneshima, H. S., Schultz, L. D., Lieberman, M., and Weissman, I. L. (1988). *Science* **241,** 1632–1639.

Michel, C., Boitard, C., and Bach, J. F. (1989). *Clin. Exp. Immunol.* **75,** 457–460.

Miller, B. J., Appel, M. C., O'Neil, J., and Wicker, L. S. (1988). *J. Immunol.* **140,** 52–58.

Milner, P., Lovelidge, C. A., Taylor, W. A., and Hughes, R. A. C. (1987). *J. Neurol. Sci.* **79,** 275–285.

Miyagawa, J., Yamamoto, K., Hanafusa, T., Itoh, N., Nakagawa, C., Otsuka, A., Katsura, H., Yamagata, K., Miyazaki, A., Kono, N., and Tarri, S. (1990). *Diabetologia* **33,** 503–505.

Miyazaki, A., Hanafusa, T., Yamada, K., Miyagawa, J., Fujino-Kurihara, H., Nakajima, H., Nonaka, K., and Tarui, S. (1985). *Clin. Exp. Immunol.* **60,** 622–630.

Miyazaki, T., Uno, M., Uehira, M., Kikutani, H., Kishimoto, T., Kimoto, M., Nishimoto, H., Miyazaki, J., and Yamamura, K. (1990). *Nature* **345,** 722–724.

Moeller, G. (1983). *Immunol. Rev.* **84,** 1–143.

Morahan, G., Allison, J., and Miller, J. F. A. P. (1989a). *Nature* **339,** 622–624.

Morahan, G., Brennan, F. E., Bhathal, P. S., Allison, J., Cox, K. O., and Miller, J. F. A. P. (1989b). *Proc. Natl. Acad. Sci. U.S.A.* **86,** 3782–3786.

Morel, P. A., Dorman, J. S., Todd, J. A., McDevitt, H. O., and Trucco, M. (1988). *Proc. Natl. Acad. Sci. U.S.A.* **85,** 6111–6115.

Mori, Y., Suko, M., Okudaira, H., Matsuba, I., Tsuruoka, A., Sasaki, A., Yokoyama, H., Tanase, T., Shida, T., Nishimura, M., Terada, E., and Ikeda, Y. (1986). *Diabetologia* **29,** 244–247.

Mori, Y., Fukuma, K., Adachi, Y., Shigeta, K., Kannagi, R., Tanaka, H., Sakai, M., Kuribayashi, K., Uchino, H., and Masuda, T. C. (1989). *Gastroenterology* **97,** 364–375.

Moriyama, T., Guilhot, S., Klopchin, K., Moss, B., Pinkert, C. A., Palmiter, R. D., Brinster, R. L., Kanagawa, O., and Chisari, F. V. (1990). *Science* **248,** 361–364.

Morris, S. C., Cheek, R. L., Cohen, P. L., and Eisenberg, R. A. (1990). *J. Exp. Med.* **171,** 503–517.

Mosier, D. E., Galizea, R. J., Baird, S. M., and Wilson, D. B. (1988). *Nature* **335,** 256–259.

Mundlos, S., Mackay, I. R., Frazer, I. H., and Rowley, M. (1990). *J. Immunol. Methods* **127,** 279–284.

Munoz, J. J., Bernard, C. C. A., and Mackay, I. R. (1984). *Cell. Immunol.* **83,** 92–100.

Nagata, M., Yokono, K., Hayawaka, M., Kawase, Y., Hatamori, N., Ogawa, W., Yonezawa, K., Shii, K., and Baba, S. (1989a). *J. Immunol.* **143,** 1155–1162.

Nagata, M., Yokono, K., Hatamori, N., Shii, K., and Baba, S. (1989b). *Clin. Immunol. Immunopathol.* **53,** 171–180.

Nagler-Anderson, C., Dober, L. A., Robinson, M. E., Siskind, G. W., and Thorbecke, G. J. (1986). *Proc. Natl. Acad. Sci. U.S.A.* **83,** 7443–7446.

Nakajima, H., Yamada, K., Hanafusa, T., Fujino-Kurihara, H., Miyagawa, J., Miyazaki, A., Saitoh, R., Minami, Y., Kono, N., Nonaka, K., Tochino, Y., and Tarui, S. (1986). *Immunol. Lett.* **12,** 91–94.

Nakhooda, A. F., Like, A. A., Chappel, C. I., Murray, F. T., and Marliss, E. B. (1977). *Diabetes* **26,** 100–112.

Neilson, E. G., and Phillips, S. M. (1982). *J. Exp. Med.* **155,** 179–189.

Newcombe, J., Glynn, P., and Cuzner, M. L. (1982). *J. Neurochem.* **38,** 1192–1194.

Nikolic-Zugic, J., and Bevan, M. J. (1990). *Nature* **344,** 65–67.

Nishimoto, H., Kikutani, H., Yamamura, K.-I., and Kishimoto, T. (1987). *Nature* **328,** 432–434.

Nishizuka, Y., and Sakakura, T. (1969). *Science* **166,** 753–755.

Nussenblatt, R. B., Caspi, R. R., Mandi, R., Chan, C.-C., Roberge, F., Lider, O., and Weiner, H. L. (1990). *J. Immunol.* **144,** 1689–1695.

Nomikos, I. N., Wang, Y., and Lafferty, K. J. (1989). *Immunol. Cell. Biol.* **67,** 85–87.

Offner, H., Hashim, G. A., Celnik, B., Galang, A., Li, X., Burns, F. R., Shen, N., Heber Katz, E., and Vandenbark, A. A. (1989). *J. Exp. Med.* **170,** 355–367.

Ogawa, M., Maruyama, T., Hasegawa, T., Kanaya, T., Kobayashi, F., Tochino, Y., and Uda, H. (1985). *Biomed. Res.* **6,** 103–105.

Oksenberg, J. R., Sherritt, M., Begovich, A. B., Erlich, H. A., Bernard, C. C. A., Cavalli-Sforza, L. L., and Steinman, L. (1989). *Proc. Natl. Acad. Sci. U.S.A.* **86,** 988–992.

Oksenberg, J. R., Stuart, S., Begovich, A. B., Bell, R. B., Erlich, A., Steinman, L., and Bernard, C. C. A. B. (1990). *Nature* **345,** 344–346.

Oldendorf, W. H., and Towner, H. F. (1974). *J. Neuropath. Exp. Neurol.* **33,** 616–631.

Oldstone, M. B. A., Ahmed, R., and Salvato, M. (1990). *J. Exp. Med.* **171,** 2091–2100.

Oldstone, M. B. A. (1990). *J. Exp. Med.* **171,** 2077–2089.

Oldstone, M. B. A. (1988). *Science* **239,** 500–503.

Olerup, O., Hillert, J., Fredrikson, S., Olsson, T., Kam-Hansen, S., Moller, E., Carlsson, B., and Wallin, J. (1989). *Proc. Natl. Acad. Sci. U.S.A.* **86,** 7113–7117.

Orian, J. M., Mackay, I. R., Tamakoshi, K., Lee, C. S., and Brandon, M. R. (1991). *In* "Viral Hepatitis—1990" (B. Hollinger, S. M. Lemon, and S. Margolis, eds.). Williams & Wilkins, Baltimore, Maryland (in press).

Ota, K., Matsui, M., Milford, E. L., Mackin, G. A., Weiner, H. L., and Hafler, D. A. (1990). *Nature* **346,** 183–186.

Parham, P. (1988). *Nature* **333,** 500–503.

Paterson, P. Y. (1972). *In* "Multiple Sclerosis, Immunology, Virology and Ultrastructure" (F. Wolfgram, G. W. Ellison, J. G. Stevens, and J. M. Andrew, eds.), pp. 539–567. Academic Press, N.Y.

Paterson, P. Y. (1979). *Rev. Infect. Dis.* **1,** 468–482.

Penhale, W. J., Farmer, A., and Irvine, W. J. (1975). *Clin. Exp. Immunol.* **21,** 362–375.

Penhale, W. J., Irvine, W. J., Inglis, J. R., and Farmer, A. (1976). *Clin. Exp. Immunol.* **25,** 6–16.

Peterson, J. E., and Jago, M. V. (1977). *Aust. J. Exp. Biol. Med. Sci.* **55,** 233–244.

Pettinelli, C. B., and McFarlin, D. E. (1981). *J. Immunol.* **127,** 1420–1423.

Pfister, C., Chabre, M., Pluet, J., Tuyen, V. V., de Kozak, Y., Faure, J. P., and Kuhn, H. (1985). *Science* **228,** 891–893.

Pontesilli, O., Carotenuto, P., Gazda, L. S., Pratt, P. F., and Prowse, S. J. (1987). *Clin. Exp. Immunol.* **70,** 84–93.

Pontesilli, O., Carotenuto, P., Hayward, A. R., and Prowse, S. J. (1989). *J. Clin. Lab. Immunol* **28,** 161–168.

Powrie, F., and Mason, D. (1990). *J. Exp. Med.* **172,** 1701–1708.

Prineas, J. W. (1985). *In* "Handbook of Clinical Neurology, Vol. 3 (47): Demyelinating Diseases" (J. C. Koetsier, ed.), pp. 213–257. Elsevier Science Publishers B. V., New York.

Prochazka, M., Leiter, E. H., Serreze, D. V., and Coleman, D. L. (1987). *Science* **237,** 286–289.

Pucetti, A., Koizumi, T., Migliorini, P., Andre-Schwartz, J., Barrett, K. J., and Schwartz, R. S. (1990). *J. Exp. Med.* **171,** 1919–1930.

Qin, S., Cobbold, S., Tighe, H., Benjamin, R., and Waldmann, H. (1987). *Eur. J. Immunol.* **17,** 1159–1165.

Raine, C. S. (1984). *Lab. Invest.* **50,** 608–635.

Reddy, S., Bibby, N. J., and Elliott, R. B. (1988). *Diabetologia* **31,** 322–328.

Reich, E.-P., Scaringe, D., Yagi, J., Sherwin, R. S., and Janeway, C. A., Jr. (1989b). *Diabetes* **38,** 1647–1651.

Reich, E.-P., Sherwin, R. S., Kanagawa, O., and Janeway, C. A., Jr. (1989a). *Nature* **341,** 326–328.

Rivers, T. M., Sprunt, D. H., and Berry, G. P. (1933). *J. Exp. Med.* **58,** 39–54.

Robinson, C. J. G., Balazs, T., and Egorov, I. K. (1986). *Toxicol. Appl. Pharmacol.* **86,** 159–169.

Roman, L. M., Simons, L. F., Hammer, R. E., Sambrook, J. F., and Gething, M.-J. H. (1990). *Cell* **61,** 383–396.

Rossert, J., Pelletier, L., Pasquer, R., and Orvet, P. (1988). *Eur. J. Immunol.* **18,** 1761–1766.

Rossini, A. A., Williams, R. M., Appel, M. C., and Like, A. A. (1978). *Nature* **276,** 182–184.

Rubin, D., Weiner, H. L., Fields, B. N., and Greene, M. I. (1981). *J. Immunol.* **127,** 1697–1701.

Saito, T., Ebina, T., Koi, M., Yamaguchi, T., Kawade, Y., and Ishida, N. (1982). *Cell Immunol.* **68,** 187–192.

Saitoh, T., Ikarashi, Y., Ito, S., Watanabe, H., Fujiwara, M., and Asakura, H. (1990). *J. Immunol.* **145,** 3268–3275.

Sakaguchi, S., and Sakaguchi, N. (1988). *J. Exp. Med.* **167,** 1479–1485.

Sakaguchi, S., Fukuma, K., Kuribayashi, K., and Masuda, T. (1985). *J. Exp. Med.* **161,** 72–87.

Sakaguchi, S., Takahashi, T., and Nishizuka, Y. (1982a). *J. Exp. Med.* **156,** 1565–1576.

Sakaguchi, S., Takahashi, T., and Nishizuka, Y. (1982b). *J. Exp. Med.* **156,** 1577–1586.

Sakai, K., Namikawa, T., Kunishita, T., Yamanouchi, K., and Tabira, T. (1986). *J. Immunol.* **137,** 1527–1532.

Sakai, K., Sinha, A. A., Mitchell, D. J., Zamvil, S. S., Rothbard, J. B., McDevitt, H. O., and Steinman, L. (1988a). *Proc. Natl. Acad. Sci. U.S.A.* **85,** 8608–8612.

Sakai, K., Zamvil, S. S., Mitchell, D. J., Lim, M., Rothbard, J. B., and Steinman, L. (1988b). *J. Neuroimmunol.* **19,** 821–832.

Sakai, K., Zamvil, S. S., Mitchell, D. J., Hodgkinson, S., Rothbard, J. B., and Steinman, L. (1989). *Proc. Natl. Acad. Sci. U.S.A.* **146,** 9470–9474.

Sarvetnick, N., Liggitt, D., Pitts, S. L., Hansen, S. E., and Stewart, T. A. (1988). *Cell* **52,** 773–782.

Sarvetnick, N., Shizuru, J., Liggitt, D., Martin, L., McIntyre, B., Gregory, A., Parslow, T., and Stewart, T. (1990). *Nature* **346,** 844–845.

Satoh, J., Rikiishi, H., Nagahashi, M., Ohuchi, E., and Kumagai, K. (1980). *Cell Immunol.* **56,** 1–15.

Satoh, J., Seino, H., Abo, T., Tanaka, S., Shintani, S., Ohna, S., Tamura, K., Sawai, T., Nobunaga, T., Oteki, T., Kumagai, K., and Toyota, T. (1989). *J. Clin. Invest.* **84,** 1345–1348.

Satoh, J., Sakai, K., Endoh, M., Koike, F., Kunishita, T., Namikawa, T., Yamamura, T., and Tabira, T. (1987). *J. Immunol.* **138,** 179–184.

Schluesener, H. J., Sobel, R. A., Linington, C., and Weiner, H. L. (1987). *J. Immunol.* **139,** 4016–4021.

Schlomchik, M., Mascelli, M., Shan, H., Radic, M. Z., Pisetsky, D., Marshak-Rothstein, A., and Weigert, M. (1990). *J. Exp. Med.* **171,** 265–297.

Schoenfeld, M., and Mozes, E. (1990). *FASEB J.* **4,** 2646–2651.

Schwerer, B., Kitz, K., Lassmann, H., and Bernheimer, H. (1984). *J. Neuroimmunol.* **7,** 107–119.

Scolding, N. J., Frith, S., Linington, C., Morgan, B. P., Campbell, A. K., and Compston, D. A. S. (1989). *J. Neuroimmunol.* **22,** 169–176.

Scott, J. S., Maddison, P. J., Taylor, P. V., Esscher, E., Scott, O., and Skinner, R. P. (1983). *N. Engl. J. Med.* **309,** 209–212.

Scott, F. W., Mongeau, R., Kardish, M., Hatina, G., Trick, K. D., and Wojcinski, Z. (1985). *Diabetes* **34,** 1059–1062.

Seemayer, T. A., Oligny, L. L., Tannenbaum, G. S., Goldman, H., and Colle, E. (1980). *Am. J. Pathol.* **101,** 485–488.

Serreze, D. V., and Leiter, E. H. (1988). *J. Immunol.* **140,** 3801–3807.

Serezze, D. V., Leiter, E. H., Kuff, E. L., Jardieu, P., and Ishizaka, K. (1988a). *Diabetes* **37,** 351–358.

Serreze, D. V., Leiter, E. H., Worthen, S. M., and Shulz, L. D. (1988b). *Diabetes* **37,** 252–255.

Serreze, D. V., Hamaguchi, K., and Leiter, E. H. (1990). *J. Autoimmunity* **2,** 759–776.

Sette, A., Buus, S., Colon, S., Smith, J. A., Miles, C., and Grey, H. M. (1987). *Nature* **328,** 395–399.

Sha, W. C., Nelson, C. A., Newberry, R. D., Kranz, D. M., Russell, L. H., and Loh, D. Y. (1988). *Nature* **336,** 73–76.

Shin, H.-C., McFarlane, E. F., Pollard, J. D., and Watson, E. G. S. (1989). *Neurosci. Lett.* **102,** 309–312.

Shizuru, J., Taylor-Edwards, C., Banks, B. A., Gregory, A. K., and Fathman, C. G. (1988). *Science* **240,** 659–662.

Sibley, R. K., Sutherland, D. E. R., Goetz, F. D., and Michael, A. F. (1985). *Lab. Invest.* **53,** 132–144.

Sibley, R. K., and Sutherland, D. E. R. (1988). *Am. J. Pathol.* **128,** 151–170.

Siegel, R. M., Yui, K., Tenenholz, D. E., Kubo, R., and Greene, M. I. (1990). *Eur. J. Immunol.* **20,** 753–757.

Signore, A., Cooke, A., Pozzilli, P., Butcher, G., Simpson, E., and Beverley, P. C. L. (1987). *Diabetologia* **30,** 902–905.

Signore, A., Pozzilli, P., Gale, E. A. M., Andreani, D., and Beverley, P. C. L. (1989). *Diabetologia* **32,** 282–289.

Silverman, D. A., and Rose, N. R. (1974). *Science* **184,** 162–163.

Simmons, R. D., Bernard, C. C. A., Kerlero de Rosbo, N., and Carnegie, P. R. (1984). *In* "Experimental Allergic Encephalomyelitis: A Useful Model for Multiple Sclerosis" (E. C. Alvord, M. W. Kies, and A. J. Suckling, eds.), pp. 23–29. Alan R. Liss, New York.

Simmons, R. D., Bernard, C. C. A., Singer, G., and Carnegie, P. R. (1982). *J. Neuroimmunol.* **3,** 307–318.

Simmons, R. D., Bernard, C. C. A., Ng, K. T., and Carnegie, P. R. (1981). *Brain Res.* **215,** 103–114.

Slattery, R. M., Kjer-Nielsen, L., Allison, J., Charlton, B., Mandel, T. E., and Miller, J. F. A. P. (1990). *Nature* **345,** 724–726.

Smith, H., Chen, I.-M., Kubo, R., and Tung, K. S. K. (1989). *Science* **245,** 749–752.

Smith, M. E. (1966). *Nature* **209,** 1031–1032.

Sobel, R. A., and Colvin, B. (1985). *J. Immunol.* **134,** 2333–2337.

Sriram, S., and Steinman, L. (1983). *J. Exp. Med.* **158,** 1362–1367.

Stauffacher, W., Burr, I., Gutzeit, A., Beaven, D., Veleminsky, J., and Renold, A. E. (1970). *Proc. Soc. Exp. Biol. Med.* **133,** 194–200.

Steinman, L., Rosenbaum, J., Sriram, S., and McDevitt, H. O. (1981). *Proc. Natl. Acad. Sci. U.S.A.* **78,** 7111–7114.

Storb, R. (1989). *Prog. Immunol.* **7,** 1177–1184.

Suenaga, K., and Yoon, J.-W. (1988). *Diabetes* **37,** 1722–1726.

Taguchi, O., and Nishizuka, Y. (1980). *Clin. Exp. Immunol.* **42,** 324–331.

Taguchi, O., Nishizuka, Y., Sakakura, T., and Kojima, A. (1980). *Clin. Exp. Immunol.* **40,** 540–553.

Taguchi, O., and Nishizuka, Y. (1981). *Clin. Exp. Immunol.* **46,** 425–434.

Tait, B. (1990). *Today's Life Sci.* **2,** 30–40.

Takeoka, T., Shinohara, Y., Furumi, K., and Mori, K. (1983). *J. Neurochem.* **41,** 1102–1108.

Tanaka, Y., Tsukada, N., Koh, Ch-S., and Yanagisawa, N. (1987). *J. Neuroimmunol.* **17,** 49–59.

Teitelbaum, D., Webb, C., Bree, M., Meshorer, A., Arnon, R., and Sela, M. (1974). *Clin. Immunol. Immunopathol.* **3,** 256–262.

Terada, M., Salzler, M., Lennartz, K., and Mullen, Y. (1988). *Transplantation,* **45,** 622–627.

Theofilopoulos, A. N., Kofler, R., Singer, P. A., and Dixon, F. J. (1989). *Adv. Immunol.* **46,** 61–109.

Thompson, H. S. G., and Staines, N. A. (1986). *Clin. Exp. Immunol.* **64,** 581–586.

Tighe, H., Silverman, G. J., Kozin, F., Tucker, R., Gulizia, R., Peebles, C., Lotz, M., Rhodes, G., Machold, K., Mosier, D. E., and Carson, D. A. (1990). *Eur. J. Immunol.* **20,** 1843–1848.

Timsit, J., Debray-Sachs, M., Boitard, C., and Bach, J. F. (1988). *Clin. Exp. Immunol.* **73,** 260–264.

Timsit, J., Savino, W., Boitard, C., and Bach, J. F. (1989). *J. Autoimmunity* **2** (Suppl.), 115–129.

Titus, R., and Chiller, J. (1981). *Int. Arch. Allergy Appl. Immunol.* **65,** 323–338.

Tiwari, J., and Terasaki, P. (1985). "HLA and Disease Associations." Springer-Verlag, New York.

Tochino, Y. (1986). *In* "Insulitis and Type I diabetes. Lessons from the NOD mouse" (S. Tarui, Y. Tochino, and K. Nanaka, eds.), pp. 3–10. Academic Press, Tokyo.

Todd, J. A., Bell, J. I., and McDevitt, H. O. (1987). *Nature* **329,** 599–604.

Toh, B.-H., Gleeson, P. A., Simpson, R. J., Moritz, R. L., Callaghan, J. M., Goldkorn, I., Jones, C. M., Martinelli, T. M., Mu, F.-T., Humphris, D. C., Pettitt, J. M., Mori, Y., Masuda, T., Sobieszczuk, P., Weinstock, J., Mantamadiotis, T., and Baldwin, G. S. (1990). *Proc. Natl. Acad. Sci. U.S.A.* **87,** 6418–6422.

Tokioka, T. (1973). *Okajimas Fol. Anat. Jap.* **50,** 133–182.

Tournade, H., Pelletier, L., Pasquier, R., Vial, M.-C., Mandet, C., and Druet, P. (1990a). *J. Immunol.* **144,** 2985–2991.

Tournade, H., Pelletier, L., Pasquier, R., Vial, M.-C., Mandet, C., and Druet, P. (1990b). *Clin. Exp. Immunol.* **81,** 334–338.

Townsend, A. R. M., Rothbard, J., Gotch, F. M., Bahadur, G., Wriath, D., McMichael, A. J. (1986). *Cell* **44,** 959–968.

Townsend, A. R. M., Oehlen, C., Bastin, J., Ljunggren, H.-G., Foster, L., and Karre, K. (1989). *Nature* **340,** 443–448.

Toyka, K. V., Drachman, D. B., Griffin, D. E., Fishbech, K. H., Kao, I., Prstronk, A., and Windelstein, J. A. (1977). *N. Engl J. Med.* **296,** 125–131.

Toyota, T., Satoh, J., Oya, K., Shintani, S., and Okano, T. (1986). *Diabetes* **32,** 496–499.

Traugott, U., McFarlin, D. E., and Raine, C. S. (1986). *Cell. Immunol.* **99,** 395–410.

Trentham, D. E., Townes, A. S., and Kang, A. H. (1977). *J. Exp. Med.* **146,** 857–868.

Tsukada, N., Inoue, A., Yanagisawa, N., Behan, W. M. H., and Behan, P. O. (1986). *J. Neuroimmunol.* **12,** 89–97.

Tsukada, N., Koh, Ch.-S., Yanagisawa, N., Okano, A., Behan, W. M. H., and Behan, P. O. (1987). *Acta Neuropathol.* **73,** 259–266.

Tsukada, N., Koh, Ch.-S., Yanagisawa, N., Okano, A., and Taketomi, T. (1988). *Acta Neuropathol.* **77,** 39–46.

Tsukada, N., Tanaka, Y., Miyagi, K., Yanagisawa, N., and Okano, A. (1989a). *J. Neuroimmunol.* **24,** 41–46.

Tsukada, N., Tanaka, Y., and Yanagisawa, N. (1989b). *J. Neurol. Sci.* **90,** 33–42.

Tung, K. S. K., Smith, S., Teusscher, C., Cook, C., and Anderson, R. E. (1987a). *Am. J. Pathol.* **126,** 293–302.

Tung, K. S. K., Smith, S., Matzner, P., Kasai, K., Oliver, J., Feuchter, F., and Anderson, R. E. (1987b). *Am. J. Pathol.* **126,** 303–314.

Tuohy, V. K., Lu, Z., Sobel, R. A., Laursen, R. A., and Lees, M. B. (1989). *J. Immunol.* **142,** 1523–1527.

Urban, J. L., Horvath, S. J., and Hood, L. (1989). *Cell* **59,** 257–271.

Urban, J. L., Kumar, V., Kono, D. H., Gomez, D., Horvath, S. J., Clayton, J., Ando, D. G., Sercarz, E. E., and Hood, L. (1988). *Cell* **54,** 577–592.

van der Veen, R. C., Trotter, J. L., Hickey, W. F., and Kapp, J. A. (1990). *J. Neuroimmunol.* **26,** 139–145.

Vandenbark, A., Hashim, G., and Offner, H. (1989). *Nature* **341,** 541–543.

Villarroya, H., Dalix, A. M., Paraut, M., and Oriol, R. (1990). *Autoimmunity* **6,** 47–60.

von Boehmer, H. (1988). *Annu. Rev. Immunol.* **6,** 309–326.

Wakasugi, H., Kasahara, T., Minato, N., Hamuro, J., Miyata, M., and Morioka, Y. (1982). *J. Natl. Cancer Inst.* **69,** 807–812.

Waksman, B. H. (1989). *Curr. Opin. Immunol.* **1,** 733–739.

Waldor, M. K., Sriram, S., Hardy, R., Herzenberg, L. A., Lanier, L., Lim, M., and Steinman, L. (1985). *Science* **227,** 415–417.

Wang, Y., Hao, L., Gill, R. G., and Lafferty, K. J. (1987). *Diabetes* **36,** 535–538.

Wang, Y., McDuffie, M., Nokimos, I. N., Hao, L., and Lafferty, K. J. (1988). *Transplantation* **46** (Suppl.), 101S–106S.

Welch, P., Rose, N. R., and Kite, J. H. (1973). *J. Immunol.* **110,** 575–577.

Whittingham, S. F., Mackay, I. R., and Tait, B. D. (1990). *In* "The Immunogenetics of Autoimmune Disease" (N. Farid, ed.), pp. 215–227. CRC Press, Boca Raton, Florida.

Wick, G., Brezinschek, H. P., Hala, K., Dietrich, H., Wolf, H., and Kroemer, G. (1989). *Adv. Immunol.* **47,** 433–500.

Wicker, L. S., Miller, B. J., Fischer, P. A., Pressey, A., and Peterson, L. B. (1989). *J. Immunol.* **142,** 781–784.

Wicker, L. S., Miller, B. J., and Mullen, Y. (1986). *Diabetes* **35,** 855–960.

Wicker, L. S., Miller, B. J., Coker, L. Z., McNally, S. E., Scott, S., Mullen, Y., and Appel, M. C. (1987). *J. Exp. Med.* **165,** 1639–1654.

Williams, R. M., and Moore, M. J. (1973). *J. Exp. Med.* **138,** 775–783.

Williams, R. M., Lees, M. B., Cambi, F., and Macklin, W. B. (1982). *J. Neuropathol. Exp. Neurol.* **41,** 508–521.

Wisniewski, H. M., Schuller-Levis, G. B., Mehta, P. D., Madrid, R. E., and Lassmann, H. (1985). *Concepts Immunopathol.* **2,** 128–150.

Witebsky, E., and Rose, N. R. (1956). *J. Immunol.* **76,** 408.

Yamada, K., Nonaka, K., Hanafusa, T., Miyazaki, A., Toyoshima, H., and Tarui, S. (1982). *Diabetes* **31,** 749–753.

Woollam, D. H. M., and Millen, J. W. (1955). *J. Neurol. Neurosurg. Psychiatry* **18,** 97–102.

Wraith, D. C., Smilek, D. E., Mitchell, D. J., Steinman, L., and McDevitt, H. (1989). *Cell* **59,** 247–255.

Wucherpfennig, K. W., Ota, K., Endo, N., Seidman, J. G., Rosenzweig, A., Weiner, H. L., and Hafler, D. A. (1990). *Science* **248,** 1016–1019.

Yamada, K., Nonaka, K., Hanafusa, T., Miyazaki, A., Toyoshima, H., and Tarui, S. (1982). *Diabetes* **31,** 749–753.

Yamada, M., Zurbriggen, A., and Fujinami, R. S. (1990). *J. Exp. Med.* **171,** 1893–1907.

Yamamoto, H., and Okamoto, H. (1980). *Biochem. Biophys. Res. Commun.* **95,** 474–481.

Yamamura, T., Namikawa, T., Endoh, M., Kunishita, T., and Tabira, T. (1986). *J. Neuroimmunol.* **12,** 143–153.

Yasunami, R., Bach, J.-F. (1988). *Eur. J. Immunol.* **18,** 481–484.

Yokono, K., Shii, K., Hari, J., Yaso, S., Imamura, Y., Ejiri, K., Ishihara, K., Fujii, S., Kazumi, T., Taniguchi, H., and Baba, S. (1985). *Diabetologia* **26,** 379–385.

Yoshida, S., Castles, J. J., and Gershwin, M. E. (1990). *Semin. Arthritis Rheum.* **19,** 224–242.

Yoshimura, T., Kunishita, T., Sakai, K., Endoh, M., Namikawa, T., and Tabira, T. (1985). *J. Neurol. Sci.* **69,** 47–58.

Young, L. H. Y., Peterson, L. B., Wicker, L. S., Persechini, P. M., and Young, J. D. (1989). *J. Immunol.* **143,** 3994–3999.

Zaller, D. M., Osman, G., Kanagawa, O., and Hood, L. (1990). *J. Exp. Med.* **171,** 1943–1955.

Zamvil, S. S., and Steinman, L. (1990). *Annu. Rev. Immunol.* **8,** 579–621.

Zamvil, S. S., Nelson, P., Mitchell, D., Knobler, R., Fritz, R., and Steinman, L. (1985b). *J. Exp. Med.* **162,** 2107–2124.

Zamvil, S. S., Mitchell, D., Powell, M. B., Sakai, K., Rothbard, J. B., and Steinman, L. (1988b). *J. Exp. Med.* **168,** 1181–1186.

Zamvil, S. S., Mitchell, D. J., Lee, N. E., Moore, A. C., Waldor, M. K., Sakai, K., Rothbard, J. B., McDevitt, H. O., Steinman, L., and Acha-Orbea, H. (1988a). *J. Exp. Med.* **167,** 1586–1596.

Zamvil, S. S., Mitchell, D. J., Moore, A. C., Kitamura, K., Steinman, L., and Rothbard, J. (1986). *Nature* **324,** 258–260.

Zamvil, S. S., Nelson, P., Trotter, J., Mitchell, D., Knobler, R., Fritz, R., and Steinman, L. (1985a). *Nature* **317,** 355–358.

Zamvil, S. S., and Steinman, L. (1990). *Annu. Rev. Immunol.* **8,** 579–621.

Zhang, Z. J., Lee, C. S. Y., Lider, O., and Weiner, H. L. (1990). *J. Immunol.* **145,** 2489–2493.

Ziegler, A. G., Vardi, P., Ricker, A. T., Hattori, M., Soeldner, S. J., and Eisenbarth, G. S. (1989). *Diabetes* **38,** 358–363.

Zinkernagel, R. M., Callahan, G. N., Althage, A., Cooper, S., Klein, P. A., and Klein, J. (1978). *J. Exp. Med.* **147,** 882–896.

CHAPTER **4**

Pathogenesis of Multisystem Autoimmunity—SLE as a Model

CLARA M. PELFREY
ALFRED D. STEINBERG
Cellular Immunology Section
Arthritis and Rheumatism Branch,
National Institute of Arthritis and Musculoskeletal and Skin Diseases
National Institutes of Health
Bethesda, Maryland

I. PATHOGENIC FACTORS IN SYSTEMIC LUPUS ERYTHEMATOSUS

Systemic lupus erythematosus (SLE) is an autoimmune syndrome that results from the secretion of autoantibodies of a number of specificities. Although the etiology of the spontaneously occurring disorder is incompletely understood, both genetic and environmental factors are believed to contribute. Insights into the pathogenesis of murine lupus have been effectively applied to human lupus (Table I). Moreover, therapeutic approaches currently being used in life-threatening disease have been verified in murine models (Steinberg, 1987; Steinberg and Steinberg, 1991). Therefore, this chapter emphasizes studies of murine lupus that provide insights applicable to human SLE. Since autoantibodies appear to initiate the pathology found in both murine and human lupus, we will emphasize processes believed to be important in the induction of pathogenic autoantibodies.

Mechanisms that may underlie the initiation of pathogenic autoantibody production include impaired self-tolerance, excess helper T-cell function, molecular mimicry, and induction of antiidiotype antibodies that bind to nonimmunoglobulin self-antigens. In addition, abnormal (polyclonal) stimulation of natural autoantibody-producing cells could favor the development of pathogenic

TABLE I

Common Features of Murine and Human Lupus

Genetics
Polygenic
No unique MHC type
Single genes may modify: a subset of mice and people carry a Y chromosome-accelerating gene
Incomplete penetrance: lack of concordance in identical twins and variability among genetically identical mice
Clinical
Autoantibody production, especially antinuclear
Immune complex glomerulonephritis with premature death
Antibodies to formed elements of the blood may lead to cytopenias
Immune
Polyclonal B-cell activation early in disease
T cell- and antigen-dependent selection of B cells later in disease
Abnormalities of and/or responsiveness to cytokines
Impaired responsiveness to immunization late in disease or with marked disease activity
Hormonal
Female sex hormones accelerate disease, and androgens retard disease (in mice this holds even when there is a Y chromosome-accelerating factor)

autoantibodies. It is possible that more than one process contributes to disease, and that different ones may be responsible for disease in different individuals.

Autoantibodies can be induced by immunization to a foreign antigen that is cross-reactive with a self-antigen (Krisher and Cunningham, 1985; Dale and Beachey, 1982). Such *molecular mimicry* involves runs of amino acid sequences or structural epitopes that are shared by both a foreign and a self-protein. This type of mimicry has been implicated in several diseases, most notably acute rheumatic fever (Krisher and Cunningham, 1985).

In addition to foreign proteins, another potential source of antigen in molecular mimicry is self-immunoglobulin. Immunoglobulins that have undergone somatic mutation provide a large potential source of neoantigens. Responses to immunoglobulin determinants follow immunization to foreign antigens—the resultant antibodies are called antiidiotypic antibodies. If one of the idiotypes mimicked a nucleic acid determinant, the resultant antiidiotypic antibodies might simultaneously be antinuclear antibodies (Agnello, 1981). Therefore, both foreign cross-reactive antigens and self-immunoglobulins may induce autoantibodies.

Since many self-determinants cross-react with foreign antigens, the immune system must recognize large numbers of foreign epitopes while preventing self-recognition. Considerable evidence indicates that deletion of self-reactive lymphocytes within the thymus plays a major role in the development of self versus foreign recognition (Blackman *et al.*, 1990; Ramsdell and Fowlkes, 1990). It is likely that clonal deletion within the thymus eliminates primarily T cells reactive with high avidity to self-epitopes that are strongly bound to class II MHC, called dominant epitopes (Steinberg *et al.*, 1990). Nondeleted thymocytes would be allowed to mature and ultimately would constitute the T-cell repertoire. It should be emphasized that the nondeleted cells would include those able to react with nondominant epitopes of self-proteins. Nondominant epitopes would be those not well presented by class II MHC in the thymus.

As a result of the maturation processes, T cells that recognize nondominant epitopes of self-antigens represent a pool of potentially self-reactive cells that could be stimulated by cross-reactive epitopes on foreign antigens (Steinberg *et al.*, 1990). To prevent such anti-self immunity, peripheral mechanisms of self-tolerance must function to complement intrathymic deletion. Defects in such peripheral tolerance may predispose to generalized autoimmunity.

A. Genetic Factors: Lessons from Murine Lupus

Human and murine lupus share many clinical features (Steinberg *et al.*, 1984). In addition, genetic factors predispose to lupus in mice and in humans. The genetic predisposition to human lupus will be covered in another chapter. Lupus-prone NZB mice have several (approximately six) independently segregating *background genes* that underlie disease (Raveche *et al.*, 1981; Miller *et al.*, 1984). The background genes include those that regulate (1) immune activation, (2) stem cell function, (3) tolerance, and (4) the quantity of autoantibodies. There is an autoimmunity-accelerating gene on the Y chromosome of BXSB mice (Murphy and Roths, 1979); this gene accelerates disease on an autoimmune genetic background but does not induce disease on a normal genetic background (Steinberg *et al.*, 1986; Hudgins *et al.*, 1985). The background genes of NZB mice and the Y chromosome accelerating gene have counterparts in humans (Steinberg *et al.*, 1984).

Other types of genes are capable of inducing abnormalities even on a non-autoimmune genetic background. For example, the recessive genes, *lpr* or *gld*, lead to hypergammaglobulinemia and a marked increase in numbers of T cells in otherwise normal mouse strains (Murphy and Roths, 1979; Theofilopoulos and Dixon, 1981; Davidson *et al.*, 1986). However, much more severe lupuslike disease is found when the *lpr* or *gld* genes are bred onto an autoimmune background such as MRL or NZB (Gause *et al.*, 1988).

Although the *gld* gene has been mapped (Seldin *et al.*, 1987), none of the genes predisposing to murine lupus has been cloned. Moreover, no protein products have been found; therefore, the mechanisms by which the genetic predisposition leads to disease are unknown. Nevertheless, a possible clue to a common final pathway of disease is the observation that all of the single genes (*lpr/lpr, gld/gld,* and BXSB-Y) lead to polyclonal B-cell activation (Ishigatsubo *et al.,* 1988; Klinman *et al.,* 1990).

B. Stem Cells

Reconstitution studies suggest an initiating role for the hemopoietic stem cell in murine lupus. Bone marrow cells from young lupus-prone NZB mice, when transplanted into normal lethally irradiated DBA/2 or BALB/c recipients, gave rise to antinuclear antibodies within 2 months of transfer (Morton and Seigel, 1974a,b). Similarly, (NZB × NZW) F_1 bone marrow transferred elevated anti-DNA titers, increased proteinuria, and decreased survival, compared with recipients of normal marrow (Akizuki *et al.,* 1978). Autoimmune potential has also been transferred with marrow from several other strains (Eisenberg *et al.,* 1980; Schultz *et al.,* 1983).

Reciprocal reconstitution experiments also have been performed. Lupus-prone strains that were lethally irradiated and reconstituted with marrow from normal mice were protected from the autoimmune syndrome (Morton and Seigel, 1974a). Thus, host cells remaining after irradiation are not able to induce the syndrome, and stem cells are necessary and sufficient for induction.

In NZB mice, at least one of the background genes underlying disease leads to increased stem-cell activity (Miller *et al.,* 1984). All of the lupus-prone mouse strains studied have a marked excess in numbers of stem cells or their immediate progeny following stress, which encourages stem-cell expansion (Scribner and Steinberg, 1988; Steinberg, 1979). Thus, murine lupus appears to be characterized by an increase in the number of stem cells, or in their proliferative capacity, or in the proliferation of their immediate offspring. Whether such activity represents an intrinsic stem-cell abnormality or results from the action of stimulatory factors made by other cell types is unknown.

The bone marrow cells of lupus-prone NZB mice have been compared with those of nonautoimmune control mice. NZB marrow differentiated into cells able to produce much more immunoglobulin than normal (Kastner and Steinberg, 1988). In view of the similar expansion of normal and NZB B cells in common *in vivo* environments (see B-cell section), it is possible that bone marrow stromal cells contribute importantly to the excess B-cell maturation in NZB mice. Since such maturation can occur in *in vitro* marrow cultures, the excess B-cell maturation pathway may not depend on factors extrinsic to the marrow.

Recent studies have mapped abnormalities of NZB thymocytes to a bone marrow pre-T cell (Krieg *et al.,* 1991). Therefore, both the tolerance defects and the abnormal retroviral expression of NZB mice may be attributable to a defect encoded in the stem cell. Similarly, studies of MRL-*lpr/lpr* and C57BL/6-*lpr/lpr* mice have mapped abnormal antibody production and T-cell proliferation to the

T- and B-cell progeny of *lpr*/*lpr* bone marrow (Katagiri *et al.*, 1988; Sobel *et al.*, 1991).

In summary, since autoimmune bone marrow cells can transfer autoimmunity in all the above cases and since the other defects found in lupus (both T cell and B cell) could derive from a defect in the progenitor cells in the marrow, it is likely that hemopoietic cells contain the genetic program for autoimmunity. Thus, the stem cells are not completely dependent on the milieu of the surrounding tissue in which they expand. However, the pace and severity of immune abnormalities and disease could be dependent on the local milieu as well as on the programmed maturation of the stem cell progenies.

C. Cytokines

Many lymphocyte functions are mediated by or facilitated by soluble stimulatory factors. Excess or deficient production of, or responsiveness to, such factors could predispose to generalized autoimmunity. B cells from lupus-prone (NZB × NZW) F_1 and BXSB mice respond excessively to T cell-derived cytokines (Prud'homme *et al.*, 1984). In contrast, lupus-prone MRL-*lpr*/*lpr* mice were found to have excess production of T cell-derived stimulatory factors (Prud'homme *et al.*, 1984). In addition, reduced responsiveness of B cells to T-cell helper signals was associated with abrogation of murine lupus by the *xid* gene (Feiser *et al.*, 1984).

Whereas older autoimmune mice have been found to manifest decreased production of cytokines in response to various stimuli (Santoro *et al.*, 1983, 1984), younger mice usually do not have such deficits and may have increased spontaneous production (Jyanouchi *et al.*, 1985). Moreover, interleukin (IL)-2 can function as a growth factor for B cells from New Zealand mice (Lehman *et al.*, 1986), probably because such B cells have increased numbers of IL-2 receptors (Chused *et al.*, 1987).

Several studies have suggested a possible role for IL-4 in the pathogenesis of B-cell hyperactivity in lupus-prone strains. Supernatants from MRL-*lpr*/*lpr* T-cell lines have shown Ia-inducing capacity, which is abrogated by anti-IL-4 antibody (Rosenberg *et al.*, 1986). In addition, *in vivo* treatment of MRL-*1pr*/*1pr* mice with anti-IL-4 has decreased their autoimmune manifestations (Rosenberg *et al.*, 1986). NZB mice had marked stimulation of their B cells by IL-4, whereas control mice required additional signals (Guitierrez *et al.*, 1986). The New Zealand mice also hyperrespond to IL-5; however, such hyperresponsiveness appears to be a manifestation of their increased percentages of CD5+ B cells (Umland *et al.*, 1989). Several autoimmune-prone strains produce circulating interferon with onset after polyclonal B-cell activation is observed.

Patients with SLE also produce serum interferon during active disease. Whether or not this serves to limit the B-cell activation is unclear. Like the mice with lupus, patients have impaired production of IL-2 in response to mitogenic stimuli (Santoro *et al.*, 1984); however, they have been reported to have increased unstimulated IL-2 production (Murakawa *et al.*, 1985 and Huang *et al.*, 1988).

D. T Cells in Murine Lupus

T cells are necessary for production of pathogenic autoantibodies in murine lupus. T cells provide critical help for autoantibody production *in vitro,* and *in vivo* elimination of CD4+ T cells prevents or retards disease (Kotzin *et al.*, 1989; Laskin *et al.*, 1982, 1983, 1986; Mihara *et al.*, 1988; Wofsy and Seaman, 1987). However, it is not entirely clear whether lupus T cells represent a primary abnormality or merely serve as a necessary factor in autoantibody production.

One study found that with increasing age, NZB mice had a progressive loss of helper and suppressor T cells, but an increase in amplifier cells (Baker *et al.*, 1986). Although the B cells were resistant to inhibitory effects of suppression, they responded to the stimulatory effects of amplifier T cells. Thus, combined immune defects may contribute to increased antibody production.

The *lpr/lpr* and *gld/gld* genotypes lead to a marked increase in T-cell mass and features of autoimmunity. Therefore, it is possible that the excess T-cell numbers may underlie the induction of polyclonal B-cell activation and the autoimmune phenomena. On the other hand, those genotypes may also be associated with abnormalities in non-T-cell lineages, perhaps as a result of an abnormality common to several cell types—for example, from a stem-cell abnormality, as discussed above. [In fact, there is strong evidence of B-cell abnormalities in such mice (Sobel *et al.*, 1991).] The cells that are most increased in *lpr/lpr* mice are CD 4−, CD 8− T cells with unusual surface markers. It has been suggested that these T cells are relatively inert. Studies from this laboratory have demonstrated that the lymph node T cells of *lpr/lpr* mice are heterogeneous, raising the possibility that the *abnormal* double negative cells may differentiate into single positive cells or vice versa (Gause *et al.*, 1988). Therefore, the increase in T cells in *lpr/lpr* mice could underlie the observed hypergammaglobulinemia and excess autoantibody production.

Studies of T-cell deletion within the thymuses of normal and autoimmune mice have not demonstrated gross abnormalities associated with autoimmunity. However, one group has found apparent expansion, later in life, of *forbidden clones* in the periphery of autoimmune mice (Adams *et al.*, 1990). This observation requires further study.

1. T-Cell Abnormalities and Anti-T-Cell Antibodies

The prevalence of anti-T-cell antibodies in murine and human lupus complicates the studies of lupus T cells (Steinberg *et al.*, 1981; Klassen *et al.*, 1977). Anti-T-cell antibodies may eliminate T-cell subsets with a resultant imbalance in normal immune regulation. This process has been described for patients with lupus (Morimoto *et al.*, 1984; Sakane *et al.*, 1979; Kumagai *et al.*, 1981a). In addition, anti-T-cell antibodies may stimulate T cells to release helper factors. In such a manner, anti-T-cell antibodies might induce or contribute to polyclonal immune stimulation. They could even serve as a positive feedback for such stimulation. Thus, a B-cell product (anti-T-cell antibody) could lead to a T-cell abnormality that superficially appeared to be an intrinsic T-cell defect driving polyclonal hyperimmunity. For example, lupus-prone NZB mice produce, from birth, antibodies reactive with self-thymocytes and T cells. NZB anti-T-cell antibodies lead to immune stimulation and contribute to accelerated disease and death when given chronically to young male (NZB × NZW) F_1 mice (Klassen *et al.*, 1977; Huston *et al.*, 1980).

Although T cells in general may be important for disease, antigen-specific T cells may be critical by directly recognizing autoantigen (or an antigen cross-reactive with an autoantigen). These might or might not include the *forbidden clones* of T cells expanded in some autoimmune mice (Adams *et al.*, 1990). In addition, antigen-specific T cells may recognize a common environmental antigen and, in being stimulated, produce cytokines that contribute to the activation of autoantibody-producing B cells.

2. Tolerance

We indicated in the introduction that deletion of self-reactive cells in the thymus provided a first defense against autoimmune diseases. The second line of defense consists of mechanisms that maintain self-tolerance despite the presence of some self-reactive cells. Various mechanisms have been included under the names of suppression, anergy, and tolerance.

Experimental tolerance involves presenting an antigen to the immune system in a nonimmunogenic form such that it renders the immune system specifically hyporesponsive to subsequent attempts at immunization with the antigen in immunogenic form. Several studies have demonstrated impaired experimental tolerance in many of the strains of mice predisposed to lupus: NZB, (NZB × NZW) F_1, BXSB, and MRL-*lpr*/*lpr* (Laskin *et al.*, 1981). Since lupus involves a loss of self-tolerance to certain self-antigens, a defect in experimental tolerance could represent a fundamental abnormality.

Our laboratory studied the response of NZB mice to the toleragen deaggregated bovine gamma globulin or BGG. Included were studies involving reconstitution of neonatally thymectomized and lethally irradiated adult (NZB × DBA/2) F_1 mice with marrow and thymocytes from parent mice in all combinations (Table II). The data suggested that the tolerance abnormality of NZB mice (to deaggregated BGG) results from an abnormality of NZB thymocytes. More-

TABLE II

Tolerance to Deaggregated Bovine Gamma Globulin[a]

Donor cells			
Thymus	Marrow	Sex/manipulation[b]	Tolerance in recipients
DBA	DBA	M or F	++++
DBA	NZB	M or F	++++
NZB	DBA	M	++++
NZB	DBA	F	0
NZB	DBA	M castrated	0
NZB	DBA	F + androgens	++++
DBA + NZB	DBA	F	0
NZB	NZB	M or F	0

[a]In neonatally thymectomized, lethally irradiated (DBA/2 × NZB) F_1 recipients. Mice were irradiated (950 rads) and reconstituted with T cell-depleted bone marrow cells plus thymocytes from 1-month-old NZB or DBA/2 mice (Laskin *et al.*, 1982). One month later, they were injected with 10 mg deaggregated BGG; 12 days later, mice were challenged with BGG in adjuvant; they were assayed for serum anti-BGG 2 weeks after challenge. Tolerance is shown semi-quantitatively, with 0, no tolerance; and ++++, tolerance observed in intact DBA/2 mice.

[b]Designation of recipient: F, unmanipulated female; M, unmanipulated male. Females treated with androgen capsules showed the same effect of androgens whether or not they were castrated.

over, whereas the combination of DBA thymocytes plus DBA marrow led to tolerance, the addition of NZB thymocytes to DBA marrow plus DBA thymocytes did not. Thus, NZB thymocytes were not simply unable to become tolerant; rather, they interfered with the normal tolerance expected of DBA cells. This active interference with tolerance may be mediated by secretion of cytokines.

Recent studies from our lab (Scott, D. E. and Steinberg, A. D., manuscript in preparation) suggest that $CD4^+$ T cells from (NZB × NZW) F_1 and MRL-*lpr*/*lpr* mice are normally deleted by the superantigen SEB. Thus, peripheral tolerance may be impaired in these murine lupus strains only when a T cell–B cell interaction is involved.

E. Sex Hormone Effects

It is well known that the majority of patients with lupus are female. Moreover, androgen administration from very early in the life of (NZB × NZW) F_1 lupus-prone female mice can turn a rapid-onset renal disease pattern into a slower male pattern (Steinberg *et al.*, 1981; Nelson and Steinberg, 1987). Conversely, castration of males in the first 2–3 weeks of life turns the slow male pattern into a rapid-onset female pattern. The possible cellular basis of some of the hormone effects was studied in the tolerance system (Laskin *et al.*, 1981). As shown in Table II, when only DBA cells were administered to recipients, both males and females were tolerant. Gender also was irrelevant when only NZB cells were given—there was no tolerance in either males or females. Of note, with the combination of NZB thymus and DBA marrow, males were tolerant, and females were not. The gender effect was demonstrated to result from sex hormone effects. Androgen treatment of females gave a male pattern of tolerance, and castration of males gave a female pattern of nontolerance. These studies suggest the possibility that a single NZB defect (presence of NZB thymocytes) is sufficient to make females susceptible to abnormalities in self-tolerance that might allow disease development. In contrast, males, by virtue of their suppressive androgens, are not predisposed to such abnormalities when a single cellular defect is present. It should be noted that androgens are not able to protect males in the face of two NZB cellular defects. Thus, with a modest genetic/cellular predisposition to lupus, androgens may be able to retard or prevent disease. With a stronger genetic/cellular predisposition to disease, androgens are less able to suppress disease.

The murine tolerance studies may help to explain gender distribution in human lupus. For example, if a minority of people destined to develop lupus have a great predisposition to disease, androgens would not protect them, and approximately half would be male. If all others susceptible to lupus manifested only a modest predisposition, most of this second group would be females (the males would be protected). This formulation could explain the presence of severe disease in males with lupus, even though they are in the minority. Alternatively, a number of the males may have Y chromosome factors that predispose them to severe disease.

F. B-Cell Studies

1. Polyclonal B-Cell Expansion

When their immune systems are polyclonally stimulated, autoimmune-prone mouse strains show accelerated disease (Steinberg, 1979; Steinberg *et al.*, 1969, 1981; Hang *et al.*, 1985). In addition, normal mice subjected to the combination of polyclonal B-cell activators and neonatal thymectomy manifest anti-DNA antibody production (Lane *et al.*, submitted for publication; Smith and Steinberg, 1983). Finally, autoimmune disease is induced by the combination of polyclonal B-cell activation and challenge with common environmental pathogens (Lane *et al.*, submitted for publication; Smith and Steinberg, 1983). Thus, polyclonal immune activation could contribute to autoimmunity. Supporting this concept is the observation of polyclonal B-cell expansion in the several lupus-prone strains of mice (Moutsopoulos *et al.*, 1977; Manny *et al.*, 1979; Theofilopoulos and Dixon, 1985; Klinman *et al.*, 1988a).

All lupus-prone mice, compared with nonautoimmune-prone strains, have increased numbers of splenic immunoglobulin-producing cells (Moutsopoulos *et al.*, 1977; Manny *et al.*, 1979; Theofilopoulos and Dixon, 1985; Klinman *et al.*, 1988a). When one considers both the increased percentage of immunoglobulin-secreting cells and the increased number of spleen cells, lupus-prone mice may have a 30-fold increase in absolute numbers of antibody-secreting cells. The repertoires of such mice could be compared by expressing the percentage of the immunoglobulin-secreting cells reactive with different specificities. When this assessment was carried out, it was found that the percentages of B cells secreting antibodies able to bind conventional antigens [the trinitrophenyl hapten (TNP), ovalbumin, sheep erythrocytes] and autoantigens (DNA, myosin, T cell-surface antigens) were quite similar. The data (summarized in Table III) indicate that early B-cell activation in lupus is polyclonal in nature. This result was obtained for autoimmune NZB, MRL-*lpr*/*lpr*, C3H-*gld*/*gld*, BXSB, and backcross mice (Ishigatsubo *et al.*, 1988; Klinman and Steinberg, 1987a,b; Klinman *et al.*, 1988a,b, 1990).

The early polyclonal expansion of B cells in murine lupus could result from a primary defect in B cells or maturation of B cells in a stimulatory environment. This question was studied by transferring B cells from autoimmune-prone mice to MHC-compatible nonautoimmune hosts carrying the *xid* gene and vice versa (Klinman and Steinberg, 1987a; Klinman *et al.*, 1988a). These studies showed that the expansion of autoantibody-producing cells was associated with the internal milieu of the recipient rather than the origin of the B cells.

The concept of polyclonal expansion of B cells in autoimmune-prone strains of mice is supported by studies of immunoglobulin heavy chain variable-region gene usage. There is no restriction in immunoglobulin gene usage for autoantibodies (Perkins *et al.*, 1990; Behar and Sharff, 1988; Kofler *et al.*, 1985;

TABLE III
Summary of B-Cell Studies in Murine Lupus[a]

Increase in absolute numbers of B cells
Increase in percentage of spleen cells that are producing Ig
Normal repertoire on a percentage basis in the first several months
Transfer of NZB or control DBA/2 B cells to the same type of *xid* recipient leads to the same degree of anti-DNA production
Transfer of NZB or control DBA/2 B cells to NZB.*xid* recipients leads to a marked increase in anti-DNA, whereas transfer to DBA/2.*xid* recipients leads to very little anti-DNA

[a]From Klinman and Steinberg (1987a,b); Klinman *et al.* (1988a,b, 1990); Ishigatsubo *et al.* (1988).

Dersimonian *et al.*, 1987). Moreover, there is no bias in the use of IgVH genes by autoimmune mice (Kastner *et al.*, 1989). Other studies have suggested a resistance of NZB B cells to suppressive signals (Baker *et al.*, 1986) pointing to a generalized B cell abnormality. These also are consistent with the cytokine experiments (Gutierrez *et al.*, 1986).

In murine lupus, there is, in addition to polyclonal B-cell activation, evidence for T cell-dependent and antigen-dependent selection of B cells destined to produce pathogenic autoantibodies. Some investigators have rigidly divided the pathogenetic processes such that evidence of B-cell selection is regarded as evidence against polyclonal effects (Steinberg, 1989). Nevertheless, it is obvious that polyclonal activation and selection may both occur in murine lupus. Moreover, it is possible that prior polyclonal B-cell activation in lupus may interfere with regulatory mechanisms so as to allow antigen-dependent expansion of B cells that produce pathogenic autoantibodies (Steinberg, 1987; 1989; Klinman *et al.*, 1990).

2. Antigen-Specific B-Cell Expansion Late in Disease

With increasing age, individual autoimmune mice express unique repertoires characterized by the expansion of B cells producing antibody that binds to a limited set of autoantigens. A similar process occurs in normal mice, but to a lesser extent and at a slower rate (Klinman *et al.*, 1988b; Eisenberg *et al.*, 1987a). Therefore, with age, clonal expansion begins to emerge from the background of polyclonal activation. Evidence for antigen dependence of autoantibody-producing B cells was obtained in the transfer system in which NZB B cells were given to unmanipulated NZB.*xid* recipients: autoantibody-producing cells expanded preferentially relative to B cells producing anti-TNP (Table IV). Immunization of recipient mice (not able to respond to TNP-Ficoll) led to marked expansion of TNP-specific *donor* B cells. Such data suggest that the *spontaneous* expansion of the autoantibody-producing cells was driven by the presence of self-antigen. The idea presented is compatible with the suggestion that somatic mutation followed

TABLE IV
Increase in Antibody-Forming Cells in NZB.*xid* Recipients[a]

Specificity	Fold increase
DNA	19
T cells	18
TNP-KLH	2
TNP-KLH after immunization with TNP-Ficoll	52

[a]Five weeks after transfer of 1 million NZB B cells. From Klinman and Steinberg (1987a); Klinman *et al.*, (1988a).

by antigen-driven selection underlies expansion of anti-DNA producing cells (Schlomchik *et al.*, 1987a, 1987b; Marion *et al.*, 1989) as well as the concept of T-cell dependence of antinuclear autoantibody production (Datta *et al.*, 1987; Bennett *et al.*, 1987).

Recent studies of [NZB × (NZB × NZW)] F_1 backcross mice have shown a significant correlation ($P < 0.001$) between the presence of polyclonal activation in mice under 3 months of age with the subsequent development of lupus glomerulonephritis (Klinman, 1990). Of note, there was no correlation between the development of disease and early production of specific autoantibodies. All of the data together suggest that polyclonal B-cell activation is a characteristic of murine lupus from early in life. This initial abnormality may favor subsequent T-cell and antigen-dependent processes. It also has been noted that certain autoantibodies, most dramatically the anti-Sm antibodies of MRL mice, do not correlate with disease (Eisenberg *et al.*, 1987b). Such a finding points to the general predisposition to oligoclonal B-cell expansion as an important pathogenic event; whether or not this leads to pathology depends on the properties of the antibodies produced by the expanded clones.

3. Does Autoreactive B-Cell Expansion Represent a Primary B-Cell Defect?

In order to determine whether the hyperactivity of NZB B cells results from an intrinsic B-cell defect or from the milieu in which they develop, transfer studies were performed. Autoimmune NZB and normal DBA/2 B cells expanded at similar rates when transferred to (DBA/2 × NZB) F_1.*xid* recipients (Klinman and Steinberg, 1987a, Klinman, *et al.*, 1988a). Cells from both NZB and DBA/2 donors expanded much more rapidly in NZB.*xid* recipients than in DBA/2.*xid* recipients (Klinman *et al.*, 1988a). These results indicate that at least one NZB defect leading to B-cell hyperactivity resides not in the NZB B cell but in the stimulatory milieu in which that B cell lives.

Whether the stimulatory environment results from T cell-derived helper effects, macrophage stimulation, or nonimmune factors remains to be determined. However, there is some evidence suggesting that a bone marrow stromal element may be important in some aspects of NZB B-cell hyperactivity (Kastner and Steinberg, 1988). Since transfer studies had suggested that the NZB B cells were not uniquely responsible for excess antibody production, the marrow culture result pointed to marrow stromal elements as potentially critical to the hypergammaglobulinemia of NZB mice.

4. Active Human Systemic Lupus Manifests Augmented Activity throughout the B-Cell Maturation Pathway

A number of studies performed at The National Institutes of Health (Sakane *et al.*, 1978, 1981; Kumagai *et al.*, 1982; Glinski *et al.*, 1976; Becker *et al.*, 1981;

TABLE V
Summary of B Cell-Pathway Studies of SLE Patients

	Active SLE	Controls
Numbers of bone marrow cells after a week in Dexter culture	148	38
B-cell colonies/10^5	28	6
Proliferation of B-enriched PMBC[a] (cpm $\times$ 10^{-3}) in the first 18 hr of culture	4.3	0.8
Cells producing antibodies to 12 chemical haptens/10^5 PBMC	61	2
Total Ig-secreting cells/10^5 PBMC	320	30

[a]PBMC, peripheral blood mononuclear cells.

Blaese *et al.*, 1980) and elsewhere indicate that patients with active multisystem SLE have elevated numbers of cells throughout the B-cell generation pathway (Table V). Patients have increased numbers of autoantibody-producing cells that, undoubtedly, are responsible for the serum autoantibodies that underlie both diagnostic tests and disease. However, the patients also have increased numbers of lymphocytes producing antibodies to nonautoantigens (such as chemical haptens). Thus, polyclonal B-cell activation may contribute to increased antibody production in some patients with active lupus. Moreover, the greatest degree of polyclonal activation generally is observed in those patients with the most active multisystem disease. If human lupus is analogous to murine lupus, much of the polyclonal B-cell expansion would be expected to occur before symptomatic disease onset. However, our studies have not included very many individuals very early in their disease, and especially before disease onset, individuals needed to fully test the hypothesis. Nevertheless, the data suggest that polyclonal B-cell expansion is most apparent during the early stages of multisystem lupus. After the disease process becomes established, B cells producing specific autoantibodies usually are increased selectively, consistent with autoantigen and T cell-dependent immune stimulation.

II. DISCUSSION

Polyclonal B-cell expansion is a consistent finding early in the course of murine lupus. Notably, such polyclonal effects are found before more specific expansion of B cells producing pathogenic autoantibodies. Subsequent to the polyclonal effects (and perhaps encouraged by them), T cell-dependent and antigen (or idiotype)-driven immunity apparently leads to the production of the bulk of the pathogenic autoantibodies. Although the evidence is less secure, comparable processes to those found in murine lupus may underlie disease in many patients with SLE, as summarized in Fig. 1.

Antigen-nonspecific stimulatory factors, such as bystander help from T cells,

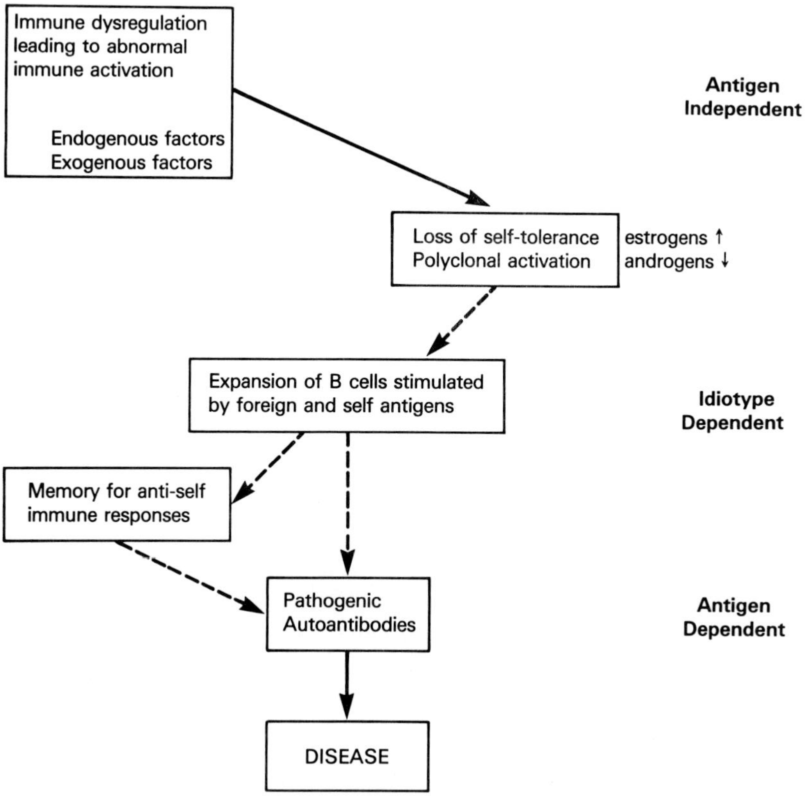

FIG. 1 Processes we believe to be important in the pathogenesis of lupus are shown in schematic form. An early immune dysregulation may be attributable to a defect in bone marrow stem cells or factors regulating them, in T cells or other factors that regulate B cells, or in B cells themselves. In some people, endogenous abnormalities may be of paramount importance, whereas in others, exogenous stimuli may be critical.

Polyclonal immune activation is shown to be an early and fundamental abnormality. This polyclonal immune stimulation may be caused by a genetic predisposition comprising hyperresponsiveness to factors that stimulate B-cell proliferation/differentiation or hyperproduction of such factors. In addition, exogenous activators (e.g., viral or bacterial) may stimulate B cells. Such factors serve also to break self-tolerance mechanisms. These effects are largely independent of specific self-antigens. The polyclonal effects tend to be suppressed by androgens and enhanced by estrogens.

In the absence of adequate down-regulating control elements, autoimmune reactions progress. These are largely antigen- and/or idiotype-dependent and give rise to pathogenic autoantibodies. For example, idiotypic determinants on self-immunoglobulin may induce helper T cells to stimulate B cells capable of producing anti-DNA antibodies. The resulting inflammation leads to the release of self-antigens, which further stimulate the process. It should be noted that the development of memory for anti-self responses reduces the threshold for a disease flare relative to that required for initial induction of disease.

immunostimulatory infections, and/or defective regulation of induced stimulation may be important in certain individuals. It is also possible that polyclonal stimulation itself may impair normal regulatory processes so as to circumvent self-tolerance mechanisms and allow immunization to self-antigens. Since polyclonal immune activators are able to break tolerance as well as interfere with its development (Weigle, 1973), those factors that stimulate polyclonal B-cell expansion should also be able to subvert normal tolerance (Steinberg *et al.*, 1990; Steinberg *et al.*, 1981; Smathers *et al.*, 1984). Thus, defects in tolerance and B-cell stimulation could be caused by the same process(es).

Thymocytes and spleen cells from lupus-prone New Zealand mice produce more stimulatory and fewer suppressive factors than do cells from non-autoimmune-prone strains (Ranney and Steinberg, 1976; Morton *et al.*, 1976). Such cells also fail to become tolerant to deaggregated bovine gamma globulin by a process of active interference with tolerance. The increased *help* and decreased *suppression* observed in murine lupus could well be different aspects of the same problem (Steinberg *et al.*, 1971, 1981) and result from excess stimulatory-factor production by autoimmune cells. A related possibility is that since graft-versus-host disease (GVH) can lead to a lupuslike illness, an endogenous GVH-like disorder, perhaps triggered by B cells, might induce autoimmunity (Rosenberg *et al.*, 1984).

Several lines of evidence support the hypothesis that bone marrow stem cells, or their immediate progeny, manifest the defects characteristic of murine lupus. Transplantation of autoimmune marrow can transfer disease to nonautoimmune recipients (Morton and Seigel, 1974a; Akizuki *et al.*, 1978). In addition, studies of NZB mice have mapped the defect in experimental tolerance to the pre-T stem cell. How the lupus stem cells promote abnormalities observed in mature lymphocytes remains to be determined. It is possible that several different cellular abnormalities present in the stem cell may be expressed in cells of several different lineages. Such a defect might help to explain abnormalities in a number of cell types.

Interference with T-cell function ameliorates murine lupus (Taurog *et al.*, 1981; Wofsy *et al.*, 1985; Marion *et al.*, 1989; Wofsy and Seaman, 1987). Thus, T-cell help must be critical for substantial autoantibody production. However, the requirement for T cells does not imply a T-cell abnormality: there could be increased responsiveness of B cells to normal T-cell signals. On the other hand, there might be increased T-cell help, cognate or bystander.

Since much autoantibody production ultimately is both T-cell and antigen dependent, the nature of the stimulatory antigens must be considered. It seems likely that several of the many endogenous and exogenous molecules cross-reacting with or mimicking self-antigens could stimulate autoantibody production. Combinations of molecules may be immunogenic, whereas neither alone is. For example, the binding of DNA to collagen could produce an immunogenic combinatorial molecule. Some drug-induced lupus also could result from such an effect. In addition, the large number of immunoglobulin molecules present in the body provides an excellent source of cross-reactive antigens (Mendlovic *et al.*, 1989). Since the antibody response to many antigens is stochastic, the expanded repertoire of each individual would vary. This might help to explain variability in autoantibody repertoire among individuals with lupus, especially genetically related individuals such as identical twins and members of an inbred mouse strain.

Production of large amounts of pathogenic autoantibodies may require several processes. Even if polyclonal activation is the immune abnormality that initiates the disease process, additional antigen or idiotype and T cell-dependent processes may be critical. Since the pathogenic autoantibodies lead to disease, the initiating polyclonal activation might not ultimately correlate with measures of disease in specific organs or with mortality (Steinberg *et al.*, 1971, 1991).

EDITORS' NOTE

Murine models of "multisystem" autoimmunity have been studied since 1960, beginning with the NZB mouse with autoimmune hemolytic anemia. The hybrid with NZW (NZB/W) was the first of the "lupus mice," so-called because nuclear autoantibodies were dominant, and the mice died from a glomerulonephritis that simulated the nephritis seen in human SLE. Later other types of lupus mice were established by hybridization of either of two autosomal recessive mutations associated with lymphoproliferation, lpr or gld, onto an appropriate background, e.g. MRL. The lpr and gld genes are associated with marked B cell hyperactivity. Although these lupus mouse models do not truly fulfil the revised ARA criteria for human SLE, they do illustrate the potentially lethal consequences of uncontrolled formation of autoantibodies to accessible antigenic epitopes of erythrocytes (NZB), or DNA (NZB/W, MRLlpr, etc.).

What do the lupus mouse models tell us? They do not point to any unifying "lesion of autoimmunity" because, as Pelfrey and colleagues indicate, there appear to be multiple genetic components which in combination create an immunologic disaster scenario. One such component gives rise to hyperfunctional B lymphocytes which initially are susceptible to polyclonal activation, but later become focused and (auto)antigen-dependent. A second component results in T lymphocytes that provide excessive helper signals. A third component influences a bone marrow stromal element and may operate through a stimulatory effect on B cells. A fourth component predisposing to autoimmunity has been identified in hemopoietic stem cells, and may operate also in the NOD mouse (see chapter 10). A fifth component, residing in the MHC, provides NZB mice with the genetic capacity to present DNA in an immunogenic form to T cells; this may operate peripherally, and/or influence repertoire selection in the thymus. Additionally there are constitutional modifying factors, particularly sex hormones. Pelfrey and colleagues emphasize one similarity between murine and human lupus, this being elevated numbers and function of B cells throughout the entire B-cell generation pathway. Is this the essential lesion of autoimmunity in the mouse models and in human SLE, and are the other genetic anomalies merely facilitatory to this? If so, this lesion of autoimmuity would be different from that operative in organ-specific autoimmune diseases, for which the main responsibility is carried by the $CD4^+$ helper T cell.

REFERENCES

Adams, S., Zordan, T., Sainis, K., and Datta, S. K. (1990). *Eur. J. Immunol.* **20,** 1435–1443.

Agnello, V., Arbetter, A., Ibanez de Kasep, G., Powell, R., Tan, E. M., and Joslin, F. (1981). *J. Exp. Med.* **151,** 1514–1527.

Akizuki, M., Reeves, J. P., and Steinberg, A. D. (1978). *Clin. Immunol. Immunopathol.* **10,** 247–250.

Baker, P. J., Fauntleroy, M. B., Stashak, P. W., McCoy, K. L., and Chused, T. M. (1986). *Immunobiol.* **171,** 400–411.

Becker, T. M., Lizzio, E. F., Merchant, B., Reeves, J. P., and Steinberg, A. D. (1981). *Intl. Arch. Aller. Appl. Immunol.* **66,** 293–303.

Behar, S. M., and Scharff, M. D. (1988). *Proc. Natl. Acad. Sci. U.S.A.* **85,** 3970–3974.

Bennett, R. M., Kotzin, B. L., and Merritt, M. J. (1987). *J. Exp. Med.* **166,** 850–863.

Blackman, M., Kappler, J., and Marrack, P. (1990). *Science* **248,** 1335–1393.

Blaese, R. M., Grayson, J., and Steinberg, A. D. (1980). *Am. J. Med.* **69,** 345–350.

Chused, T. M., McCoy, K. L., Lal, R. B., Malek, T. R., Brown, E. M., Edison, L. J., Baker, P. J. (1987). "Autoimmune Disease in New Zealand Mice" (Smolen, J. and Zielinski, N., eds.), pp. 50–59. Springer, Berlin.

Dale, J. B., and Beachey, E. H. (1982). *J. Exp. Med.* **156,** 1165–1176.

Datta, S. K., Patel, H., and Berry, D. (1987). *J. Exp. Med.* **165,** 1252–1268.

Davidson, W. F., Dumont, F., Bedigian, H. G., Fowlkes, B. J., and Morse, H. C., III. (1986). *J. Immunol.* **137,** 4075–4089.

Dersimonian, H., Schwartz, R. S., Barrett, K. J., and Stoller, B. D. (1987). *J. Immunol.* **139,** 2496–2501.

Eisenberg, R. A., Izui, S., MaConahey, P. J., Hang, L., Peters, C. J., Theofilopoulos, A. M., and Dixon, F. J. (1980). *J. Immunol.* **125,** 1032–1036.

Eisenberg, R. A., Craven, S. Y., and Cohen, P. L. (1987a). *J. Immunol.* **139,** 728–733.

Eisenberg, R. A., Craven, S. Y., Warren, R. W., and Cohen, P. L. (1987b). *J. Clin. Invest.* **80,** 691–697.

Feiser, T. M., Gershwin, M. E., Steinberg, A. D., Dixon, F. J., and Theofilopoulos, A. N. (1984). *Cell. Immunol.* **87,** 708–713.

Gause, W. C., Steinberg, A. D., and Mountz, J. D. (1988). *Concepts Immunopathol.* **6,** 89–118.

Glinski, W., Gershwin, M. E., Budman, D. R., and Steinberg, A. D. (1976). *Clin. Exp. Immunol.* **26,** 228–238.

Gutierrez, C., Howard, M., Gaspar, M. L., and Raveche, E. S. (1986). *Clin. Immunol. Immunopathol.* **39,** 319–328.

Hang, L., Aguado, M. T., Dixon, F. J., and Theofilopoulos, A. N. (1985). *J. Exp. Med.* **161,** 423–428.

Huang, Y. P., Perrin, L. H., Miescher, P. A., and Zubler, R. H. (1988). *J. Immunol.* **141,** 827–833.

Hudgins, C. C., Steinberg, R. T., Klinman, D. M., Reeves, J. P., and Steinberg, A. D. (1985). *J. Immunol.* **134,** 3849–3854.

Huston, D. P., Raveche, E. S., and Steinberg, A. D. (1980). *J. Immunol.* **124,** 1635–1641.

Ishigatsubo, Y., Steinberg, A. D., and Klinman, D. M. (1988). *Eur. J. Immunol.* **18,** 1089–1094.

Jyanouchi, H., Kimmel, M. D., Lee, G., Kincade, P. W., and Good, R. A. (1985). *J. Immunol.* **135,** 1891–1899.

Kastner, D. L., McIntyre, T. M., Mallett, C. P., Hartman, A. B., and Steinberg, A. D. (1989). *J. Immunol.* **143,** 2761–2767.

Kastner, D. L., and Steinberg, A. D. (1988). *Concepts Immunopathol.* **6,** 22–88.

Katagiri, T., Cohen, P. L., and Eisenberg, R. A. (1988). *J. Exp. Med.* **167,** 741–751.

Klassen, L. W., Krakauer, R. S., and Steinberg, A. D. (1977). *J. Immunol.* **119,** 830–837.
Klinman, D. M., and Steinberg, A. D. (1987a). *J. Immunol.* **139,** 2284–2289.
Klinman, D. M., and Steinberg, A. D. (1987b). *J. Exp. Med.* **165,** 1755–1760.
Klinman, D. M., Ishigatsubo, Y., and Steinberg, A. D. (1988a). *J. Immunol.* **141,** 801–806.
Klinman, D. M., Ishigatsubo, Y., and Steinberg, A. D. (1988). *Cell. Immuno.* **117,** 360–368.
Klinman, D. M., Eisenberg, R. A., and Steinberg, A. D. (1990). *J. Immunol.* **144,** 506–511.
Klinman, D. M. (1990). *J. Clin. Invest.* **86,** 1249–1254.
Kofler, R., Noonan, D. J., Levy, D. E., Wilson, M. C., Moller, N. P. H., Dixon, F. J., and Theofilopoulos, A. N. (1985). *J. Exp. Med.* **161,** 805–815.
Kotzin, B. L., Kappler, J. W., Marrack, P. C., and Herron, L. R. (1989). *J. Immunol.* **143,** 89–94.
Krieg, A. M., Gourley, M. F., and Steinberg, A. D. (1991). *J. Immunol.* **146,** 3002–3005.
Krisher, K., and Cunningham, M. W. (1985). *Science* **227,** 413–415.
Kumagai, S., Steinberg, A. D., and Green, I. (1981a). *J. Clin. Invest.* **67,** 605–614.
Kumagai, S., Steinberg, A. D., and Green, I. (1981b). *J. Immunol.* **128,** 258–262.
Lane, J. R., Neumann, D. A., LaFond-Walker, A., Herskowitz, A., and Rose, N. R. (submitted for publication).
Laskin, C. A., Taurog, J. D., Smathers, P. A., and Steinberg, A. D. (1981). *J. Immunol.* **127,** 1743–1747.
Laskin, C. A., Smathers, P. A., Reeves, J. P., and Steinberg, A. D. (1982). *J. Exp. Med.* **155,** 1025–1036.
Laskin, C. A., Smathers, P. A., Lieberman, R., and Steinberg, A. D. (1983). *J. Immunol.* **131,** 1121–1125.
Laskin, C. A., Haddad, G., and Soloninka, C. A. (1986). *J. Immunol.* **137,** 1867–1873.
Lehman, K. R., Kotzin, B. L., Portanova, J. P., and Santoro, T. J. (1986). *Eur. J. Immunol.* **16,** 1105–1110.
Manny, N., Datta, S. K., and Schwartz, R. S. (1979). *J. Immunol.* **122,** 1220–1227.
Marion, T. N., Bothwell, A. L. M., Briles, D. E., and Janeway, C. A., Jr. (1989). *J. Immunol.* **142,** 4269–4274.
Mendlovic, S., Fricke, H., Shoenfeld, Y., and Mozes, E. (1989). *Eur. J. Immunol.* **19,** 729–734.
Mihara, M., Ohsugi, Y., Saito, K., Miyai, T., Togashi, M., Ono, S., Murakami, S., Dobashi, K., Hirayama, F., and Hamaoka, T. (1988). *J. Immunol.* **141,** 85–90.
Miller, Raveche, E. S., Laskin, C. A., Klinman, D. M., and Steinberg, A. D. (1984). *J. Immunol.* **133,** 1325–1331.
Morimoto, C., Reinherz, E. L., Distaso, J. A., Steinberg, A. D., and Schlossman, S. F. (1984). *J. Clin. Invest.* **73,** 689–700.
Morton, J. I., and Siegel, B. V. (1974a). *Proc. Natl. Acad. Sci. U.S.A.* **71,** 2162–2165.
Morton, J. I., and Seigel, B. V. (1974b). *Transplantation* **17,** 624–626.
Morton, R. O., Goodman, D. G., Gershwin, M. E., Derkay, C., Squire, R. A., and Steinberg, A. D. (1976). *Arthritis Rheum.* **19,** 1347–1350.
Moutsopoulos, H. M., Boehm-Truitt, M., Kassan, S. S., and Chused, T. M. (1977). *J. Immunol.* **119,** 1639–1644.
Murakawa, Y., Takada, S., Ueda, Y., Suzuki, N., Hoshino, T., and Sakane, T. (1985). *J. Immunol.* **134,** 187–193.
Murphy, E. D., and Roths, J. B. (1979). *Arthritis Rheum.* **22,** 1188–1191.
Nelson, J. L., and Steinberg, A. D. (1987). *In* "Hormones and Immunity" (I. Berczi and K. Kobazs, eds.), pp. 93–119. M. P. Press, Lancaster, Pennsylvania.
Perkins, D. L., Glaser, R. M., Mahon, C. A., Michaelson, J., and Marshak-Rothstein, A. (1990). *J. Immunol.* **145,** 549–555.

Prud'homme, G. J., Fieser, T. M., Dixon, F. J., and Theofilopolous, A. N. (1984). *Immunol. Rev.* **78,** 159–183.

Ramsdell, F., and Fowlkes, B. J. (1990). *Science* **248,** 1342–1348.

Ranney, D. F., and Steinberg, A. D. (1976). *J. Immunol.* **117,** 1219–1225.

Raveche, E. S., Novotny, E. A., Hansen, C. T., Tijo, J. H., and Steinberg, A. D. (1981). *J. Exp. Med.* **153,** 1187–1197.

Rosenberg, Y., Steinberg, A. D., Santoro, T. (1984). *Immunol. Today* **5,** 64–67.

Rosenberg, Y. *et al.,* (1986). *Ann. N.Y. Acad. Sci.* **475,** 251.

Sakane, T., Steinberg, A. D., and Green, I. (1978). *Arthritis Rheum.* **21,** 657–664.

Sakane, T., Steinberg, A. D., Reeves, J. P., and Green, I. (1979). *J. Clin. Invest.* **63,** 954–965.

Santoro, T. J., Malek, T. R., Rosenberg, Y. L., Morse, H. C., III, and Steinberg, A. D. (1984). *J. Mol. Cell. Immunol.* **1,** 347–356.

Santoro, T. J., Luger, T. A., Ravache, E. S., Smolen, J. S., and Steinberg, A. D. (1983). *Eur. J. Immunol.* **13,** 601–4.

Schlomchik, M. J., Marshak-Rothstein, A., Wolfowicz, C. B., Rothstein, T. L., and Weigert, M. G. (1987a). *Nature* **328,** 805–811.

Schlomchik, M. J., Aucoin, A. H., Pisetsky, D. S., and Weigert, M. G. (1987b). *Proc. Natl. Acad. Sci. U.S.A.* **84,** 9150–9154.

Scribner, C. L., and Steinberg, A. D. (1988). *Clin. Immunol. Immunopathol.* **49,** 133–142.

Seldin, M. F., Conroy, J., Steinberg, A. D., D'Hoosteleare, L. A., and Raveche, E. S. (1987). *J. Exp. Med.* **166,** 1585–1590.

Schultz, L. D., Bailey, C. L., and Coman, D. R. (1983). *Exp. Hematol.* **11,** 667–680.

Smathers, P. A., Santoro, T. J., Chused, T. M., Reeves, J. P., and Steinbèrg, A. D. (1984). *J. Immunol.* **133,** 1955–1961.

Smith, H. R., and Steinberg, A. D. (1983). *Annu. Rev. Immunol.* **1,** 175–210.

Sobel, E. S., Katagiri, T., Katagiri, K., Morris, S. C., Cohen, P. L., and Eisenberg, R. A. (1991). *J. Exp. Med.* 1441–1449.

Steinberg, A. D., Baron, S., and Talal, N. (1969). *Proc. Natl. Acad. Sci. U.S.A.* **63,** 1102–1107.

Steinberg, A. D., Kaltreider, H. B., Staples, P. J., Goetzl, E. J., Talal, N., and Decker, J. L. (1971). *Ann. Intern. Med.* **75,** 165–171.

Steinberg, A. D., Huston, D. P., Taurog, J. D., Cowdery, J. S., and Raveche, E. S. (1981). *Immunol. Rev.* **55,** 121–154.

Steinberg, A. D., Raveche, E. S., Laskin, C. A., Smith, H. R., Santoro, T. J., Miller, M. L., and Plotz, P. H. (1984). *Ann. Intern. Med.* **100,** 714–727.

Steinberg, A. D., Krieg, A. M., Gourley, M. F., and Klinman, D. M. (1990). *Immunol. Rev.* **118,** 129–163.

Steinberg, A. D., Triem, K., Smith, H. A., Laskin, C. A., Rosenberg, Y. J., Klinman, D. K., Mushinski, J. F., and Mountz, J. D. (1986). *Ann. N.Y. Acad. Sci.* **475,** 200–218.

Steinberg, A. D. (1979). *Ann. Intern. Med.* **91,** 587–604.

Steinberg, A. D. (1980). *In* "Strategies of Immune Regulation" (E. E. Sercarz, ed.), pp. 377, 503. Academic Press, New York.

Steinberg, A. D. (1987). *Ann. Intern. Med.* **106,** 709–794.

Steinberg, A. D. (1989). *J. Immunol.* **143,** 3858–3863.

Steinberg, A. D., and Steinberg, S. C. (1991). *Arthritis Rheum.* **34,** 945–950.

Steinberg, A. D., Gourley, M. F., Klinman, D. M., Tsokos, G. C., Scott, D. E., and Krieg, A. M. (1991). *Ann. Intern. Med.* **115,** 548–549.

Taurog, J. D., Raveche, E. S., Smathers, P. A., Glimcher, L. H., Huston, D. P., Hansen, C. J., and Steinberg, A. D. (1981). *J. Exp. Med.* **153,** 221–234.

Theofilopoulos, A. N., and Dixon, F. J. (1985). *Adv. Immunol.* **37,** 269–390.

Theofilopoulos, A. N., and Dixon, F. J. (1981). *Immunol. Rev.* **55,** 179–211.
Umland, S. P., Go, N. F., Cupp, J. E., and Howard, M. (1989). *J. Immunol.* **142,** 1528–1535.
Weigle, W. O. (1973). *Adv. Immunol.* **16,** 122.
Wofsy, D., Ledbedder, J. A., and Hendler, P. L. *et al.* (1985). *J. Immunol.* **134,** 852–857.
Wofsy, D., and Seaman, W. E. (1987). *J. Immunol.* **138,** 3247–3253.

CHAPTER **5**

Molecular Genetics of Autoimmunity

GERALD T. NEPOM
PATRICK CONCANNON
Immunology and Diabetes Research Programs
Virginia Mason Research Center
Department of Immunology
University of Washington School of Medicine
Seattle, Washington

I. THE HUMAN LEUKOCYTE ANTIGEN COMPLEX

A. Introduction

Structural genes for human leukocyte antigen (HLA) molecules lie within the major histocompatibility complex on the chromosome 6. The HLA class I loci (HLA-A, HLA-B, HLA-C, HLA-E, HLA-F, HLA-G) encode glycoproteins which, when complexed with β2 microglobulin, form an intact HLA class I molecule (Koller *et al.*, 1987). The HLA-A, HLA-B, HLA-C molecules are the major transplantation antigens in man, and are highly polymorphic (Parham *et al.*, 1988). In other words, multiple allelic variants occur in the population for each of these three loci, accounting for much of the genetic diversity responsible for histoincompatibility. Class I molecules are found on the cell surface of all nucleated cells; in normal and autoimmune responses, the class I molecules act as restriction elements essential for co-recognition by CD8-positive T lymphocytes.

There are 14 HLA class II loci, which cluster into three regions, known as DR, DQ, and DP (Bodmer, 1984). Each of these regions contains at least one α gene and one β gene, each of which encodes a class II polypeptide. The intact class II molecule is a dimer consisting of the products of one α gene and one β gene, expressed as a membrane-bound protein (Kaufman *et al.*, 1984). Class II molecules are found on B lymphocytes, monocytes, activated T cells, and, with appropriate induction, on nonhematopoietic cells such as vascular endothelium, thyroid epithelium, glial cells, and numerous other tissues (Lee, 1989). The potential of class II molecules to be aberrantly expressed on nonlymphoid tissues is often thought to play a role in organ-specific autoimmunity.

Most of the class II loci are highly polymorphic. Allelic variation between class II molecules of different individuals accounts for the functional differences revealed by HLA typing specificities, allograft reactivity, and, most important, differential ability to bind antigenic peptides (McDevitt, 1986; Buus *et al.*, 1987; Nepom, 1989b). When expressed on the surface of antigen-presenting cells, the class II molecules present such peptides to CD4-positive T lymphocytes.

B. HLA and Disease Associations

A comprehensive listing published in 1985 identified 76 diseases, mostly autoimmune syndromes, associated with different HLA specificities (Tiwari and Terasaki, 1985). Each HLA specificity (i.e., B27, DR3, DR4) is a serologically defined marker present on one or more HLA molecules. Therefore, when a disease is associated with a particular HLA specificity, actually a number of genes are potentially responsible for the association. In order to discriminate between different genes that encode serologically cross-reactive HLA molecules, various molecular techniques have been successfully employed. Restriction fragment length polymorphism (RFLP) analysis provides a detailed catalog of linked polymorphic markers that can, in most cases, discriminate among haplotypes (Bidwell and Jarrold, 1986; Robinson *et al.*, 1988; Cox *et al.*, 1989). More recently, specific oligonucleotide probes have become widely used in hybridization analysis to discriminate specific polymorphic genes (Gorman *et al.*, 1982; Angelini *et al.*, 1986; LeGall *et al.*, 1986; Nepom *et al.*, 1986a; Amar *et al.*, 1987). The combination of oligonucleotide hybridization and gene amplification using the polymerase chain reaction brings this specific technology within reach of most laboratories (Saiki *et al.*, 1986; Horn *et al.*, 1988; Erlich *et al.*, 1990; Todd *et al.*, 1987; Morel *et al.*, 1988).

Since each HLA haplotype contains an entire set of closely linked genes, identifying a disease-associated polymorphism in one of those genes links susceptibility only with a cluster of HLA genes on that haplotype. Additional genetic analysis is then required to pinpoint actual susceptibility genes within such a linked cluster. Thus, analysis of HLA associations with disease proceeds in a step-wise progression: First, a serological or RFLP marker identifies an association with a disease; second, the haplotypes that carry that marker are defined; and third, individual HLA genes within the implicated haplotypes are sought as candidates contributing to pathogenesis. This process is illustrated for several of the best-studied examples of HLA associations with autoimmune disease. As will be discussed, individual HLA susceptibility genes are indeed known in a few autoimmune diseases; this new level of precision is important not only for identifying individuals at risk, but also because of the opportunity to test the functional role of these susceptibility gene products in models of disease.

C. Genetic Determinants of HLA Genes Associated with Autoimmunity

Figure 1 lists 20 of the most common class II HLA haplotypes in Caucasian populations. As illustrated, each haplotype can be defined by a unique set of linked alleles spanning the DQ and DR loci. The combination of specific alleles on a given haplotype defines a linkage group, which encodes class II molecules responsible for the associated HLA specificities. Each allele has a unique numerical designation, defined by an HLA nomenclature adopted in 1990; Fig. 1 lists the unique combinations of these linked alleles that define the basic HLA class II haplotypes.

These linkage relationships pose a problem for the analysis of HLA associations with disease. For example, autoimmune diseases such as Graves' disease, systemic lupus erythematosus, myasthenia gravis, celiac disease, and type I diabetes are all associated with the HLA-DR3(Dw3) specificities. As shown in Fig. 1, only one major Caucasian haplotype carries these specificities, made up of the linked DQ alleles, DQB1*0201, DQA1*0501, DRB1*0301. Which one of these genes is actually the responsible susceptibility gene for any of these diseases, however, is not known. Indeed, an as yet unidentified gene elsewhere on this haplotype linked to the DQ-DR cluster may well be responsible for the HLA-DR3 association with disease.

On the other hand, comparisons among linked genes on different haplotypes can also provide important insight into the actual molecular basis for HLA and disease associations. As can be seen from Fig. 1, most of the HLA specificities (i.e., DR2, DR4, DR6, DR7, DR8) occur on products of multiple haplotypes. Even within a single specificity, such as DR4, there may be six or more different haplotypes, each of which encodes a class II molecule that types as HLA-DR4 (Nepom, B. *et al.*, 1983; Nepom, G. *et al.*, 1984). In the case of HLA-DR4, the serologically defined DR4 epitope is a product of alleles at the DRB1 locus. The different DRB1 alleles that encode DR4-positive products are called *subtypes* of DR4, and include the *0401, *0402, *0403, *0404, and *0405 alleles. These DR4-positive DRB1 alleles differ from each other by between one and five amino acids, sufficient to account for major differences in immune recognition and disease associations (Gregersen *et al.*, 1986; Nepom *et al.*, 1986b). In addition, they are linked to other DQA1 and DQB1 genes as shown, providing further diversity within the DR4 family of haplotypes (Nepom, G. *et al.*, 1984; Nepom *et al.*, 1986c).

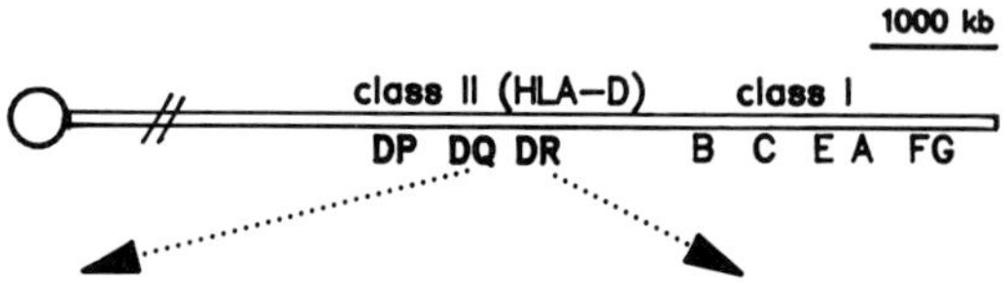

DQB 1	DQA 1	DRB 1	Associated HLA–DR specificity
0501	0101	0101(Dw1)	DR1
0602	0102	1501(Dw2)	
0601	0103	1502(Dw12)	DR2
0502	0102	1601(Dw21)	
0201	***0501***	0301(Dw3)	DR3
0301	0301	***0401 (Dw4)***	
0302	0301	***0401 (Dw4)***	
0302	0301	***0404 (Dw14)***	DR4
0301	0301	0403(Dw13)	
0302	0301	***0402 (Dw10)***	
0401	0301	0405(Dw15)	
0503	0101	1401(Dw9)	
0603	0103	1301(Dw18)	DR6
0604	0102	1302(Dw19)	
0301	***0501***	1101(Dw5)	DR5
0201	0201	0701(Dw7)	DR7
0303	0201	0701(Dw11)	
0402	0401	0801(Dw8)	DR8
0601	0103	0803(Dw8)	
0303	0301	0901(Dw23)	DR9
0501	0301	1001	DR10

FIG. 1 HLA class II haplotypes associated with autoimmunity. Linked genes within the HLA-DQ/DR interval define a series of discrete class II haplotypes. Several haplotypes are often associated with a single HLA serological specificity. Individual alleles within each haplotype are illustrated, using a consensus nomenclature adopted in 1990; the predominant Caucasian haplotypes are shown. As discussed in the text, the identification of an HLA-DR specificity associated with a disease is the first step in determining which specific haplotypes account for that disease association. Genes within those haplotypes can often then be pinpointed as the primary determinants of susceptibility. For several autoimmune diseases, individual alleles within specific haplotypes are directly implicated in disease susceptibility, some of which are highlighted in the figure: The DRB1 alleles *0401, *0404 (and possibly *0405) are candidate susceptibility genes in rheumatoid arthritis; the DRB1 allele *0402 and the DQB1 allele *0503 are candidate susceptibility genes in pemphigus vulgaris; the DQB1 allele *0302 is the predominant susceptibility gene in type I diabetes; and the DQA1 and DQB1 alleles that encode a DQw2 dimer, DQA1*0201 and DQB1*0501, are implicated in celiac disease.

These linkage relationships can be used to implicate specific genes in disease susceptibility. For instance, characterization of the DR and DQ linkage groups associated with type I diabetes has implicated both the DR3, Dw3 haplotype and also several of the DR4-positive haplotypes. However, all of the DR4-positive haplotypes associated with insulin-dependent diabetes mellitus (IDDM) carry a single allele at the DQB1 locus, the DQB1*0302 gene (previously termed DQ3.2). There are two DR4,Dw4-positive haplotypes, which differ only at the DQB1 locus. They are identical at DQA1 and DRB1 (Fig. 1). Since only the haplotype carrying the DQB1*0302 allele is associated with IDDM, this provided early evidence for the notion that, on DR4-positive haplotypes, the DQβ locus and not the DR locus was the primary determinant of genetic susceptibility (Holbeck and Nepom, 1988; Nepom, 1988).

It is important to note that the analysis of genetic associations with disease progresses from the identification of the specificity to the identification of a haplotype, and then to the characterization of individual susceptibility loci on that haplotype. Recognition of this progression reinforces the point that associations are haplotype specific. Thus, although the DQβ locus appears to account for the primary association of diabetes with HLA-DR4, it is completely unknown what locus accounts for the primary association of diabetes on other haplotypes, such as HLA-DR3. The best example of the haplotype-specific nature of genetic associations comes from the study of an autoimmune dermatologic disorder, pemphigus vulgaris. Pemphigus vulgaris is associated with both HLA-DR4 and HLA-DR6 (Szafer *et al.*, 1987; Scharf *et al.*, 1989). The DR4 association appears to be owing to genes within the DQ-DR linkage cluster on the DR4, Dw10 haplotype, but not on other DR4-positive haplotypes. Since the only class II gene within this cluster that is unique to the DR4,Dw10 haplotype is the DRB1*0402 gene, this is likely to be the important susceptibility gene on that haplotype (Scharf *et al.*, 1989). In contrast, the DR6 association with pemphigus is probably not attributable to genes at the DRB1 locus. Among the DR6-positive haplotypes, only the DR6,Dw9 DQ-DR linkage cluster is associated with this disease. Furthermore, detailed analysis of subtypes within the DR6, Dw9 cluster shows that only the DQB1*0503 allele predominates in DR6 patients. Thus, a likely interpretation is that the DQB1*0503 gene and the DRB1*0402 gene are independent susceptibility genes associated with pemphigus vulgaris. This example could establish an important lesson for other associations with autoimmune disease, namely that different loci on different haplotypes may account for susceptibility to the same disease.

The HLA class II molecule is a heterodimer, composed of one α and one β chain, which are encoded by distinct α and β genes, respectively. Thus, it is not surprising that, in some cases, susceptibility appears to be the result of combinations of α and β loci inherited together. Because HLA alleles are co-dominantly expressed, the α and β loci do not necessarily need to be linked on the same haplotype in order to form a class II heterodimer. The most straightforward example of this phenomenon appears to be the HLA-association with celiac disease (CD), a gluten enteropathy with autoimmune characteristics. It has been known for some time that most CD patients carry the DR3,Dw3 haplotype. Recently, several investigators have noted that the majority of non-DR3 patients with CD are heterozygous for DR5 and DR7 (Kagnoff *et al.*, 1989; Sollid *et al.*, 1989). Analysis of these DR5 and DR7 haplotypes has shown that, within the DQ/DR linkage cluster, the combination of a DR5,Dw5 and a DR7,Dw7 haplotype reconstitutes an intact αβ combination which is also found on DR3,Dw3 haplotypes. In other words, the same DQα and β chains that are encoded in cis on a DR3 haplotype (DQA1*0501, DQB1*0201) also occur in trans in a DR5/7 heterozygote, where the DR5 haplotype contributes the α chain, and the DR7 haplotype contributes the β chain. Taking this observation into account, more than 90% of the patients with celiac disease contain this one DQ heterodimer, suggesting that this indeed is a candidate susceptibility molecule potentially encoded by multiple haplotypes.

More subtle trans-associated effects are also seen in other autoimmune diseases. In type I diabetes, as mentioned above, the predominant class II gene accounting for the association with HLA-DR4 is a DQβ allele called DQB1*0302(DQ3.2). When this gene occurs on a DR4,Dw4 haplotype, it confers a relative risk for diabetes of 9.8. However, when the same gene occurs on this haplotype in a heterozygote who also carries a DR3,Dw3 haplotype, the relative risk for this heterozygous combination is 20 (Bertrams and Baur, 1984). This remarkable synergy occurs only in this particular combination of haplotypes, and has led to the notion that trans-associated DQ molecules may contribute synergistic risk for IDDM; in this view, the DQ3.2 β chain would pair in a dimer with a DQα chain from the DR3 haplotype, a pairing combination that indeed has been shown to form readily in heterozygous cells (Nepom *et al.*, 1987; Kwok *et al.*, 1988). A converse example is found in DR4/2 heterozygotes, who actually have a reduced relative risk for IDDM compared to that of the DR4 association alone (Thomson *et al.*, 1988). Although the mechanism for this relative protection is obscure (see the following sections), it emphasizes the level of detailed genetic analysis necessary to fully evaluate complex HLA associations with disease.

D. Candidate Susceptibility Genes

Most HLA genes have been sequenced, and comparison between susceptible and nonsusceptible alleles provides a useful method for focusing on the important structural elements within a gene that are associated with disease. This approach has been most extensively used for three well-known genetic associations: the association of HLA-B27 with ankylosing spondylitis, the association with DRβ genes in DR4-positive rheumatoid arthritis, and the association of DQβ genes in DR4-positive type I diabetes. Some of the important general features derived from these studies will be briefly reviewed here.

The major functional repercussions of the extreme allelic variability of HLA genes are seen in the ability of a given HLA molecule to bind and present an antigenic peptide. Many of the structural requirements for this peptide-binding function are now understood, based on the x-ray crystallographic analysis of the HLA-A2 and HLA-Aw68 class I molecules, derived in the laboratories of Wiley and Strominger (Bjorkman *et al.*, 1987). The most remarkable feature of the molecule is the presence of a deep 10 × 25 Ångstrom peptide-binding cleft, bordered on two sides by alpha-helical loops and supported by a *floor* consisting of a β-pleated sheet platformlike structure. Amino acid residues within the class I heavy chain (which lie on the alpha-helical loops bordering the peptide-binding cleft or which lie on the β-pleated sheet platform directly below the peptide-binding cleft) are likely to contact the antigenic fragment directly, and therefore may play a major role as genetic determinants of peptide interaction. In addition to peptide binding, polymorphic determinants on class I molecules also occur at sites responsible for associative recognition by the T-cell receptor. This suggests a direct mechanistic basis for the association of specific genetic polymorphisms with disease. On the one hand, disease-susceptibility alleles are predicted to contain specific amino acid polymorphisms, which restrict autoantigenic peptide binding. On the other hand, susceptibility alleles are predicted to contain specific amino acid polymorphisms that preferentially trigger autoreactive T cells. There is yet a third possibility, that the specific polymorphic sequences on susceptibility alleles mimic antigenic structures foreign to the immune system and can function as autoantigenic targets.

In the case of B27-associated disease, it is not known which of these mechanisms is most likely to play a major role. All of the HLA-B alleles that carry the B27 specificity carry a cysteine at residue 67 and a lysine at amino acid 70. These two substitutions are unique to the B27-positive alleles (Parham *et al.*, 1989). It is highly likely that these residues account for the serologic B27 specificity associated with these molecules and potentially for unique functional characteristics as well. At least six different B locus alleles carry these polymorphisms and are members of the B27 family of genes (Vega *et al.*, 1986). B27.1, B27.2, and B27.3 all differ from each other in the specific amino acid at codon 77. B27.4 differs from these other members of the B27 family at codons 114 and 116. Such substitutions can be functionally significant; T-cell clones that differentially recognize each of these different B27 alleles have been identified. Each of the B27 subtypes studied to date is associated with ankylosing spondylitis in different population groups; therefore, it is likely that the common genetic feature associated with disease is the B27 epitope itself, rather than any structural variation that distinguishes among the different B27-positive alleles (Breur-

Vriesendorp *et al.*, 1987). As already mentioned, this points to the region around residue 67 to 70 as a critical determinant of susceptibility. This corresponds to a region of the molecule located on the alpha-helical loop of the α1 domain, positioned to contact both peptide and T-cell receptor. It has also been pointed out that sequences within this region share considerable homology with proteins encoded by several bacteria, including some Klebsiella strains that have been epidemiologically linked to ankylosing spondylitis (Keat, 1986; Ewing *et al.*, 1990).

The same kind of structural analysis has been performed for class II molecules associated with some autoimmune diseases, notably the DRβ molecules associated with rheumatoid arthritis and the DQβ3.2 gene associated with type I diabetes. In the case of rheumatoid arthritis, there is once again a striking sequence homology in the region of amino acid 67 through 71 (of the DRB1 gene), which is implicated in disease susceptibility. A particular acidic sequence motif of Gln-Lys-Arg-Ala-Ala or Gln-Arg-Arg-Ala-Ala (QK/RRAA) occurs on disease-associated alleles at this position. DR4 subtypes that contain such a QK/RRAA sequence in this region are associated with rheumatoid arthritis (RA), whereas DR4 subtypes with amino acid variability in this region are not (Nepom *et al.*, 1986b; Nepom *et al.*, 1989a; Gregersen *et al.*, 1987). As with the B27-specific polymorphisms, however, the exact functional significance of these sequences is not known, since residues within this 67 to 71 region are likely to contact both peptide and T-cell receptor. This QK/RRAA epitope has been shown to function as a discrete T-cell recognition element in its ability to stimulate alloreactive T-cell clones, and site-directed mutagenesis within this region ablates T-cell reactivity (Seyfried *et al.*, 1987; Hiraiwa *et al.*, 1990).

Another striking feature of this epitope sequence suggests that it is the primary HLA genetic unit associated with RA. This QK/RRAA sequence occurs not only on the RA-associated subtypes of DR4, but also on two other unrelated DRB1 alleles, which also occur in patients with RA. These are the DRB1*0101 allele, found on some DR1,Dw1 haplotypes (Schiff *et al.*, 1982), and the DRB1*1402 allele, found on the DR6,Dw16 haplotype, which is very rare in Caucasians, but prevalent among Native American populations (Willkens *et al.*, 1990). Remarkably, when populations that have a low incidence of HLA-DR4 are studied for the incidence of RA, HLA genetic associations are indeed found, and these HLA associations are to the HLA-DR1 and/or HLA-DR6, Dw16 haplotypes. In other words, the QK/RRAA epitope sequences are associated with RA not only in DR4-positive haplotypes but also in non-DR4-positive haplotypes.

It is tempting, but not always possible, to apply the same kind of sequence-comparison analysis to other HLA susceptibility genes. In the case of type I diabetes, the most prevalent susceptibility gene is the DQB1*0302(DQ3.2) allele. This allele differs in six amino acids from a closely related gene, DQB1*0301, which is not associated with IDDM. Four of these amino acid changes occur in positions within the polymorphic first domain of the molecule, at codons 13, 26, 45, and 57 (Holbeck and Nepom, 1988; Michelsen and Lernmark, 1987). These sites of amino acid polymorphism are scattered, and are likely to function not as a discrete epitope but as a coordinated set of structural determinants of peptide binding. One of these specific polymorphic amino acids, at codon 57, has been proposed as a primary determinant of susceptibility to IDDM: The *Codon 57 hypothesis* proposes that the presence of an aspartic acid at codon 57 of the DQβ gene protects individuals from IDDM (Todd *et al.*, 1987). This hypothesis is extrapolated from the observation that haplotypes that carry a DQβ allele positive for an aspartic acid at codon 57 are negatively associated with IDDM. Several studies have confirmed this finding in some Caucasian haplotypes, although not in Oriental diabetics (Awata *et al.*, 1990). However, even among Caucasians, many patients with IDDM carry at least one Asp-57-positive *protective* allele (Rønningen *et al.*, 1989; Baisch *et al.*, 1990; Erlich *et al.*, 1990). Thus, in contrast to the QK/RRAA epitope association with RA discussed above, there are many exceptions to the codon 57 association with IDDM. Furthermore, in family studies analyzed for segregation of Asp-57-positive DQβ alleles, an equal number of affected and unaffected siblings shared such haplotypes, inconsistent with the hypothesis that dominant protection is conferred by an Asp-57-positive DQ gene (Nepom and Robinson, 1990). The most likely interpretation that reconciles the codon 57 hypothesis with the combined data set is to treat the presence of an aspartic acid at DQβ codon 57 as a linked marker, albeit within the coding region, for certain haplotypes. Since haplotypes that lack Asp-57-DQβ include DR4,DQ3.2, and DR3,DQw2, this codon 57 polymorphism is a convenient marker that identifies most of the known susceptible haplotypes in Caucasians; however, it is apparent that the residue at codon 57 does not itself account for genetic susceptibility to IDDM. Using site-directed mutagenesis, Kwok *et al.* (1990) have shown that recognition by T-cell clones specific for DQ3.2 is heavily influenced by multiple polymorphic sites on the β chain. In these studies, the residue at codon 57 contributes in a significant way to interactions between polymorphic DQα chains and recognition of specific sites on the β chain. Thus, a likely mechanistic interpretation would be that the residue at codon 57, in concert with other polymorphic sites in the class II molecule, forms a composite class II recognition element permissive for IDDM.

The role of specific class II polymorphisms present in IDDM-associated alleles, such as codon 57, may be quite different from the role of other polymorphisms more directly implicated in disease susceptibility, such as the QK/RAA sequence in RA. In the latter case, the disease-associated sequence is a linear epitope recognized directly by T cells; in contrast, the DQβ polymorphisms associated with IDDM predominantly influence peptide recognition and DQ α/β dimer interchain interactions. This difference suggests that the genetically mediated pathways of disease susceptibility may differ in these two diseases, and helps identify important mechanistic considerations involving T-cell receptors and/or peptides involved in pathogenesis.

As these examples illustrate, the detailed structural features of individual class II molecules provide important clues that reflect the functional properties of each allele. Immunological models to explain how these structural details lead to disease susceptibility rely on the binding of an autoantigenic peptide and/or the triggering of autoreactive T-cell clones; Thus, the class II molecule is but one element of an intermolecular interaction that needs to be more fully understood, and whose specific contribution to pathogenic events is likely to differ for different diseases. In the next section we shall examine the second key genetic element in this interaction, the T-cell receptor.

II. T-CELL RECEPTOR GENES AND AUTOIMMUNE DISEASE

A. The α/β T-Cell Receptor

The human T-cell receptor (TcR) responsible for HLA-restricted antigen recognition is a disulfide-linked heterodimer made up of α and β chains, each of approximately 45 kDa molecular mass. The receptor is present on the surface of greater than 90% of human peripheral T cells and is expressed as part of a receptor complex that includes the various subunits of the CD3 molecule as well as accessory molecules such as CD4 or CD8 (for review, see Allison and Lanier 1987; Clevers *et al.*, 1988). However, despite the large number of molecules involved in making up this complex, DNA transfection studies clearly demonstrate that the specificity of a given T cell is conferred exclusively by the structure of the TcR α and β chains that it expresses (Dembic *et al.*, 1986). In light of the specificity of the immune response characteristic of many autoimmune diseases, the known HLA associations, and the necessity of physical interaction between HLA molecules and TcR in an immune response, knowledge of the nature of the repertoire of TcR molecules in patients with autoimmune disease may be of critical importance in understanding the disease processes.

B. Organization of the TcR Genes

In contrast to HLA molecules, which display great diversity at the population level as a result of extensive polymorphism, TcR molecules must be capable of tremendous structural diversity within a single organism in order to recognize the diverse world of potential foreign antigens. To generate this diversity, TcRs employ many of the molecular mechanisms first observed in studies of immunoglobulins. TcR α and β chains have specialized amino terminal variable (V) regions involved in antigen recognition, and carboxyl terminal constant (C) regions involved in membrane anchoring and signal transduction. The genes that encode the TcR chains are arranged in germline DNA as discontinuous gene segments, which are juxtaposed to create a functional TcR gene through a process of specific chromosomal rearrangement during T-cell ontogeny. A functional TcRα gene is assembled from a single variable gene segment (Vα), a joining gene segment (Jα), and a constant region gene (Cα). Likewise, a functional TcRβ gene is assembled from one variable gene segment (Vβ), a diversity gene segment (Dβ), a joining gene segment (Jβ), and a constant region gene. In addition to the combinatorial possibilities available through recombining a wide variety of gene segments, somatic mechanisms, such as N-region and junctional diversification, act to provide an additional level of diversity to TcR molecules. Owing in part to the action of these somatic mechanisms, it is likely that every individual in the population, even identical twins, will have slightly different repertoires of TcR specificities (for review, see Wilson *et al.*, 1988).

1. The TcRβ Gene Complex

The human TcRβ chain genes are encoded in a complex on chromosome 7 band q35 (Isobe *et al.*, 1985). There are an estimated 80 Vβ gene segments scattered over most of the 1000 kilobases (kb) included in the complex (Kimura *et al.*, 1987; Lai *et al.*, 1988). The two Dβ gene segments, 13 functional Jβ gene segments, and two Cβ genes are clustered in a region of less than 20 kb at the 3′ end of the TcRβ complex (Toyonaga *et al.*, 1985).

Nucleotide sequences corresponding to more than 80 different human Vβ gene segments have been reported, and these sequences can be divided into 24 different subfamilies based on the criteria of 75% or greater shared nucleotide sequence homology (Ikuta *et al.*, 1985; Jones *et al.*, 1985; Yanagi *et al.*, 1985; Concannon *et al.*, 1986; Duby and Seidman, 1986; Kimura *et al.*, 1986; Leiden and Strominger, 1986; Siu *et al.*, 1986; Tillinghast *et al.*, 1986; Kimura *et al.*, 1987; Ferradini *et al.*, 1991; Robinson, 1991). Subfamilies are designated Vβ1-Vβ24 with individual member gene segments identified by a number after the decimal point (e.g., the Vβ2 subfamily contains two members, Vβ2.1 and Vβ2.2). A physical map of the TcRβ complex generated from deletion mapping, field inversion gel analysis, and cosmid walking has been constructed and contains approximately one half of the known Vβ gene segments (Lai *et al.*, 1988). Within the complex, gene segments of different subfamilies and of varying levels of sequence homology are highly interspersed. Therefore, members of a particular Vβ subfamily that share a high degree of sequence homology and might be expected to serve analogous functions in the immune response may not necessarily map near to each other.

2. The TcRα Complex

The human TcRα genes are encoded in a complex on chromosome 14 bands q11–12 (Croce *et al.*, 1985). There are 65 known Vα gene segments (although estimates indicate there may be as many as 100), 61 known Jα gene segments scattered over approximately 80 kb, and a single Cα gene (Jones *et al.*, 1985; Yanagi *et al.*, 1985; Yoshikai *et al.*, 1985; Yoshikai *et al.*, 1986; Kimura *et al.*, 1987; Klein *et al.*, 1987; Roman-Roman *et al.*, 1991). In addition, the genes encoding the delta chain of a second type of TcR, the gamma/delta receptor, are also encoded within the TcRα complex, between the Vα and Jα gene segments (Lai *et al.*, 1989).

Vα gene segments are also classified into subfamilies, according to the same criteria described above for Vβ gene segments, and utilize a similar nomenclature. There are 29 known human Vα subfamilies, but they contain relatively fewer gene segments than do comparable Vβ subfamilies, and presumably a number of Vα subfamilies remain, as yet, unidentified. A physical map of the TcRα complex comparable to that derived for the TcRβ complex has not yet been constructed. Data from pulsed-field gel analysis indicates that the gene complex must span approximately 1000 kb (Griesser *et al.*, 1988; Lai *et al.*, 1989). Only limited information derived from deletion mapping is available to map the physical relationships of the various Vα gene segments within the complex (Wilson *et al.*, 1988; Lai *et al.*, 1989).

C. Variation in the Germline TcR Gene Repertoire

Polymorphism of genes in the HLA complex was originally detected with serologic reagents that identified variants later subjected to detailed molecular analysis. Unfortunately, it has proven more difficult to develop antibodies directed against TcR variable regions in order to carry out a similar analysis. Only one antibody, which detects a polymorphic determinant on a particular human V gene segment, has been described. Subsequent nucleotide sequence analysis has mapped this determinant to one of two amino acid substitutions in the Vβ6.7 gene segment (Li *et al.*, 1990). In the absence of serologically defined alleles, molecular approaches will be necessary in order to carry out a thorough assessment of germline polymorphism of TcR genes. Given the potentially large numbers of V gene segments, such analysis represents a formidable task.

There are a number of possible sources of immunologically significant polymorphism of TcR genes, and, as with HLA, additional combinatorial diversity is available because of the heterodimeric nature of the molecule. One simple source of variation in the germline repertoire of V gene segments might be through variation in the number of gene segments as a result of deletions or duplications.

For example, in studies of laboratory and wild mice, deletions of Vα and Vβ gene segments have been reported in a number of strains (Behlke *et al.*, 1986; Klotz *et al.*, 1989; Jouvin-Marche *et al.*, 1989). However, Southern blotting studies utilizing gene-segment probes representative of 14 Vβ and 10 Vα subfamilies to probe human genomic DNA from large numbers (>100) of individuals have failed to reveal more than a few isolated examples of variation in the number of human V gene segments (Concannon *et al.*, 1987; Wright, Hood, and Concannon, in press, 1991).

Such an analysis by Southern blotting is effective for detecting variation in gene segment number but is relatively insensitive to polymorphism resulting from nucleotide substitutions within the coding regions of gene segments. Nevertheless, simple coding region substitutions may have important structural and immunological consequences. Some molecular studies to assess the level of sequence polymorphism in individual V genes have been carried out. Nucleotide sequence analysis of alleles of the Vβ1 gene has revealed an amino acid substitution that is tightly linked to a TaqI RFLP (Robinson, 1989). Similarly, nucleotide sequence analysis of the Vα21 gene segment has identified a rare variant containing a nonsense mutation as well as several common alleles that differ because of silent nucleotide substitutions (Wright, Hood, and Concannon, in press). These isolated examples suggest that, while variation in gene segment number appears to be uncommon in human populations, there exists some level of coding-region polymorphism, not well characterized as yet, which can contribute to genetic differences in the TcR repertoire between individuals in human populations.

By far the most common form of polymorphism observed in the human TcR gene complexes is RFLPs. In general, these polymorphisms lie outside of known coding regions. Nevertheless, they provide useful markers for following the genetic inheritance of these immunologically important loci, and allow the construction and characterization of haplotypes even in the absence of knowledge of specific V gene polymorphism.

D. Disease Association Studies with TcR RFLPs

1. Population-Based Studies

HLA molecules with their bound peptide antigens and the variable regions of TcR molecules must physically interact in the course of an immune response. As indicated in Section I of this chapter, polymorphism of HLA molecules can play an important role in susceptibility to autoimmune diseases. However, in many cases, inheritance of predisposing HLA alleles cannot account for all of the genetic susceptibility to a particular disease. These observations, among others, have led a number of investigators to test the hypothesis that genetic variation in the germline TcR repertoire might play a similar predisposing role in autoimmune disease.

The association between HLA alleles and susceptibility to certain autoimmune diseases was first observed in population-based disease-association studies. In these studies, the frequencies of alleles at a given locus are measured in a disease population and compared to those from a matched healthy control group. Depending on the degree of linkage disequilibrium between the polymorphic locus studied and other loci in the region, the marker does not necessarily have to be the gene responsible for disease susceptibility, but could serve simply as a marker for other genes being carried on a particular haplotype. Strong linkage disequilibrium between alleles at different loci in the HLA complex has been a hallmark of disease-association studies with HLA genes, and has necessitated an approach in which whole haplotypes are considered, as discussed in Section I. Therefore, by analogy to HLA, the existence of RFLPs among, but not necessarily within, the TcRα and TcRβ genes suggests the opportunity to test for possible genetic associations between autoimmune diseases and TcR genes. Some of the diseases that have been studied for TcR gene associations include ankylosing spondylitis (Durand *et al.*, 1988), autoimmune hyperthyroidism (Weetman *et al.*, 1987), Graves' disease (Demaine *et al.*, 1987; Weetman *et al.*, 1987), IDDM (Hoover *et al.*, 1987; Martell *et al.*, 1987; Millward *et al.*, 1987; Ito *et al.*, 1988; Sheehy *et al.*, 1989; Concannon *et al.*, 1990; Niven *et al.*, 1990), membranous nephropathy (Demaine *et al.*, 1988; Niven *et al.*, 1990), multiple sclerosis (MS) (Martell *et al.*, 1987; Oksenberg *et al.*, 1988, 1989; Beall *et al.*, 1989; Seboun *et al.*, 1989; Fugger *et al.*, 1990), myasthenia gravis (Smith *et al.*, 1987; Oksenberg *et al.*, 1988, 1989), rheumatoid arthritis (Gao *et al.*, 1988), and systemic lupus erythematosus (Fronek *et al.*, 1986; Wong *et al.*, 1988; Perl *et al.*, 1989). Two of the most extensively studied of these disorders are MS and IDDM. Table I summarizes the results of population-association studies of these two diseases, which are typical of results obtained for many of the others cited above.

The results in Table I are difficult to interpret for a number of reasons. First, there are conflicting results arising from different investigations. This is not unexpected in population studies, which are, in general, only suggestive of the existence of disease-susceptibility genes. Differences from one study to another may be attributable to a variety of causes, including clinical heterogeneity or the use of different sets of RFLP markers by different groups. Second, negative results from such studies must be treated cautiously, since they might reflect either the absence of a nearby disease-susceptibility locus, or simply the absence of sufficient linkage disequilibrium to detect such a locus. Third, these studies are of relatively limited resolution compared to analogous HLA studies. This is because most of the TcR RFLPs studied to date are biallelic or rarely triallelic. By contrast, HLA genes and their products are highly polymorphic and, therefore, carry a higher information content in genetic studies. Fourth, because of the

TABLE I
TcR Disease Associations

	Disease			
Disease	HLA association	TcR marker	Assocation	Study
Multiple sclerosis	DR2	Vβ	+	Beall *et al.* (1989)
		Vβ	−	Fugger *et al.* (1990)
		Cβ	−	Martell *et al.* (1987)
		Cβ	−	Oksenberg *et al.* (1988)
		Vα	+	Oksenberg *et al.* (1989)
		Cα	+	Martell (1987)
Insulin-dependent diabetes mellitus (IDDM)	DR3,DR4	Cβ	+	Hoover *et al.* (1987)
		Cβ	+	Millward *et al.* (1987)
		Cβ	+	Ito *et al.* (1988)
		Cβ	−	Martell *et al.* (1987)
		Cβ	−	Niven *et al.* (1990)
		Cα	−	Hoover *et al.* (1987)

known HLA associations for many autoimmune diseases, it may be necessary to stratify the TcR marker data by HLA type in order to see an association.

2. Multiple Sclerosis

An examination of the studies in Table I highlights many of the difficulties with population-based disease-association studies involving TcR genes. In the case of MS, four studies have been reported utilizing markers in the TcRβ locus. Two studies, by Beall *et al.* (1989) and Fugger *et al.* (1990) employ the same set of Vβ markers but yield different results. However, the studies may not be comparable for clinical reasons, as one study focuses on patients diagnosed as chronic progressive MS and the other, on relapsing–remitting MS patients. The study by Beall *et al.* (1989) also demonstrates an effect of stratification by HLA type, as the reported TcR association is stronger in DR2-positive MS patients. Two additional studies utilize only Cβ markers (Martell *et al.*, 1987; Oksenberg *et al.*, 1988). These studies are negative, and, therefore, are at odds with the Vβ study of Beall *et al.* (1989). The use of RFLPs detected with the Cβ probe in these studies and in many of the other cited disease studies raises an important question. Since the constant region is unlikely to be involved directly in antigen recognition and therefore in disease pathogenesis, it must be assumed that this marker is serving as a haplotype marker via linkage disequilibrium with the nearby V genes. However, in the case of the TcRβ complex, for which mapping data is available, many of the Vβ gene segments are physically far removed from

Cβ and might not be expected to be in linkage disequilibrium with the Cβ RFLPs.

Confirmation of the presence of a disease-susceptibility gene in the TcRα or TcRβ complexes requires a formal demonstration of linkage between the TcR complex and the disease of interest. Classically, this requires family studies. A limited number of such studies have been carried out with regard to the TcRα and TcRβ genes. These studies have employed the method of affected-sib-pair analysis as was previously used to confirm HLA associations with various autoimmune diseases. In such a study, the investigator uses one or several markers that allow the independent identification of each of the four parental haplotypes in a family. The segregation of these haplotypes is followed in multiplex disease families, and statistical tests are applied to determine whether affected siblings preferentially share parental haplotypes for the markers in question. Such studies have a number of significant advantages for studying the inheritance of the TcR gene complexes. First, it is not necessary to specify the mode of inheritance in advance. Second, these studies assay haplotype sharing without regard to the exact nature of the haplotype itself. Therefore, in a case such as the TcRβ gene complex, the investigator can use multiple genetic markers in order to make most of the families studied informative. These data can then be pooled, since the chances of encountering a recombinant in the complex in one of the families under study is relatively low ($\leqslant 1\%$). In contrast, in a population study, even such low levels of recombination would be sufficient to randomly assort the alleles of different markers within the gene complex. Using affected-sib-pair analysis, Seboun *et al.* (1989) were able to avoid many of the pitfalls of the population studies cited in Table I, and provide strong evidence for an MS-susceptibility gene in or near the TcRβ complex. In addition, one particular TcRβ haplotype was observed to be over-represented in MS patients compared to their unaffected sibs and provides an important target for future investigations.

3. Insulin-Dependent Diabetes Mellitus

Table I also summarizes the results of population-based association studies with TcR genes in another autoimmune disease, IDDM. All of the studies reported use RFLPs detected with C gene probes, five with Cβ and one with Cα. The positive associations reported for Cβ in three of the studies, Hoover *et al.* (1987), Millward *et al.* (1987), and Ito *et al.* (1988), were revealed by stratification of the TcR data according to HLA type. In at least one case, Niven *et al.* (1990), negative results were also obtained from a data set stratified by HLA type. Because of the consistent use of C gene probes, all of these studies are open to the question of whether this choice of marker is suitable to infer information regarding V gene inheritance.

In order to test the hypothesis that inheritance of TcRα or TcRβ genes is involved in the pathogenesis of IDDM, affected-sib-pair studies in multiplex IDDM families have been carried out. Contrary to the results of the population studies in Table I, neither the TcRα (Sheehy *et al.*, 1989; Concannon *et al.*, 1990) nor TcRβ (Concannon *et al.*, 1990) gene complexes show a statistically significant association with IDDM in family studies. Therefore, in IDDM, unlike MS, family studies were unable to confirm population-based associations. Furthermore, in only two of the studies of MS or IDDM was there concordance between data collected in population studies with a Cβ probe and the results of family studies.

4. TcR Haplotypes

Many of these issues hinge on the question of the extent of linkage disequilibrium that exists between various RFLP markers within the TcRα and TcRβ complexes. If linkage disequilibrium is strong, then a limited number of haplotypic combinations of markers will exist, and the use of one or a limited number of markers in a population-based disease-association study would be justified. Conversely, if the alleles at various marker loci are randomly associated with each other such that there are many haplotypic combinations in the population, then the testing of many markers will be required, and the ability to exclude association greatly reduced. While it is possible to use studies of multiplex disease families, as in the cited examples of MS and IDDM, to avoid this problem, the resources to carry out such studies may not be available for all autoimmune diseases.

One way to address this issue is to directly determine the frequencies of particular haplotypes by segregation studies of markers in normal families. This information can then be used to guide the selection of markers for population-based disease-association studies. An initial step toward defining the haplotypic relationships between various TcRβ RFLP markers has been taken by Charmley and co-workers (Charmley *et al.*, 1990). In their studies they tested the segregation of eight different RFLPs in the TcRβ complex, six defined by different Vβ gene segment probes, and two defined by Cβ gene probes. The segregation patterns of these RFLPs were followed in 40 large families of predominantly northern European Caucasian ancestry containing a total of 530 members. The results of these studies have important implications for disease-association studies of the TcRβ complex. First, they concluded that the vast majority of Vβ gene segments are not in linkage disequilibrium with the known Cβ RFLPs. Therefore, population-based studies utilizing Cβ RFLPs alone are unlikely to detect disease associations to the TcRβ complex and are incapable of excluding them. Second, they observed statistically significant linkage disequilibrium only between physically adjacent pairs of Vβ RFLP marker loci. Therefore, it should be possible to carry out a systematic search for population-based disease associations with genes in the TcRβ complex by utilizing a panel of well-spaced markers of known linkage relationship. Such a study would then have a strong likelihood of detecting an association if it existed or of excluding one if it did not. Similar results might be expected from an analysis of the TcRα locus, since in a study of Vα RFLP markers in normal families, Robinson (1987) observed a variety of different haplotypes, suggesting frequent genetic recombination within the TcRα complex.

In addition to examining the frequencies of alleles at a panel of individual marker loci in disease studies, haplotypes can also be constructed in the absence of segregation data for individuals homozygous for all but one of a panel of linked markers studied. The frequencies of haplotypes in affected individuals can then be compared to the frequencies for normal individuals derived from segregation analysis, as previously described. While this approach can lead to a large reduction in the number of informative affected individuals in the study by excluding those that are heterozygous at multiple marker loci, it can sometimes reveal associations not detectable through the analysis of individual markers. For example, Beall *et al.* (1989), in their previously cited study of TcRβ complex RFLPs in MS patients, observed statistically significant differences only in TcRβ haplotype frequencies between their MS patient population and controls but not in the frequencies of alleles for any individual marker.

E. Summary

Compared to the study of HLA genes and disease, the study of TcR gene polymorphism and its impact on autoimmunity is in its infancy. While a great deal of basic information regarding TcR gene polymorphism remains to be determined, the tools are available to begin to assess the role of germline TcR repertoire variation in autoimmunity. Already these studies have provided strong evidence for a role of the TcRβ complex in susceptibility to multiple sclerosis, but many other putative associations remain to be investigated. It should be remembered, however, that the TcR repertoire is shaped by many factors that may not show direct genetic linkage to the TcR gene complexes themselves. Section III suggests some other possible roles for the TcR repertoire in autoimmune diseases.

III. HLA–T-CELL RECEPTOR INTERACTIONS

A. The Normal Immune Response

Disease-association studies such as those cited in Sections I and II have been instrumental in identifying inherited components of autoimmune disease susceptibility in the HLA complex and, to a lesser extent, in the TcR complexes.

Mechanisms of pathogenesis involving these gene complexes, however, remain unknown. Since a large number of HLA class II–associated autoimmune diseases are mediated by T cells, there are several opportunities for the products of HLA genes and of TcR genes to interact, at various biological sites, with important consequences for disease susceptibility.

The most obvious interaction between TcR and HLA molecules occurs in HLA-restricted antigen recognition, where an accessory cell such as a B cell or monocyte presents a complex of an HLA class II molecule with its bound peptide antigen to a mature T cell bearing a receptor specific for that HLA–antigen complex. This event occurs in the peripheral immune system, perhaps in the target organ itself, long after genetic and somatic factors have acted to shape the TcR repertoire of the individual. Presumably, in autoimmune diseases that are T-cell dependent, this event is the trigger for the autoimmune process. There is a requirement for great specificity at this step, based on the use of specific Vβ and Vα gene segments in the TcR; therefore, it provides a critical opportunity for therapeutic interruption of the disease process. Recent attempts at specific immunosuppression in experimental autoimmune diseases are based on this sort of *anti-Vβ therapy,* with promising results (Acha-Orbea *et al.*, 1988; Urban *et al.*, 1988; Zaller *et al.*, 1990).

A second type of interaction between HLA and TcRs occurs earlier, during the development of the immune system in a given individual, and results in a biasing or shaping of the T-cell repertoire in favor of T cells expressing receptors that can effectively recognize the complex of self-HLA and antigen in the periphery. This shaping of the repertoire represents a compromise between the dual needs of an individual to be able to respond effectively to all potential antigen challenges, and to avoid self-reactivity, that is, to be self-tolerant. As described in Section II, the potential repertoire of TcR specificities in an individual is dependent on the rearrangement of germline-encoded V, D, J, and C elements. The rearrangement of these gene segments occurs in immature T cells in the thymus, which subsequently express a mature TcR heterodimer on their cell surface. T cells expressing the α/β TcR heterodimer then undergo a selection process in the thymus based on their ability to interact with self-HLA molecules (or self-antigens bound to self-HLA) expressed on thymic epithelial cells. These self-HLA molecules, of course, are determined by the HLA haplotypes present in that individual; hence, this selection process results in a phenotype of a specific TcR repertoire, but is genetically dependent on HLA type.

Two types of selection events are thought to occur as T cells transit the thymus. First, T cells that are autoreactive and recognize self-antigens in the thymus with high affinity are deleted in a primary selection event known as negative selection (Kappler *et al.*, 1987; Marrack *et al.*, 1988). These cells fail to mature into functional T cells, and undergo a programmed cell death. Therefore, this negative selection plays a critical role in establishing self-tolerance. Second, T cells that are not deleted, but whose receptors still maintain the ability to interact with self-HLA molecules, are positively selected to differentiate and mature (Kisielow *et al.*, 1988; Teh *et al.*, 1988). It is these cells that ultimately exit the thymus and establish the peripheral T-cell repertoire. Both these negative and positive selection events, because of their dependence on specific HLA recognition, are potentially key factors in the generation of autoreactive TcR specificities contributing to autoimmune disease.

B. Autoimmune Disease

Both of the levels at which TcR and HLA can interact, thymic selection and peripheral recognition, are fundamental to our understanding of disease susceptibility. It is possible that in different autoimmune diseases, the critical HLA–TcR interactions may be entirely different. In some cases, the important recognition event may occur in the thymus, while in others, it may be in the peripheral lymphoid organs. Perhaps even more intriguing is the possibility that diseases which display multiple HLA associations, both positive and/or negative, may reflect the additive contributions of each of these types of HLA–TcR interaction. Consider, for example, the case of IDDM. As discussed in Sections I and II, IDDM is associated with the DQ3.2 molecule encoded on the DR4 haplotype and shows no apparent association with TcR alleles. Analysis of the relative risk for IDDM in individuals stratified according to the second HLA haplotype they carry (besides the DR4 DQ3.2 *susceptible haplotype*) clearly indicates that some haplotypes, such as DR3, have a synergistic effect in combination with DR4, while others, such as DR2Dw2, have a dominant protective effect (Thomson *et al.*, 1988).

In the context of HLA genes, *dominant protection* means that one HLA haplotype or gene, present in a heterozygote, prevents the expression of a disease-susceptibility phenotype attributed to the other HLA haplotype. The protective effect of DR2 in IDDM is such an example: Although individuals with the DQ3.2 gene have a relative risk of disease of approximately 8.0, DR2/DQ3.2 heterozygotes have a relative risk less than 1.0 (Baisch *et al.*, 1990). In considering HLA–TcR interactions, this dominant effect of certain HLA alleles might result from the negative selection of T cells described above. Therefore, it is appealing to hypothesize that the protective effect of DR2 in DR2/4 heterozygous individuals may reflect the elimination of potentially autoreactive T-cell clones during thymic maturation in the presence of HLA class II molecules expressed on the DR2 haplotype.

The enhancing effect of the DR3 haplotype in DR3/4 heterozygotes might also reflect HLA-TcR interactions during thymic selection events. On the one hand, a hypothesis consistent with negative selection is that regulatory T cells, capable of controlling potentially autoreactive T-cell clones, are eliminated during thymic maturation in the presence of molecules encoded on the DR3 haplotype. The role of the DQ3.2 molecule might then be in direct presentation of an islet cell antigen to autoreactive T cells, perhaps as a result of its aberrant expression on islet cells. On the other hand, there could be some specific interaction between DR3- and DR4-encoded molecules in the thymus that acts to positively select for autoreactive T cells, which are later stimulated in the periphery in association with a sequestered or occult antigen, basically increasing the precursor frequency of pathogenic T cells (and therefore the susceptibility) compared to a DR4/non-DR3 individual.

In each of these interaction models, although the key genetic event is the loss or gain of T cells expressing a particular class of TcR, the effect maps to the HLA locus, not the TcR loci. This is because the specificity of the interaction is dependent on the polymorphic sites of HLA molecules that account for self–nonself discrimination. This is an important consideration, and challenge, in the study of autoimmunity, since it identifies an important developmental pathway predisposing to disease susceptibility. This is not an isolated example, as other autoimmune diseases display multiple HLA associations, both positive and negative, similar to IDDM. For example, rheumatoid arthritis is positively associated with DR4 but negatively associated with DR2, while pemphigus vulgaris is positively associated with independent alleles at the DRβ and DQβ loci.

C. Future Directions

The nature of interactions involving HLA and TcR molecules discussed above suggests two different potential lines of investigation to elucidate the mechanisms of autoimmunity by working backward from genetically associated elements. First, in diseases where peripheral antigen recognition is the primary inciting event, a detailed understanding of the way in which the associated HLA and/or TcR molecules interact, even in the absence of knowledge of the relevant antigen, may help to identify critical structural features of the molecules involved in pathogenesis. Identification of a critical TcR, for example, might provide a specific site for clinical intervention with anticlonotypic antibodies (Acha-Orbea *et al.*, 1988; Urban *et al.*, 1988; Zaller *et al.*, 1990). Alternatively, knowledge of important HLA residues involved in peptide binding by a susceptible allele might facilitate the development of high-affinity peptide antigens that could block the critical HLA–TcR interaction that triggers disease (Urban *et al.*, 1989; Wraith *et al.*, 1989). Second, in diseases where thymic selection appears to play a critical role, comparisons of the use of specific TcR V genes in individuals carrying susceptible and protective HLA genotypes might allow the identification of the critical TcR(s) whose deletion results in dominant protection. Such considerations provide an opportunity to open a new door to intervention therapies based on specific blocking of HLA–TcR interactions.

EDITORS' NOTE:

Nepom and Concannon have provided a coherent account of the association of MHC class II determinants with autoimmune disease. There is no doubt that this work is a landmark in the understanding of the genetics of autoimmunity. It has already raised new possibilities for treatment and may well lead to new opportunities for prevention of autoimmune diseases by identifying individuals at great risk of future disease. It is dealt with in more detail in chapter 17.

REFERENCES

Acha-Orbea, H., Mitchell, D. J., Timmermann, L., Wraith, D. C., Tausch, G. S., Waldor, M. K., Zamuil, S. S., McDevitt, H. O., and Steinman, L. (1988). *Cell* **54,** 263–273.

Allison, J. P., and Lanier, L. L. (1987). *Annu. Rev. Immunol.* **5,** 503–540.

Amar, A., Holbeck, S. L., and Nepom, G. T. (1987). *Transplantation* **44,** 831–835.

Angelini, G., dePreval, C., Gorski, J., and Mach, B. (1986). *Proc. Natl. Acad. Sci. U.S.A.* **83,** 4489–4493.

Awata, T., Kuzuya, T., Matsuda, A., Iwamoto, Y., Kanazawa, Y., Okuyama, M., and Juji, T. (1990). *Diabetes* **39,** 266–269.

Baisch, J. M., Weeks, T., Giles, T., Hoover, M., Stastny, P., and Capra, J. D. (1990). *N. Engl. J. Med.* **322,** 1836–1841.

Beall, S. S., Concannon, P., Charmley, P., McFarland, H. F., Gatti, R. A., Hood, L. E., McFarlin, D. E., and Biddison, W. E. (1989). *J. Neuroimmunol.* **21,** 59–66.

Behlke, M., Chou, H., Huppi, K., and Loh, D. (1986). *Proc. Natl. Acad. Sci. U.S.A.* **83,** 767–771.

Bertrams, J., and Baur, M. (1984). *In* "Insulin-Dependent Diabetes Mellitus" (E. Albert, M. Baur, and W. Mayer, eds.), pp. 348–358. Springer-Verlag, Berlin.

Bidwell, J. A., and Jarrold, E. A. (1986). *Mol. Immunol.* **23,** 1111–1116.

Bjorkman, P. J., Saper, M. A., Samraoui, B., Bennett, W. S., Strominger, J. L., and Wiley, D. C. (1987). *Nature* **329,** 506–518.

Bodmer, W. F. (1984). *In* "The HLA system 1984" (E. D. Albert, M. P. Baur, and W. R. Mayr, eds.), pp. 11–22. Springer-Verlag, Berlin.

Breur-Vriesendorp, B. S., Dekker-Saeys, A. J., and Ivany, P. (1987). *Ann. Rheum. Dis.* **46,** 353–356.

Buus, S., Sete, A., Colon, S. M., Miles, C., and Grey, H. M. (1987). *Science* **235,** 1353–1358.

Charmley, P., Chao, A., Concannon, P., Hood, L., and Gatti, R. A. (1990). *Proc. Natl. Acad. Sci. U.S.A.* **87,** 4823–4827.

Clevers, H. C., Alarcon, B., Wileman, T. E., and Terhorst, C. (1988). *Annu. Rev. Immunol.* **6,** 629–662.

Concannon, P., Pickering, L., Kung, P., and Hood, L. (1986). *Proc. Natl. Acad. Sci. U.S.A.* **83,** 6598–6602.

Concannon, P., Gatti, R. A., and Hood, L. E. (1987). *J. Exp. Med.* **165,** 1130–1140.

Concannon, P., Wright, J. A., Wright, L. G., Sylvester, D. R., and Spielman, R. S. (1990). *Am. J. Hum. Genet.* **47,** 45–52.

Cox, N. J., Gogolin, K. J., Horvath, V. J., Barker, D. F., Wright, E., Tran, T., Skolnick, M. H., Boehm, B. O., Fehsel, K., Bertrams, J., Hodge, T. W., Acton, R. T., McGill, J., Elbein, S. C., Permutt, M. A., de Preval, C., Avoustin, P., Cambon-Thomsen, A., Robinson, D. M., Holbeck, S. L., Nepom, G. T., Schneider, P. M., Rittner, C., Toyoda, H., Rotter, J. I., and Spielman, R. (1989). *Genet. Epidemiol.* **6,** 21–26.

Croce, C., Isobe, M., Palumbo, A., Puck, J., Ming, J., Tweardy, D., Erikson, J., Davis, M., and Rovera, G. (1985). *Science* **227,** 1044–1047.

Demaine, A., Welsh, K. I., Hawe, B. S., and Farid, N. R. (1987). *J. Clin. Endocrinol. Metab.* **65,** 643–646.

Demaine, A. G., Vaughan, R. W., Taube, D. H., and Welsh, K. I. (1988). *Immunogenetics* **27,** 19–23.

Dembic, Z., Haas, W., Weiss, S., McCubrey, J., Kiefer, H., von Boehmer, H., and Steinmetz, M. (1986). *Nature* **320,** 232–238.

Duby, A., and Seidman, J. (1986). *Proc. Natl. Acad. Sci. U.S.A.* **83,** 4890–4894.

Durand, J. P., El-Zaatari, F. A. K., Krieg, A. M., and Taurog, J. D. (1988). *J. Rheumatol.* **15,** 1115–1118.

Erlich, H. A., Bugawan, T. L., Scharf, S., Nepom, G. T., Tait, B., and Griffith, R. L. (1990). *Diabetes* **39,** 96–103.

Ewing, C., Ebringer, R., Tribbick, G., and Geysen, H. M. (1990). *J. Exp. Med.* **171,** 1635–1647.

Ferradini, L., Roman-Roman, S., Azocar, J., Michalaki, H., Triebel, F., and Hercend, T. (1991). *Eur. J. Immunol.* **21,** 935–942.

Fronek, Z., Lents, D., Berliner, N., Duby, A. D., Klein, K. A., Seidman, J. G., and Schur, P. H. (1986). *Arthritis Rheum.* **29,** 1023–1025.

Fugger, L., Sandberg-Wollheim, M., Morling, N., Ryder, L. P., and Svejgaard, A. (1990). *Immunogenetics* **31,** 278–280.

Gao, X. J., Ball, E. J., Dombrausky, L., Olsen, N. J., Pincus, T., Khan, M. A., Wolfe, F., and Stastny, P. (1988). *Am. J. Med.* **85,** 14–16.

Gorman, C. M., Moffat, L. F., and Howard, B. H. (1982). *Mol. Cell. Biol.* **2,** 1044–1051.

Gregersen, P. K., Shen, M., Song, Q. L., Merryman, P., Degar, S. S., Seki, T., Maccari, J., Goldberg, D., Murphy, H., Schwenzer, J., and Wang, C. (1986). *Proc. Natl. Acad. Sci. U.S.A.* **83,** 2642–2646.

Gregersen, P. K., Silver, J., and Winchester, R. J. (1987). *Arthritis Rheum.* **30,** 1205–1213.

Griesser, H., Champagne, E., Tkachuk, D., Takihara, Y., Lalande, M., Ballie, E., Minden, M., and Mak, T. W. (1988). *Eur. J. Immunol.* **18,** 641–644.

Hiraiwa, A., Yamanaka, K., Kwok, W. W., Mickelson, E. M., Masewicz, S., Hansen, J. A., Radka, S. F., and Nepom, G. T. (1990). *Proc. Natl. Acad. Sci. U.S.A.* **87,** 8051–8055.

Holbeck, S. L., and Nepom, G. T. (1988). *Hum. Immunol.* **21,** 183–192.

Horn, G., Bugawan, T., Long, C., and Erlich, H. (1988). *Proc. Natl. Acad. Sci. U.S.A.* **85,** 6012–6016.

Hoover, M. L., Angelini, G., Ball, E., Stastny, P., Marks, J., Rosenstock, J., Raskin, P., Ferrara, G. B., Tosi, R., and Capra, J. D. (1987). *Cold Spring Harbor Symp. Quant. Biol.* **51,** 803–808.

Ikuta, K., Ogura, T., Shimizu, A., and Honjo, T. (1985). *Proc. Natl. Acad. Sci. U.S.A.* **82,** 7701–7705.

Isobe, M., Erikson, J., Emanuel, B., Nowell, P., and Croce, C. (1985). *Science* **228,** 580–582.

Ito, M., Tanimoto, M., Kamura, H., Yoneda, M., Morishima, Y., Takatsuki, K., Itatsu, T., Takatsuki, K., and Saito, H. (1988). *Diabetes* **37,** 1633–1636.

Jones, N., Leiden, J., Dialynas, D., Fraser, J., Clabby, M., Kishimoto, T., and Strominger, J. L. (1985). *Science* **227,** 311–314.

Jouvin-Marche, E., Trede, N. S., Bandeira, A., Tomas, A., Loh, D. Y., and Cazenave, A. (1989). *Eur. J. Immunol.* **19,** 1921–1926.

Kagnoff, M. F., Harwood, J. I., Bugawan, T. L., and Erlich, H. A. (1989). *Proc. Natl. Acad. Sci. U.S.A.* **86,** 6274–6278.

Kappler, J. W., Wade, T., White, J., Kushner, E., Blackman, M., Bill, J., Roehm, N., and Marrack, P. (1987). *Cell* **49,** 263–271.

Kaufman, J., Auffrey, C., Korman, A., Shackleford, D., and Strominger, J. (1984). *Cell* **36,** 1–13.

Keat, A. (1986). *Immunol. Today* **7,** 144–148.

Kimura, N., Toyonaga, B., Yoshikai, Y., Du, R.-P., and Mak, T. W. (1987). *Eur. J. Immunol.* **17,** 375–383.

Kimura, N., Toyonaga, B., Yoshikai, Y., Triebel, F., Debre, P., Minden, M., and Mak, T. (1986). *J. Exp. Med.* **164,** 739–750.
Kisielow, P., Teh, H. S., Blüthmann, H., and von Boehmer, H. (1988). *Nature* **335,** 730–733.
Klein, M., Concannon, P., Everett, M., Kim, L., Hunkapiller, T., and Hood, L. (1987). *Proc. Natl. Acad. Sci. U.S.A.* **84,** 6884–6888.
Klotz, J., Barth, R. K., Kiser, G. L., Hood, L. E., and Kronenberg, M. (1989). *Immunogenetics* **29,** 191–201.
Koller, B. H., Geraghty, D., Orr, H. T., Shimizu, Y., and DeMars, R. (1987). *Immunol. Res.* **6,** 1–10.
Kwok, W. W., Schwarz, D., Nepom, B., Thurtle, P., Hock, R., and Nepom, G. T. (1988). *J. Immunol.* **141,** 3123–3127.
Kwok, W. W., Mickelson, E., Masewicz, S., Milner, E. C. B., Hansen, J., and Nepom, G. T. (1990). *J. Exp. Med.* **171,** 85–95.
Lai, E., Concannon, P., and Hood, L. (1988). *Nature* **331,** 543–546.
Lai, E., Wilson, R. K., and Hood, L. E. (1989). *Adv. Immunol.* **46,** 1–59.
Lee, J. S. (1989). *In* "Immunobiology of HLA" (B. Dupont, ed.), pp. 49–62. Springer-Verlag, New York.
LeGall, I., Millasseau, P., Dausset, J. L., and Cohen, D. (1986). *Proc. Natl. Acad. Sci. U.S.A.* **83,** 7836–7840.
Leiden, J., and Strominger, J. (1986). *Proc. Natl. Acad. Sci. U.S.A.* **83,** 4456–4460.
Li, Y., Szabo, P., Robinson, M. A., Dong, B., and Posnett, D. N. (1990). *J. Exp. Med.* **171,** 221–230.
Marrack, P., Lo, D., Brinster, R., Palmiter, R., Burkly, L., Flavell, R. H., and Kappler, J. (1988). *Cell* **53,** 627–634.
Martell, M., Marcadet, A., Strominger, J., Dausset, J., and Cohen, D. (1987). *C. R. Acad. Sci. Paris* **304,** 105–110.
McDevitt, H. O. (1986). *Clini. Res.* **34,** 163–175.
Michelsen, B., and Lernmark, A. (1987). *J. Clin. Invest.* **79,** 1144–1152.
Millward, B. A., Welsh, K. I., Leslie, R. D. G., Pyke, D. A., and Demaine, A. G. (1987). *Clin. Exp. Immunol.* **70,** 152–157.
Morel, P. A., Dorman, J. S., Todd, J. A., McDevitt, H. O., and Trucco, M. (1988). *Proc. Natl. Acad. Sci. U.S.A.* **85,** 8111–8115.
Nepom, B. S., Nepom, G. T., Mickelson, E., Antonelli, P., and Hansen, J. A. (1983). *Proc. Natl. Acad. Sci. U.S.A.* **80,** 6962–6966.
Nepom, B. S., Schwarz, D., Palmer, J. P., and Nepom, G. T. (1987). *Diabetes* **36,** 114–117.
Nepom, G. T., Nepom, B. S., Antonelli, P., Mickelson, E., Silver, J., Goyert, S. M., and Hansen, J. A. (1984). *J. Exp. Med.* **159,** 394–404.
Nepom, G. T., Seyfried, C. E., Holbeck, S. L., Wilske, K. R., and Nepom, B. S. (1986a). *Lancet* **ii,** 1002–1005.
Nepom, G. T., Hansen, J., and Nepom, B. (1986b). *J. Clin. Immunol.* **7,** 1–7.
Nepom, G. T., Palmer, J., and Nepom, B. S. (1986c). *In* "Immunology of Diabetes Mellitus" (M. Jaworski, *et al.*, eds.), pp. 9–20. Elsevier Publishers, New York.
Nepom, G. T. (1988). *In* "Genetic Basis of Autoimmune Disease [Concepts in Immunopathology]" (J. M. Cruse and R. Lewis, eds.), Vol. 51, pp. 80–105. S. Karger AG, Basel, Switzerland.
Nepom, G. T., Byers, P., Seyfried, C., Healey, L. A., Wilske, K. R., Stage, D., and Nepom, B. S. (1989a). *Arthritis Rheum.* **32,** 15–21.
Nepom, G. T. (1989b). *Immunol. Res.* **8,** 16–38.
Nepom, G. T., and Robinson, D. M. (1990). *In* "The Molecular Biology of Autoimmune Disease" (A. G. Demaine and A. McGregor, eds.), pp. 251–262. Springer-Verlag, Berlin, Heidelberg.

Niven, M. J., Caffrey, C., Moore, R. H., Sachs, J. A., Mohan, V., Festenstein, H., Hoover, M. L., and Hitman, G. A. (1990). *Hum. Immunol.* **27,** 360–367.

Oksenberg, J. R., Gaiser, C. N., Cavalli-Sforza, L. L., and Steinman, L. (1988). *Hum. Immunol.* **22,** 111–121.

Oksenberg, J. R., Sherritt, M., Begovich, A. B., Erlich, H. A., Bernard, C. C., Cavalli-Sforza, L. L., and Steinman, L. (1989). *Proc. Natl. Acad. Sci. U.S.A.* **86,** 988–992.

Parham, P., Lomen, C. E., Lawlor, D. A., Ways, J. P., Holmes, N., Coppin, H. L., Salter, R. D., Wan, A. M., and Ennis, P. D. (1988). *Proc. Natl. Acad. Sci. U.S.A.* **85,** 4005–4009.

Parham, P., Lawlor, D. A., Salter, R. D., Lomen, C. E., Bjorkman, P. J., and Ennis, P. D. (1989). *In* "Immunobiology of HLA" (B. Dupont, ed.), pp. 10–32. Springer-Verlag, New York.

Perl, A., Divincenzo, J. P., Gergely, P., Condemi, J. J., and Abraham, G. N. (1989). *Immunology* **67,** 135–138.

Robinson, D. M., Holbeck, S., Seyfried, C., Byers, P., Palmer, J., and Nepom, G. T. (1988). *Genet. Epidemiol.* **6,** 27–30.

Robinson, M. A. (1987). *Proc. Natl. Acad. Sci. U.S.A.* **84,** 9089–9193.

Robinson, M. A. (1989). *Proc. Natl. Acad. Sci. U.S.A.* **86,** 9422–9426.

Robinson, M. A. (1991). *J. Immunol.* **146,** 4392–4397.

Roman-Roman, S., Ferradini, L., Azocar, J., Genevée, C., Hercend, T., and Triebel, F. (1991). *Eur. J. Immunol.* **21,** 927–933.

Rønningen, K. S., Iwe, T., Halstensen, T. S., Spurkland, A., and Thorsby, E. (1989). *Hum. Immunol.* **26,** 215–225.

Saiki, R. K., Bugawan, T. L., Horn, G. E., Mullis, K. B., and Erlich, H. (1986). *Nature* **324,** 163–166.

Scharf, S. J., Freidmann, A., Steinman, L., Brautbar, C., and Erlich, H. A. (1989). *Proc. Natl. Acad. Sci. U.S.A.* **86,** 6215–6219.

Schiff, B., Mizrachi, Y., Orgad, S., Yaron, M., and Gazit, I. (1982). *Ann. Rheum. Dis.* **41,** 403–404.

Seboun, E., Robinson, M. A., Doolittle, T. H., Ciulla, T. A., Kindt, T. J., and Hauser, S. L. (1989). *Cell* **57,** 1095–1100.

Seyfried, C. E., Nepom, B. S., Gregersen, P. T., and Nepom, G. T. (1987). *Mol. Immunol.* **24,** 471–477.

Sheehy, M. J., Meske, L. M., Emler, C. A., Rowe, J. R., Neme de Jimenez, M. H., Ingle, C. A., Chan, A., Trucco, M., Mak, T. W. (1989). *Hum. Immunol.* **26,** 261–271.

Smith, C. I., Borgonovo, L., Carlsson, B., Hammarstrom, L., and Rabbits, T. H. (1987). *Ann. N.Y. Acad. Sci.* **505,** 388–397.

Sollid, L. M., Markussen, G., Ek, J., Gjerde, H., Vartdal, F., and Thorsby, E. (1989). *J. Exp. Med.* **169,** 345–350.

Sui, G., Strauss, E., Lai, E., and Hood, L. (1986). *J. Exp. Med.* **164,** 1600–1614.

Szafer, F., Chaim, B., Tzfoni, E., Frankel, G., Sherman, L., Cohen, I., Hacham-Zadeh, S., Aberer, W., Tappeiner, G., Holubar, K., and Steinman, L. (1987). *Proc. Natl. Acad. Sci. U.S.A.* **84,** 6542–6545.

Teh, H. S., Kisielow, P., Scott, B., Kishi, H., Uematsu, Y., Blüthmann, H., and von Boehmer, H. (1988). *Nature* **335,** 229–233.

Thomson, G., Robinson, W. P., Kuhner, M. K., Joe, S., MacDonald, M. J., Gottschall, J. L., Barbosa, J., Rich, S. S., Bertrams, J., Baur, M. P., Partanen, J., Tait, B. D., Schober, E., Mayr, W. R., Ludbigsson, J., Lindblom, B., Farid, N. R., Thompson, C., and Deschamps, I. (1988). *Am. J. Hum. Genet.* **43,** 799–816.

Tillinghast, J., Behlke, M., and Loh, D. (1986). *Science* **233,** 879–883.

Tiwari, J., and Terasaki, P. (1985). "HLA and Disease Associations." Springer-Verlag, New York.

Todd, J. A., Bell, J. I., and McDevitt, H. O. (1987). *Nature* **329,** 599–604.

Toyonaga, B., Yoshikai, Y., Vadasz, V., Chin, B., and Mak, T. W. (1985). *Proc. Natl. Acad. Sci. U.S.A.* **82,** 8624–8628.

Urban, J. L., Kumar, V. K., Kono, D. H., Gomez, C., Horvath, S. J., Clayton, J., Ando, D. G., Sercarz, E. E., and Hood, L. (1988). *Cell* **54,** 577–592.

Urban, J. L., Horvath, S. J., and Hood, L. (1989). *Cell* **59,** 259–271.

Vega, M. A., Bragado, R., Ivanyi, P., Pelaez, J. L., and Lopez de Castro, J. A. (1986). *J. Immunol.* **137,** 3557–3565.

Weetman, A. P., So, A. K., Roe, C., Walport, M. J., and Foroni, L. (1987). *Hum. Immunol.* **20,** 167–173.

Willkens, R. F., Nepom, G. T., Marks, C. R., Nettles, J. W., and Nepom, B. S. (1991). *Arthritis Rheum.* **34,** 43–47.

Wilson, R. K., Lai, E., Concannon, P., Barth, R. K., and Hood, L. E. (1988). *Immunol. Rev.* **101,** 149–172.

Wong, D. W., Bentwich, Z., Martinez-Tarquino, C., Seidman, J. G., Duby, A. D., Quertermous, T., and Schur, P. H. (1988). *Arthritis Rheum.* **31,** 1371–1376.

Wraith, D. C., Smilek, D. E., Mitchell, D. J., Steinman, L., and McDevitt, H. O. (1989). *Cell* **59,** 247–255.

Yanagi, Y., Chan, A., Chin, B., Minden, M., and Mak, T. (1985). *Proc. Natl. Acad. Sci. U.S.A.* **82,** 3430–3434.

Yoshikai, Y., Clark, S., Taylor, S., Sohn, U., Wilson, B., Minder, M., and Mak, T. (1985). *Nature* **316,** 837–840.

Yoshikai, Y., Kimura, N., Toyonaga, B., and Mak, T. (1986). *J. Exp. Med.* **164,** 90–103.

Zaller, D. M., Osman, G., Kanagawa, O., and Hood, L. (1990). *J. Exp. Med.* **171,** 1943–1955.

CHAPTER 6

Molecular Mimicry

ROBERT S. FUJINAMI
Department of Neurology
University of Utah School of Medicine
Salt Lake City, Utah

I. INTRODUCTION

Several mechanisms have been proposed to explain how self-tolerance is broken and autoimmune disease is initiated. Diseases with an autoimmune foundation include many of the chronic debilitating diseases of man, such as rheumatoid arthritis, diabetes, systemic lupus erythematosus, autoimmune kidney, skin, heart, and thyroid diseases, as well as multiple sclerosis. While these diseases can involve many organ systems, all have been associated with infectious agents either initiating or exacerbating the various conditions.

Thoughts toward microbial initiation of autoimmune responses have been studied for many years. The idea that organisms have cross-reacting determinants and induce immune responses to self is the basis for one of the mechanisms explaining microbial pathogenesis of autoimmunity. While this concept of cross-reacting determinants has existed for many decades, the term molecular mimicry was first ascribed to microbes or infectious agents and host-cell components in the early 1960s (Damian, 1964). For the next 20 years, the term disappeared and was forgotten. However, in the 1980s, the term molecular mimicry reemerged as new and better techniques were developed to study this phenomenon at a molecular level (Fujinami *et al.*, 1983). While these new approaches have been established, i.e., the use of synthetic peptides, computer-aided protein and nucleic acid database analyses, and identification of the major histocompatibility complex (MHC) and T-cell receptor molecules, the basic mechanisms involved in tissue injury remain the same.

Immune responses are generated by the host in response to invading microbes.

If the organism shares a common immunologic determinant with the host, a cross-reactive immune response is generated. The immune response to the invading organism can then be directed toward the host-cell component that shares the epitope, and limited to a particular tissue or systemic element. This can occur at the level of antibodies or T cells. What is important is that the cross-reacting immune response must take place between a disease-inducing region or site on a self-molecule, i.e., encephalitogenic site (Fujinami and Oldstone, 1985). For example, a cross-reacting immune response must be generated to an encephalitogenic site in a genetically susceptible animal in order for experimental allergic encephalomyelitis involving inflammation and demyelination to occur in the central nervous system. Both specific and nonspecific recognition of the target molecules are associated with disease. If the induced immune response is to a cross-reacting site that is not a disease-inducing region, autoantibodies may be produced. However, no overt disease would result with any significant pathologic consequences.

In the example above, T cells to critical disease-inducing epitopes from myelin basic protein are involved in the pathology. In other instances, antibody may initiate tissue injury via complement activation, and/or antibody-dependent cell-mediated lysis. Various combinations of T cells and antibody-effector mechanisms can be involved in the recognition of self that leads to disease.

This chapter will in most instances deal with articles published within the past several years. Unfortunately, all references relating to the subject cannot be included. Selected articles are included to make certain points. For additional articles on the subject from prior years, the reader is referred to Fujinami and Oldstone (1989).

II. STREPTOCOCCUS AND HEART —EARLY MODEL

Some of the earliest associations between microbes and autoimmune disease have been studied in the streptococcus organism. Here, various streptococcal cell wall and membrane components have been found to have common or shared determinants with heart (Unny and Middlebrooks, 1983). The group A streptococcus can initiate an acute myocarditis, which later, with subsequent infections or by autostimulation with heart valve antigen(s), leads to chronic rheumatic heart disease (Williams, 1985). Several antigens have been implicated in disease. For example, M protein associated with the streptococcal cell wall and a heart muscle determinant have been studied. An epitope similarity between group A streptococcal M protein and myosin has been demonstrated by Cunningham *et al.* (1989). Cross-reacting immune responses to this determinant may contribute to the presence of heart-reactive antibodies in acute rheumatic fever.

These investigators (Cunningham *et al.*, 1989) found that human and mouse antibodies to a particular sequence found in M protein bound to heart tissue.

Other streptococcal antigens include complexes of mucopeptide and polysaccharide antigens, which can generate cross-reacting immune responses that can lead to myocardial and valvular lesions in animals. Mucopeptide composed of *N*-acetylglucosamine and *N*-acetylmuramic acid associated with a particular tetrapeptide provoked potent cardiac lesions in susceptible animals (reviewed in Unny and Middlebrooks 1983). The streptococci–heart models have been and still are important systems for understanding the molecular basis of autoimmune disorders.

III. EXPERIMENTAL ALLERGIC ENCEPHALOMYELITIS

Experimental allergic encephalomyelitis (EAE) is an autoimmune disease of the central nervous system, which can be induced in susceptible animals by injection with myelin components, particularly myelin basic protein and more recently proteolipid protein. The antigen, myelin basic protein, has been sequenced and the encephalitogenic (disease-inducing) regions have been well established for a wide variety of animal species. This is an animal model for multiple sclerosis and the postinfectious encephalopathies. Several years ago we made the observation that viruses share common determinants with host-cell proteins and reestablished the term molecular mimicry (Fujinami *et al.*, 1983). In extending these observations, additional experiments were conducted. First, computer comparisons were made with known sequenced viral proteins and the encephalitogenic regions of myelin basic protein for various species of animals (Fujinami and Oldstone, 1985). Several similarities were uncovered. These included the nucleoprotein and hemagglutinin of influenza virus; the coat protein of polyoma virus; the core protein of adenovirus; the polyprotein of Rous avian sarcoma, and Abelson leukemia viruses; the polyprotein of poliomyelitis virus; and the EC-LF2 protein of Epstein–Barr virus. At that time the best *fit* was with the hepatitis B virus polymerase and the encephalitogenic region of myelin basic protein for the rabbit. Since this region was the rabbit encephalitogenic site, rabbits were immunized once with the viral peptide. Three questions were addressed: first, whether autoantibodies could be generated; second, whether cellular reactivity to myelin basic protein could be observed; and third, whether disease could be produced. In most of the animals, autoantibodies to myelin basic protein were generated. In half of the rabbits immunized with the viral peptide, peripheral blood mononuclear cells from the animals proliferated in response to myelin basic protein. Central nervous system tissue taken from some of these rabbits had a histologic picture resembling EAE (Fujinami and Oldstone 1985). These seminal experiments demonstrated that a viral determinant could trigger the production of autoantibodies and self-reactive mononuclear cells by molecular mimicry, and under suitable conditions, pathologic changes in the target organ could result. Further, these experiments suggested that tissue injury resulting from autoimmune responses could take place in the absence of the infectious agent that initiated or generated the cross-reacting immune response.

More recently, Weise and Carnegie (1988) found, using computer search, sequence similarities between myelin basic protein and several viral proteins. Sequence similarities with visna and vaccinia viruses and myelin basic protein were found, as well as mimicry between P2 protein (found in peripheral nerve) and influenza A NS2 protein. These investigators suggested an association with P2 and influenza virus in Guillain-Barré syndrome. In other studies, Rubio and Cuesta (1989) could detect no cross-reaction between myelin basic protein and Theiler murine encephalomyelitis virus, SV5, and measles virus by an antibody radioimmunoassay. In these instances, conformational determinants not recognized by these antibodies were not studied, nor were T-cell epitopes critical for the induction of pathologic changes in Theiler's virus infection or measles virus encephalomyelitis where the necessity for CD4+ T cells has been reported.

IV. UVEITIS

An interesting model for autoimmune disease is experimental autoimmune uveitis. This experimental autoimmune disease can be produced by the injection of a soluble retinal protein, known as S antigen, into a susceptible host. This animal disease model serves as an experimental correlate for human ocular inflammation. Singh *et al.* (1989b) found a region of the S antigen that had an amino acid sequence similar to the yeast histone protein, H3. The common determinant was found to reside in a 15-amino-acid peptide covering residues 106–121. The yeast histone H3 peptide as well as the native yeast histone could induce an inflammatory uveitis in Lewis rats when animals were immunized with histone antigen and adjuvant. Lymph node cells from such animals immunized with the peptide M (uveitopathogenic peptide from S antigen), histone H3 peptide, or native histone proliferated when cultured in the presence of histone or S antigen preparations. Lymph node cells from these rats could also transfer the disease to naive rats. In other experiments, Singh *et al.* (1989a) induced experimental autoimmune uveitis using another synthetic peptide corresponding to a common region from an *Escherichia coli* protein and the uveitopathogenic site in human S antigen (peptide M). The disease induced in rats by the *E. coli* peptide was similar to that produced by the injection of peptide M. Lymph node cells from animals immunized with either peptide (*E. coli* or peptide M) proliferated in response to one or the other peptide. In additional studies, Singh *et al.* (1990)

described another system in which the S antigen has a cross-reactive determinant with several viruses. These investigators demonstrated that hepatitis B virus DNA polymerase, gag-pol polyprotein of baboon endogenous retrovirus, and a similar protein from AKV murine leukemia virus had an amino acid segment similar to that of the disease-inducing region from the S antigen (peptide M). Proliferative responses to the viral peptides could be generated when animals were injected with peptide M. Thus, tissue injury due to infection with several different and diverse agents having a cross-reacting determinant with the peptide M potentially could induce autoimmune eye injury. One of the key issues or questions is to understand what regulatory mechanisms or modulating factors, such as MHC contributions, are involved in disease induction. For example, *E. coli* is a common inhabitant of the host's normal flora yet is not associated with spontaneous eye disease. Additional factors are necessary to generate a cross-reacting response that attains a certain threshold resulting in injury to the host.

V. SYSTEMIC LUPUS

This autoimmune disease expresses itself as a systemic vasculitis of many organ systems. While this disease entity has been investigated for many decades, the etiology is still unclear. Several new approaches have recently been used. For example, advances in molecular biology have allowed Query and Keene (1987) to construct a cDNA library from brain. Using autoantibodies from patients with connective tissue disease, these investigators were able to isolate a 70-kDa protein associated with U1 snRNP. This complex is an autoantigen often associated with this autoimmune disorder. A region from the 70-kDa protein had a domain similar to that of the gag protein from type C retroviruses. Synthetic peptides to this region were constructed, and these peptides could inhibit the binding of the patients' autoantibodies. Immunization of animals with the p30 gag from retrovirus could induce antibodies that bound to the U1 snRNP. Query and Keene (1987) suggest that immune responses to such a cross-reacting epitope from a retrovirus could play a role in generation of autoantibodies involved in disease.

In a similar system, Guldner *et al.* (1990) studied autoantibodies from patients with connective tissue disease and systemic lupus erythematosus. Their sera contained antibodies that bound to the snRNP-specific p68 protein as determined by enzyme-linked immunosorbent assay (ELISA) and Western blotting. In addition, these antibodies were found to bind to the M1 matrix protein of influenza B viruses. They further narrowed the determinant in common between the p68 protein from snRNP and influenza M1 protein to a stretch of five amino acids (ERKRR), using synthetic peptides and fusion proteins produced in *E. coli*. Such a common determinant from influenza B virus could play a role in the initiation of the p68 protein response and anti-RNP autoimmune responses in this disorder.

Argov *et al.* (1989) have examined sera from patients with both visceral and cutaneous leishmaniasis. They found that antibodies from these patients contained specificities to nine nuclear antigens. These antigens are common with those binding with antibodies from lupus patients. Particularly, these were anti-Sm, RNP, SS-A, and SS-B autoantibodies. In one patient with visceral leishmaniasis, serum was obtained that reacted with all of these antigens by Western blotting. These same antigens were recognized by serum from a patient with systemic lupus erythematosus. The binding of the leishmaniasis serum to the Sm, RNP, SS-A, and SS-B determinants could be inhibited by prior incubation of the serum with either a membrane preparation or intact cells from four species of Leishmania indicating common determinants with the parasite and ribonucleoproteins. Thus, not only viruses but also parasites have common determinants with self-antigens implicated in systemic lupus. These cross-reacting epitopes, associated with the B-cell hyperresponsiveness, may be key components in the syndrome called lupus.

VI. ARTHRITIS

Several experimental models have been developed to study this human disease. Two experimental autoimmune systems entail the immunization of susceptible animals with either collagen or derivatives of mycobacteria in adjuvant.

Studies involving adjuvant-induced arthritis have been expanded by van Eden *et al.* (1989). This is an experimentally induced autoimmune disease in which joints are affected; it is initiated in susceptible animals by the injection of mycobacteria. There appears to be a common epitope, that is recognized by T cells, present on a 65-kDa heat-shock protein in mycobacteria. This determinant is found on a cartilage-associated molecule found in the joints. These investigators (van Eden *et al.*, 1989) provide evidence that rheumatoid arthritis patients have immunological reactivity to the 65-kDa heat-shock protein, and this is involved in human disease.

Dudani and Gupta (1989) have determined that a human mitochondrial protein, P1, has sequence similarity to the 65-kDa mycobacterial heat-shock antigen as well. They have developed several monoclonal antibodies (MAbs) to the 65-kDa protein from *Mycobacterium leprae*. Some of these MAbs stained mitochondria and reacted with the human P1 protein. These investigators also demonstrated common elements between other bacterial and viral proteins. They suggested that some of these cross-reacting determinants are involved in rheumatoid arthritis.

In another model, Munk *et al.* (1989) found that in normal human subjects, peripheral blood mononuclear cells activated *in vitro* to killed *Mycobacterium tuberculosis* could kill autologous target cells. Target cells could be primed with *M. tuberculosis* or tryptic fragments but not with the intact 65-kDa protein. To determine whether the reactivity could be targeted to self, synthetic peptides from various regions of the 65-kDa protein in common with bacterial and human sequences were constructed and used to prime targets. Cytotoxic T cells generated with killed *M. tuberculosis* lysed autologous target cells primed with the peptide derived from the human 65-kDa protein. In addition, these investigators (Munk *et al.*, 1989) used HLA-DR transfected murine L cells as targets, and found that killing took place in the context of class II; that is, killing was class II restricted. This demonstrated that a cross-reacting determinant at the T-cell level could result in tissue injury.

Similarly, Koga *et al.* (1989) found that the 65-kDa human protein could be induced in macrophages by gamma interferon or viral infection. Such treated or infected human macrophages were recognized by CD8+ T cells specific for the bacterial heat-shock protein. This suggests that self-heat-shock proteins are processed in host cells and that epitopes shared by heat-shock proteins of bacterial and host origin can be presented in the context of class I molecules and recognized by class I-restricted T cells. From these two reports it appears that the host 65-kDa protein can be recognized and presented either in the context of class I or II MHC determinants.

Lewis rats are susceptible to an autoimmune arthritis induced by the injection of streptococcal cell walls or by mycobacteria (as described above). DeJoy *et al.* (1989) have demonstrated that lymph node cells from such animals proliferate in response to streptococcal cell walls or *M. tuberculosis*. T-cell lines generated from animals with streptococcal cell wall–induced arthritis were able to transfer the disease to naive recipients. These T-cell lines proliferated in response to cell-wall antigens derived from either mycobacteria or streptococci. The T-cell lines did not response to the 65-kDa protein from mycobacteria, suggesting that the determinants involved in this model are distinct from those of the mycobacterial-induced heat-shock model, and that other antigens play a role in arthritis induction. In contrast, van Den Broek *et al.* (1989) reported that streptococcal cell wall–induced arthritis in rats could be prevented by prior treatment of the rats with the 65-kDa heat-shock protein from mycobacteria. These investigators administered four injections of the 65-kDa protein to Lewis rats before immunization with the streptococcal cell-wall preparation. Both the clinical and histopathologic signs of the polyarthritis were suppressed or prevented. This suppression could be transferred to naive recipients using splenic T cells. Further experiments defining the roles of various antigens and specificities should clarify this point.

Two developing arthritis models involve mycoplasma and viral agents. Fernsten *et al.* (1987) have developed a MAb to a 46-kDa polypeptide, which is specific for *Mycoplasma hyorhinis,* an organism associated with arthritis. This protein has a common determinant with a host cellular protein(s) of 24 kDa (doublet) in size, as determined by Western blotting.

Along this line, Sulitzeanu and Anafi (1989) found a sequence similarity with the major Epstein–Barr nuclear antigen (EBNA)-1 protein from Epstein–Barr virus and collagen and keratin. Thus far these investigators have made a prediction only from sequence comparisons and are determining whether anticollagen and keratin antibodies cross-react with EBNA-1 peptides. Their suggestion is that Epstein–Barr virus may be involved in the pathogenesis of arthritis. Further study as to how these epitopes are involved in the actual pathogenesis will prove provocative.

VII. ANKYLOSING SPONDYLITIS AND REITER'S SYNDROME

A common feature of patients with ankylosing spondylitis and reactive arthritis is that most have the HLA-B27 haplotype. Ogasawara *et al.* (1986) found that an anti-HLA-B27 MAb, M2, reacted with several bacteria, some of which are associated with chronic inflammation observed in this syndrome. By Western blotting two protein antigens (60 and 80 kDa molecular mass) from *Klebsiella pneumoniae* were visualized using the MAb. Seven other gram-negative bacteria were also tested, and no reactivity was observed. Antibodies generated to the 80-kDa protein were found to bind to HLA-B27-positive cells.

Schwimmbeck *et al.* (1987), using a computer search for comparisons of HLA-B27 and various microbes, found that the *Klebsiella pneumoniae* nitrogenase had six consecutive amino acids, residues 188–193, in common with the HLA-B27.1 antigen residues (amino acid 72–77). In testing sera from patients, 53% of Reiter's syndrome patients had reactivity to this region, as did approximately 30% of patients with ankylosing spondylitis. Only 1 of 22 sera from HLA-B27-positive control individuals with no disease had reactivity to the common epitope. In other studies Schwimmbeck and Oldstone (1988) found that antibodies against the HLA-B27.1 region also reacted with the peptide from Klebsiella and vice versa. The antibodies bound to articular tissues from HLA-B27-positive patients with ankylosing spondylitis.

Previous investigations have identified several bacterial envelope proteins that were reactive with the MAb B27.M1 and M2 (von Bohemen *et al.* 1984). Yong *et al.* (1989) have performed binding studies with an MAb to HLA-B27 and bacterial envelope proteins. Using synthetic peptides to B27, these investigators were not able to identify the common determinant between the envelope protein and HLA. Yong *et al.* (1989) have derived an MAb, which they call Ye-2, that reacts with a synthetic peptide derived from amino acids 63–84 of HLA-B27.1. This region was found to have a sequence similarity with the bovine carbonic anhydrase (amino acids 230–238). These authors are attempting to further assess whether this region shares immunological cross-reactivity with the bacterial envelope proteins. Yu *et al.* (1989) discuss a bacterial protein region of six amino acids in length. Sera from some patients with reactive arthritis bind to this peptide. It is implied that in a subset of patients this cross-reactive determinant is involved in the pathogenesis (reviewed in Yu *et al.* 1989).

Chen *et al.* (1987) have developed an MAb against HLA-B27 and used it to screen various bacterial species. They found two strains of *Yersinia pseudotuberculosis* bound the MAb. The Yersinia protein that contained the epitope was found to be a 19-kDa molecule by Western blotting. This Yersinia 19-kDa protein was purified, and rabbits were immunized. The antibodies generated reacted with HLA-B27. Synthetic peptides derived from HLA-B27.1 indicated that the cross-reactive epitope was contained in residues 69–83. This area of the HLA-B27 is responsible for the allotypic specificity of the molecule.

A sterile inflammatory polyarthropathy is associated with HLA-B27 and various gram-negative bacteria. Interestingly, Stieglitz *et al.* (1988) have identified a 2-megadalton plasmid (virulence factor) specific to the arthritogenic bacterial strains. This plasmid was found to encode a number of small peptides that could be affiliated with the development of reactive arthritis (Stieglitz *et al.*, 1989). The plasmid, pHS-2, contained a DNA sequence encoding a 22-amino-acid polypeptide, encompassing a pentapeptide homologous to part of the polymorphic region of the alpha-1 domain of HLA-B27. Immune responses to the determinant encoded by the bacterial plasmid found in arthritogenic Shigella strains could play a role in the induction of the polyarthropathy.

Besides the determinant ascribed by the 2-megadalton plasmid, Raybourne *et al.* (1988) isolated two MAbs from Reiter's syndrome patients. These MAbs were studied for their reactivity to the envelope proteins from *Shigella flexneri*. Proteins of 36 and 23 kDa were found to react with MAbs. By ELISA the two MAbs bound to whole Shigella envelope preparations, and these envelopes could inhibit the binding of the MAbs to B27-positive cell lines as determined by flow cytometry. The presence of the cross-reactive proteins was not related to the presence of the virulence-associated plasmid (described previously), since two *Shigella sonnei* isolates, not connected with Reiter's syndrome or reactive arthritis, had a similar cross-reactive protein pattern. These investigators hypothesize that other factors besides the plasmid can play a role in the induction of arthritis in B27-positive individuals.

The role of HLA-B27 is still unclear in the pathogenesis. Bluestein (1988) speculated that the widespread distribution of B27 in the cells of the body versus the restricted anatomic distribution of the pathology of the spondyloarthritis remains a major problem in explaining the association. He suggests investigations focusing on other etiologic factors and tropism for connective tissue at fibromuscular and fibroskeletal junctions. Viitanen *et al.* (1988) described studies finding no sequence homology between *Yersinia enterocolitica* O:3 and HLA-B27 at the DNA level. They suggest a conformational determinant(s) may be involved in the pathogenesis. Other factors such as lymphokine production in restricted sites of the body, such as the joints, may lead to the up-regulation of class I or II HLA molecules, leading to targeting of immune cells to specific areas. This may help localize or target an inflammatory response to a particular tissue.

VIII. MYASTHENIA GRAVIS

This disease entity is an immune-mediated disorder affecting neuromuscular transmission. Antibodies to the acetylcholine receptor (AChR) are found in most patients with autoimmune myasthenia gravis. Schwimmbeck *et al.* (1989) have found using synthetic peptides to the human AChR that antibodies from the sera of patients react with the alpha-subunit, amino acid residues 160–167. This region of the human AChR shares a homologous domain with herpes simplex virus glycoprotein D. Human antibodies isolated by affinity chromatography from myasthenia gravis patients also reacted with the herpes simplex glycoprotein D and to native AChR protein. These investigators predict that herpes simplex virus may be associated with the initiation of myasthenia in certain susceptible individuals. In further experiments Dyrberg *et al.* (1990) have found that antisera made by immunizing rabbits with synthetic peptides representing the herpes simplex virus glycoprotein D (amino acids 286–296) bound to the AChR peptide, while another antiserum made from another similar region of the herpes simplex virus glycoprotein D (381–388), sharing a similarly high degree of amino acids homology, did not bind to the AChR peptide. The antibody reactivity was further defined to an important amino acid residue, leucine, in the herpes simplex glycoprotein D, which was responsible for the antibodies' ability to bind or not bind to the AChR. These studies demonstrate the importance of critically specific residues or conformations for the development of disease.

IX. HIV AND AUTOIMMUNITY

An interesting connection has been growing between acquired immunodeficiency syndrome (AIDS) and autoimmunity, and some of the pathogenic features of the disease. Beretta *et al.* (1987) found a common determinant between the env gp 120 protein from human immunodeficiency virus (HIV) and a host cell-surface protein using an MAb to the virus. This cellular antigen is 80 kDa in size and is found on a small percentage of mononuclear cells in peripheral blood and in lymph nodes. The protein is present on monocytes and may be an activation antigen. The MAb to the virus could inhibit proliferation of lymphocytes in antigen-presentation assays. Further, the 80-kDa protein was found in small amounts on a T-lymphoblastoid cell line, H9, and was not up-regulated by gamma interferon. HIV-positive individuals have no detectable antibodies in their serum to the 80-kDa protein but have antibodies to gp 120. Beretta and associates propose that both viral and cellular structures recognized by the MAb are involved in interactions with CD4+ cells and may be relevant to the pathology of HIV infection.

Parravicini *et al.* (1988) provide evidence for a cross-reaction between p18 protein of HIV I and follicular dendritic cells in lymph nodes in HIV-infected individuals and epithelial cells of the skin, the thymus, tonsils, and astrocytes. The common determinants were demonstrated using MAbs to p18 protein. Four MAbs were used in the study. These investigators related the importance of these common determinants to the pathophysiology of HIV infection.

Golding *et al.* (1988, 1989) have demonstrated highly conserved homologous regions located in the carboxy terminus of the HIV I gp41 protein and the amino-terminal region of the beta chain of HLA class II antigens. MAbs to the homologous regions bound peptides and native gp 160 and HLA class II molecules. Approximately one third of patients with HIV I infection had antibodies in their sera that reacted to both gp41 and HLA class II-derived peptides. These sera, which contained the cross-reacting antibodies, could inhibit proliferative responses of CD4+ T cells to specific antigen such as tetanus toxoid. In addition, allogeneic stimuli responses were markedly reduced. In other experiments, they found that sera from HIV I-infected individuals with the cross-reacting antibodies could lyse HLA class II-bearing cells by antibody-dependent cellular cytotoxicity. Affinity-purified antibodies from the patients' sera had similar effects as described above.

AIDS dementia complex is one of the most common syndromes with neurologic complications of infection with HIV I. Recent studies of AIDS dementia complex brains have demonstrated that HIV I infection of brain was found only in a subset of patients and was rarely observed in neuronal cells, suggesting that pathogenesis of the dementia is unlikely to be simply attributed to direct HIV I infection of the central nervous system. We have generated MAbs to an immunodominant 12-amino-acid region from gp 41. These MAbs react with astrocytes in the human and rodent central nervous systems. By Western blotting, the MAbs bound to a 43-kDa protein. Antibodies to astrocytes were detected in cerebrospinal fluid from AIDS dementia patients but not in control HIV patients. These results indicate that gp41 contains a common epitope with astrocytes and that production of the antibodies could initiate immunopathologic responses to astrocytes. Astrocytes regulate the environment for neuronal function, and astrocyte hyperactivity (gliosis) is a common feature in the central nervous system of AIDS patients. These antibody-induced events on astrocytes could lead to the dementia observed in AIDS dementia (Yamada *et al.*, 1991).

X. MOLECULAR MIMICRY AND MHC

We have synthesized a peptide, amino acid residues 82–96, from the immediate-early region of human cytomegalovirus (HCMV) (Fujinami *et al.*, 1988a). This region shares five identical amino acids in tandem with the HLA-DR beta chain. By computer analysis, both were hydrophilic and had beta turn potential. The cytomegalovirus immediate-early 2 region peptide induced antibodies that recognized the human DR beta chain as determined by Western blotting. The reaction could be inhibited using viral-specific peptide. These findings suggest a scenario of how HCMV could partake in rejection of a renal or bone marrow graft. Immunologic attack against HLA molecules up-regulated in local regions by cytokine release could lead to alloreactions and tissue rejection. Various allodeterminants can be recognized by antibodies and T cells induced during infection. Interestingly, Todd *et al.* (1988) have identified this region to be important in the development of diabetes.

Marchitto *et al.* (1986) found that class I MHC and *Treponema pallidum* have a common immunologic determinant. By immunostaining procedures using an MAb to murine H-2K^b, they found reactivity with the surface of *T. pallidum* and rabbit MHC-containing tissues. MAb for HLA class I was reactive against the spirochetes, whereas anti-HLA class II was negative. These authors predict an association or common epitope between class I and the Treponema parasite.

Nagy *et al.* (1989) have presented molecular mimicry in an interesting role. It is considered to be the driving force for MHC diversification. They suggest that it actually increases the number (polymorphism) and selectivity of peptide-binding sites. This is reviewed in Nagy *et al.* (1989) and will not be discussed in further detail.

XI. CHAGAS' DISEASE

Trypanosoma cruzi has been associated with the induction of a disease known as Chagas' disease. Part of the immunopathology of the disease appears to be autoimmune, or immune mediated. Data suggest that the host could mount a T cell-mediated and antibody response against cross-reacting antigens of *T. cruzi* and nervous tissue. Van Voorhis and Eisen (1989) have cloned a DNA from *T. cruzi* that expresses a 160-kDa protein, which is present on the surface of the parasite. Antibodies to this 160-kDa protein react with a 48-kDa nervous system protein that is found in sciatic nerve, brain, and myenteric plexi of gut. The myenteric plexi are areas of inflammation characteristic of Chagas' disease. These investigators predict that this determinant is involved in the pathogenesis of this disease entity.

XII. DIABETES

The nonobese diabetic (NOD) mouse is a model for autoimmune insulin-dependent diabetes. This is in contrast to the diabetes-resistant strain or nonobese normal (NON) mice. Serreze *et al.* (1988) found that NOD mice developed much higher autoantibody titers to insulin than did the NON mice. Antibodies to C type and intracisternal type A retroviral antigens were also investigated. The type C retrovirus antibodies in the NOD mice peaked just after mice were weaned, whereas autoantibodies against insulin or the type A viral antigens were present shortly before or at the time of the development of hyperglycemia. They suggested that the appearance of antiinsulin antibodies and antiviral p73 antibodies (type A) were associated with tissue damage of the beta cells. Absorption studies indicated that anti-p73 antibodies recognized a common determinant with insulin and that an immune response to the region was one of the contributing factors in the development of diabetes in the NOD mouse. This observation, linked with the inherited defect of B-cell regulation resulting in the hyperproduction of natural autoantibodies (Lehuen *et al.*, 1990), could drive the system over a threshold for disease production. This defect could potentiate antibodies to endogenous retroviruses as well.

For other additional cross-reactions relating to diabetes the reader is referred to Dyrberg (1989).

XIII. POLYMYOSITIS

Induction of autoimmune muscle disease has also been associated with molecular mimicry. Walker and Jeffrey (1986) found amino acid sequences of the histidyl-tRNA synthetase and alanyl-tRNA synthetase were identified as autoantigens in polymyositis. These investigators found that various sequences of viral and muscle proteins had similar regions.

More recently, Walker and Jeffrey (1988) have found that the Jo-I antigen of polymyositis, the host histidyl-tRNA synthetase, shares a sequence similarity with the polyprotein of encephalomyocarditis virus. The shared determinant was with the capsid protein vp-1 of encephalomyocarditis virus. They found that vp-1 also had some sequence similarity with several muscle proteins. This virus has been associated with polymyositis. The investigators made various three-dimensional predictions as to the potential antibody-binding sites between the capsid protein vp-1 and the histidyl-tRNA synthetase. From such predictions these investigators suggested that this provides evidence for the origin of the antibodies that react with the histidyl-tRNA synthetase antigen in polymyositis.

XIV. EPSTEIN–BARR VIRUS AND MOLECULAR MIMICRY

During Epstein–Barr virus infection, many autoantibodies can be detected. Besides polyclonal activation of B cells as a mechanism for the generation of these antibodies, for which Epstein–Barr virus is well known, Rhodes *et al.* (1987) have determined that the Epstein–Barr nuclear antigen shares a common determinant with at least nine nonviral host-tissue proteins. The cross-reacting determinant appears to span a repeating region of glycine and alanine. The reactivity was determined by IgM autoantibodies. Surprisingly, after the IgG switch that occurs during the maturation of an immune response, the reactivity to normal tissues could not be demonstrated. The disappearance of reactivity to self following an isotype switch may be involved in the transient nature of some forms of autoimmune events.

XV. LYME DISEASE

Aberer *et al.* (1989) have found an antigenic determinant shared between *Borrelia burgdorferi* and discrete human cell types associated with the pattern of disease. This organism is involved in Lyme disease such that infection can result in clinical manifestations; however, the mechanism by which the disease is initiated is not clear. These investigators have developed an MAb that reacts with a 41-kDa Borrelia flagella protein and human myelinated fibers found in peripheral nerve. In addition, this MAb bound to heart, muscle cells, and certain epithelial cells, including those found in joint synovia. These authors propose that this determinant is involved in the pathogenesis of Lyme borreliosis, particularly the chronic organ manifestations; thus, it is implied that the disease is immunopathogenic.

XVI. HOST INCORPORATION

Molecular mimicry can take two forms or occur on two levels. First, the microorganism can encode for the cross-reacting determinant, many examples of which have been discussed above. Second, the microbe can incorporate a host protein or component into its structure. Three examples follow.

In an experimental model for demyelination, Theiler's murine encephalomyelitis virus can induce a chronic inflammatory demyelinating disease in mice. The lesions appear very similar to those found in EAE and acute lesions of multiple sclerosis. During Theiler's virus infection, antibodies are produced to viral components but also to central nervous system myelin constituents (Yamada *et al.*, 1990). We have generated an MAb to Theiler's virus, which also cross-

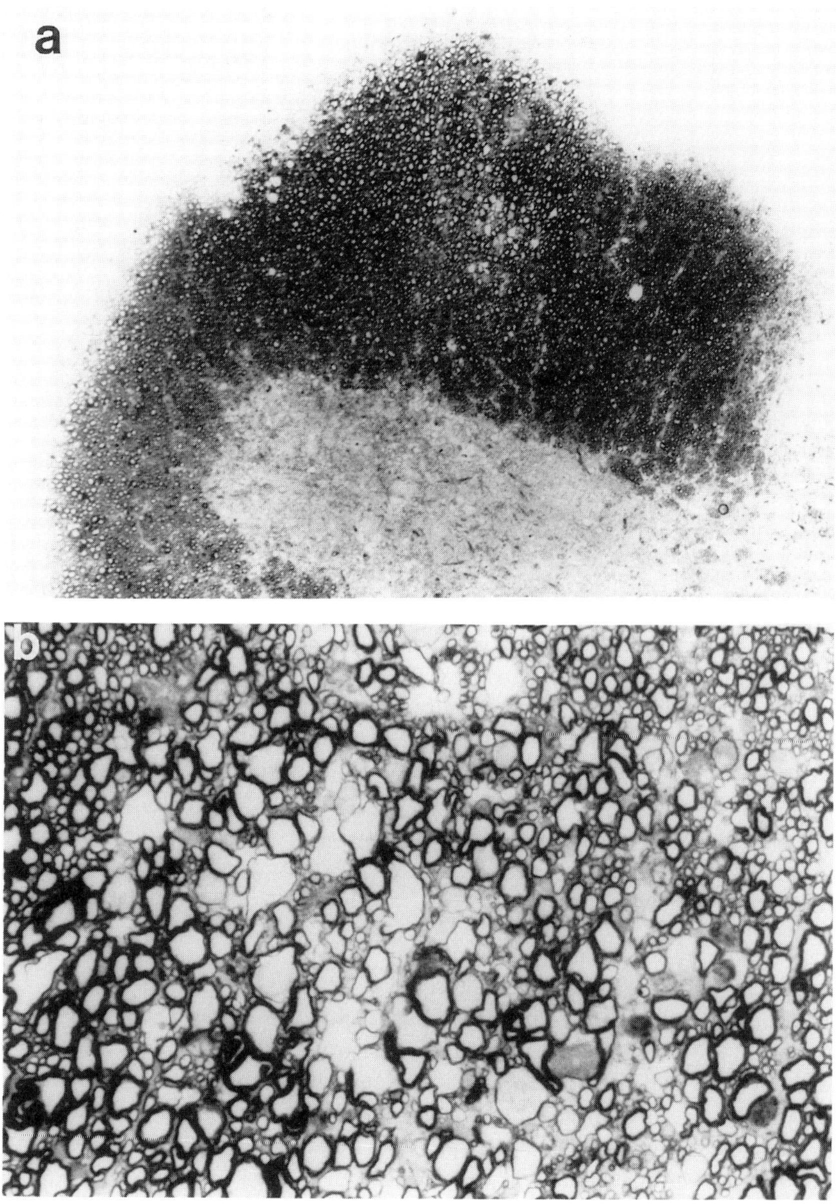

FIG. 1 (a) Low-power magnification of animal treated with MAb to Theiler's virus and galactocerebroside. Note significant areas of demyelination. (Original magnification 40.) (b) High-power magnification of above section demonstrating primary demyelination. From Yamada *et al.*, 1990. (Original magnification 400.)

reacts with galactocerebroside (Fujinami *et al.*, 1988b). By Western blotting the MAb reacted with vp-1, one of the major capsid proteins of the virus. The MAb has the ability to neutralize Theiler's virus. In looking for biologic activity of the MAb involved in the pathogenesis of the disease, newborn mouse brain cell cultures were initiated. In these cultures the MAb bound to oligodendrocytes (Fujinami *et al.*, 1988b; Yamada *et al.*, 1990), the cells that produce myelin and galactocerebroside. Interestingly, this MAb *in vivo* could potentiate the demyelination by almost 10-fold when injected into mice with EAE (see Fig. 1A and B). This is the first example of an immune response potentiating a demyelinating disease *in vivo* (see Yamada *et al.*, 1990). Thus, the initiating virus need not be present for enhanced pathologic consequences to occur in the host, generated in order to eliminate the invading pathogen.

In a totally different system, Hayunga *et al.* (1989) found that the strobilocerci of *Taenia taeniaeformis* in a rat model contain rat IgG. Using Western blot analysis of cyst fluid and parasite homogenates, various bands were detected that were consistent with degradation products from immunoglobulin. These investigators claimed that the pattern of reactivity discounted nonspecific adsorption of IgG to the parasite. They suggested that the observed bands represent a common determinant with IgG found in the parasite or enzymatic cleavage of IgG, which is bound to the tegument of the organism.

McClure and Shearer (1988) found the presence of antiactin antibodies in many patients with various viral infections and autoimmune diseases. They have proposed that the antiactin antibodies were generated to cross-reactivity determinants through molecular mimicry. We have demonstrated previously that many viruses can cross-react with intermediate filaments or actinlike structures within host cells (Fujinami *et al.*, 1983; Dales *et al.*, 1983).

XVII. SUMMARY

Many microbes share various determinants with host cells. In many instances these organisms are facultative intracellular parasites, i.e., viruses. It is not unreasonable that various viral proteins have common features or conformational structures with host-cell proteins such as intermediate filaments. Viruses are assembled and mature in discrete compartments within infected cells. By having common regions with host-cell proteins, viral proteins could be targeted using the same intracellular signals as host proteins to the appropriate cellular compartments for assembly and maturation.

Gorby *et al.* (1988) have suggested that parasites could have molecules on their surfaces that mimic or resemble natural host ligands for which the cells have a receptor. By binding to the host ligand, the organism could be endocytosed and gain entry into the cell. Such interactions have been demonstrated for a variety of viruses.

Another possibility is that viruses that mimic the host either by incorporating host determinants or by coding for similar regions may not provoke an immune response to critical regions necessary for vital functions on viral proteins. These regions would be necessary for viral replication and/or persistence. An effective immune response may not be invoked, allowing the virus to persist and not be eliminated. In addition, by mimicking class I or II MHC molecules, viruses could potentially modulate the immune response. Aberrant expression of these MHC molecules could lead to induction of autoimmune disease or immune responses to these molecules. Antibodies could modulate these proteins from the surface of antigen-presenting cells (Fujinami and Oldstone, 1980) and/or regulate their expression via idiotypic networks. In a similar fashion, T cells may regulate other T cells bearing these molecules. Such alterations in the immune system could lead to either suppression of an immune response or the enhancement or potentiation of an existing one, in the former instance, allowing for viral persistence, and in the latter, autoimmunity.

EDITORS' NOTE:

It is worth reiterating Fujinami's final comment that molecular mimicry is a two-edged sword. Where the rules of self/nonself discrimination prevail, parasites (including viruses) presenting antigens that simulate host antigens may well avoid an immune response, thereby permitting the agent to persist. It would not seem to be in the interest of the parasite to kill or sicken its host with autoimmune disease. This important decisive point, autoimmune disease *vs.* persistence of the parasite, may well depend upon the context of antigen presentation, the degree of homology, and the conjunction of accessory factors.

Another point to emphasize is that most of the examples of mimicry studied thus far relate to induction of cross-reactivity on the T-cell or B-cell level. There are still very few examples where autoimmune disease is actually produced by such an immunological cross-reaction.

ACKNOWLEDGMENTS

We thank Peggy Farness, Susan McClanahan, and Pamela Lewis for their excellent technical skills, and Jan Richards for manuscript preparation. This research is supported by The National Multiple Sclerosis Society Grant Numbers RG 2087-A-4 and RG 1780-B-3 and The National Institutes of Health Grant Number NS 23162. Dr. Robert S. Fujinami is a Javits Neuroscience Scholar.

REFERENCES

Aberer, E., Brunner, C., Suchanek, G., et al. (1989). *Ann. Neurol.* **26,** 732–737.

Argov, S., Jaffe, C. L., Krupp, M., Slor, H., and Shoenfeld, Y. (1989). *Clin. Exp. Immunol.* **76,** 190–197.

Beretta, A., Grassi, F., Pelagi, M., et al. (1987). *Eur. J. Immunol.* **17,** 1793–1798.

Bluestein, H. G. (1988). *J. Rheumatol. (Suppl.* 16) 29–32.

Chen, J. H., Kono, D. H., Yong, Z., Park, M. S., Oldstone, M. M., and Yu, D. T. (1987). *J. Immunol.* **139,** 3003–3011.
Cunningham, M. W., McCormack, J. M., Fenderson, P. G., Ho, M. K., Beachey, E. H., and Dale, J. B. (1989). *J. Immunol.* **143,** 2677–2683.
Dales, S., Fujinami, R. S., and Oldstone, M. B. A. (1983). *J. Immunol.* **131,** 1546–1553.
Damian, R. T. (1964). *Am. Nat.* **98,** 129–149.
DeJoy, S. Q., Ferguson, K. M., Sapp, T. M., Zabriskie, J. B., Oronsky, A. L., and Kerwar, S. S. (1989). *J. Exp. Med.* **170,** 369–382.
Dudani, A. K., and Gupta, R. S. (1989). *Infect. Immunol.* **57,** 2786–2793.
Dyrberg, T. (1989). *Curr. Top. Microbiol. Immunol.* **145,** 117–125.
Dyrberg, T., Petersen, J. S., and Oldstone, M. B. A. (1990). *Clin. Immunol. Immunopathol.* **54,** 290–297.
Fernsten, P. D., Pekny, K. W., Harper, J. R., and Walker, L. E. (1987). *Infect. Immunol.* **55,** 1680–1685.
Fujinami, R. S., Nelson, J. A., Walker, L., and Oldstone, M. B. A. (1988a). *J. Virol.* **62,** 100–105.
Fujinami, R. S., and Oldstone, M. B. A. (1980). *In* "Animal Virus Genetics" (B. Fields, R. Jaenisch, and C. F. Fox, eds.), pp. 769–790. Academic Press, New York.
Fujinami, R. S., and Oldstone, M. B. A. (1985). *Science* **230,** 1043–1045.
Fujinami, R. S., and Oldstone, M. B. A. (1989). *Immunol. Res.* **8,** 3–15.
Fujinami, R. S., Oldstone, M. B. A., Wroblewska, Z., Frankel, M. E., and Koprowski, H. (1983). *Proc. Natl. Acad. Sci. U.S.A.* **80,** 2346–2350.
Fujinami, R. S., Zurbriggen, A., and Powell, H. C. (1988b). *J. Neuroimmunol.* **20,** 25–32.
Golding, H., Robey, F. A., Gates, F. T., III, et al. (1988). *J. Exp. Med.* **167,** 914–923.
Golding, H., Shearer, G. M., Hillman, K., et al. (1989). *J. Clin. Invest.* **83,** 1430–1435.
Gorby, G. L., Robinson, E. N., Jr., Barley, L. R., Clemens, C. M., and McGee, Z. A. (1988). *Can. J. Microbiol.* **34,** 507–512.
Guldner, H. H., Netter, H. J., Szostecki, C., Jaeger, E., and Will, H. (1990). *J. Exp. Med.* **171,** 819–829.
Hayunga, E. G., Sumner, M. P., and Letonja, T. (1989). *J. Parasitol.* **75,** 638–642.
Koga, T., Wand-Wurttenberger, A., DeBruyn, J., Munk, M. E., Schoel, B., and Kaufmann, S. H. E. (1989). *Science* **245,** 1112–1116.
Lehuen, A., Bendelac, A., Back, J. F., and Carnaud, C. (1990). *J. Immunol.* **144,** 2147–2151.
Marchitto, K. S., Kindt, T. J., and Norgard, M. V. (1986). *Cell. Immunol.* **101,** 633–642.
McClure, J. E., and Shearer, W. T. (1988). *Mol. Cell Probes* **2,** 305–319.
Munk, M. E., Schoel, B., Modrow, S., Karr, R. W., Young, R. A., and Kaufmann, S. H. E. (1989). *J. Immunol.* **143,** 2844–2849.
Nagy, Z. A., Lehmann, P. V., Falcioni, F., Muller, S., and Adorini, L. (1989). *Immunol. Today* **10,** 132–138.
Ogasawara, M., Kono, D. H., and Yu, D. T. (1986). *Infect. Immunol.* **51,** 901–908.
Parravicini, C. L., Klatzmann, D., Jaffray, P., Costanzi, G., and Gluckman, J. C. (1988). *AIDS* **2,** 171–177.
Query, C. C., and Keene, J. D. (1987). *Cell* **51,** 211–220.
Raybourne, R. B., Bunning, V. K., and Williams, K. M. (1988). *J. Immunol.* **140,** 3489–3495.
Rhodes, G., Rumpold, H., Kurki, P., Patrick, K. M., Carson, D. A., and Vaughan, J. H. (1987). *J. Exp. Med.* **165,** 1026–1040.
Rubio, N., and Cuesta, A. (1989). *Mol. Immunol.* **26,** 663–668.
Schwimmbeck, P. L., Dyrberg, T., Drachman, D. B., and Oldstone, M. B. A. (1989). *J. Clin. Invest.* **84,** 1174–1180.
Schwimmbeck, P. L., and Oldstone, M. B. (1988). *Am. J. Med.* **85,** 51–53.
Schwimmbeck, P. L., Yu, D. T., and Oldstone, M. B. (1987). *J. Exp. Med.* **166,** 173–181.

Serreze, D. V., Leiter, E. H., Kuff, E. L., Jardieu, P., and Ishizaka, K. (1988). *Diabetes,* **37,** 351–358.

Singh, V. K., Kalra, H. K., Yamaki, K., Abe, T., Donoso, L. A., and Shinohara, T. (1990). *J. Immunol.* **144,** 1282–1287.

Singh, V. K., Yamaki, K., Abe, T., and Shinohara, T. (1989a). *Cell Immunol.* **122,** 262–273.

Singh, V. K., Yamaki, K., Donoso, L. A., and Shinohara, T. (1989b). *J. Immunol.* **142,** 1512–1517.

Stieglitz, H., Fosmire, S., and Lipsky, P. (1989). *Arthritis Rheum.* **32,** 937–946.

Stieglitz, H., Fosmire, S., and Lipsky, P. E. (1988). *Am. J. Med.* **85,** 56–58.

Sulitzeanu, D., and Anafi, M. (1989). *Immunol. Lett.* **20,** 89–91, 93, 95.

Todd, J. A., Acha-Orbea, H., Bell, J. I., Chao, N., Fronek, Z., Jacob, C. O., McDermott, M., Sinha, A. A., Timmerman, L., and Steinman, L. (1988). *Science* **240,** 1003–1009.

Unny, S. K., and Middlebrooks, B. L. (1983). *Microbiol. Rev.* **47,** 97–120.

van Eden, W., Hogervorst, E. J., van der Zee, R., van Embden, J. D., Hensen, E. J., and Cohen, I. R. (1989). *Rheumatol. Int.* **9,** 187–191.

Van Voorhis, W. C., and Eisen, H. (1989). *J. Exp. Med.* **169,** 641–652.

Van Bohemen, C., Grumet, F. C., and Zanen, H. C. (1984). *Immunology* **52,** 607–609.

Van DenBroek, M. F., Hogervorst, E. J. M., VanBruggen, M. C. J., VanEden, W., VanDerZee, R., and VanDenBerg, W. B. (1989). *J. Exp. Med.* **170,** 449–466.

Viitanen, A. M., Lahesmaa-Rantala, R., Weiss, E., and Toivanen, A. (1988). *J. Rheumatol.* **15,** 1123–1125.

Walker, E. J., and Jeffrey, P. D. (1986). *Lancet* **2,** 605–607.

Walker, E. J., and Jeffrey, P. D. (1988). *Med. Hypotheses* **25,** 21–25.

Weise, M. J., and Carnegie, P. R. (1988). *N. Neurochem.* **51,** 1267–1273.

Williams, R. C., Jr. (1985). *Clin. Rheum. Dis.* **11,** 573–590.

Yamada, M., Zurbriggen, A., Oldstone, M. B. A., and Fujinami, R. S. (1991). *J. Virol.* **65,** 1370–1376.

Yamada, M., Zurbriggen, A., and Fujinami, R. S. (1990). *J. Exp. Med.* **171,** 1893–1907.

Yong, Z., Zhang, J. J., Schaack, T., Chen, S., Nakayama, A., and Yu, D. T. (1989). *Clin. Exp. Rheumatol.* **7,** 513–519.

Yu, D. T., Choo, S. Y., and Schaack, T. (1989). *Ann. Intern. Med.* **111,** 581–591.

CHAPTER 7

B-Cell Epitopes in Natural and Induced Autoimmunity

ROBERT L. RUBIN
ENG M. TAN
W. M. Keck Autoimmune Disease Center
Department of Molecular & Experimental Medicine
The Scripps Research Institute
La Jolla, California

I. INTRODUCTION

Circulating autoantibodies are a characteristic feature of most autoimmune diseases. A strict definition of autoantibodies requires demonstration of reactivity with cellular or secreted macromolecules or organelles derived from the serum donor. In practice, autoantibodies not only display relatively uniform binding to antigens derived from all members of the species (i.e., allogeneic reactivity), but also tend to bind quite well to homologous antigens obtained from phylogenetically disparate species. This xenogeneic binding property of autoantibodies has practical significance because it allows the use of nonhuman sources of antigens for detecting human autoantibodies. In addition and more significantly, cross-species reactivity of autoantibodies may suggest that major epitopes targeted by these antibodies are evolutionarily conserved regions of structural or functional importance. As discussed later, this concept has direct experimental support and has important implications in the origin of autoantibodies.

Epitope maps of autoantigens may help to formulate concepts on the structure, form, and composition of the putative immunogens driving the autoimmune response. The size of an epitope based on peptide-binding studies was considered to be approximately four to six amino acids (Fieser *et al.*, 1987), but the amino acid side-chains within an epitope are not necessarily derived from a continuous sequence and also may require a stringent secondary structure to facilitate proper side-chain contacts with the antibody combining site (Berzofsky, 1985). Furthermore, x-ray crystallographic studies of antigen–antibody complexes demonstrated that the complete epitope is much larger, consisting of 15–22 amino acid side-chains (Laver *et al.*, 1990), and usually a discontinuous sequence. Molecular-biology techniques offer great potential to identify minimal epitopes derived from a continuous sequence of amino acids, but epitopes determined by the conformation of the polypeptide backbone (secondary structure), protein folding (tertiary structure), or intermolecular interactions (quaternary structure) are difficult to characterize and have not been systematically evaluated. In this chapter we shall describe our own experiences, supporting the view that natural autoepitopes are generally determined by higher order, conformational structures on the target antigen.

II. EPITOPES IN DRUG-INDUCED AUTOIMMUNITY

A syndrome resembling systemic lupus erythematosus (SLE) can arise as a side effect of therapy with a wide variety of drugs. This is a milder form of the idiopathic disease, and it generally resolves after discontinuation of therapy with the implicated agent. Unlike SLE, drug-induced lupus (DIL) displays a highly restricted immune response largely limited to antihistone and anti-denatured-DNA antibodies. At commonly used doses, procainamide has the highest association with DIL (up to 20% of patients treated for > 1 yr), and hydralazine-induced lupus occurs in approximately 5–10% of treated patients. Other drugs show a much lower risk for development of DIL, but individual case reports of lupus induced by practolol, D-penicillamine, isoniazid, quinidine, propylthiouracil, chlorpromazine, acebutolol, and methyldopa are generally convincing because discontinuation of therapy is associated with resolution of symptoms and signs. In addition, many of these drugs, especially procainamide and chlorpromazine, induce antihistone and anti-denatured-DNA antibodies without accompanying symptomatic disease. These antihistone antibodies are also autoantibodies because they react with nuclei, but, as described later, have a fine specificity and isotype distinguishable from antihistone antibodies associated with symptomatic DIL.

A. Antibodies to Individual Histones Induced by Procainamide

The antinuclear antibody reactivity in procainamide-induced lupus sera can be largely accounted for by histone-reactive antibodies. Total histones consist of five major proteins. By polyacrylamide gel electrophoresis and Western blot techniques using procainamide-induced lupus sera, patterns of reactivity with individual histone have been reported. However, the significance of these observations is unclear, because there was little agreement in the predominant antigenic targets (H1, H2A and H2B) in Gohill *et al.* (1985); H3, H2B, and H2A in Portanova *et al.* (1987); and H2B, H1 and H4 in Craft *et al.* (1987). While these studies did suggest that accessible regions in chromatin are commonly antigenic for antibodies in procainamide-induced lupus sera, the apparent interstudy variation and the different patterns of autoantibody reactivity with individual histones in Western blot formats, failed to provide a clear picture of the nature of the putative immunogen underlying autoantibody elicitation.

B. Interpolypeptide Chain (Quaternary) Interactions Enhance Antigenicity of Histones in Procainamide-Induced Lupus

Isolation of individual histones by preparative scale biochemical techniques allowed application of these proteins to quantitative solid-phase immunoassay formats. In addition, the capacity of certain histones to interact with each other to form stable complexes facilitated comparison of individual histones and histone–histone complexes for differences in antigenicity. An example of this type of analysis is shown in Fig. 1 for IgM and IgG antihistone antibodies in four patients with procainamide-induced lupus syndrome. Although there appears to be considerable patient-to-patient variability in histone profiles, a common denominator linking these profiles is the presence of elevated reactivity on the H2A–H2B complex. This tends to be mainly IgG antibodies and cannot be

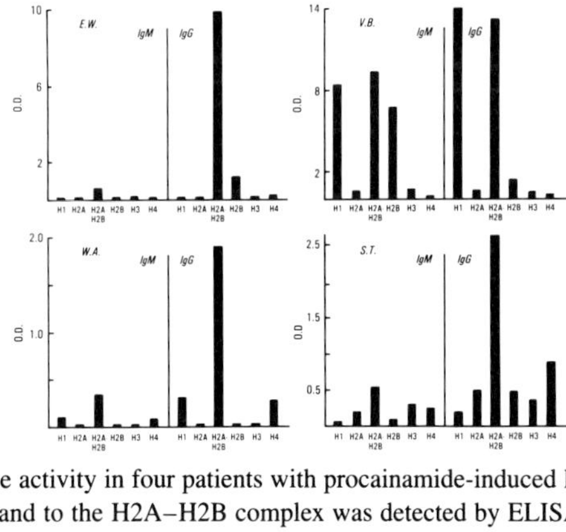

FIG. 1 Antihistone activity in four patients with procainamide-induced lupus. Antibody binding to individual histones and to the H2A–H2B complex was detected by ELISA with either antihuman IgM or antihuman IgG. From Rubin *et al.* (1985), with permission.

TABLE I

Antibody to the H2A–H2B Complex and Its Component Histones H2A and H2B[a]

		IgG reactivity to antigen (O.D.)			
		H2A–H2B Complex			
Patient status	Patient Number	Native	Denatured	H2A	H2B
Symptomatic	10	5.52	1.81	0.17	0.06
	8	2.98	0.81	0.19	0.07
	16	5.85	1.62	0.13	0.04
	13	4.34	1.70	0.16	0.21
Asymptomatic	21	1.80	1.68	1.85	1.74
	22	1.28	1.11	0.90	1.80
	23	1.77	1.40	0.33	2.99
	24	1.12	0.51	0.66	2.88

[a]In procainamide-induced autoimmunity. From Totoritis *et al.* (1988), with permission.

accounted for by reactivity on individual histones H2A and/or H2B. As shown in Table I, if the H2A–H2B complex was subsequently denatured by heating in sodium dodecyl sulfate, substantial loss in antigenicity for antibodies in patients with symptomatic procainamide-induced lupus occurred, although reactivity above that shown by the component monomers was still apparent, even with

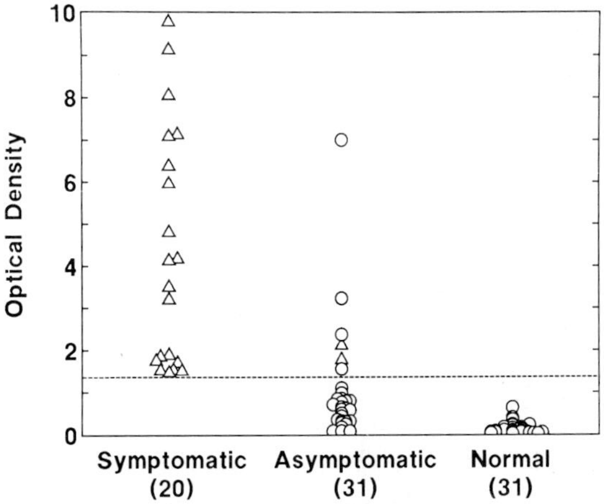

FIG. 2 Prevalence of IgG antibodies to the H2A–H2B complex in patients treated with procainamide. Triangles indicate serum samples with antibody activity against H2A–H2B that decreased at least twofold when tested against H2A–H2B complex denatured in sodium dodecyl sulfate. Circles represent sera with similar activity on the native H2A–H2B complex and the denatured antigen. The broken line at 1.4 optical density units defines an arbitrary cutoff value for a positive reaction characteristic of serum from patients with symptomatic procainamide-induced lupus. From Totoritis *et al.* (1988), with permission.

denatured H2A–H2B complex. That dimer complex requirement was not an assay artifact was demonstrated by the fact that patients treated with procainamide who remained asymptomatic, but developed antihistone antibodies, often had reactivity with individual component histones H2A and/or H2B. This activity was not enhanced by association of these histones in a dimer complex whether native or denatured (Table I). This observation also points to the diagnostic utility of this observation in that IgG anti-H2A-H2B is a relatively specific marker for symptomatic procainamide-induced lupus; the few nonsymptomatic patients who display reactivity with the H2A–H2B complex can usually be accounted for by a similar level of reactivity with the individual component histones H2A and/or H2B (Fig. 2). These results indicate that a special immune response develops in patients displaying lupuslike symptoms induced by procainamide in which the epitope requires higher order structures, presumably amino acid residues from both histones H2A and H2B, for stable antibody binding. The uniform association of this antibody activity with a specific disease syndrome suggests that this immune response is driven by an autoimmunogen with discrete and stable structural features.

C. Antigenicity of the (H2A-H2B)-DNA Subnucleosome Particle in Drug-Induced Lupus

The predominant reactivity of the H2A–H2B complex for antibodies in procainamide-induced lupus suggests that some form of this histone–histone complex may underlie the immune response in these patients. The H2A–H2B complex is a component of the nucleosome core particle, one each of these dimers flanking the kernel of the core particle, the H3–H4 tetramer. DNA wraps around this tripartite structure, making phosphate salt bridges with basic amino acid side-chains on the histones (Fig. 3). The ionic bonds between DNA and the H2A–H2B dimer are stable below an NaCl concentration of 0.6 *M*, and a nucleoprotein particle can be reconstituted by annealing the H2A–H2B dimer with DNA *in vitro*.

Comparison of the antigenicity of the (H2A–H2B)–DNA complex with its macromolecular components, the H2A–H2B dimer and DNA is shown in Table II. DNA enhanced from 2- to 10-fold the antigenicity of the H2A–H2B dimer for all sera from patients with procainamide-induced lupus. Increased antibody binding to the (H2A-H2B)–DNA complex was not owing to a separate population of antibodies to DNA, as the sera did not react with DNA bound to the solid phase via another basic protein (methylated albumin).

Of particular interest was the finding that sera from patients with lupus induced by drugs other than procainamide also had pronounced reactivity with the (H2A–H2B)–DNA complex. As shown in Table II, three patients with

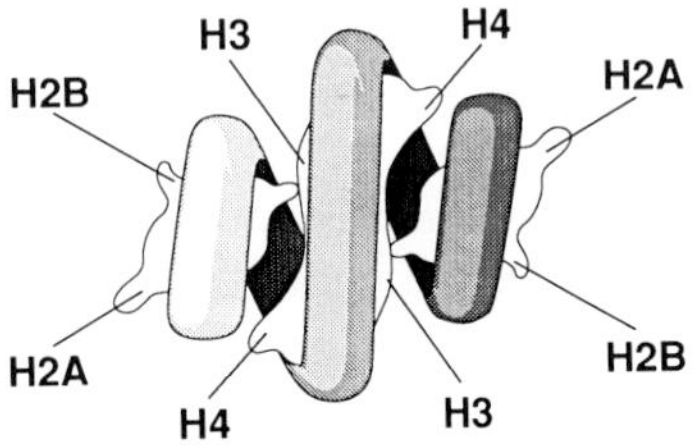

FIG. 3 Diagramatic representation of the nucleosome core particle. Approximately 146 base pairs of DNA wrap around an octamer of histones consisting of 2 H2A–H2B dimers flanking an H3–H4 tetramer. The dimers are shown artificially separated from the tetramer for clarity, but the native core particle is a compact structure stabilized by noncovalent bonds between residues in the tetramer and the dimer. This model is based on Richmond *et al.* (1984) and Burlingame *et al.* (1985).

quinidine-induced lupus and one patient with penicillamine-induced lupus had highly elevated reactivity with this antigen. Interestingly, these sera did not bind the H2A–H2B dimer in the absence of DNA. Thus, unlike procainamide-induced lupus antibodies, the antihistone antibodies in lupus induced by quinidine and penicillamine required both DNA and the H2A–H2B dimer for detectable antibody binding, whereas procainamide-induced lupus antibodies also displayed considerable binding to the H2A–H2B dimer in the absence of DNA. The remarkably high antigenicity of the dimer–DNA complex was observed in essentially all patients with procainamide-induced lupus, 50% of patients with quinidine-induced lupus, and in occasional patients with lupus induced by penicillamine, isoniazid, acebutalol, and α-methyldopa (manuscripts submitted). Since these antibodies also bound well to chromatin, it appears likely that chromatin or a degradation product containing the (H2A-H2B)–DNA subnucleosome particle may drive the autoimmune response in lupus induced by various drugs.

TABLE II
Effect of DNA on the Antigenicity of the H2A–H2B Complex[a]

Diagnosis	Patient Number	1gG reactivity to antigen (O.D.)		
		H2A–H2B	(H2A–H2B)–DNA	DNA
Procainamide-induced lupus	1	4.1	9.3	0.1
Procainamide-induced lupus	2	2.3	8.9	0.1
Procainamide-induced lupus	3	1.8	14.1	0.3
Procainamide-induced lupus	4	0.4	4.2	0.1
Quinidine-induced lupus	5	0.2	4.1	0.0
Quinidine-induced lupus	6	0.1	13.1	0.0
Quinidine-induced lupus	7	0.0	1.5	0.0
Penicillamine-induced lupus	8	0.1	5.0	0.2

[a]In drug-induced lupus.

III. CHARACTERISTICS OF MURINE EXPERIMENTAL ANTIHISTONE ANTIBODIES

Antihistone antibodies appear spontaneously in autoimmune NZB/NZW F_1 (Gioud *et al.*, 1983) and MRL/lpr/lpr (Costa and Monier, 1986) mice and arise during experimental murine SLE-like systemic autoimmune disease accompanying chronic graft-versus-host (GVH) disease in C57Bl/6 × DBA/2 F_1 mice (Portanova *et al.*, 1988). These are natural autoantibodies, and their induction may give insights into antihistone antibodies in human drug-induced and idiopathic SLE. If these autoantibodies are driven by endogenous histone, it may be of interest to compare the fine specificity of antihistone antibodies accompanying murine autoimmune disease with antibodies induced by deliberate immunization of otherwise normal mice with immunogenic forms of histones.

Soluble antigens are generally nonimmunogenic, but even autoantigens can be made to elicit an immune response if adsorbed to 0.4-μm diameter latex beads and injected intraperitoneally into mice (Rubin *et al.* 1990). This experimental model allowed us to explore the effect of different forms of histone in the induction of antihistone antibodies and to compare the fine specificity of these antibodies to those that arise during murine GVH disease in the same strain of mice.

Chromatin, the most native form of isolatable nucleoprotein, was nonimmunogenic when immobilized onto latex beads, but histone beads elicited a robust antihistone response. Figure 4 shows the average immune response of mice to immunization with histone beads and compares it to the autoantibody response of the same strain of mice undergoing a GVH reaction due to injection of parental lymphocytes. Both responses were characterized by antibodies capable of binding total histones in solid-phase enzyme-linked immunosorbent assay (ELISA), but antihistone antibodies elicited by beads were exclusively IgM, whereas GVH-induced antibodies were predominantly IgG in isotype. More important, antibodies in GVH animals displayed good reactivity with chromatin, but chromatin was a relatively poor antigen for experimentally induced antihistone antibodies. These results were consistent with absorption studies in which more than ten times as much chromatin was needed to remove the antihistone activity elicited by deliberate immunization with histone beads compared to the natural antihistone response accompanying GVH disease (Rubin *et al.*, 1990).

Further examination of the fine specificity of antihistone antibodies in these two experimental murine systems revealed additional differences. The H2A–H2B dimer was a good antigen for both groups of mice, although the enhanced antigenicity compared to the monomeric components H2A and H2B as observed in human procainamide-induced lupus was not apparent. However, as shown in Table III, when DNA was complexed to the H2A–H2B dimer, experimentally

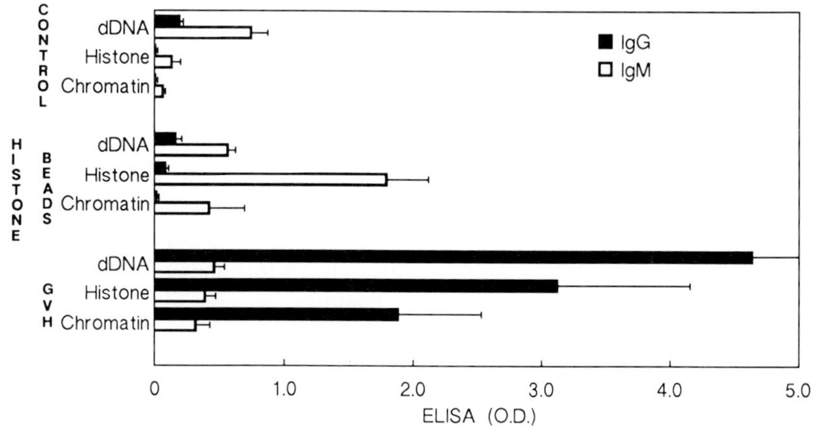

FIG. 4 Antibodies in GVH disease and in histone-immunized C57B1/6xDBA/2 F_1 mice. Sera were collected 6 weeks after the initiation of the immunization procedure or after injection of DBA/2 lymphocytes to induce GVH disease. Antibodies were measured by ELISA on three antigens using immunoglobulin class-specific detecting reagents as shown. From Rubin *et al.* (1990), with permission.

induced antihistone antibodies no longer reacted, whereas antihistone antibodies in GVH mice retained and even increased reactivity to H2A-H2B in the presence of DNA. The dramatic suppression of the antigenicity of the H2A–H2B dimer when complexed to DNA indicates that either experimentally induced antihistone antibodies bind to regions on the H2A–H2B dimer that overlap with the DNA binding sites on the dimer, or an indirect effect of DNA on the epitope conformation occurs. These results are consistent with the antigenicity of other (H2A-H2B)-containing DNA–histone complexes such as chromatin and nuclei in which good binding was observed with GVH but not with bead-elicited antihistone antibodies.

TABLE III
Effect of DNA on the Antigenicity of the H2A–H2B Complex[a]

Group	N	Antibody activity (O.D. ± S.D.)		
		nDNA	H2A–H2B	(H2A–H2B)–DNA
Unimmunized	9	0.29 ± 0.23	0.40 ± 0.13	0.08 ± 0.14
Histone bead immunized	10	0.26 ± 0.21	4.19 ± 3.88	0.22 ± 0.53
GVH disease	10	0.33 ± 0.24	1.91 ± 2.57	2.53 ± 4.39

[a]In murine GVH disease and in histone-immunized mice. From Rubin *et al.* (1990), with permission.

Thus, antihistone antibodies accompanying GVH disease are true autoantibodies, capable of binding native forms of histone, nucleoprotein, and nuclei. In contrast, antihistone antibodies elicited by deliberate immunization are pseudoautoantibodies, binding histones only to regions that are inaccessible in native chromatin. Unlike antihistone antibodies accompanying murine GVH disease and human drug-induced lupus, immunogenic forms of histone coated on beads do not give rise to antibodies of the same specificities as those in natural autoimmunity.

IV. CHARACTERISTICS OF NATURAL EPITOPES IN NONHISTONE NUCLEAR ANTIGENS

Important insights concerning epitopes on nuclear antigens in natural autoimmunity have also come from studies of the nonhistone nuclear protein antigens. The majority of patients with SLE have antibodies to DNA, histones, Sm and/or SS-A, with antibodies to DNA and Sm being of greatest diagnostic specificity for SLE. However, antibodies to a variety of other nuclear antigens such as SS-B, nuclear and ribosomal RNP, and PCNA (proliferating cell nuclear antigen) are occasionally observed in individual patients. Anti-SS-B is also found in a high percentage of patients with Sjögren's syndrome (SS) and is the basis for the abbreviation that signifies Sjögren's syndrome B antigen.

A. Evolutionary Conservation of Autoepitopes

1. SS-B

SS-B/La is a nuclear protein of 46 to 48 kDa, which is one of the target antigens of autoantibodies in the sera of patients with lupus and Sjögren's syndrome [reviewed in Chapter 8 and in Tan (1989)]. This nuclear protein is transiently associated with a number of RNA species, especially those transcribed by RNA polymerase III, such as precursors of tRNA and 5S RNA, 4.5 RNA, 7S RNA, the so-called Y RNAs and U6 RNA. SS-B forms complexes with pol III-transcribed precursor RNAs and other RNAs to form ribonucleoprotein particles.

Calf thymus SS-B antigen was obtained by affinity column purification, using IgG fraction of a human serum containing the cognate antibody. This purified SS-B antigen was used to immunize BALB/c mice, and hybridomas producing antibodies were isolated from splenocytes of a mouse with high-titer antibody. Five murine monoclonal antibodies were generated in this fashion, and the reactivities of these monoclonal antibodies were analyzed by comparison with the reactivities of human anti-SS-B antibodies (Chan and Tan, 1987). Figure 5

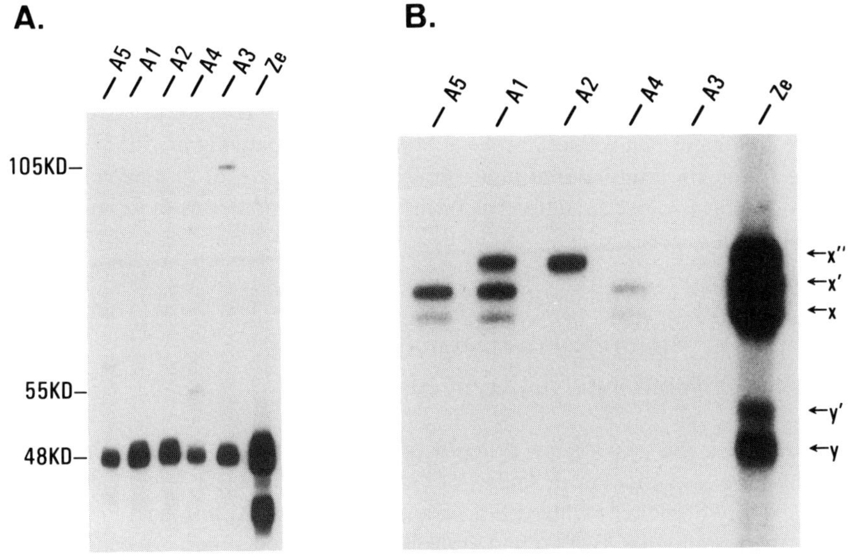

FIG. 5 Immunoblotting analysis of the reactivities of monoclonal antibodies (A1–A5) using HeLa cell extract (A) and HeLa cell extract partially digested with S. aureus V8 protease (B).

illustrates the Western blot analysis of the five monoclonal antibodies A1 to A5 compared with human serum Ze. Differences in reactivity were clearly apparent, with the murine monoclonal antibodies immunoblotting the 48-kDa complete SS-B protein, and the human antibody blotting, in addition, a degradation product of the whole protein with which the monoclonal antibodies were nonreactive. Figure 5B illustrates a study in which the SS-B protein was partially digested with *Staphylococcus aureus* V8 protease, resulting in three fragments, X, X′ and X″ and two smaller fragments designated Y and Y′, which were recognized by human serum Ze. The reaction of the murine monoclonals was quite diverse, with A3 and A4 showing little or no reactivity with any of the digestion products, and others showing incomplete spectrum of reaction with the X products and no reaction with the Y products.

Another method for analyzing the reactivity of these antibodies was immunoprecipitation of the SS-B ribonucleoprotein particle and analysis of the RNAs that were coprecipitated. This study is illustrated in Fig. 6, showing immunoprecipitation of ^{32}P-labeled HeLa cell extracts with mouse monoclonal antibodies and serum Ze. RNA was extracted from the immunoprecipitate with phenol and analyzed on urea/polyacrylamide gels. Human serum Ze and monoclonal antibodies A1, A2, and A3 were all capable of immunoprecipitating precursor tRNAs complexed to SS-B. However, monoclonal antibodies A4 and A5 did not immunoprecipitate tRNAs. It could be deduced from this experiment

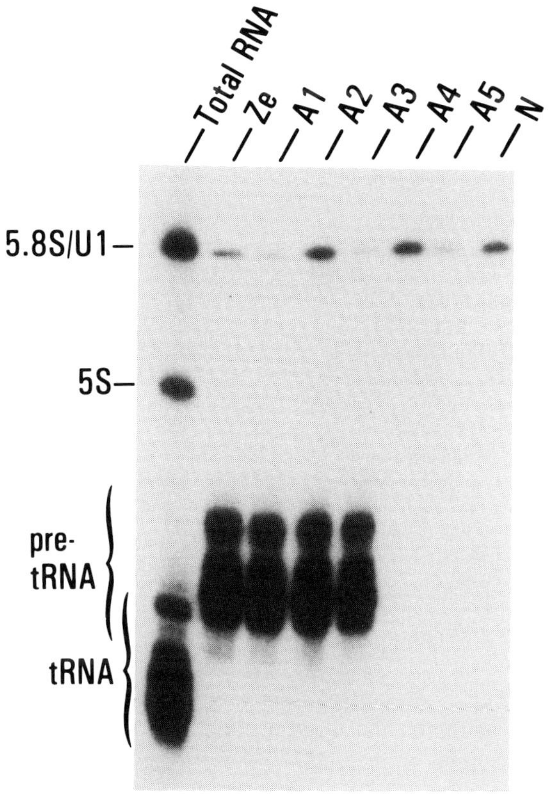

FIG. 6 Immunoprecipitation of ^{32}P-phosphate-labeled HeLa cell extracts with mouse monoclonal antibodies and human serum Ze. RNA was extracted from the immunoprecipitate with phenol, precipitated with ethanol, and analyzed on 7 *M* urea/8% polyacrylamide gel.

that A4 and A5 were reacting with epitopes present only in denatured SS-B protein, as demonstrated by their reactivity in Western blots, but these epitopes were not present in the native ribonucleoprotein particle.

Human antibodies to SS-B react by immunofluorescence with a nuclear antigen that is present in a wide variety of species. This method of analysis was applied to the murine monoclonal antibodics and the reference human serum used in these studies (Table IV). Human serum Ze reacted with SS-B nuclear antigen in tissues ranging from human to rat kangaroo. In contrast, monoclonal antibodies A4 and A5, which were nonreactive in immunoprecipitation, were also nonreactive with the nuclear antigen in immunofluorescence. Monoclonal antibodies A1, A2, and A3 were reactive with SS-B nuclear antigen in tissues of man, monkey, rabbit, and bovine species, but were nonreactive with hamster,

TABLE IV
Species-Specific Reactivities of MAbs to SS-B

		Immunofluorescence[a]					
		Murine MAbs					Human serum
Species	Cell-line origin	A1	A2	A3	A4	A5	ZE+[b]
Human	HEp-2, larynx	+	+	+	−	−	+
Human	HeLa, cervix	+	+	+	−	−	+
Human	Raji, Burkitt's lymphoma	+	+	+	−	−	+
Monkey	Vero, kidney	+	+	+	−	−	+
Rabbit	R9ab, lung	+	+	+	−	−	+
Bovine	MDBK, kidney	+	+	+	−	−	+
Hamster	BHK-21, kidney	−	−	−	−	−	+
Rat	6m2, kidney	−	−	−	−	−	+
Mouse	3T3, fibroblasts	−	−	−	−	−	+
Rat kangaroo	PtK2, kidney	−	−	−	−	−	+

[a]Cells were grown in Lab-Tek tissue culture chambers and fixed in a mixture of acetone and methanol (3 : 1) at −20°C for 2 min.

[b]Ze serum is the CDC reference serum for anti-SS-B/La specificity.

rat, mouse, and rat kangaroo. The evidence that epitopes recognized by monoclonal A1 to A5 were not the same targets of human autoantibodies was supported by additional evidence from blocking experiments, showing that human serum Ze failed to inhibit the reactivity of monoclonal antibodies with SS-B either in Western blots or in ELISA. These experiments showed that human autoantibodies were recognizing epitopes different from those of five murine monoclonal antibodies produced by experimental immunization, and more important, that human autoantibodies targeted more highly conserved epitopes.

2. PCNA, Sm, and Fibrillarin

The conserved nature of the SS-B epitope recognized by human autoantibodies is by no means unique to this autoimmune system. PCNA was originally identified as a 36-kDa nuclear protein antigen present in proliferating cells and was detected by autoantibodies from a subset of human patients with lupus (Miyachi *et al.*, 1978). PCNA was shown by immunofluorescence and autoradiography to colocalize with sites of DNA synthesis in the nuclei of proliferating mammalian tissue culture cells (Bravo, 1986). It has been shown that PCNA is the auxiliary protein of DNA polymerase δ (Mathews *et al.*, 1984), whose function is identified with leading-strand synthesis at the DNA replication fork (Prelich and Stillman, 1988). In the ciliated protozoan, *Euplotes eurystomus*, DNA replication as determined by uptake of labeled thymidine has been shown to take place at the rear zone of the replication band in macronuclei. Using human anti-PCNA antibody, this zone of DNA replication in the macronucleus is reactive with anti-PCNA antibody in immunofluorescence (Olins *et al.*, 1989). Conditions such as starvation or heat shock that reduce macronuclei replication also resulted in a decrease of PCNA in the replication bands. The epitopes on PCNA recognized by human antibody have now been observed in a wide range of species including human, rat, amphibian, yeast, and ciliated protozoa. The highly conserved character of epitopes recognized by human autoantibodies has also been shown for the Sm antigen. In the case of fibrillarin, a 34-kDa protein antigen of the nucleolus, human autoantibodies can be used to detect fibrillarin in plant cells.

B. Functional Roles of Autoepitopes

The conserved characteristic of epitopes recognized by natural autoantibodies suggests that these epitopes could be related to structures that have been preserved in evolution in order to subserve important or perhaps essential structural or functional roles in the biology of the cell. There are many instances of autoantibodies that inhibit important functions. These include autoantibody to Sm, which inhibits precursor mRNA splicing; autoantibody to RNA polymerase 1, which inhibits RNA pol 1 transcription; autoantibody to DNA topoisomerase 1, which inhibits relaxation of supercoiled DNA; and autoantibody to transfer RNA synthetases, which inhibits aminoacylation of tRNAs. Two such studies were especially revealing in that they compared the reactivities of natural antibodies to induced experimental antibodies.

1. Threonyl-tRNA Synthetase

Certain patients with polymyositis produce antibodies to threonyl-tRNA synthetase. Antibodies to tRNA synthetases are described further in Chapter 8 of this volume. The reactions of natural autoantibody were compared with an antibody induced by immunization of rats with purified threonyl-tRNA synthetase (Dang *et al.*, 1988). The human autoantibody reacted with the native but not the denatured form of threonyl-tRNA synthetase. This was demonstrated in immunoblots in which SDS-treated and gel-electrophoresed tRNA synthetase was analyzed in the standard Western blotting technique. The human antibody was not reactive with this form of threonyl-tRNA synthetase. On the other hand, if the tRNA synthetase was not subjected to Western blotting but was directly applied to cellulose nitrate in a dot-blot assay, human antibody was fully reactive. In contrast, the experimentally induced rat antibody to threonyl-tRNA synthetase was reactive in both Western blots and dot blots. This study suggested that the epitope recognized by human antibody was at least conformational in nature and that the conformational epitope was destroyed in the Western blotting procedure. This conclusion received further support in a functional assay in which human autoantibody was able to inactivate threonyl-tRNA synthetase, whereas the rat antibody was inactive.

2. PCNA

Experiments with PCNA also illustrated the functional nature of the epitope recognized by naturally occurring antibodies (Tan *et al.*, 1987). Two experimentally induced murine monoclonal antibodies to PCNA and a rabbit polyclonal antibody raised against an *N*-terminal peptide were compared with a human autoantibody to PCNA by examining the effect of these antibodies on DNA polymerase δ function. Human antibody was capable of neutralizing DNA pol δ function based on its ability to inhibit the activity of the auxiliary protein (PCNA), which is required by pol δ in template/primer systems containing high template:primer ratios, poly(dA)/oligo(dT) (20:1). Immunoprecipitation comparing these antibodies also showed that whereas human autoantibodies recognized native auxiliary protein, the epitopes recognized by both the antipeptide antibody and monoclonal antibodies were not accessible in the native protein. These two studies emphasize the important feature that the epitopes on autoantigens recognized by natural antibodies frequently include the active or functional sites of these proteins. In contrast, experimentally induced antibodies appear to recognize other antigenic sites on these proteins, some of which appear to be denatured regions of the target molecules.

V. Structure of Natural Autoepitopes— Discontinuous Sequences in PCNA

Insights into the structure of epitopes recognized by natural antibodies have been obtained from the study of recombinant products of cDNA clones that encode PCNA (Huff *et al.*, 1990). In this study, the strategy was to produce deletion mutants of PCNA cDNA and to analyze the reactivity of recombinant proteins by immunoprecipitation of transcription–translation products and by Western blotting of fusion proteins. As a preliminary approach, 15-mer synthetic peptides that spanned the entire sequence of the full-length protein were used in ELISA to determine reactivity of two murine monoclonals raised against purified PCNA and a rabbit polyclonal antibody raised against an *N*-terminus synthetic peptide. These experimentally induced antibodies reacted with expected synthetic peptides, whereas none of 14 human lupus sera-containing antibodies to PCNA were reactive. This result by itself denoted that the epitopes recognized by human antibodies were not present in continuous-sequence 15-mer peptides of linearized PCNA.

Deletion mutants of PCNA were constructed as shown in Fig. 7. IVPs 1–6 represented *in vitro* transcription–translation products, and fusion products (FPs)

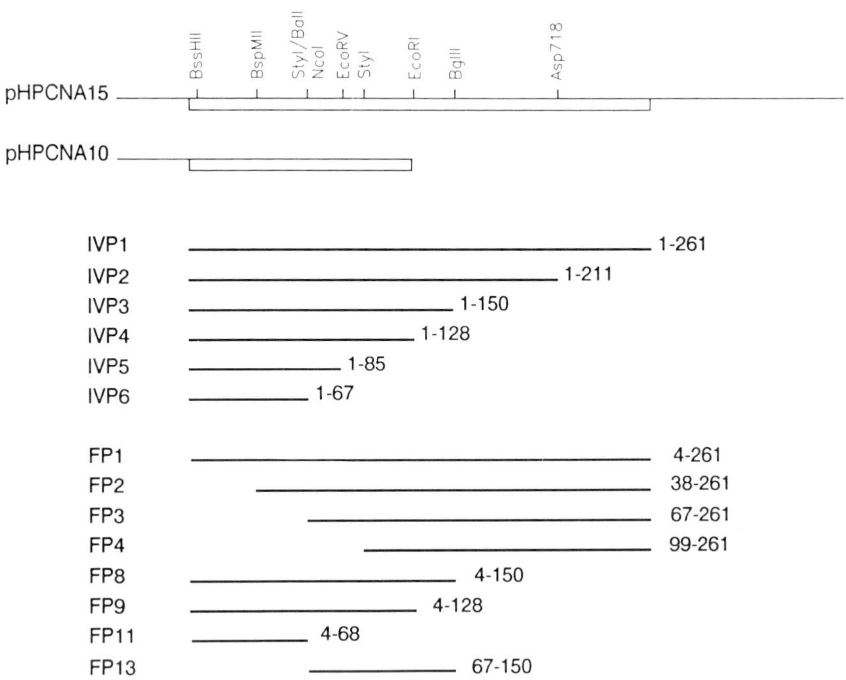

FIG. 7 cDNA restriction enzyme map of PCNA and the cDNA constructs that were used to generate recombinant protein products. IVP1–IVP6 were *in vitro* transcription and translation products, and FP1–FP13 were fusion proteins. These recombinant protein products were used in immunoprecipitation (IVP1–IVP6) and in Western blotting (FP1–FP13) to map fragments reactive with antibodies.

1–13 represented fusion products of the deletion mutants generated by restriction enzymes. Again, experimentally induced antibodies, i.e., rabbit polyclonal antibody to amino-terminal peptide and two murine monoclonal antibodies induced by immunization with purified PCNA reacted by both immunoprecipitation and Western blotting with expected protein products. The 14 lupus sera demonstrated a variety of reactivities (Table V). All 14 human sera immunoprecipitated the full-length translation product IVP1, but had different reactivities with truncated products. In Western blotting, nine human sera failed to react with any fusion proteins, whereas five others were reactive in different patterns. In general, the lupus sera could be divided into four subgroups as depicted in Table V. By a process of deduction analysis, the epitopes recognized by the 14 human lupus sera could be mapped as illustrated in Fig. 8. Lupus group II sera (top left) were reactive only by immunoprecipitation, and the regions necessary for reactivity could be localized to the stippled and hatched areas. On the other hand, lupus

TABLE V

Immunoreactivity of *In Vitro* Protein Products and Fusion Proteins of PCNA

		Reactivity with antibodies															
				SLE I					SLE II				SLE III			SLE IVA / SLE IVB	
Protein product	Aa sequence	RAPab	MoAb 19A2	AI	YK	MI	KU	JO	CR	OD	CA	EB	PT	AL	YO	NE	FL
IVP—Immunoprecipitation																	
IVP 1	1-261	+	+	+	+	+	+	+	+	+	+	+	+	+	+	+	+
IVP 2	1-211	+	+	−	−	−	−	−	+	−	−	−	−	−	−	+	−
IVP 3	1-150	+	+	−	−	−	−	−	+	−	−	−	−	−	−	+	−
IVP 4	1-128	+	−	−	−	−	−	−	+	+	+	+	−	−	−	−	+
IVP 5	1-85	+	−	−	−	−	−	−	−	+	+	+	−	−	−	−	+
IVP 6	1-67	+	−	−	−	−	−	−	−	−	−	−	−	−	−	−	−
FP— Immunoblotting																	
FP-1	4-261	+	+	−	−	−	−	−	−	−	−	−	+	+	+	+	+
FP-2	38-261	−	+	−	−	−	−	−	−	−	−	−	+	+	+	+	+
FP-3	67-261	−	+	−	−	−	−	−	−	−	−	−	+	+	+	+	+
FP-4	99-261	−	+	−	−	−	−	−	−	−	−	−	+	+	+	+	+
FP-8	4-150	+	+	−	−	−	−	−	−	−	−	−	+	+	+	+	+
FP-9	4-128	+	+	−	−	−	−	−	−	−	−	−	−	+	+	+	+
FP-11	4-68	+	−	−	−	−	−	−	−	−	−	−	−	−	−	−	−
FP-13	67-150	−	+	−	−	−	−	−	−	−	−	−	−	+	−	−	+

group III sera (top right) were nonreactive in immunoprecipitation with truncated translation products but were reactive with fusion proteins, and the regions necessary for reactivity were mapped to the shaded areas. The minor groups IVA and IVB are shown in the bottom left and right frames, respectively, and they incorporated properties of both groups II and III.

This analysis, taken together with the total lack of reactivity of human autoantibodies with synthetic peptides, demonstrates the striking difference between epitopes recognized by induced antibodies and by natural antibodies. It was also quite remarkable that nine of 14 lupus sera failed to immunoblot recombinant fusion proteins, although they were all capable of immunoprecipitating full-length translation product. These observations strongly suggest that epitopes recognized by naturally occurring human antibodies comprise higher-order conformational structures that are not represented in the synthetic peptides. This type of conformational structure may be formed by amino acid residues from two or more regions of the molecule that are brought into proximity with one another by protein folding (tertiary conformation). If the epitope recognized by natural antibodies was from discontinuous sequences, it appears that none of the PCNA synthetic peptides contains sufficient portions of the epitope for stable antibody binding. These observations further emphasize the special features of *native*

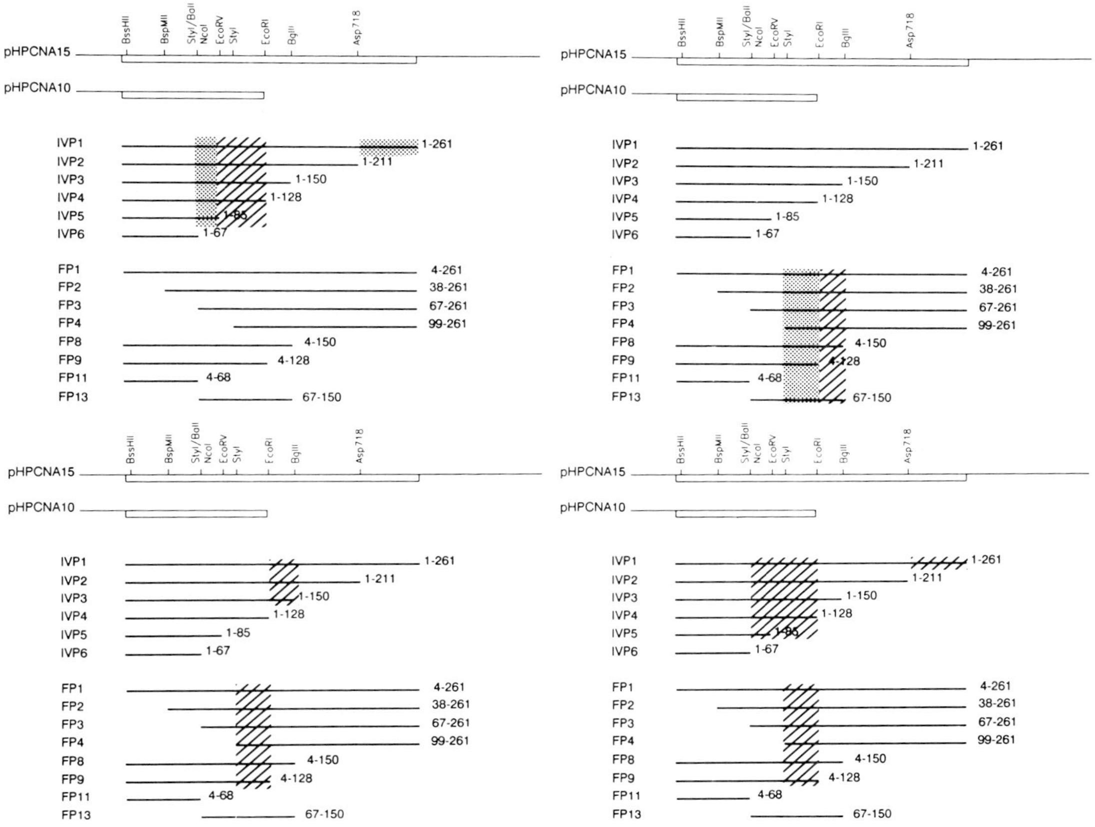

FIG. 8 Epitope mapping of reactive regions in PCNA deduced by subtraction analysis of data derived from immunoprecipitation and Western blotting (see Table V). SLE group II sera (top left) were reactive only by immunoprecipitation, and the regions necessary for reactivity could be localized to the stippled and hatched areas. SLE group III sera (top right) were nonreactive with truncated translation products but were reactive with FPs, and the regions necessary for reactivity were mapped to the shaded areas. The reactivities of group IVA are shown in bottom left of the figure, and those of group IVB, in bottom right of the figure.

epitopes of intranuclear antigens that are recognized by autoantibodies. These features may be related to protein folding or to association of the antigen with other intranuclear proteins or nucleic acids, as might occur with antigens that are components of subcellular particles. Geysen *et al.* (1986) have analyzed the reactivity of a monoclonal antibody directed against a discontinuous antigenic determinant in foot-and-mouth disease virus. They showed that a linear hexapeptide with the appropriate stereochemistry could mimic an epitope that was deduced to be derived from three separate regions of the protein. This approach may also be useful in identifying discontinuous autoepitopes.

VI. SUMMARY AND CONCLUSIONS

The data discussed in the preceding sections focus on the dichotomy between natural and immunization-induced autoantibodies. These observations derive from studies on the fine specificity of both polyclonal and monoclonal antibodies to a diversity of macromolecules that are often targets of autoantibodies including PCNA, threonyl-tRNA synthetase, SS-B, and histones. Detection of natural autoantibodies generally required assays that presented antigens in a nativelike form, such as whole cells as substrates in immunofluorescence assays, aqueous cell extracts in immunoprecipitation assays, or solid-phase immunoassays using purified intact proteins or particles consisting of protein–protein and/or protein–nucleic acid complexes. These autoantibodies apparently recognize quaternary, tertiary, and possibly secondary structures native to the target antigen, but rarely show reactivity with oligopeptides, even those of sufficient size to encompass a minimal epitope. Autoantibodies are not species specific, reacting with epitopes that are often conserved across phyla and even kingdoms. In contrast, antibodies induced by deliberate immunization are often specific to the species from which the immunogen was derived and almost never react with the homologous antigen in the host. These pseudo-autoantibodies may react with denatured epitopes in the immunogen or with components present only in the form of the antigen used in the assay. Induced antibodies frequently react with linear sequences of amino acids as found in peptides, deletion mutants, or fusion proteins of the parent molecules. Although some exceptions to this dichotomy between natural autoantibodies and induced antibodies are implied by some reports, rigorous scrutiny of their fine specificity may yet reveal significant distinctions.

One conclusion that follows the observation that higher-order structures are required for antigenicity is that the *in vivo* immunogen putatively driving the autoimmune response is a native, probably particulate form of self material. The observation that autoantibodies stand out as reacting with functional regions or active sites of the targeted particle may have at least two interpretations: (1) the predominant autoimmune response is directed to these active functional sites, or (2) the autoimmune response is directed to immunodominant regions of the particle, some of which include important structural and/or functional regions. Rigorous distinction between these alternative explanations is not easy, requiring careful absorption and/or affinity purification studies in order to determine the polyclonality of the autoimmune response.

The observation that immunization-induced antibodies usually reacted with non-native epitopes may also have two interpretations: (1) isolation of the particle and preparation of the immunogen may cause extensive denaturation, directing the bulk of the immune response toward those non-native structures, or (2) the immune response of an inherently normal animal permits recognition of only those regions of the immunogen that are different from the animal's own self material. If the immunogen is derived from syngeneic tissue, an immune response to only the physically and/or chemically denatured regions may develop. Distinguishing these possibilities is hampered by not knowing what happens to the immunogen once it is introduced into the host animal and the fact that methodology for assaying antibodies cannot readily distinguish between binding to native versus denatured epitopes in the test antigen.

Despite these difficulties in interpretation of experimental observations, some speculation as to the significance of each interpretation might be permitted. Based on the first series of interpretations, the normal failure to develop autoimmunity may be attributable to absence of native, potentially immunogenic particles *in vivo*. Normally potential autoimmunogens may not encounter the immune system because they are sequestered within the cell. After cell death, intracellular contents may normally be quickly disposed of by the reticuloendothelial system and therefore not delivered in a native form to lymphocytes possessing autoantigen receptors. Using this argument, autoimmunity could be a sequence of abnormal cell death or abnormal processing of cell debris, allowing native forms such as functionally active cellular organelles or subcellular particles to encounter the immune system.

Alternatively, there may normally be an active mechanism preventing an immune response to self material, even if it is present in potentially immunogenic forms. An autoimmune response would then occur when this immune-tolerance mechanism breaks down. Loss of immune tolerance to specific macromolecules would permit particulate cellular debris containing these macromolecules to initiate and sustain an autoimmune response, modulated by immunodominant features in the immunogen.

These speculations are intended to provide the framework for interpreting previous and future studies on this challenging problem in immunology.

REFERENCES

Berzofsky, J. A. (1985). Intrinsic and extrinsic factors in protein antigenic structure. *Science* **229**, 932–940.

Bravo, R. (1986). Synthesis of the nuclear protein cyclin (PCNA) and its relationship with DNA replication. *Exp. Cell Res.* **163,** 287–293.

Burlingame, R. W., Love, W. E., Wang, B.-C., Hamlin, R., Xuong, N.-H., and Moudrianakis, E. N. (1985). Crystallographic structure of the octameric histone core of the nucleosome at a resolution of 3.3 Å. *Science* **228,** 546–553.

Chan, E, K. L., and Tan, E. M. (1987). Human autoantibody-reactive epitopes on SS-B/La are highly conserved in comparison with epitopes recognized by murine monoclonal antibodies. *J. Exp. Med.* **166,** 1627–1640.

Costa, O., and Monier, J. C. (1986). Antihistone antibodies detected by micro-ELISA and immunoblotting in mice with lupus-like syndrome (MRL/l, MRL/n, PN, and NZB strains). *Clin. Immunol. Immunopathol.* **40,** 276–282.

Craft, J. E., Radding, J. A., Harding, M. W., Bernstein, R. M., and Hardin, J. A. (1987). Autoantigenic histone epitopes: A comparison between procainamide- and hydralazine-induced lupus. *Arthritis Rheum.* **30,** 689–694.

Dang, C. V., Tan, E. M., and Traugh, J. A. (1988). Myositis autoantibody reactivity and catalytic function of threonyl-tRNA synthetase. *FASEB J.* **2,** 2376–2379.

Fieser, T. M., Tainer, J. A., Geyson, H. M., Houghten, R. A., and Lerner, R. A. (1987). Influence of protein flexibility and peptide conformation on reactivity of monoclonal antipeptide antibodies with a protein α-helix. *Proc. Natl. Acad. Sci. U.S.A.* **84,** 8568–8572.

Geysen, H. M., Rodda, S. J., and Mason, T. J. (1986). *A priori* delineation of a peptide which mimics a discontinuous antigenic determinant. *Mol. Immunol.* **27,** 709–715.

Gioud, M., Kotzin, B. L., Rubin, R. L., Joslin, F. G., and Tan, E. M. (1983). *In vivo* and *in vitro* production of anti-histone antibodies in NZB/NZW mice. *J. Immunol.* **131,** 269–279.

Gohill, J., Cary, P. D., Couppez, M., and Fritzler, M. J. (1985). Antibodies from patients with drug-induced and idiopathic lupus erythematosus react with epitopes restricted to the amino and carboxyl termini of histone. *J. Immunol.* **135,** 3116–3121.

Huff, J. P., Roos, G., Peebles, C. L., Houghten, R., Sullivan, K. F., and Tan, E. M. (1990). Insights into native epitopes of proliferating cell nuclear antigen using recombinant DNA protein products. *J. Exp. Med.* **172,** 419–429.

Laver, W. G., Air, G. M., Webster, R. G., and Smith-Gill, S. J. (1990). Epitopes on protein antigens: Misconceptions and realities. *Cell* **61,** 553–556.

Mathews, M. B., Bernstein, R. M., Franza, B. R., Jr., and Garrels, J. I. (1984). Identity of the proliferating cell nuclear antigen and cyclin. *Nature (Lond.)* **309,** 374–376.

Miyachi, K., Fritzler, M. J., and Tan, E. M. (1978). Autoantibody to a nuclear antigen in proliferating cells. *J. Immunol.* **121,** 2228–2234.

Olins, D. E., Olins, A. L., Cacheiro, L. H., and Tan, E. M. (1989). Proliferating cell nuclear antigen/cyclin in the ciliate *Euplotes eurystomus:* Localization in the replication band and in micronuclei. *J. Cell Biol.* **109,** 1399–1410.

Portanova, J. P., Arndt, R. E., and Kotzin, B. L. (1988). Selective production of autoantibodies in graft-vs-host-induced and spontaneous murine lupus. *J. Immunol.* **140,** 755–760.

Portanova, J. P., Arndt, R. E., Tan, E. M., and Kotzin, B. L. (1987). Anti-histone antibodies in idiopathic and drug-induced lupus recognize distinct intra-histone regions. *J. Immunol.* **138,** 446–451.

Prelich, G., and Stillman, B. (1988). Coordinated leading and lagging strand synthesis during SV40 DNA replication *in vitro* requires PCNA. *Cell* **53,** 117–126.

Richmond, T. J., Finch, J. T., Rushton, B., Rhodes, D., and Klug, A. (1984). Structure of the nucleosome core particle at 7 Å resolution. *Nature* **311,** 532–537.

Rubin, R. L., McNally, E. M., Nusinow, S. R., Robinson, C. A., and Tan, E. M. (1985). IgG antibodies to the histone complex H2A-H2B characterize procainamide-induced lupus. *Clin. Immunol. Immunopathol.* **36,** 49–59.

Rubin, R. L., Tang, F.-L., Tsay, G., and Pollard, K. M. (1990). Pseudoautoimmunity in normal mice: Anti-histone antibodies elicited by immunization versus induction during graft-vs-host reaction. *Clin. Immunol. Immunopathol.* **54,** 320–332.

Tan, E. M. (1989). Antinuclear antibodies: Diagnostic markers for autoimmune diseases and probes for cell biology. *Adv. Immunol.* **44,** 93–151.

Tan, C.-K., Sullivan, K., Li, X., Tan, E. M., Downey, K. W., and So, A. G. (1987). Autoantibody to the proliferating cell nuclear antigen neutralizes the activity of the auxiliary protein for DNA polymerase delta. *Nucleic Acids Res.* **15,** 9299–9308.

Totoritis, M. C., Tan, E. M., McNally, E. M., and Rubin, R. L. (1988). Association of antibody to histone complex H2A-H2B with symptomatic procainamide-induced lupus. *N. Engl. J. Med.* **318,** 1431–1436.

CHAPTER 8

Disease-Specific Autoantibodies in the Systemic Rheumatic Diseases

MORRIS REICHLIN
Arthritis/Immunology Program
Oklahoma Medical Research Foundation
Department of Medicine
Oklahoma University Health Sciences Center
Oklahoma City, Oklahoma

I. INTRODUCTION

Systemic rheumatic diseases are characterized by the presence of families of specific autoantibodies. These autoantibodies not only have diagnostic utility but they also partition patients into subsets, each with a varying course and prognosis. They were first recognized by two major techniques: double diffusion in agar by the method of Ouchterlony and by their reactions with specific subcellular organelles in indirect immunofluorescence. In the past 10 years, direct biochemical purification and characterization, Western blotting, protein and tRNA immunoprecipitation with appropriately labeled cell extracts, and most recently, cloning of cDNAs encoding their antigenic proteins, have led to a rich picture of their structure.

This chapter will focus on such disease-specific antibodies in four diseases: poly- and dermatomyositis, progressive systemic sclerosis or scleroderma, systemic lupus erythematosus, and primary Sjögren's syndrome. The emphasis will be on the biochemical definition of the antigenic targets and their association with disease subsets. As all these diseases are of unknown etiology, it is tantalizing to think that these disease-specific autoantibodies are clues to their causes. Detailed clinical information about these diseases can be found in the initial edition of *The Autoimmune Diseases* (1985) and in standard textbooks of rheumatology.

II. POLY- AND DERMATOMYOSITIS

Polymyositis (PM) is an inflammatory muscle disease in which there is a progressive destruction of muscle fibers characterized by a mononuclear cell infiltrate, suggesting a direct cytotoxic attack of lymphocytes on the muscle cell. Other issues not related to disease-specific antibodies are dealt with in Chapter 13. This process results in weakness varying from mild to profound, and the disease is usually chronic. In dermatomyositis (DM), the muscle disease is accompanied by a characteristic inflammatory erythematous skin disease, which has a typical clinical distribution on the extensor surfaces of the extremities and the eyelids, in which a violaceous discoloration is present and is called heliotrope. It is widely believed that, because of immunogenetic and pathological differences, as well as differences in the inflammatory infiltrates in the muscle, PM and DM are different diseases. The frequency of the various autoantibodies to be described in this chapter lend further support to this view. The autoantibody specificities that are strongly associated with PM and DM are listed in Table I.

A. Antibodies to tRNA Synthetases

The first antibody that was found to be a marker for PM was the anti-Jo_1 system described by the reaction of sera with a concentrated extract of calf thymus tissue. This precipitin was found in about 30% of patients with PM and was rarely found in DM patients (Nishikai and Reichlin, 1980a). Rosa *et al.* (1983) showed that anti-Jo_1 sera bound only histidyl tRNA, but that an unidentified protein was the antigenic target, since the histidyl tRNA did not bind directly to the antibody. Mathews and Bernstein (1983) suggested that the antigenic target was the cognate enzyme histidyl tRNA synthetase since anti-Jo_1 effectively inhibited the aminoacylation of histidine but not any of the other 19 amino acids.

TABLE I
Myositis-Specific Autoantibodies

	Autoantigenic target	Clinical associations
Jo_1	Histidyl tRNA synthetase	Polymyositis with interstitial lung disease
PL-7	Threonyl tRNA synthetase	
PL-12	Alanyl tRNA synthetase, alanyl tRNA	
OJ	Isoleucyl tRNA synthetase	
EJ	Glycyl tRNA synthetase	
KJ	Unknown translation factor	
Signal recognition particle		Polymyositis
Mi-2 nuclear protein		Dermatomyositis
PM-Scl nucleolar protein		PM/DM, PSS, PM/PSS overlap
U_2RNP, U_1RNP		PM overlap with SLE, PSS

Subsequent work directly proved this point, since the Jo_1 antigen eluted from anti-Jo_1 IgG affinity columns had aminoacylation activity only for histidine (Targoff and Reichlin, 1984).

Subsequent work has shown that the threonyl (Mathews *et al.*, 1984) and alanyl tRNA synthetases (Bunn *et al.*, 1986) are less-frequent targets of autoantibodies in polymyositis patients and that a few PM patients with antialanyl tRNA synthetase also produce antibodies to the alanyl tRNA. Production of antibodies to the tRNA itself is thus far unique to the alanyl tRNA.

Targoff (1990) has shown that rare PM patients produce antibodies to either the isoleucyl or the glycine enzymes.

Quantitative studies with individual sera show that there is no overlap of specificity between antibodies to the various synthetase enzymes (Targoff and Reichlin, 1987). Moreover, PM patients produce antibodies to one enzyme at a time, and thus far, no patients have been described who produce appreciable amounts of autoantibody to a second synthetase. Another point of interest is that in all instances, antibodies to the synthetases are very active in inhibiting the enzyme activity. This suggests that the functional site of the enzyme is somehow involved in the immunization process.

The clinical aspects of this autoantibody are that the patients frequently also have interstitial lung disease (ILD) as well as Raynaud's phenomenon and polyarthritis. This has been referred to as the Jo_1 syndrome, in which the major clinical manifestations are the PM and ILD and less frequently Raynaud's phenomenon plus polyarthritis (Wasicek *et al.*, 1984; Yoshida *et al.*, 1983; Bernstein *et al.*, 1984).

B. Antibody to Translation Factor

Of great interest is the report that antibodies to a translation factor KJ (Targoff *et al.*, 1989), which is not a tRNA synthetase, have been found in two patients with PM with ILD, i.e., the Jo_1 syndrome. Thus the clinical picture is related not only to antibodies to tRNA synthetases but to other biochemical components of the translation apparatus. These findings have stimulated speculation that an RNA virus may be the etiological trigger in these diseases, since RNA viruses parasitize the host cell by commandeering the host's translation apparatus to produce viral rather than host proteins. As yet no RNA virus has been found that can be held responsible for these diseases.

C. Antibody to Signal-Recognition Particle

A second cytoplasmic component that has been found to be a target for autoimmunity is the signal-recognition particle or SRP. This particle binds the signal sequence of nascent secretory, membrane, and lysosomal proteins, and directs them to the endoplasmic reticulum (Reeves *et al.*, 1986; Targoff *et al.*, 1990). SRP is a ribonucleoprotein (RNP) particle with a unique RNA (7SL) and a series of six proteins of molecular mass 9, 14, 19, 54, 68, and 72 kDa. The 54-kDa protein component is the most frequent target of autoimmunity, but the 68- and 72-kDa components are also reactive with some sera. The clinical interest is that antibodies to SRP occur in patients with PM without ILD. Thus, this antibody is not associated with the Jo_1 syndrome, and its occurrence is associated with a different clinical subset of the disease.

Another rare but defined autoantibody reacts with elongation factor 1a (Efla), which was found in a single patient with nodular polymyositis (Targoff and Hanas, 1989).

D. Antibodies to Nuclear Components

There are four important myositis specific autoantibody specificities in which the antigenic target resides in the nucleus. These are the PM-Scl, Ku, U_2RNP and Mi_2 antigens. Three of these are proteins, and U_2RNP is an RNP particle related to the other URNP particles (U_1, U_4, U_5, and U_6) discussed in the section on disease-specific antibodies in systemic lupus erythematosus.

E. Antibodies to PM-Scl

PM-Scl is a complex of proteins that are nucleolar in origin, and all sera with anti-PM-Scl bind the nucleolus in indirect immunofluorescence (IFA). The proteins are not reactive by Western blotting and are defined in immunoprecipitation with ^{35}S methionine-labeled HeLa cell extracts, in which a complex of 11 proteins is seen. It is not known precisely which of the proteins is (are) antigenic.

Sera with precipitins designated anti-PM-Scl stain both the nucleus and the nucleolus in IFA. Either there is a second antibody in these sera or PM-Scl is represented in both the nucleus and the nucleolus. Interestingly, specific antibody isolated from immune precipitates made with sera that stain both the nucleus and the nucleolus bind only the nucleolus in IFA (Targoff and Reichlin, 1985a). This result favors the first hypothesis.

The clinical specificity of these antibodies is that they occur most frequently in patients with scleroderma–myositis overlap, but also occur in isolated DM and PM.

F. Antibodies to Ku and U_2RNP

Two other antigen–antibody reactions are also seen in scleroderma–polymyositis overlap patients; these are the Ku and the U_2RNP systems. Ku is a complex of nuclear proteins with 70- and 80-kDa components and binds to internucleosomal segments of DNA (Reeves, 1985, Mimori *et al.*, 1986). Antibodies to Ku occur more commonly in Japanese patients with scleroderma–myositis overlap than in U.S. Caucasians, in which this reactivity is rare (Mimori *et al.*, 1981). Antibodies to Ku probably occur more frequently in SLE patients than in patients with myositis. cDNAs for the 70- and 80-kDa proteins have been cloned and sequenced, and the epitopes are being defined (Mimori *et al.*, 1988; Reeves and Sthroeger, 1989). The human proteins are the preferred targets, and this species specificity is strong evidence for the immune response being antigen driven by the human protein (Porges and Reeves, 1989).

A small group of sera have been recognized that immunoprecipitate only U_1 and U_2 RNAs but not U_4, U_5, and U_6 RNAs. These sera are directed at two proteins, the A′ and B″ components of the U_2 particle and are thus referred to as antibodies to the U_2RNP particle. As B″ and the A protein of the U_1RNP particle are structurally related (as will be discussed in the section on SLE); such sera invariably immunoprecipitate U_2 and U_1 RNAs. Almost all patients with antibodies to U_2RNP have scleroderma-myositis (Mimori *et al.*, 1984; Craft *et al.*, 1988). As will be discussed, patients with anti-U_1RNP also may have scleroderma–myositis overlap.

It is unclear why the syndrome of scleroderma–myositis overlap should be so serologically heterogeneous and have antibodies to either PM-Scl, Ku, U_2RNP, or U_1RNP.

G. Antibodies to Mi_2

In the original studies of sera with anti-Mi, two precipitins were found, designated Mi_1 and Mi_2 (Nishikai and Reichlin, 1980b). Mi_1 proved to be bovine IgG, and antibodies to the antigen were also found in SLE. Anti-Mi_2 has proven to be specific for DM, and the antigen is a nuclear complex of proteins of molecular mass 205, 196, 151, 54, and 50 kDa (Nilasena and Targoff, 1990). The protein has been found in the nucleus of all cells thus far examined, including HEp2 cells, HeLa cells, mouse kidney and liver, rat liver, and bovine liver, spleen, and thymus. Its function is unknown.

Anti-Mi_2 occurs in about 20% of DM patients and in all clinical subsets of DM including adult and juvenile forms, DM with malignancy, and DM overlapped with other connective tissue diseases (Targoff and Reichlin, 1985b).

H. Antibodies to the 56-kDa Protein

Antibodies to a 56-kDa component of heterogeneous RNP particles purified from Syrian Hamster cells have been demonstrated by Western blot in sera from myositis patients (Arad-Dunn *et al.*, 1987). This antibody occurs in a high proportion of all subsets of myositis sera tested, but the further molecular definition of the antigenic target and its subcellular location are unknown, as is its relationship to any of the other myositis antigens.

It is clear that there is great heterogeneity in the autoimmune response of patients with PM and DM, but equally clear that part of this heterogeneity has been resolved by the biochemical definition of the antigenic targets and the recognition that certain autoantibody specificities are tightly associated with clinical subsets of the disease.

III. PROGRESSIVE SYSTEMIC SCLEROSIS: SCLERODERMA

The frequent presence of antinuclear antibodies has long been recognized in progressive systemic sclerosis (PSS), and in the past decade, many antigenic targets have been defined at the molecular level.

A. Antibodies to Nuclear Antigens

Three antigens have a nuclear distribution. Antibodies to these targets occur in large numbers of patients with PSS and are associated with clinical subsets of the disease.

The first antigen, designated Scl_{70}, was initially defined by gel diffusion and thereafter by Western immunoblotting; this suggested that the reactive antigen had a molecular mass of 70 kDa (Douvas *et al.*, 1979). Subsequent work demonstrated that the molecular identity of this antigen was the enzyme DNA topoisomerase I (topo I), and its native molecular mass was shown to be 100 kDa (Shero *et al.*, 1986; Guldner *et al.*, 1986; Maul *et al.*, 1986). The sensitive Western immunoblotting method with HeLa cell nuclear extracts results in a slightly higher prevalence than does gel diffusion.

The second antigen, P-100, is a molecule apparently distinct from topoisomerase I since it is demonstrated by Western immunoblotting with *Xenopus laevis* oöcyte extracts in numerous sera negative by gel diffusion for anti-Scl_{70} (Thomas *et al.*, 1988). In addition, absorption experiments with rabbit thymus extracts (RTE) as a source of topo I and xenopus extracts (XE) as a source of P-100 provide further evidence for their distinct antigenicity, since RTE absorbs anti-topo I activity without affecting reactivity with P-100, and contrariwise, XE absorbs anti-P-100 activity without affecting reactivity with topo I in appropriately selected sera from PSS patients (Thomas *et al.*, 1988).

The third antigen, to the centromeric region of chromosomes, gives a nuclear large, speckled pattern of fluorescence, and can be recognized as chromosome associated in chromosome spreads (Moroi *et al.*, 1980). Subsequent molecular and cellular localization studies have revealed that three polypeptides of molecular mass 17, 80, and 140 kDa, which reside in the kinetochore, are the antigenic targets (Brenner *et al.*, 1981; Cox *et al.*, 1983; Guldner *et al.*, 1985; Earnshaw *et al.*, 1986). A partial cDNA clone for the 80-kDa protein, the most prevalent antigen, has been isolated and sequenced (Earnshaw *et al.*, 1987).

B. Antibodies to Nucleolar Antigens

The remainder of the recognized characterized antigens reactive with PSS sera are nucleolar, and antibodies of these specificities occur in small numbers of scleroderma sera. A proportion (8 to 25%) of PSS sera contain antibodies that bind nucleolar antigens (Reimer *et al.*, 1988). The most frequent antigenic target is the 34-kDa protein fibrillarin, rich in N^GN^G dimethylarginine, which is the protein moiety of the U_3 RNA protein particle (Lischwe *et al.*, 1985). Antibodies to this antigen are associated with a clumpy pattern of nucleolar staining in IFA on HEp2 cells. Antibodies to RNA polymerase I (Reimer *et al.*, 1987) and PMScl (Reichlin *et al.*, 1984; Targoff and Reichlin, 1985a) are equally prevalent nucleolar targets and occur in 1 to 5% of PSS sera. These latter two specificities have distinctive patterns in IFA: antibodies to RNA polymerase I are associated with a discrete speckled pattern restricted to the nucleolus, whereas antibodies to PmScl are associated with homogeneous nucleolar staining as well as more general nucleoplasmic staining. Finally, two rare nucleolar targets reactive with PSS sera are To, a 40-kDa protein complexed to 7-2 and 8-2 RNAs (Hashimoto and Steitz, 1983; Reddy *et al.*, 1983) and Nor 90 (Tan, 1989), a 90-kDa protein localized to the nucleolar organizing region.

C. Clinical Associations

Table II lists the clinical subsets that have been associated with these specific autoantibodies. The clearest association is that of antibodies to centromere with a

TABLE II

Scleroderma-Specific Autoantibodies

Autoantigenic target	Clinical subset
Nuclear	
Centromere	CREST and/or limited cutaneous involvement
DNA topoisomerase I	Diffuse systemic sclerosis
P-100	Diffuse systemic sclerosis
Nucleolar	
RNA polymerase I	Diffuse systemic sclerosis
PM-Scl	Scleroderma-polymyositis overlap
Fibrillarin	CREST and diffuse systemic sclerosis

subset of PSS patients with limited disease and the CREST (calcinosis, Raynaud's phenomenon, esophageal motility disturbances, sclerodactyly, and telangiectasia) syndrome. Centromere antibodies occur almost exclusively in patients with limited cutaneous disease and/or CREST, and in several series occur in 43 to 98% of such patients. Antibodies to topo I, P-100, and RNA polymerase I appear to be markers for patients with diffuse disease, while antibodies to PM-Scl occur most frequently in patients with polymyositis–scleroderma overlap, as discussed in an earlier section of this chapter. Antibodies to the other nucleolar specificities occur too infrequently to determine their clinical specificity.

IV. SYSTEMIC LUPUS ERYTHEMATOSUS

Patients with systemic lupus erythematosus (SLE) produce a rich array of autoantibodies and, as described in the previous sections, such autoantibodies tend to associate with, if not define, clinical subsets. Antibodies to histone 1 and PCNA are discussed in Chapter 7. Information about antibodies to DNA is provided by the initial edition of *The Autoimmune Diseases* (1985) (Mackworth *et al.*, 1988; Pisetsky *et al.* (1990).

This section will focus on immune responses to a family of RNA protein antigens that occur in two overlapping pairs. Precipitating antibodies to one or more of these specificities occur in 85% of SLE patients, and these are called U_1RNP, Sm, Ro/SS-A, and La/SS-B. Almost all patients who produce anti-Sm also produce anti-U_1RNP, while anti-U_1RNP can occur alone or in combination with anti-Sm antibodies. In an analogous manner, all patients who produce anti-La/SS-B also produce anti-Ro/SS-A, and a substantial proportion of patients produce anti-Ro/SS-A alone. These associations have been documented and discussed elsewhere (Wasciek and Reichlin, 1982; Harley *et al.*, 1986; Reichlin, 1987; Hamilton *et al.*, 1988; Reichlin *et al.*, 1989).

A. Antibodies to U_1RNP and Sm

Molecular definition of Sm and U_1RNP as RNA protein particles was reported by Lerner and Steitz (1979), and a combination of Western blotting, protein immunoprecipitation, and chemical isolation methods (Takano *et al.*, 1980; Takano *et al.*, 1981; Lerner *et al.*, 1981c; Douvas, 1982) has revealed the size and the antigenicity of the protein moieties.

The particle bound by anti-U_1RNP is composed of an RNA component designated U_1 (U for uridine rich) complexed to at least seven proteins varying in molecular mass from 12 to 65 kDa; Sm particles are composed of the same seven proteins as well as U_2, U_1, U_4, U_5, and U_6 RNAs containing 196, 171, 145, 120, and 95 nucleotides, respectively. Thus, anti-Sm binds five different U RNA-containing particles, each with a distinctive RNA and seven common proteins. Gel precipitation reactions of U_1RNP with its antibody require the whole particle, both RNA and protein. Protein alone is sufficient for the precipitation of Sm with anti-Sm. The consensus that has emerged from several laboratories is that anti-U_1 RNP antibodies react with epitopes on three polypeptides (unique to the U_1 particle) of 70, 33, and 22 kDa. The 33- and 22-kDa proteins are also designated the A and C peptides. Antibodies to Sm react with two proteins of 28 and 16 kDa common to all the U-containing RNP particles, designated the B and D proteins. B protein is also designated B/B′, since it occurs as a doublet of 29 and 28 kDa, respectively. Antibodies against the RNA component of U_1RNP have recently been shown to occur with some frequency (van Venrooijh *et al.*, 1990).

There are also three smaller polypeptides of 12, 11, and 9 kDa, designated E, F, and G. There is considerable overlap in the distribution of these specificities in sera containing various combinations of anti-U_1RNP and anti-Sm precipitins. It is common for anti-U_1RNP sera that immunoprecipitate only U_1RNA and have a single RNAse-sensitive precipitin line to strongly bind the B/B′ bands in Western blot analysis (Habets *et al.*, 1985; Combe *et al.*, 1989). Whereas there may be a frequent occurrence of antibodies to B/B′ in sera with anti-Sm precipitins, the only common specific reactivity characteristic of the *anti-Sm* specificity is reactivity to the D peptide. Less frequently, antibodies to the E peptide are also found in anti-Sm sera (Petterson *et al.*, 1984; Petterson *et al.*, 1986). The striking findings are that there are antigenic relationships between the A and C polypeptides characteristic of the U_1RNP and anti-Sm sera, and this is reflected in shared amino acid sequences (Habets *et al.*, 1989). Thus the antigenic polypeptides of the Sm and U_1RNP specificities are not only found on the same particles, but also share a primary amino acid sequence.

It is also of interest that despite the sharing of antigenic epitopes between B/B′ and D, their primary amino acid sequences are entirely different (Rokeach *et al.*, 1988; Rokeach *et al.*, 1989), which indicates the shared epitope is conformational.

Autoantibodies specific to the U_2 particle have been described, and these are directed to two unique polypeptides of 33 kDa (A′) and 28 kDa (B″).

Sera with anti-U_2RNP always are accompanied by antibodies that immunoprecipitate the U_1 particle as well. Thus anti-U_2RNP sera characteristically immunoprecipitate U_1 + U_2 RNAs, anti-U_1RNP sera immunoprecipitate U_1RNA alone, and anti-Sm sera immunoprecipitate all five U RNAs, 1, 2, 4, 5, and 6 (Mimori *et al.*, 1984; Craft *et al.*, 1988). The basis of this *cross-reactivity* is the sequence homology between the A protein of the U_1 particle and the B″ protein of the U_2 particle (Habets *et al.*, 1989). The fine specificity of these anti-SnRNP antibodies is listed in Table III.

TABLE III
Antigenic Relationships of SnRNPs

Antibody specificities	Antigenic targets
Anti-U_1RNP	70 kDa, A (33 kDa) and C (22 kDa)
Anti-Sm	B/B′ (29, 28 kDa), D (16 kDa)
Anti-U_2RNP	A′ (33 kDa) and B″ (28 kDa)

B. Clinical Associations of Anti-U_1RNP and Anti-Sm

Antibodies to Sm with or without anti-U_1RNP occur in SLE, and antibodies to U_1RNP alone occur in SLE and in the overlap syndrome mixed connective tissue disease (MCTD), which consists of various mixtures of SLE, PM, and PSS (Sharp *et al.*, 1971; Sharp *et al.*, 1972). Much work has centered on the identification of a specific immunochemical marker of MCTD, and two groups have reported the high specificity of anti-70 kDa for MCTD (Habets *et al.*, 1983; Petterson *et al.*, 1986). However, subsequent studies with a recombinant 70-kDa protein found an almost uniform presence of anti-70-kDa protein antibodies in SLE sera (Netter *et al.*, 1988; Guldner *et al.*, 1988). An additional study employing subfragments of recombinant 70-kDa protein has shown that there are multiple epitopes, and the pattern of reactivity of sera from SLE and MCTD sera is very similar if not identical (Cram *et al.*, 1990). The search for a specific immunochemical marker for MCTD (as distinct from SLE) remains elusive.

One of the most intriguing clinical associations of these antibodies is their relationship to nephritis. Patients with only anti-U_1RNP have a low frequency of renal disease (Sharp *et al.*, 1971; Sharp *et al.*, 1972; Reichlin and Mattioli, 1972; Parker, 1973). This problem has been recently reinvestigated by studying the distribution of anti-U_1RNP and anti-Sm by quantitative enzyme-linked immunosorbent assay (ELISA) and Western blotting sera from patients with lupus nephritis. If the antibody reacted with an RNA-protein antigen with a ratio of U_1RNP to Sm of less than 200, nephritis was likely, whereas ratios of 200 or greater were never associated with nephritis. While antibodies to the 70-kDa protein were present in 83% of those without nephritis, they were also present in 23% of patients with nephritis. Thus the quantitative preponderance of the U_1RNP to Sm response was a better indication of a low risk of nephritis than was the presence or absence of antibodies to the 70-kDa particle (Reichlin and van Venrooij, in press). Some clinical and serological associations are listed in Table IV.

Antibodies to the U_2RNP were almost invariably associated with overlap disease, with a very high prevalence of myositis among these patients (Craft *et al.*, 1988).

TABLE IV
SLE-Associated Autoantibodies

Autoantigenic target	Clinical association
U_1RNP	Mild SLE when it occurs alone and/or overlap with PSS and PM
Ro/SS-A	Subacute cutaneous lupus erythematosus, neonatal LE, lupus of homozygous C_2 and C_4 deficiency, vasculitis of Sjögren's syndrome, photosensitivity, interstitial lung disease, SLE–Sjögren's syndrome overlap

Increasing knowledge of the fine specificity of the autoimmune response to the U RNA protein particle should enhance our ability to relate these autoantibodies to clinical phenomena.

C. Structure of Ro/SS-A and La/SS-B

The RNA component of Ro/SS-A is known as hY RNA for human (h) cytoplasmic (Y) RNA (Lerner *et al.*, 1981). It is uridine rich and, in humans, is composed of at least four unique RNA species between 83 and 112 bases, of which three of the RNA species have been sequenced. Helical regions near the 3′ and 5′ ends are protected from RNAse digestion when the hY RNA is complexed with the Ro/SS-A protein (Wolin and Steitz, 1984). The genes for hY1 and hY3 RNAs are adjacent on the human genome (Wolin and Steitz, 1983).

The La RNAs are more complicated. In many cells, there are RNA species termed 4.5 S RNA, which bind the La/SS-B protein. Although 4.5 S appears to be the major RNA in mice (Hendrick *et al.*, 1981) and 5.0 S in humans (Rinke and Steitz, 1982), 4.5 S RNA is partially homologous to the Alu DNA family, which is composed of highly repetitive interspersed sequences found in mammalian genomes (Jelinik *et al.*, 1980). The 5.0 S RNA has been shown to be a precursor form of ribosomal RNA (Rinke and Steitz, 1982). There are, however, many other RNAs also immunoprecipitated by anti-La/SS-B, largely between 80 and 120 nucleotides (Lerner *et al.*, 1981a). Some of these have been shown to be precursor tRNA molecules, leading to the hypothesis that all RNA polymerase III transcripts are at least initially associated with the La/SS-B protein. The common structural feature of the RNA that binds it to the La/SS-B protein is an oligouridylate stretch found at the 3′ end of the polymerase III transcripts (Stefano, 1984).

Viral-encoded RNAs also have been shown to complex with the La/SS-B protein. In particular, two adenovirus RNAs and two Epstein–Barr virus RNAs containing 160–173 nucleotides bind the La/SS-B protein (Lerner *et al.*, 1981a; Lerner *et al.*, 1981b; Rosa *et al.*, 1981).

The La/SS-B protein is a single polypeptide of 50 kDa (Lerner *et al.*, 1981a), which is easily degraded to an antigenically active 29 kDa, after which it loses antigenicity (Venables *et al.*, 1983). A cDNA for La/SS-B has been cloned and sequenced, and a major antigenic epitope has been localized to the COOH terminal region (McNeilage *et al.*, 1990). Epitope definition has been accomplished by studies of the reactivity of human recombinant fusion proteins with autoimmune sera. Multiple epitopes were demonstrable and were reproducibly reactive with multiple patient sera and spanned the length of the molecule (St. Clair *et al.*, 1988a; St. Clair *et al.*, 1988b; Bini *et al.*, 1990). Thus far, no isoforms of La/SS-B have been identified. The La/SS-B protein appears to function as a termination factor for RNA polymerase III, which accounts for its binding to numerous polymerase III transcripts. It has also been identified as an enzyme, a nucleic acid-dependent ATPase/dATPase with melting properties (Bachman *et al.*, 1990).

D. Heterogeneity of Ro/SS-A and Anti-Ro/SS-A

The first Ro/SS-A protein characterized was a 60-kDa protein (Venables *et al.*, 1983; Wolin and Steitz, 1984; Yamagata *et al.*, 1984). It is now known to exist in at least two distinctive molecular forms with two isoforms of each in the lymphocyte and red blood cell. There are two 60-kDa forms: one in nucleated cells, and the other in red blood cells (Rader *et al.*, 1989a). There is a 52-kDa form in lymphocytes (Ben Chetrit *et al.*, 1988) and an analogous 54-kDa form in red blood cells (Rader *et al.*, 1989a). Red cell Ro/SS-A binds only the hY_1 and hY_4 RNAs. Affinity elution studies and frequency analysis of antibodies to these various Ro/SS-A molecules reveal that the two 60-kDa forms are distinctive but related, while the lymphocyte 52-kDa and red cell 54-kDa forms are likewise distinctive but related (Itoh *et al.*, 1990). Antibodies to one of the pairs do not cross-react with members of the other pair and vice versa. Cloned cDNAs for the Ro lymphocyte 60-kDa form have been sequenced (Deutscher *et al.*, 1988; Ben Chetrit *et al.*, 1989).

This heterogeneity of the Ro/SS-A antigen is also reflected in the autoimmune response. Patients with different precipitin profiles have anti-Ro/SS-A that differs in fine specificity. This has been demonstrated with two different immunochemical properties of the Ro/SS-A/anti-Ro/SS-A system (Rader *et al.*, 1989b). One is based on the observation that anti-Ro/SS-A is preferentially reactive with the human Ro/SS-A particle (Reichlin *et al.*, 1989; Reichlin and Wolfson-Reichlin, 1989), and the other reflects the differing pattern of antibodies to the various Ro/SS-A isoforms in sera from patients with differing precipitin profiles. Thus, disease sera with anti-Ro/SS-A alone have the highest fraction of antibody remaining reactive with human Ro/SS-A after absorption with bovine Ro/SS-A, compared with patient sera with anti-Ro/SS-A and anti-La/SS-B, and anti-Ro/SS-A and anti-nRNP, respectively. Thus anti-Ro/SS-A alone sera have the largest fraction of antibody exclusively reactive with human Ro/SS-A, whereas sera with anti-Ro/SS-A and nRNP have the smallest fraction of such human-specific antibody (Rader *et al.*, 1989b). Western blot analysis with red cell hemolysates cleared of hemoglobin was the other procedure applied to these sera, and this also distinguished the three groups. The most homogeneous were the sera with anti-Ro/SS-A and anti-nRNP, in which 16 of 17 reacted exclusively with the RBC 60-kDa isoform of Ro/SS-A. The seventeenth serum reacted with both the RBC 60-kDa and the 54-kDa isoform of Ro/SS-A. Sera with both anti-Ro/SS-A and anti-La/SS-B precipitins reacted uniformly with the RBC 54-kDa molecule and always more strongly than the RBC 60-kDa Ro/SS-A. In this property, anti-Ro/SS-A sera were more heterogeneous but resembled anti-Ro/SS-A and anti-La/SS-B sera more closely than did anti-Ro/SS-A and anti-nRNP sera. Thus, it is clear that not only is there heterogeneity in the profile of autoimmune reactants (e.g., anti-DNA, antihistone, anti-U_1RNP, anti-Ro/SSB, etc.), but also, at least with respect to the anti-Ro/SS-A response, there is considerable heterogeneity within that response.

E. Clinical Associations with the Anti-Ro/SS-A Response

A number of lupus disease subsets are closely associated with the anti-Ro/SS-A response. These include the following: subacute cutaneous lupus erythematosus (SCLE), neonatal lupus erythematosus, the lupus of homozygous deficiency of the complement components C2 and C4, and the vasculitis of primary Sjögren's syndrome (Reichlin, 1986). In addition, the clinical finding of photosensitivity (Mond *et al.*, 1989) and ILD (Hedgpeth and Boulware, 1988) are also closely related to the presence of anti-Ro/SS-A within the SLE population.

The clinical specificity of antibodies to Ro/SS-A and La/SS-B is restricted to SLE and Sjögren's syndrome. This point is emphasized by the occurrence of a subset of patients with an overlap of Sjögren's syndrome and SLE, in which the most prominent feature of the SLE component is extensive SCLE (Provost *et al.*, 1988a; Provost *et al.*, 1988b).

It is suspected but unproven that the association of anti-Ro/SS-A with clinical subsets depends on the direct involvement of antibodies to Ro/SS-A in the clinical expression of disease. As these studies are performed, it is obvious that the great heterogeneity of the Ro/SS-A antigen and its cognate antibodies will have to be considered. One might suspect that various subpopulations of anti-Ro/SS-A would be differentially involved in the different clinical subsets.

V. SUMMARY

Much has been learned in the past decade about the biochemical definition of numerous autoantigen targets in systemic rheumatic disease. This progress has been greatly facilitated by the powerful tools of molecular biology.

It is clear that disease-specific autoimmune responses exist, and that each disease is characterized by a family of autoantibodies. Emerging clinical data suggest that heterogeneity of disease (subsets) is accompanied and mirrored by a heteogeneous autoimmune response; i.e., clinical subsets are associated with autoantibodies of a relatively narrow specificity.

The frontier areas are several. The etiology of all these diseases is still unknown. It would be surprising if, in these diseases, specific autoimmune responses were not intimately related in a mechanistic way to the finally determined etiologies. At present, the role of these autoantibodies in the pathogenesis of the tissue damage remains obscure and will require a renewed effort for definition.

EDITOR'S NOTE:

Reichlin's analysis of the rapid developments in knowledge of the non-DNA antigens in the multisystem autoimmune diseases, including the fine specificities of the antibodies, raises two expectations. (1) There can be an improved classification of these diseases into categories with relevance to nosology, treatment, and outcome: This has been, in part at least, fulfilled. (2) There will be clues into the trigger factors that set these diseases in train. This expectation is not yet fulfilled. However, it is clear that the autoantigenic molecules tend to be enzymes, and that functional sites on the enzymes represent autoepitope sites, with the capacity of autoimmune sera to inhibit specifically the function of the enzyme being increasingly noted. Of interest the La/SS-B protein is now identified as an enzyme molecule, a "nucleic acid dependent ATPase with melting properties" (*Cell* **60**: 85–93, 1990).

However, the tantalizing enigma remains: is there any connection between the specificity of the autoantibody and the expression of the disease? The anti-TRNA synthetase activity characteristic of polymyositis is held to represent the footprint of an antecedent virus infection with an autoimmune process supervening on this. But a clinical type of polymyositis can complicate treatment with D-penicillamine, which would have a completely different antigenic configuration.

In scleroderma there is such a high frequency of accompanying autoantibodies of one type or another, antitopoisomerase 1, anticentromere or antinucleolar, with the latter attracting increasing attention. We are certainly now more comfortable with autoimmunity as a pathogenetic component in scleroderma but, certainly now as with the other multisystem autoimmune diseases, the link between symptoms serology remains as mysterious as ever.

Reichlin emphasizes the insights that molecular biology has provided into the amino acid sequences of autoantigens and the mapping of the autoepitopes, at least for B cells. The existence of multiple epitopes and cross-reactivities between discrete sequences with no evident structural homology points to the likelihood that epitopes are complex structures encompassing discontinuous regions of a conformationally organized molecule. If this has implications for pathogenesis, it would suggest that the antigen drive is derived from the autoantigen itself.

Questions always arise on the SLE-Sjögren's syndrome (SS) connection. Can the overlap be explained simply by formation of immune complexes in both diseases? Certainly when "pedigree" examples are taken, SLE segregates with anti-DNA and anti-Sm, and Sjögren's syndrome segregates with anti-La and anti-Ro. But then anti-Ro turns up, without anti-La, as an autoantibody for an SLE subset! And why should Ro and La be "immunologic fellow-travellers" when these polypeptides have a different cellular location. Whatever the uncertainties, we commend Reichlin, a specialist on the Ro particle, on his informative discussion on the puzzling heterogeneity of the Ro polypeptide and the serologic responses to it.

Reichlin refers to the "unknown etiology" of the multisystem autoimmune diseases. Perhaps the "etiology" is the autoimmune state itself, with a native autoantigen providing both the trigger and the drive for self-perpetuation in subjects with a peculiar derangement of tolerance that we do not yet fully understand.

REFERENCES

Arad-Dann, H., Isenberg, D. A., Shoenfeld, T., Offen, D., Sperling, J., and Sperling, R. (1987). *J. Immunol.* **138,** 2463–2468.

Bachman, M., Pfeifer, K., Schroder, H. C., and Müller, W. E. G. (1990). *Cell* **60,** 85–93.

Ben Chetrit, E., Chan, E. K. L., Sullivan, K. F., and Tan, E. M. (1988). *J. Exp. Med.* **167,** 1560–1571.

Ben Chetrit, E., Gandy, B. J., Tan, E. M., and Sullivan, K. F. (1989). *J. Clin. Invest.* **83,** 1284–1292.

Bernstein, R. M., Morgan, S. H., and Chapman, J. (1984). *Br. Med. J.* **289,** 151–152.

Bini, P., Chu, J. L., Okolo, C., and Elkon, K. (1990). *J. Clin. Invest.* **85,** 325–333.

Brenner, S., Pepper, D., Berus, M. W., Tan, E. M., and Brinkley, B. R. (1981). *J. Cell. Biol.* **91,** 95–102.

Bunn, C. C. Bernstein, R. M., and Matthews, M. B. (1986). *J. Exp. Med.* **163,** 1281–1291.

Combe, B., Rucheton, M., Graafland, H., Lussiez, V., Brunel, G., and Sany, G. (1989). *Clin. Exp. Immunol.* **75,** 18–24.

Cox, J. V., Schenk, E. A., and Olmstead, J. B. (1983). *Cell* **35,** 331–339.

Craft, J., Mimori, T., Olsen, T. L., and Hardin, J. A. (1988). *J. Clin. Invest.* **81,** 1716–1724.

Craig, D. S., Fisicaro, N., Coppel, R. L., Whittingham, S., and Harrison, L. C. (1990). *J. Immunol.* **145,** 630–635.

Cram, D., Fisicaro, N., Coppel, R. L., Whittingham, S., and Harrison, L. C. (1990). *J. Immunol.***145,** 630–635.

Deutscher, S. L., Harley, J. B., and Keene, J. D. (1988). *Proc. Natl. Acad. Sci. U.S.A.* **85,** 9479–9483.

Douvas, A. S. (1982). *Proc. Natl. Acad. Sci. U.S.A.* **79,** 5401–5405.

Earnshaw, W. C., Bordwell, B. J., Morris, C., and Rothfield, N. F. (1986). *J. Clin. Invest.* **77,** 426–430.

Earnshaw, W. C., Sullivan, K. F., and Maehlin, P. S., Cooke, C. A., Kaiser, D. A., Pollard, T. D., Rothfield, N. F., and Cleveland, D. W. (1987). *J. Cell. Biol.* **104,** 817–829.

Guldner, H. H., Lakomek, H. S., and Bautz, F. A. (1985). *Clin. Exp. Immunol.* **58,** 13–20.

Guldner, H. H., Szostecki, C., Vosberg, H. P., Lakomilk, H. J., Penner, E., and Bautz, F. A. (1986). *Chromosome* **94,** 132–138.

Guldner, H. H., Netter, H. J., Szostecki, C., Takomek, H. J., and Hill, H. (1988). *J. Immunol.* **141,** 469–475.

Habets, W. J., deRooij, D. J., Saldew, M. H., Verhagen, A. P., Van Eckellew, C. A., Van de Putte, L. B., and Van Venrooij, W. J. (1983). *Clin. Exp. Immunol.* **54,** 265–276.

Habets, W. J., deRooij, D. J., Hoet, M. H., Van de Putte, L. B. A., and Van Venrooij, W. J. (1985). *Clin. Exp. Immunol.* **59,** 457–466.

Habets, W. J., Sillikens, P. T. G., Hoet, M. H., McAllister, G., Lerner, M. R., and Van Venrooij, W. J. (1989). *Proc. Natl. Acad. Sci. U.S.A.* **86,** 4674–4678.

Hamilton, R. G., Harley, J. B., Bias, W. B., Roebber, H., Reichlin, M., Hochberg, M. C., and Arnett, F. C. (1988). *Arthritis Rheum.* **31,** 496–505.
Harley, J. B., Alexander, E., Bias, W. B., Fox, O. F., Provost, T. T., Reichlin, M., Yamagata, H., and Arnett, F. C. (1986). *Arthritis Rheum.* **29,** 196–206.
Hashimoto, C., and Steitz, J. A. (1983). *J. Biol. Chem.* **258,** 1379–1382.
Hedgpeth, J. J., and Boulware, D. W. (1988). *Arthritis Rheum.* **31,** 545–548.
Hendrick, J. P., Wolin, S., Rinke, J., Lerner, M. R., and Steitz, J. A. (1981). *Mol. Cell. Biol.* **1,** 1138–1149.
Itoh, Y., Rader, M. D., and Reichlin, M. (1990). *Clin. Exp. Immunol.* **81,** 45–51.
Jelinek, W. R., Toomey, T. P., Leinwand, L., Duncan, C. H., Biro, P. A., Chondary, P. A., Weissman, S. M., Rubin, C. M., Deininger, P. L., and Schmidt, C. W. (1980). *Proc. Natl. Acad. Sci. U.S.A.* **77,** 1398–1402.
Lerner, M. R., Boyle, J. A., Hardin, J. H., and Steitz, J. A. (1981a). *Science* **211,** 400–402.
Lerner, M. R., Andrews, N. C., Miller, G., and Steitz, J. A. (1981b). *Proc. Natl. Acad. Sci. U.S.A.* **78,** 805–809.
Lerner, E. A., Lerner, M. R., Janeway, C. A., Jr., and Steitz, J. A. (1981c). *Proc. Natl. Acad. Sci. U.S.A.* **78,** 2737–2741.
Lischwe, M. A., Odis, R. L., Reddy, R., Cook, R. G., Yeoman, L. C., Tan, E. M., Reichlin, M., and Busch, H. (1985). *J. Biol. Chem.* **260,** 14304–14310.
Mackworth-Young, C., and Schwartz, R. S. (1988). *CRC Crit. Rev.* **8,** 147–173.
Mathews, M. B., and Bernstein, R. M. (1983). *Nature* **304,** 177–179.
Mathews, M. B., Reichlin, M., Hughes, G. R. V., and Bernstein, R. M. (1984). *J. Exp. Med.* **160,** 420–434.
Maul, G. G., Freud, B. T., Van Venrooij, W. J., and Jiminez, S. A. (1986). *Proc. Natl. Acad. Sci. U.S.A.* **83,** 5145–5149.
McNeilage, L. J., MacMillan, E. M., and Wittingham, S. F. (1990). *J. Immunol.* **145,** 3829–3835.
Mimori, T., Akizuki, M., Yamagata, H., Inada, S., Yoshida, S., and Homma, M. (1981). *J. Clin. Invest.* **68,** 611–620.
Mimori, T., Hinterberger, M., Petterson, I., and Steitz, J. A. (1984). *J. Biol. Chem.* **259,** 560–565.
Mimori, T., Hardin, J. A., and Steitz, J. A. (1986). *J. Biol. Chem.* **261,** 2274–2278.
Mimori, T., Hama, N., Suwa, A., Akizuki, M., and Homma, M. (1988). *Arthritis Rheum.* **31,** S13 (Abstr.).
Mond, C. B., Peterson, M. G. E., and Rothfield, N. F. (1989). *Arthritis Rheum.* **32,** 202–204.
Moroi, Y., Peebles, C., Fritzler, M. J., Steigerwald, J., and Tan, E. M. (1980). *Proc. Natl. Acad. Sci. U.S.A.* **77,** 1627–1631.
Netter, H. J., Guldner, H. H., Szostecki, C., Takomek, H. J., and Will, H. (1988). *Arthritis Rheum.* **31,** 616–622.
Nilasena, D. S., and Targoff, I. N. (1990). *Clin. Res.* **38,** 550A (Abstract)
Nishikai, M., and Reichlin, M. (1980a). *Arthritis Rheum.* **23,** 881–888.
Nishikai, M., and Reichlin, M. (1980b). *Mol. Immunol.* **17,** 1129–1141.
Parker, M. D. (1973). *J. Lab. Clin. Med.* **82,** 769–775.
Petterson, I., Hintemeyer, M., and Mimori, T. (1984). *J. Biol. Chem.* **259,** 5907–5911.
Petterson, I., Wang, G., Smith, E. L., Wizzell, H., Hedfors, E., Horn, J., and Sharp, G. C. (1986). *Arthritis Rheum.* **29,** 980–996.
Pisetsky, D. S., Grudier, J. P., and Gilkeson, G. S. (1990). *Arthritis Rheum.* **33,** 153–159.
Porges, A., and Reeves, W. H. (1989). *Arthritis Rheum.* **32,** S81 (Abstr.).
Provost, T. T., Talal, N., Harley, J. B., Reichlin, M., and Alexander, E. L. (1988a). *Arch. Dermatol.* **124,** 63–71.
Provost, T. T., Talal, N., Bias, W., Harley, J. B., Reichlin, M., and Alexander, E. L. (1988b). *J. Invest. Dermatol.* **91,** 369–371.

Rader, M. D., O'Brien, C., Liu, Y., Harley, J. B., and Reichlin, M. (1989a). *J. Clin. Invest.* **83,** 1293–1298.
Rader, M. D., Codding, C., and Reichlin, M. (1989b). *Arthritis Rheum.* **76,** 373–377.
Reddy, P., Tan, E. M., Henning, D., Noghen, K., and Busch, H. (1983). *J. Biol. Chem.* **258,** 1383–1386.
Reeves, W. H. (1985). *J. Exp. Med.* **161,** 18–39.
Reeves, W. H., Nigau, S. K., and Blobel, G. (1986). *Proc. Natl. Acad. Sci. U.S.A.* **83,** 9507–9511.
Reeves, W. H., and Sthroeger, Z. M. (1989). *J. Biol. Chem.* **264,** 5047–5052.
Reichlin, M., and Mattioli, M. (1972). *N. Engl. J. Med.* **286,** 908–911.
Reichlin, M., Maddison, P. J., Targoff, I. N., Bunch, T., Arnett, F. C., Sharp, G. C., Treadwell, E., and Tan, E. M. (1984). *J. Clin. Immunol.* **4,** 40–44.
Reichlin, M. (1986). *J. Clin. Immunol.* **5,** 339–348.
Reichlin, M. (1987). *In* "Mixed Connective Tissue Disease and Anti-Nuclear Antibodies" (R. Kasukaua and G. C. Sharp, eds.), pp. 85–96. Elsevier, Amsterdam.
Reichlin, M., Rader, M. D., and Harley, J. B. (1989). *Clin. Exp. Immunol.* **76,** 373–377.
Reichlin, M., and Wolfson-Reichlin, M. (1989). *J. Autoimmunol.* **2,** 359–365.
Reichlin, M., and van Venrooij, W. J. (1991). *Clin. Exp. Immunol.* **83,** 286–290.
Reimer, G., Scheer, U., Peters, J. M., and Tan, E. M. (1986). *J. Immunol.* **137,** 3802–3808.
Reimer, G., Rose, K. M., Scher, U., and Tan, E. M. (1987). *J. Clin. Invest.* **79,** 65–72.
Reimer, G., Steen, V. D., Penning, C. A., Medsger, T. A., Jr., and Tan, E. M. (1988). *Arthritis Rheum.* **31,** 525–532.
Rinke, J. and Steitz, J. A. (1982). *Cell* **29,** 149–159.
Rokeach, L. A., Haselby, J. A., and Hoch, S. O. (1988). *Proc. Natl. Acad. Sci. U.S.A.* **85,** 4832–4836.
Rokeach, L. A., Jannatipour, U., Haselby, J. A., and Hoch, S. O. (1989). *J. Biol. Chem.* **264,** 5024–5030.
Rosa, M. D., Gottlieb, E., Lerner, M. R., and Steitz, J. A. (1981). *Mol. Cell. Biol.* **1,** 785–796.
Rosa, M. D., Hendrick, J. R., Jr., Lerner, M. R., Steitz, J. A., and Reichlin, M. (1983). *Nucleic Acids Res.* **11,** 853–870.
St. Clair, E. W., Pisetsky, D. S., Reich, C. F., Chambers, J. C., and Keene, J. D. (1988a). *Arthritis Rheum.* **31,** 506–514.
St. Clair, E. W., Pisetsky, D. S., Reich, C. F., and Keene, J. D. (1988b). *J. Immunol.* **141,** 4173–4180.
Sharp, G. C., Irvin, W. S., Laroque, R. L., Velez, C., Daly, V., Kaiser, A. D., and Holman, H. R. (1971). *J. Clin. Invest.* **50,** 350–359.
Sharp, G. C., Irvin, W. S., Tan, E. M., Gould, R. G., and Holman, H. R. (1972). *Am. J. Med.* **52,** 148–159.
Shero, H. J., Bordwell, B., Rothfield, N. F., and Earnshaw, W. C. (1986). *Science* **231,** 737–740.
Stefano, J. E. (1984). *Cell* **36,** 145–154.
Takano, M., Agris, P. F., and Sharp, G. C. (1980). *J. Clin. Invest.* **65,** 1449–1456.
Takano, M., Golden, S. S., Sharp, G. C., and Agris, P. F. (1981). *Biochemistry* **21,** 5929–5935.
Tan, E. M. (1989). *J. Clin. Invest.* **84,** 1–6.
Targoff, I. N., Raghu, G., and Reichlin, M. (1982). *Clin. Exp. Immunol.* **53,** 76–82.
Targoff, I. N., and Reichlin, M. (1984). *Arthritis Rheum.* **27,** S45 (Abstr.).
Targoff, I. N., and Reichlin, M. (1985a). *Arthritis Rheum.* **28,** 226–230.
Targoff, I. N., and Reichlin, M. (1985b). *Arthritis Rheum.* **28,** 796–803.
Targoff, I. N., and Reichlin, M. (1987). *J. Immunol.* **138,** 2874–2882.
Targoff, I. N., Arnett, F. C., Berman, L., O'Brien, C., and Reichlin, M. (1989). *J. Clin. Invest.* **84,** 162–172.
Targoff, I. N., and Hanas, J. (1989). *Arthritis Rheum.* **32,** S81(Abstr.).

Targoff, I. N. (1990). *J. Immunol.* **144,** 1737–1743.
Targoff, I. N., Johnson, A. E., and Miller, F. W. (1990). *Arthritis Rheum.* **33,** 1361–1370.
Thomas, P., Rother, R. P., Pryor, T., and Reichlin, M. (1988). *Arthritis Rheum.* **520,** 57(Abstr.).
Van Venrooij, W. J., Hoet, R., Castrop, J., Hageman, B., Mattaj, I. W., and Van de Putte, L. B. (1990). *J. Clin. Invest.* **86,** 2154–2160.
Venables, P. J. W., Smith, P. R., and Maini, R. W. (1983). *Clin. Exp. Immunol.* **54,** 731–738.
Wasiek, C. A., and Reichlin, M. (1982). *J. Clin. Invest.* **69,** 835–843.
Wasicek, C. A., Reichlin, M., Montes, M., and Raghu, G. (1984). *Am. J. Med.* **76,** 538–544.
Wolin, S. L., and Steitz, J. A. (1983). *Cell* **32,** 735–744.
Wolin, S. L., and Steitz, J. A. (1984). *Proc. Natl. Acad. Sci. U.S.A.* **81,** 1996–2000.
Yamagata, H., Harley, J. B., and Reichlin, M. (1984). *J. Clin. Invest.* **74,** 625–633.
Yoshida, S., Akizuki, N., Mimori, T., Yamagata, H., Inado, S., and Homma, M. (1983). *Arthritis Rheum.* **26,** 604–611.

CHAPTER 9

Molecular Analysis of Cytoplasmic Autoantigens in Liver Disease

M. ERIC GERSHWIN
Division of Rheumatology
Allergy and Clinical Immunology
School of Medicine
University of California at Davis
Davis, California

MICHAEL P. MANNS
Department of Gastroenterology and Hepatology
Zentrum Innere Medizin und Dermatologie
Medizinische Hochschule Hannover
Hannover, Germany

IAN R. MACKAY
Centre for Molecular Biology and Medicine
Monash University
Clayton, Victoria, Australia

I. INTRODUCTION

Autoimmune diseases are characterized by a failure in the immune system to distinguish between self and nonself. Consequential to this breakdown in tolerance, there may be adverse clinical consequences that include systemic dysfunction and/or destruction of particular organs or tissues. The understanding of failure of tolerance requires knowledge of autoantigens but, until recently, the analysis of autoantigens has been slow and difficult because these may be present in low concentrations, or may be hard to purify. Moreover, autoimmune sera may contain multiple autoantibodies, some critical, and others irrelevant. All of these features have retarded our understanding of autoimmunity. However, the recent advent of molecular biology and its technologic applications have provided new insights and approaches, well exemplified by two autoimmune liver diseases, primary biliary cirrhosis and the subset of chronic active hepatitis marked by reactivity with a microsomal antigen.

II. PRIMARY BILIARY CIRRHOSIS

A. BACKGROUND

Primary biliary cirrhosis (PBC) results from an autoimmune destruction of bile ducts and eventually causes liver failure. The disease specificity for PBC of high-titer autoantibodies to a mitochondrial antigen has been long recognized (Mackay 1958; Walker *et al.*, 1965; Berg *et al.*, 1967), and the possible significance, discussed (Kaplan, 1987; Gershwin *et al.*, 1988a). These autoantibodies and certain other features have led to the description of PBC as a model autoimmune disease. However, while PBC is a paradigm for autoimmunity in some respects, it is a paradox in others (Gershwin and Mackay, 1991), in that the autoimmune attack is focused on the intrahepatic biliary ductules, yet the unique mitochondrial autoantigen is not tissue specific and, moreover, is apparently well shielded from the immune system. Earlier on, the mitochondrial autoantigens for PBC sera were found to react with trypsin-sensitive antigens in the inner mitochondrial membrane (Berg *et al.*, 1967), but further characterization was slow (Meek *et al.*, 1980; Mendel-Hartvig *et al.*, 1985). In 1985, four groups used immunoblotting to show that some five mitochondrial autoantigens could be identified with molecular masses ranging from 74 to 36 kDa, as judged by migration in gels, with minor variations depending on technical factors (Lindenborn-Fotinos *et al.*, 1985; Ishii *et al.*, 1985; Frazer *et al.*, 1985; Manns *et al.*, 1985). However, the biochemical identification of the mitochondrial antigen remained elusive.

In 1987, a cDNA for the mitochondrial 74-kDa autoantigen of PBC was cloned and sequenced (Gershwin *et al.*, 1987) by screening a rat liver cDNA library with sera from patients with PBC, and this led to the identification of the antigen as the pyruvate dehydrogenase complex (PDC) (Van de Water *et al.*, 1988a,b; Gershwin *et al.*, 1988b; Coppel *et al.*, 1988). By subcloning different fragments of this cDNA into frame-shifted expression vectors, an immunodominant polypeptide was found to be expressed by a 603-base-pair fragment, and a synthetic 20-amino-acid peptide from this polypeptide sequence absorbed the reactivity of serum with the original recombinant protein (Van de Water *et al.*, 1988a). This 20-amino-acid peptide corresponded to a peptide proposed as a candidate epitope by reason of sequence conservation, that is the lipoyl domain of dihydrolipoamide acetyltransferase, the E2 component of PDC-E2 (Coppel *et al.*, 1988; Yeaman *et al.*, 1988). Thereafter, a group of antigens associated with

PDC and related enzymes were identified and characterized, as described below. Thus, finally, the true mitochondrial antibodies of PBC have "stood up" and can be accounted for by reactivity with PDC and two closely related enzymes of the 2-oxo-acid dehydrogenase complex (2-OADC) family (Surh *et al.*, 1988b; Van de Water *et al.*, 1988; Fussey *et al.*, 1988; Van de Water *et al.*, 1989; Fregeau *et al.*, 1990). For convenience, the earlier designation, M2, is used for the 2-OADC enzyme antigens, and anti-M2, for the corresponding autoantibodies.

B. Properties of M2 Autoantibodies

The anti-M2 mitochondrial autoantibodies in PBC show some notable features. First, the major reactivity appears to be with PDC, the 74-kDa antigen, since some 95% of sera are positive by immunoblotting; the frequency of reactivity against the E2 subunits of the other enzymes, oxo-glutaric dehydrogenase complex (OGDC) and branched chain oxo-acid dehydrogenase complex (BCOADC), is lower at around 50 to 70%. Despite the fact that in PBC there is usually reactivity against two, or even all three of the 2-OADC enzymes, there is usually no serological cross-reactivity (Fregeau *et al.*, 1991); the only cross-reactivity observed among the M2 reactants is that between PDC and the protein X, which is a constituent of the same enzyme (Surh *et al.*, 1989) (*vide infra*). Moreover, in keeping with this immunologic specificity, the M2 antibodies are not cross-reactive in enzyme inhibition assays (Fregeau *et al.*, 1989), as described below.

Second, there is more than one determinant on the M2 autoantigens. For PDC, the E2 subunit contains a major site around the lipoyl-binding region, and there are other unmapped sites on the E1α and E1β subunits (Fregeau *et al.*, 1990; Fussey *et al.*, 1990). Sites on the other 2-OADC enzymes are less well characterized, but major reactivity can at least be confidently allocated to the single lipoyl-binding domains of these enzymes.

Third, there is a restriction to class (IgM) and isotype (IgG3) of autoantibodies to the M2 antigens (Surh *et al.*, 1988a). Autoantibodies in PBC are not, as was formerly believed, predominantly IgM, but this isotype is nonetheless well represented, in contrast to antibodies in other autoimmune diseases, which are predominantly IgG. Moreover, a low molecular type of IgM is present in PBC (Harris *et al.*, 1986), and has anti-M2 reactivity. Among the IgG autoantibodies, there is subclass restriction to IgG3, as seen in other autoimmune diseases, perhaps indicative of a fault in T cell-dependent class-switching of antibody isotype.

Fourth, antibodies in PBC have very potent inhibitory effects on the catalytic function *in vitro* of the enzyme with which they react; the effect is very rapid and occurs at high serum dilutions. This fits with recent findings that autoantibodies in general tend to be directed to the functional sites of their cognate antigen and exemplified by various of the antinuclear antibodies (Gershwin and Mackay,

1991). However, the M2 antibodies are of particular interest because PDC is such a well-studied enzyme with relatively simple assays available for inhibitory effects *in vitro*.

Data on the inhibitory capacity of PBC antibodies to PDC have been published from three laboratories (Van de Water *et al.*, 1988a; Uibo *et al.*, 1990; Sundin *et al.*, 1990). The enzyme-inhibitory capacity of PBC sera is specific for each enzyme, as judged by affinity purification of sera, as a further indication that there are separate populations of antibodies reactive with each of the three 2-OADC enzymes. This was established in a study based on the enzyme-inhibitory capacity of PBC sera for PDC and OGDC (Fregeau *et al.*, 1991). Thus, 73 of 188 (39%) of PDC sera reacted with OGDC-E2, as judged by immunoblotting against purified OGDC. In addition, the same PBC sera possessing OGDC-E2 reactivity specifically inhibited enzyme function of OGDC. Enzyme activity was not affected by PBC sera that contained autoantibodies to PDC-E2 and/or BCOADC-E2, but that lacked OGDC-E2 reactivity. Furthermore, affinity -purified PBC sera against OGDC-E2 inhibited only OGDC activity, but did not alter the enzyme activity of either PDC or BCOADC. Other studies on PBC sera using affinity purification were confirmatory since, when PBC sera were affinity purified on PDC-E2, the adsorbed preparation in contrast to whole serum reacted exclusively with PDC-E2 in serologic and enzyme-inhibition assays (Rowley *et al.*, 1991). Of interest, animals immunized with recombinant PDC-E2 develop antibodies that resemble those of PBC in most respects except for a lack of enzyme-inhibitory activity (Rowley *et al.*, 1991). Hence it appears that the inhibitory antibody is a highly specific serologic indication of PBC-related autoreactivity, and could well be useful in serologic diagnosis (Uibo *et al.*, 1990; Sundin, 1990). A semiautomated microassay for enzyme-inhibitory activity has been described (Teoh *et al.*, 1991).

C. Mitochondrial Autoantigens Other than M2 in PBC

It can be expected that autoantigens other than the 2-OADC enzymes will exist in mitochondria, and various of these have been identified, notably by immunofluorescence and chromatography. The series has been named M1–M9 (Berg and Klein, 1989). M1 corresponds to cardiolipin, and M3, M5, M6, and M7 are described in diseases other than PBC. The other claimed PBC-associated autoantigens are M4, identified with the chronic active hepatitis (CAH)-PBC overlap syndrome (Berg *et al.*, 1980) and as yet uncharacterized; M8, and M9 identified with benign-type disease (Berg and Klein, 1989) and characterized as glycogen phosphorylase (Klein and Berg, 1990). Given the present availability of technical procedures for characterizing polypeptide autoantigens, the lack of identification of some of the M3–M9 autoantigens brings into question their existence as independent molecules.

D. Nonmitochondrial Autoantigens in PBC

The frequency of autoantibodies to nonmitochondrial antigens in PBC reflects a clear increase above background, and includes several types of autoantibody, but reactivity to nuclear antigens stands out (Mackay and Gershwin, 1989a; Goldenstein *et al.*, 1989). The most provocative is reactivity to centromeric antigen with the same specificity as seen in scleroderma (CREST type), either with or without one or more of the clinical components of calcinosis, Raynaud's phenomenon, esophageal motility disturbances, sclerodactyly, and telangiectasia (CREST); some 12% of patients with PBC have anticentromere antibodies, and some 2% have clinically evident scleroderma (Powell *et al.*, 1987). This is especially puzzling because a cDNA for centromeric antigen has been cloned and sequenced (Earnshaw *et al.*, 1987), and no homologies with cDNAs for M2 antigens (*vide infra*) are evident. A second reactivity is with nuclear lamins, described by Wesierska-Gadek *et al.* (1989) and Courvalin *et al.* (1990). In addition, some 40–50% of PBC sera react by immunofluorescence with other nuclear antigens, with speckled patterns. A cDNA was derived for one of the nuclear antigen(s) involved, SP-100; the protein sequence showed homologies with α1 and α2 domains of major histocompatibility complex (MHC) class 1 molecules, and with several transcriptional regulatory proteins (Szostecki *et al.*, 1990).

Other autoantibodies for which there is an apparent increase in PBC include those to thyroid and gastric antigens, and liver-specific antigens; certain of these autoantibodies are increased in first-degree relatives of patients with PBC (Mackay, 1985). Among the explanations would be a general and familial defect in tolerance in PBC.

E. The M2 Autoantigens: Structural and Functional Features

The M2 autoantigens of PBC have been identified with the functionally related enzyme family, the 2-oxo-acid dehydrogenase complexes (Mackay and Gershwin, 1989b, 1990). We can summarize the structure and properties of these enzymes, PDC, BCOADC, and OGDC (Table I). The three enzymes consist of three subunits, E1, E2 and E3, each of which is nuclear encoded. The E1 subunits of PDC and BCOADC exist as two forms, E1α and E1β. After synthesis on ribosomes, the enzyme subunits are separately imported into mitochondria by a leader sequence that directs the import into, and transfer across, the inner mitochondrial membrane. Assembly of the three mature protein subunits occurs on the inner membrane, and some 30 assembled molecules are packaged as high-molecular-weight (MW) multimers. Thus, PDC has a MW of 8×10^6 and the functional enzyme exists as a very large molecular aggregate, readily visualized by electron-microscopy as a dodecahedron.

TABLE I

Molecular Weights and Functions of the 2-Oxo-Acid Dehydrogenase Complex

Enzymes	kDa	Function
Pyruvate dehydrogenase complex (PDC)		
El-α decarboxylase	41	Decarboxylates pyruvate with thiamine
El-β decarboxylase	36	pyrophosphate (TPP) as a cofactor
E2-acetyltransferase	74	Transfers acetyl group from El to coenzyme
E3-lipoamide dehydrogenase	55	A (CoA)
		Regenerates disulfide of E2 via oxidation of lipoic acid
Protein X	56	?
Branched-chain 2-oxo-acid dehydrogenase complex		
El-α decarboxylase	46	Decarboxylates α-keto acids
El-β decarboxylase	38	Derived from leucine, iso-leucine and valine with TPP as a cofactor
E2-acyltransferase	52	Transfers acyl group from El to CoA
E3-lipoamide dehydrogenase	55	Regenerates disulfide for E2 via oxidation of lipoic acid 38
2-oxoglutarate dehydrogenase, complex (OGDC)		
El-2-oxoglutarate decarboxylase	113	Decarboxylates α-ketoglutarate with TPP as a cofactor
E2-succinyl transferase	48	Transfers succinyl group from El to CoA
E3-lipoamide dehydrogenase	55	Regenerates disulfide for E2 via oxidation of lipoic acid

The 2-OADH enzymes are functionally complex. For PDC, the E1 subunit, a dehydrogenase, decarboxylates pyruvate-releasing CO_2 and an acetyl group; the E2 subunit, dihydrolipoamide, effects the reductive transfer of the acetyl group by the lipoic acid cofactor to co-enzyme A, which enters the Krebs cycle; the E3 subunit is a (FAD)-containing dihydrolipoamide that reoxidizes lipoic acid with formation of NADH, reduced nicotinamide adenine dinucleotide (NAD), a readily measurable end product of the enzyme reaction. The E2 subunits serve as the framework for the other components of PDC (E1, E3, X, kinase, and phosphorylase), which are noncovalently bound to E2 (Roche and Cate, 1977; Roche and Lawlis, 1982; Yeaman 1986). All three enzymes, PDC, OGDC, and BCOADC, have structural similarities but act on different substrates (Lawson *et al.*, 1983; Yeaman, 1986; Perham and Lowe, 1988). PDC oxidatively decarboxylates pyruvate, OGDC decarboxylates α-oxo-glutarate to form succinyl Co A, and BCOADC catalyzes the catabolism of essential amino acids, including the branched-chain amino acids, leucine, isoleucine, and valine.

F. Molecular Domains of PDC-E2

Since the E2 subunit carries the major antigenic reactivity of PDC, the 74-kDa antigen, it is appropriate to consider the four structural/functional molecular domains of PDC-E2 (Thekkumkara *et al.*, 1988). From the N-terminus, these include the lipoyl-binding domain(s), alanine-proline-rich linker regions that confer flexibility on the molecule, a site at which there is binding of the other subunits (E1 and E3) and, at the C-terminus, the catalytic site at which transfer occurs of an acetyl group to co-enzyme A. The structure of the lipoyl domains varies according to the source of the enzyme. *Escherichia coli* PDC contains three lipoyl regions, whereas mammalian PDC has two such regions, outer and inner (Fussey *et al.*, 1988); the inner appears to be more potent as an autoantigen than the outer (Surh *et al.*, 1990). The other 2-OADH enzymes have only one lipoyl-binding domain.

G. Epitope Mapping on PDC-E2

To characterize further the major PDH-E2 epitope, a set of truncated constructs of PDH-E2 were generated by progressively creating cDNA restriction fragments at the amino and the carboxyl termini (Surh *et al.*, 1990). The cDNAs were subcloned and the resultant fusion proteins analyzed by immunoblotting and ELISA, using PBC sera at a 1:500 dilution. Of the N-terminal deletion constructs, the fusion protein that contained amino acid residues 128–227 from the N terminus of the mature protein was strongly reactive, whereas the fusion protein that contained residues 136–227 was less frequently and more weakly reactive. Thus, by immunoblotting, 23 of 26 sera reacted with the 128–227 protein, but only 14 of 26 PBC reacted with the 136–227 protein. Furthermore, although serum titers by immunoblotting or ELISA against the 128–227 protein and the full-length fusion protein were similar for all of 10 sera analyzed, the titers against the 136–227 fusion protein were 100-fold lower. A similarly diminished frequency of reactivity and titer was observed against a fusion protein that contained residues 146–227, and a fusion protein that contained residues 160–227 was not reactive. From the C-terminus, only the deletion to residue 221 was permissive without any effect on the frequency or titer of reactivity with PBC sera. This indication that the smallest reactive determinant required residues 146–221 was verified by subcloning a restriction cDNA that encoded residues 146–221 to produce a fusion protein weakly reactive with PBC sera (Surh *et al.*, 1990).

In previous work, using only a partial-length rat liver cDNA clone, it was demonstrated that the immunodominant epitope of PDH-E2 was localized to the lipoic acid-binding site (Van de Water *et al.*, 1988b). Noting that human PDC-E2, in contrast to rat PDC-E2, has two lipoic acid-binding sites, and by using a full-length human cDNA for PDC-E2 and preparation of multiple overlapping recombinant fusion proteins, we can specify that at least three autoepitopes are present on human PDC-E2: the cross-reactive outer and inner lipoyl sites and a site surrounding the E1/E3-binding region. The dominant epitope is localized to the inner lipoyl site; the outer lipoyl site has only weak reactivity, and only 1 of 26 PBC sera reacted with the E1/E3-binding region sera. As indicated above, analysis of recombinant fusion proteins expressed from small restriction cDNA fragments encoding the inner lipoyl site has shown a requirement of 75 amino acids (residues 146–221) for detectable autoantibody binding, and 93 amino acids (residues 128–221) for strong binding. This requirement for such a large peptide region is of interest and indicates that a conformational autoepitope is involved. Strong evidence for this has also been obtained by Rowley *et al.* (in press) based on the reactivity of PBC sera after affinity purification on columns loaded with the PDC-E2 fusion protein or the intact PDC enzyme. The pattern of reactivity of the column eluates indicated that the conformational epitope involved is closely associated with the functional activity of the E2 subunit.

Since the lipoyl region constitutes the major antigenic site of the 2-OADC enzymes, the contribution of the lipoic acid cofactor to the antigenicity of the lipoyl domains of the 2-OADC enzymes is of interest. Three mutants in the lipoyl domain of PDC-E2 were created by site-directed *in vitro* mutagenesis (Leung *et al.*, 1990). The critical lysine residue at which lipoic acid is covalently attached was replaced by differently charged residues, glutamine or histadine, or by an aromatic amino acid, tyrosine. These variations in the charge distribution at the lipoyl-binding site of PDC-E2 did not significantly alter the reactivity of M2 antibody by immunoblotting or enzyme-linked immunosorbent assay (ELISA). Full interpretation of the data requires knowledge of whether lipoic acid is in fact present on transcripts from the cDNA for mammalian PDC-E2. This seems unlikely, since a recombinant mammalian BCOADC-E2 had no attached lipoic acid, but could be lipoylated *in vitro* in the presence of 2 m*M* adenosine triphosphate (ATP) using a mitochondrial extract (Griffin *et al.*, 1990).

However, in other studies on the reactivity of PBC sera with bacterial (*E. coli*) wild-type PDC-E2, or with genetically engineered bacterial PDC-E2, there was a requirement for the lipoic acid moiety, since reactivity was lost with an unlipoylated (lysine → glutamine) mutant (Fussey *et al.*, 1990). Also, the nonreactivity with lipoyl-deficient molecules could be partially restored if the lipoic cofactor was replaced by another group, octanoic acid, which could mimic the unique peptide–cofactor conformation within the lipoyl domain. It was found (Teoh, K.-L., Mackay, I. R., Rowley, M. J., and Fussey, S. P. M., 1991), that PBC sera inhibited the catalytic function of purified mammalian PDC but not that of purified bacterial PDC, despite the sera's being reactive with the E2 subunits of both enzymes by immunoblotting, indicative of a fine difference in the configuration of the lipoyl domains of the mammalian and bacterial enzymes. A more detailed characterization of the binding site of the PBC autoantibodies is needed.

III. AUTOIMMUNE-TYPE CHRONIC ACTIVE HEPATITIS

A. Background

Chronic active hepatitis is defined using clinical and morphological criteria. It is known that several different etiological agents or processes are responsible for this condition. Hepatitis B virus (HBV), hepatitis D virus (HDV), and hepatitis C virus (HCV) have been identified as important etiologic agents, whereas metabolic and toxic causes and drug hypersensitivities account for a small minority of cases. A decreased or ineffective response of the T-cell component of the immune system is a main contribution to the chronicity of hepatotropic virus infections, whereas a loss of tolerance against hepatocellular antigens underlies the pathogenesis of autoimmune-type chronic active hepatitis (AI-CAH). AI-CAH is characterized by a predominance of females over males (8:1), hypergammaglobulinemia (> 30 g per liter), association with particular human leukocyte antigen (HLA) alleles (B8 and DR3 among Caucasians and DR4 among Japanese), absence of markers of infection with HBV, and circulating autoantibodies against tissue antigens (Manns, 1989a and b; Mackay, 1990). Immunosuppressive treatment with corticosteroids alone or in combination with azathioprine leads to clinical, biochemical, and morphological remission associated with a prolonged survival (Kirk *et al.*, 1980). Various autoantibodies, non-tissue specific and liver specific, have been described in AI-CAH. Based on these autoantibodies as markers, subgroups of AI-CAH have been defined (Table II). The presence of these serum autoantibodies is useful in distinguishing AI-CAH from chronic hepatitis due to persistent infection with hepatotropic viruses. This is at least applicable to infection with HBV. However, for HCV, the picture is less clear in view of reports of coexistence of antibody to HCV and marker autoantibodies (Esteban *et al.*, 1989; Lenzi *et al.*, 1990; McFarlane *et al.*, 1990), although our view is that most positive tests for anti-HCV in cases otherwise fulfilling criteria for autoimmune hepatitis are spurious, and are owing to reactions with components other than HCV in the test system. An exception may be some elderly patients with type 2 AI-CAH sera positive for anti-LKM-1 (*vide infra*). The issue is clinically relevant, since in AI-CAH immunosuppressive treatment prolongs survival whereas interferons that are given for virus-induced liver diseases may be deleterious.

Classic AI-CAH was described 40 years ago in young females with hypergammaglobulinemia who responded well to corticosteroids (Waldenström, 1950). This form of chronic hepatitis was found to be associated with positive lupus erythematosus (LE) cell tests and antinuclear antibodies (ANA), which led to the term lupoid hepatitis (Mackay *et al.*, 1956). It is known that there is an array of antigens for antinuclear antibodies in AI-CAH, but these have still not been characterized at a molecular level. Whereas subtypes of AI-CAH can be

TABLE II
Heterogeneity of HBsAG-Negative Chronic Active Hepatitis (CAH)[a]

	ANA	LKM	SLA	SMA	AMA	Immunosuppressive treatment
CAH nonA, nonB (HCV)	−	−	−	−	−	−
Classic autoimmune (lupoid) CAH	+	−	−	+	−	+
LKM antibody-positive CAH	−	+	−	−	−	+
SLA antibody-positive CAH	−	−	+	+/−	+/−	+
SMA antibody-positive CAH	−	−	−	+	−	+
Primary biliary cirrhosis	−	−	−	−	+	−

[a]From Manns *et al.* (1987a).

specified, the two major types are type 1, the lupoid type, and type 2, as described in Table II. Type 1 was described in the previous edition of *The Autoimmune Diseases,* and type 2, for which there is molecular identification of the target autoantigen, will be described herein.

There are further autoantibodies associated with AI-CAH. Antibodies against a soluble liver antigen (SLA) have been characterized by radioimmunoassay (Manns *et al.*, 1987a) (Table II), and these are not detectable by immunofluorescence. They seem to characterize a third subgroup of AI-CAH and may help in distinguishing this form of autoimmune hepatitis from chronic viral hepatitis (Table II). Data suggest that liver cytokeratins 8 and 18 are the antigens recognized by autoantibodies to SLA (Wächter *et al.*, 1990).

Finally, autoantibodies against the hepatic asialoglycoprotein-receptor (ASGP-R) have been described (McFarlane *et al.*, 1986; Treichel *et al.*, 1990). Antibodies against this liver-specific membrane antigen are not restricted to any given subgroup of autoimmune liver diseases, and they occur also in a proportion of virus-induced liver diseases, and in PBC. Antibodies to ASGP-R appear to correlate with disease activity and may be a consequence of liver degradation, or represent a secondary autoimmune response that potentiates liver disease due to various primary causes.

B. Clinical Features of Type 2 Autoimmune Chronic Active Hepatitis

In 1973, antibodies against a microsomal antigen enriched in liver and kidney (LKM) were recognized by immunofluorescence (Rizzetto *et al.*, 1973) and were later found to be associated with a subgroup of AI-CAH (Smith *et al.*, 1974; Homberg *et al.*, 1987; Manns *et al.*, 1987b). In some respects type 2 AI-CAH resembles the classic lupoid type, but there are particular differences. A point worth making is that, whereas the first description of anti-LKM positive CAH was from England, this type of CAH has been accorded only minor reference in case surveys from North America, [e.g., Mayo Clinic (Czaja *et al.*, 1983)] or Australia, whereas the proportion of all cases of AI-CAH in Europe is cited as about 10% (Manns *et al.*, 1984). A detailed clinical description of type 2 AI-CAH is given by Homberg *et al.* (1987), based on 68 cases. As for type 1, there was a high preponderance of females (61:7) and a bimodal age distribution, but there was a striking frequency of cases in the 0–10-year age group (Homberg *et al.*, 1987; Manns *et al.*, 1987b). The onset was often acute (58%), and there was rapid progression to cirrhosis. As for type 1 AI-CAH, there was a striking response to prednisolone. The survival rate for untreated cases is poor, and for treated cases resembles that of type 1 AI-CAH. In 22 of the 68 cases cited by Homberg *et al.* (1987), there was an associated extrahepatic disease of autoimmune type, vitiligo, thyroid disorder, insulin-dependent diabetes mellitus, pernicious anemia, representing the organ-specific thyrogastric group, as well as various others (Homberg *et al.*, 1987; Manns *et al.*, 1987b; Sacher *et al.*, 1990). The clinical, laboratory, and histologic features resemble those of type 1 AI-CAH, apart from the frequency of low levels of immunoglobulin A in type 2 AI-CAH. HLA phenotypes, present in only 23 of the patients, showed a nonsignificant increase in HLA-A1, B8 (Homberg *et al.*, 1987); analysis of a larger case series is awaited.

There is a notable subclass restriction of LKM-1 autoantibodies for IgG1 and IgG4 (Weber *et al.*, 1988; Peakman *et al.*, 1987), which is different from the IgG3 restriction seen for mitochondrial antibodies in PBC (Surh *et al.*, 1988a; Weber *et al.*, 1988).

C. Identification of Reactant for Microsomal LKM-1 Antibodies

These antibodies were first recognized in CAH by immunofluorescence (Rizzetto *et al.*, 1973), owing to their characteristic high reactivity with the cytoplasm of hepatocytes and proximal tubules of rat kidney and liver. Subsequently, LKM antibodies were found in other diseases (Smith *et al.*, 1974; Manns *et al.*, 1989a). It was shown that the antibody bound to the rough and smooth endoplasmic reticulum (Storch *et al.*, 1977; Ballardini *et al.*, 1982). Alvarez *et al.* (1985) and Kyriatsoulis *et al.* (1987) reported that LKM sera from patients with AI-CAH recognize a 50-kDa microsomal protein by immunoblotting. The LKM antibodies in spontaneous AI-CAH were nominated as LKM-1 as opposed to LKM-2 present in drug-induced hepatitis (Table III). Different groups then found that LKM-1-positive sera reacted with preparations of several biochemically purified cytochrome P450 proteins (Manns *et al.*, 1988; Waxman *et al.*, 1988).

TABLE III
Liver-Kidney Microsomal (LKM) Autoantigens in Liver Disease

Molecular mass		Biochemical definition	Disease association
50 kDa	LKM-1	P450 dbl (IID6)	Autoimmune CAH
50 kDa	LKM-2	P450 meph (IIC9)	Drug-induced hepatitis (tienilic acid)
?	LKM-3	?	Chronic hepatitis D
50 kDa	LKM	P450 IA2	Autoimmune CAH, dihydralazine hepatitis
55 kDa	?	?	Autoimmune CAH
64 kDa	?	?	Autoimmune CAH

Thus, either the autoepitope recognized by LKM-1 antibodies was shared by different P450 proteins, or the LKM-1 antigen was an unidentified protein copurifying with these P450 enzymes.

The identification of cytochrome P-450 IID6 as major target of LKM-1 antibodies was achieved by various groups applying different experimental approaches. Zanger *et al.* (1988) immunopurified P-450 IID6 with human LKM-1 positive sera and showed specific inhibition of bufuralol-1′-hydroxilation mediated by P-450 IID6. Gueguen *et al.* (1988) isolated rat liver cDNA clones and concluded from their restriction map analysis that LKM-1 antibodies react with a class II P-450. Manns *et al.* (1989a) used immunoblots to analyze a panel of LKM-1 sera from children and adults with type 2 AI-CAH and found reactions of these sera with human microsomal antigens at 50, 55, and 64 kDa. The main antigen is 50 kDa, but some sera recognized in addition the 55-kDa or 64-kDa antigen (Manns *et al.*, 1989a). A high-titer serum reactive with both the 50-kDa and 64-kDa antigen was selected to screen a human liver cDNA library, and five immunopositive clones were isolated (Manns *et al.*, 1989a). Autoantibodies that were affinity purified on LKM-cDNA-derived fusion proteins reacted only with the 50 kDa but not with the 55-kDa or the 64-kDa liver microsomal antigen by Western blots and with the cytoplasm of proximal renal tubular epithelium in immunofluorescence. These experiments demonstrated that the isolated cDNA encodes for the 50-kDa LKM-1 antigen, which is immunologically identical in liver and kidney; however, the 64-kDa and 55-kDa antigens are immunologically distinct from the 50-kDa antigen. Nucleic acid sequence analysis revealed that the recombinant cDNA encodes for human cytochrome P-450 IID6 (Manns *et al.*, 1989a; Gueguen *et al.*, 1989). The immunodominant B-cell epitope has been localized on human cytochrome P-450 IID6 and consists of a linear sequence of 8 amino acids, which are highly conserved for class IID P-450s (Manns *et al.*, 1990a).

D. Autoantibodies to Antigens Other than LKM

The uniqueness of type 2 AI-CAH is highlighted by the serologic profile of the disease. Thus, of Homberg's 68 cases, only two had an ANA titer > 1/100, only two had SMA titers > 1/100, and none had actin antibody, which is a distinct marker for type 1 AI-CAH. By contrast, autoantibodies to thyroid microsomes/gastric parietal cells were present in 30%. This aligns this type of AI-CAH more with the thyrogastric than with the lupus-associated autoimmune diseases, but it needs to be established whether LKM-1-positive sera react with the organ-specific antigens, thyroid peroxidase, and gastric H^+K^+-ATPase.

E. Diagnostic Utility of Recombinant LKM-1 (P450 IID6) Antigen

Human recombinant LKM-1 (P450 IID6) antigen was used in diagnostic tests for LKM-1 antibodies in 46 disease sera that gave anti-LKM 1 reactions by immunofluorescence (Manns *et al.*, 1989b); 3 of the 46 sera were from patients with nonhepatic autoimmune diseases (scleroderma, Wegener's disease, idiopathic thrombocytopenia), and 43 were from patients with chronic hepatitis. Of the 46 sera, 25 reacted with a 50-kDa liver microsomal protein and 39 with the 78-kDa recombinant P450 IID6 in Western blots. From these data it became evident that approximately 10% of patients with anti-LKM-positive liver disease react with a 50-kDa microsomal protein that differs from cytochrome P450 IID6 (LKM-1). One of these rare LKM antigens has been identified as another enzyme of the cytochrome P450 supergene family, cytochrome P450 IA2 (Sacher *et al.*, 1990; Manns *et al.*, 1990b) (see the following).

F. Inhibition of Enzyme Function by Human Serum

Zanger *et al.* (1988) showed that sera positive for anti-LKM-1 inhibit bufuralol-I′-hydroxylation mediated by P450 IID6 in isolated human liver microsomes. The metabolism of the antiarrhythmic drug sparteine, also mediated by P450 IID6, is similarly inhibited by LKM-1 autoantibodies. Sparteine has a high first-pass effect; therefore, its metabolism *in vivo* is independent of hepatic blood flow. Thus sparteine can be used to study drug metabolism *in vivo* mediated by P450 IID6. Cytochrome P450 IID6 is a a drug-metabolizing enzyme known to metabolize more than 25 commonly used drugs, including those blocking β-adrenergic receptors, antiarrhythmic drugs, antihypertensive drugs, and tricyclic antidepressant drugs (Gonzales *et al.*, 1988). There exists a genetic polymorphism that is responsible for the lack of expression of cytochrome P450 IID6 enzyme in the livers of 5 to 10% of Caucasians; accordingly, such individuals have a poor capacity to metabolize these drugs. The molecular basis for this genetic polymorphism has been analyzed, and found to result from erroneously spliced P450 IID6 pre-mRNA (Gonzales *et al.*, 1988). However, patients with type 2 AI-CAH express functionally intact cytochrome P450 IID6 in their livers and hence are competent to metabolize drugs by cytochrome P450 IID6 including sparteine, etc. (Manns *et al.*, 1990c). Thus the genetic polymorphism resulting in lack of this autoantigen is not linked to the expression of the disease. Since sera of patients with type 2 AI-CAH inhibit P450 IID6 *in vitro,* yet the patients can metabolize drugs dependent on this enzyme, it appears that LKM-1 autoantibodies do not penetrate through the intact liver cell membrane to inhibit enzyme function *in vivo* (Manns *et al.*, 1990c).

G. Other Cytochrome P450 Autoantigens

There are LKM autoantigens additional to LKM-1, the reactant in type 2 AI-CAH. LKM-2 is the antigen for the microsomal antibodies detected in ticrynafen-induced hepatitis (Beaune *et al.*, 1987), and LKM-3 for the microsomal autoantibodies detected in chronic hepatitis D (delta) virus (HDV) infection (Crivelli *et al.*, 1983) (Table III).

The first cytochrome P450 that was identified as a human autoantigen was cytochrome P450 IIC9 (LKM-2) (Table III) (Beaune *et al.*, 1987; Meier and Meyer, 1987). Cytochrome P450 IIC9 metabolizes drugs that include the diuretic agent ticrynafen. The occurrence of antibodies to P450 IIC9 is linked to hepatitis induced by ticrynafen (tienilic acid) (Beaune *et al.*, 1987). Cases of hepatitis with anti-LKM-2 have been described only in France, presumably because this drug is available only in France and the United States of America. In Germany there has been no example of a serum reacting with P450 IIC9. While autoantibodies to cytochrome P450 IID6 and IA2 occur in spontaneous autoimmune hepatitis, antibodies to P450 IIC9 occur only in drug-induced hepatitis. In terms of pathogenesis, it is speculated that a reactive metabolite of tienilic acid binds to the P450 enzyme, which renders it antigenic (Beaune *et al.*, 1987).

There is a rare type of anti-LKM reactivity in which the antigen has been identified as cytochrome P450 IA2. This enzyme is dioxin(TCDD) inducible and is the main enzyme in man for the metabolism of phenacetin. Antibodies to P450 IA2 occur in spontaneous AI-CAH, and in drug-induced hepatitis related to the intake of dihydralazine (Manns *et al.*, 1990b; Bourdi *et al.*, 1990). This cytochrome is liver specific and so far has not been detected in other organs. Autoantibodies to cytochrome P450 IA2 react predominantly with perivenous hepatocytes (Sacher *et al.*, 1990; Bourdi *et al.*, 1990) in contrast to P450 IID6 (LKM-1) antibodies, which react homogeneously with the entire liver lobule. Interestingly, autoantibodies to cytochrome P450 IA2, like those reactive with P450 IID6, specifically inhibit the drug metabolism mediated by this enzyme *in vitro* (Manns *et al.* 1990b). Proof of the specificity of these autoantibodies for P450 IA2 is derived from the following experiments. First, there is increased reactivity of anti-P450 IA2 sera when microsomes are tested from rabbits pretreated with TCDD (dioxin). Second, there is strong reactivity of anti-P450 IA2 serum with lysates from COS-cells transfected with a vector carrying the full-length human cDNA for P450 IA2, whereas negative results were obtained for lysates from COS-cells transfected with a full-length human P450 IA1 cDNA, or the vector alone (Manns *et al.*, 1990b). These and other P450 autoantibodies may be useful in the future for studying specific drug metabolism mediated by individual members of related P450 subfamilies.

Autoantibodies reacting with human microsomes from liver and kidney were found by immunofluorescence in a minor proportion of patients with chronic HDV infection (Crivelli *et al.*, 1983). However, the LKM-3 antigen for these antibodies has not been identified. In addition, the 55-kDa and 64-kDa liver microsomal autoantigens detected by immunoblotting (Manns *et al.*, 1989a; Codoner-Franch *et al.*, 1989) await molecular definition (Table III). Possibly these latter microsomal antigens are also cytochrome P450 proteins.

H. Origin and Significance of Microsomal Autoantibodies

Microsomal autoantibodies in liver disease are directed against antigens located in the endoplasmic reticulum of hepatocytes, and these proteins are members of the cytochrome P450 superfamily of enzymes. These antibodies, like various other autoantibodies, inhibit the function of their cognate enzyme antigens *in vitro*, and epitopes recognized by these autoantibodies are conserved parts of the molecules. Although anti LKM-1 antibodies inhibit the function of the cytochrome P450 IID6 enzyme *in vitro*, they do not penetrate the intact liver cell membrane sufficiently to allow inhibition of the enzyme *in vivo* (Manns *et al.*, 1990c). So far, it is unknown how the immune reaction is initiated against microsomal autoantigens in type 2 AI-CAH. Metabolites of these enzymes are candidates, or as yet unidentified hepatotropic viruses (Manns *et al.*, 1990a). Antibodies against the hepatitis C virus detected by ELISA are reported in autoimmune hepatitis in some 50 and 70% of the patients (Esteban *et al.*, 1989; Lenzi *et al.*, 1990; McFarlane *et al.*, 1990), but some or even most of this reactivity may be spurious. Studies applying the polymerase chain reaction (PCR) that can directly detect HCV-specific RNA will clarify this question.

In a family with identical twins investigated by one of us (M.M.), only one of the 13-year-old female twins suffered from chronic hepatitis (Manns *et al.*, 1991). Both twins had the autoimmune haplotype B8, DR3, C4AQ0, and were extensive metabolizers; only the serum from the twin with hepatitis was positive for microsomal autoantibodies, and reacted with recombinant (LKM-1) P450

IID6, and inhibited P450 IID6 function *in vitro*. These data indicate that an environmental agent(s) may initiate this type of liver disease in patients with an appropriate genetic background. It will certainly be relevant to analyze the genetic background of anti-LKM-1 autoimmune liver disease not only at the MHC locus, but also at the locus of the autoantigen itself.

It has been reported that the LKM-1 (P450 IID6) antigen is expressed on the intact liver cell membrane (Lenzi *et al.*, 1984; Loeper *et al.*, 1989). However, it could not be demonstrated that cytochrome P450 IID6 is expressed on isolated viable normal hepatocytes in tissue culture (Gerken *et al.*, 1987). Newer techniques need to be developed to facilitate investigations on whether epitopes derived from cytochrome P450 IID6 are expressed on the liver cell surface in patients suffering from type 2 AI-CAH. The specificity of autoimmunity to cytochrome P450 IID6 in type 2 AI-CAH is supported by the fact that whereas a similar type of tissue destruction is caused by hepatitis B virus infection, and that this viral liver lesion may be associated with massive liver cell necrosis, there is no associated formation of cytochrome P450 (LKM) autoantibody. In other words, this autoantibody cannot be triggered simply as a consequence of liver destruction and release of the autoantigen.

IV. ANALOGIES BETWEEN AUTOIMMUNE LIVER DISEASES AND OTHER AUTOIMMUNE DISEASES

The application of techniques of molecular biology to autoimmune diseases has led to the cloning of cDNAs for several intracellular autoantigens and to the mapping of immunodominant epitopes for antibody (B cells), although not so far for T cells. Examples include sequential epitopes of La/SS-B (Chambers and Keene, 1985; Chan and Tan, 1987), Ro/SS-A (Chan and Tan, 1987; Deutscher *et al.*, 1988; Ben-Chetrit *et al.* 1989), cyclin (Ogata *et al.*, 1987), U1-RNP (Thiessen *et al.*, 1986), and ribosomal phosphoproteins (Coppel *et al.*, 1989). In these examples, more than one, and often several, immunodominant epitopes have been characterized. The existence of more complex conformational epitopes on these and other intracellular autoantigens has been suggested. As noted above, a major epitope on PDC-E2 (and probably the other 2-OADC enzymes) is located within a region where the functionally critical cofactor, lipoic acid, is bound, consistent with the inhibition by PBC sera of the catalytic function of these enzymes.

These observations are consistent with an emerging trend seen with a number of other autoimmune diseases for autoantibodies to be directed to functionally important sites of cognate antigens. This pertains also to the microsomal autoantigens that have been identified in type 2 autoimmune hepatitis; all LKM autoantibodies react with cytochrome P450 proteins and inhibit their function *in vitro* (Manns, 1989). Autoantibodies to tRNA synthetases in polymyositis sera inhibit tRNA aminoacylation (Mathews and Bernstein 1983; Mathews *et al.*, 1984; Dang *et al.*, 1988); antibodies to proliferating cell nuclear antigen in SLE sera inhibit *in vitro* DNA replication (Tan *et al.*, 1987); synthesis of 28S and 18S RNA is inhibited by RNA polymerase I-specific antibodies in scleroderma sera (Reimer *et al.*, 1987); autoantibodies to Sm and U1-RNP (both components of small nuclear ribonucleoproteins) inhibit splicing of early RNA sequences of adenovirus, and autoantibodies to La/SS-B interfere with the termination of transcription by an RNA polymerase (Padgett *et al.*, 1983; Gottlieb and Steitz, 1989).

Two striking themes are prominent. First, as for many of the described autoantigens, the mitochondrial antigens of PBC and the microsomal P450 antigens in autoimmune and drug-induced hepatitis are intracellular enzymes and exist not as single proteins but as components of large enzyme aggregates. Second, the autoantibodies directed against these subcellular structures, including anti-M2 and LKM, are directed against functional sites or domains and dramatically inhibit critical biological or catalytic activities of the autoantigen molecule *in vitro*. In the *model* of LKM-1-positive autoimmune hepatitis, it is also possible to study the function of the autoantigen *in vivo* (Manns *et al.*, 1990c).

The advent of cDNAs for mitochondrial autoantigens has allowed not only for more precise studies of their role in PBC but also for the development of quick and sensitive immunoassays utilizing recombinant PDC-E2 and BCOADC-E2 proteins (Van de Water *et al.*, 1989). Immunoassays with recombinant proteins have facilitated examination for Ig subclass restriction shown to exist for antibodies to both PDC-E2 and BCOADC-E2, and probably also for PDC-E1α (Surh *et al.*, 1988a). The advent of cDNAs for microsomal autoantigens is even more important, since reactivity with 50 kDa bands in immunoblotting may be owing to different antigens. More than 200 members of the cytochrome P450 supergene family have been identified, and all have a molecular mass around 50 kDa.

The availability of cloned autoantigens is a valuable resource for accurate diagnosis, and further understanding of the molecular basis of autoimmune diseases. A cloned cDNA provides for a precise characterization of autoantigens, including nucleotide sequence and amino acid sequence determination. Subcloning of cDNAs for autoantigens with epitope mapping allows for accurate definition of autoantibody-binding sites. Moreover, relatively simple assays such as ELISA based on recombinant antigens can be employed for more direct and precise diagnosis of specific diseases. Other potential uses of cloned cDNAs for autoantigens include detailed clinicoserologic correlations between autoimmune disease expression and the type of antibody response. Furthermore, LKM autoantibodies may become important tools for pharmacologists and toxicologists working with these enzymes. A good example is cytochrome P450 IA2 (Sacher *et al.,* 1990; Manns *et al.,* 1990b; Bourdi *et al.,* 1990). Whereas murine monoclonal antibodies against class I P450s react with both IA2 and IA1, the human autoantibodies predominantly react with IA2. This conclusion is derived from the observation that IA2 antibodies react with COS-cells transfected with full-length IA2 cDNA but not with COS-cells transfected with IA1 cDNA (Manns *et al.,* 1990b).

Finally, we can note the interest of experimental immunopathologists in *vaccination* against autoimmune disease using attenuated T-cell clones, and/or blocking T-cell epitopes by monoclonal antibodies or mimotopes (Vandenbark *et al.,* 1989; Wraith *et al.,* 1989; Lider *et al.,* 1987; Acha-Orbea *et al.,* 1988). The understanding of the molecular structure of autoantigens, and the identification and mapping of sites that stimulate T-cell responses, could open up new therapeutic approaches (Lider *et al.,* 1987; Acha-Orbea *et al.,* 1988) as described in Chapter 16 of this volume. The identification of autoantigens, and the autoepitopes relevant to human autoimmune diseases, consequent on the application of molecular biological techniques, is a prerequisite for these future therapeutic developments.

REFERENCES

Acha-Orbea, H., Mitchell, D. J., Timmermann, L., Wraith, D. C., Tausch, G. S., Waldor, M. K., Zamvil, S. S., McDevitt, H. O., and Steinman, L. (1988). *Cell* **54,** 263.

Alvarez, F., Bernard, O., and Homberg, J. C. (1985). *J. Exp. Med.* **161,** 1231.

Ballardini, G., Landi, P., Busachi, C. A., Bianchi, F. B., and Pisi, E. (1982). *Clin. Exp. Immunol.* **43,** 599.

Beaune, P. H., Dansette, P. M., and Mansuy, D. (1987). *Proc. Natl. Acad. Sci. U.S.A.* **84,** 551.

Ben-Chetrit, E., Gandy, B. J., Tan, E. M., and Sullivan, K. F. (1989). *J. Clin. Invest.* **83,** 1284.

Berg, P. A., Doniach, D., and Roitt, I. M. (1967). *J. Exp. Med.* **126,** 277.

Berg, P. A., and Klein, R. (1989). *Semin. Liver Dis.* **9,** 103.

Berg, P. A., Wiedmann, K.-H., and Sayers, T. J. (1980). *Lancet* **2,** 1329.

Bourdi, M., Larrey, D., Nataf, J., Bernuau, J., Pessayre, D., Iwasaki, M., Guengerich, F. P., and Beaune, P. H. (1990). *J. Clin. Invest.* **85,** 1967.

Chambers, J. C., and Keene, J. D. (1985). *Proc. Natl. Acad. Sci. U.S.A.* **82,** 2115.

Chan, E. K. L., and Tan, E. M. (1987). *J. Exp. Med.* **166,** 1627.

Codoner-Franch, P., Paradis, K., Gueguen, M., Bernard, O., Costesec, A. A., and Alvarez, F. (1989). *Clin. Exp. Immunol.* **75,** 354.

Coppel, R. L., Gershwin, M. E., and Sturgess, A. D. (1989). *Mol. Biol. Med.* **6,** 27.

Coppel, R. L., McNeilage, L. J., Surh, C. D., Van de Water, J., Spithill, T. W., Whittingham, S., Gershwin, M. E. (1988). *Proc. Natl. Acad. Sci. U.S.A.* **85,** 7317.

Courvalin, J.-C., Lassoued, K., Worman, H. J., and Blobel, G. (1990). *J. Exp. Med.* **172,** 961.

Crivelli, D., Lavarini, C., and Chiaberge, E. (1983). *Clin. Exp. Immunol.* **54,** 232.

Czaja, A. J., Davis, G. L., Ludwig, J., Baggenstoss, A. H., and Taswell, H. F. (1983). *Gastroenterology* **85,** 713.

Dang, C. V., Tan, E. M., and Traugh, J. A. (1988). *FASEB J.* **2,** 2376.

Deutscher, S. L., Harley, J. B., Keene, J. D. (1988). *Proc. Natl. Acad. Sci. U.S.A.* **85,** 9479.

Earnshaw, W. C., Machlin, P. S., Bordwell, B. J., Rothfield, N. F., and Cleveland, D. N. (1987). *Proc. Natl. Acad. Sci. U.S.A.* **84,** 4979.

Esteban, J. I., Esteban, R., Viladomiu, L. *et al.,* (1989). *Lancet* **ii,** 294.

Frazer, I. H., Mackay, I. R., Jordan, T. W., Whittingham, S., and Marzuki, S. (1985). *J. Immunol.* **135,** 1739.

Fregeau, D. R., Davis, P. A., Danner, D. J., Ansari, A., Coppel, R. L., Dickson, E. R., and Gershwin, M. E. (1989). *J. Immunol.* **142,** 3815.

Fregeau, D. R., Prindiville, T., Coppel, R. L., Kaplan, M., Dickson, E. R., and Gershwin, M. E. (1991). *Hepatology* (in press).

Fregeau, D. R., Roche, T. E., Davis, P. A., Coppel, R., and Gershwin, M. E. (1990). *J. Immunol.* **144,** 1671.

Fussey, S. P. M., Ali, S. T., Guest, J. R., James, O. F. W., Bassendine, M. F., and Yeaman, S. J. (1990). *Proc. Natl. Acad. Sci. U.S.A.* **87,** 3987.

Fussey, S. P. M., Bassendine, M. F., Fittes, D., Turner, I. B., James, O. F. W., and Yeaman, S. J. (1989). *Clin. Sci.* **77,** 365.

Fussey, S. P. M., Guest, J. R., James, O. F. W., Bassendine, M. F., and Yeaman, S. J. (1988). *Proc. Natl. Acad. Sci. U.S.A.* **85,** 8654.

Gerken, G., Manns, M., Ramadori, G., Poralla, T., Dienes, H. P., and Meyer zum Büschenfelde, K.-H. (1987). *J. Hepatol.* **5,** 65.

Gershwin, M. E., Ahmed, A., Danner, D., Fregeau, D., Van de Water, J., Leung, P., and Coppel, R. (1988b). *FASEB J.* (Abstr.) **2,** 3334, A869.

Gershwin, M. E., Coppel, R. L., and Mackay, I. R. (1988a). *Hepatology* **8,** 147.

Gershwin, M. E., and Mackay, I. R. (1991). *Gastroenterology,* **100,** 822.

Gershwin, M. E., Mackay, I. R., Sturgess, A., and Coppel, R. L. (1987). *J. Immunol.* **138,** 3525.

Goldenstein, C., Rabson, A. R., Kaplan, M. M., and Canoso, J. J. (1989). *J. Rheumatol.* **16,** 681.

Gonzalez, F. J., Skoda, R. C., and Kimura, S. (1988). *Nature* **331,** 442.

Gottlieb, E., and Steitz, J. A. (1989). *EMBO J.* **8,** 841.

Griffin, T. A., Wynn, R. M., and Chuang, D. T. (1990). *J. Biol. Chem.* **265,** 12104.

Gueguen, M., Meunier-Rotival, M., Bernard, O., and Alvarez, F. (1988). *J. Exp. Med.* **168,** 801.

Gueguen, M., Yamamoto, A. M., Bernard, O., and Alvarez, F. (1989). *Biochem. Biophys. Res. Commun.* **159,** 542.

Harris, R., Beckman, I., and Roberts-Thomson, P. J. (1986). *J. Immunol. Methods* **88,** 97.

Homberg, J. C., Abuaf, N., Bernard, O. *et al.,* (1987). *Hepatology* **7,** 1333.

Ishii, B. H., Saifuku, K., and Namihisa, T. (1985). *Immunol. Lett.* **9,** 325.

Kaplan, M. M. (1987). *Adv. Intern. Med.* **32,** 359.

Kirk, A. P., Jain, S., Pocock, S., Thomas, H. C., and Sherlock, S. (1980). *Gut* **21,** 78.

Klein, R., and Berg, P. A. (1990). *Clin. Exp. Immunol.* **81,** 65.

Kyriatsoulis, A., Manns, M., Gerken, G., Lohse, A. W., Ballhausen, W., Reske, K., and Meyer zum Büschenfelde, K.-H. (1987). *Clin. Exp. Immunol.* **70,** 53.

Lawson, R. K. G., Cook, K. G., and Yeaman, S. J. (1983). *FEBS Lett.* **157,** 54.

Lenzi, M., Ballardini, G., and Fusconi, M. (1990). *Lancet* **i,** 258.

Lenzi, M., Bianchi, F. B., Cassani, F., and Pisi, E. (1984). *Clin. Exp. Immunol.* **55,** 36.

Leung, P. S. C., Iwayama, T., Coppel, R. L., and Gershwin, M. E. (1990). *Hepatology* **12,** 1321.

Lider, O., Reshef, T., Beraud, E., Ben-Nun, A., and Cohen, I. R. (1987). *Science* **239,** 181.

Lindenborn-Fotinos, J., Baum, H., and Berg, P. A. (1985). *Hepatology* **5,** 763.

Loeper, J., Descatoire, V., Amouyal, G., Letteron, P., Larrey, D., and Pessayre, D. (1989). *Hepatology* **9,** 675.

Mackay, I. R. (1958). *N. Engl. J. Med.* **258,** 185.

Mackay, I. R. (1985). *In* "The Autoimmune Diseases" (N. R. Rose and I. R. Mackay, eds.), pp. 291–337. Academic Press, Orlando, Florida.

Mackay, I. R. (1990). *J. Gastroenterol. Hepatol.* **5,** 352.

Mackay, I. R., and Gershwin, M. E. (1989a). *Semin. Liver Dis.* **9,** 149.

Mackay, I. R., and Gershwin, M. E. (1989b). *Immunol. Today* **10,** 315.

Mackay, I. R., and Gershwin, M. E. (1990). *Springer Semin. Immunopathol.* **12,** 101.

Mackay, I. R., Taft, C. I., and Cowling, D. S. (1956). *Lancet* **ii,** 1323.

Manns, M. (1989). *J. Hepatol.* **9,** 272.

Manns, M., Gerken, G., Kyriatsoulis, A., Dienes, H. P., and Meyer zum Büschenfelde, K.-H. (1987b). *J. Clin. Lab. Analysis* **1,** 344.

Manns, M., Gerken, G., Meuer, M., Poralla, T., and Meyer zum Büschenfelde, K.-H. (1985). *J. Hepatol.* (Suppl. 1), 85.

Manns, M., Gerken, G., Kyriatsoulis, A., Staritz, M., Meyer zum Büschenfelde, K.-H. (1987a). *Lancet* **i,** 292.

Manns, M., Griffin, K. J., Quattrochi, L. C., Sacher, M., Thaler, H., Tukey, R. H., and Johnson, E. F. (1990b). *Arch. Biochem. Biophys.* **280,** 229.

Manns, M., Griffin, K. J., Sullivan, K. F., Meyer zum Büschenfelde, K.-H., and Johnson, E. F. (1990a). *Hepatology* **12,** 907.

Manns, M., Johnson, E. F., Griffin, K. J., Meyer zum Büschenfelde, K.-H., Tan, E. M., and Sullivan, K. F. (1989b). *Hepatology* **10,** 637.

Manns, M., Johnson, E. F., Griffin, I. C. J., Tan, E. M., and Sullivan, K. F. (1989a). *J. Clin. Invest.* **83,** 1066.

Manns, M., Koletzko, S., Löhr, H., Borchard, F., Ritter, C., and Meyer zum Büschenfelde, K.-H. (1991) (submitted for publication).

Manns, M., Kyriatsoulis, A., Amelizad, Z., Gerken, G., Lohse, A. W., Reske, K., Meyer zum Büschenfelde, K.-H., and Oesch, F. (1988). *J. Clin. Lab. Anal.* **2,** 245.

Manns, M., Meyer zum Büschenfelde, K.-H., Slusarcyzk, J., and Dienes, H. P. (1984). *Clin. Exp. Immunol.* **57,** 600.

Manns, M., Zanger, U., Gerken, G., Sullivan, K. F., Meyer zum Büschenfelde, K.-H., Meyer, U. A., and Eichelbaum, M. (1990c). *Hepatology* **12,** 127.

Mathews, M. B., and Bernstein, R. M. (1983). *Nature* **304,** 177.

Mathews, M. B., Reichlin, M., Hughes, G. R. V., and Bernstein, R. M. (1984). *J. Exp. Med.* **160,** 420.

McFarlane, B. M., McSorley, C. G., Vergani, D., McFarlane, I. G., and Williams, R. (1986). *J. Hepatol.* **3,** 196.

McFarlane, I. G., Smith, H. M., Johnson, J. P., Bray, G. P., Vergani, D., and Williams, R. (1990). *Lancet* **335,** 754.

Meek, F., Khoury, E. L., Doniach, D., and Baum, H. (1980). *Clin. Exp. Immunol.* **41,** 43.

Meier, U. T., and Meyer, U. A. (1987). *Biochemistry* **26,** 8466.

Mendel-Hartvig, I., Nelson, B. D., Loof, L., and Totterman, T. H. (1985). *Clin. Exp. Immunol.* **62,** 371.

Ogata, K., Ogata, Y., Takasaki, Y., and Tan, E. M. (1987). *J. Immunol.* **139,** 2942.

Padgett, R. A., Mount, S. M., Steitz, J. A., and Sharp, P. A. (1983). *Cell* **35,** 101.

Peakman, M., Lobo-Yeo, A., Mieli-Vergani, G., Davies, E. T., Mowat, A. P., and Vergani, D. (1987). *Clin. Exp. Immunol.* **15,** 331.

Perham, R. N., and Lowe, P. N. (1988). *Methods Enzymol.* **166,** 330.

Powell, F. C., Scroeter, A. L., and Dickson, E. R. (1987). *Q. J. Med.* **237,** 75.

Reimer, G., Rose, K. M., Scheer, U., and Tan, E. M. (1987). *J. Clin. Invest.* **79,** 65.

Rizzetto, M., Swana, G., and Doniach, D. (1973). *Clin. Exp. Immunol.* **15,** 331.

Roche, T. E., and Cate, R. L. (1977). *Arch. Biochem. Biophys.* **183,** 664.

Roche, T. E., and Lawlis, V. B. (1982). *Ann. N.Y. Acad. Sci.* **378,** 236.

Rowley, M. R., McNeilage, L. J., Armstrong, J. McD., and Mackay, I. R. (1991). *Clin. Immunol. Immunopathol.* **60,** 356–370.

Rowley, M. J., Maeda, T., Mackay, I. R., Loveland, B., McMullin, G., Tribbick, G., and Bernard, C. C. A. (submitted for publication).

Sacher, M., Blümel, P., Thaler, H., and Manns, M. (1990). *J. Hepatol.* **10,** 364.

Smith, M. G. M., Williams, R., and Walker, R. (1974). *Br. Med. J.* **2,** 80.

Storch, W., Cossel, L., and Dargel, R. (1977). *Immunology* **32,** 941.

Sundin, V. (1990). *Clin. Exp. Immunol.* **81,** 238.

Surh, C. D., Cooper, A. E., Coppel, R. L., Leung, P., Ahmed, A., Dickson, R., and Gershwin, M. E. (1988a). *Hepatology* **8,** 290.

Surh, C. D., Coppel, R. L., and Gershwin, M. E. (1990). *J. Immunol.* **144,** 3367.

Surh, C. D., Danner, D. J., Ahmed, A., Coppel, R. L., Mackay, I. R., Dickson, R., and Gershwin, M. E. (1988b). *Hepatology* **9,** 63.

Surh, C. D., Roche, T. E., Danner, D. J., Ansari, A., Coppel, R. L., Dickson, R., and Gershwin, M. E. (1989). *Hepatology* **10,** 127.

Szostecki, C., Guldner, H. H., Netter, H. J., and Will, H. (1990). *J. Immunol.* **145,** 4338.

Tan, C.-K., Sullivan, K., Li, X., Tan, E. M., Downey, K. W., and So, A. G. (1987). *Nucleic Acids Res.* **15,** 9299.

Teoh, K.-L., Rowley, M. J., and Mackay, I. R. (1991). *Liver* (in press).

Thekkumkara, T. J., Ho, L., Wexler, I. D., Pons, G., Liu, T., Patel, M. S. (1988). *FEBS Lett.* **240,** 45.

Thiessen, H., Etzerodt, M., Reuter, R., Schneider, C., Lottspeich, F., Argos, P., Luhrmann, R., and Philipson, L. (1986). *EMBO J.* **5,** 3209.

Treichel, U., Poralla, T., Hess, G., Manns, M., and Meyer zum Büschenfelde, K.-H. (1990). *Hepatology* **11,** 606.

Uibo, R., Mackay, I. R., Rowley, M., Humphries, P., Armstrong, J. M. C. D., and McNeilage, J. (1990). *Clin. Exp. Immunol.* **80,** 19.

Vandenbark, A. A., Hashim, G., and Offner, H. (1989). *Nature* **341,** 541.

Van de Water, J., Cooper, A., Surh, C. D., Coppel, R., Danner, D., Ansari, A., Dickson, R., and Gershwin, M. E. (1989). *N. Engl. J. Med.* **320,** 1377.

Van de Water, J., Gershwin, M. E., Leung, P., Ansari, A., and Coppel, R. L. (1988). *J. Exp. Med.* **167,** 1791.

Van de Water, J., Fregeau, D., Davis, P., Ansari, A., Danner, D., Leung, P., Coppel, R., and Gershwin, M. E. (1988). *J. Immunol.* **141,** 2321.

Wächter, B., Kyriatsoulis, A., Lohse, A. W., Gerken, G., Meyer zum Büschenfelde, K.-H., and Manns, M. (1990). *J. Hepatol.* **11,** 232.

Waldenström, J. (1950). *Dtsch. Ges. Verd. Stoffw.* **15,** 113.

Walker, J. G., Doniach, D., Roitt, I. M., and Sherlock, S. (1965). *Lancet* **1,** 827.

Waxman, D. J., Lappenson, D. P., Krishnan, M., Bernard, O., Kreibich, G., and Alvarez, F. (1988). *Gastroenterology* **95,** 1326.

Weber, M., Lohse, A. W., Manns, M., Meyer zum Büschenfelde, K.-H., and Köhler, H. (1988). *Nephron* **49,** 54.

Wesierska-Gadek, J., Penner, E., Hitchman, E., and Sauermann, G. (1989). *Immunol. Invest.* **18,** 365.

Wraith, D. C., Smilek, D. E., Mitchell, D. J., Steinman, L., and McDevitt, H. O. (1989). *Cell* **59,** 247.

Yeaman, S. J. (1986). *Trends Biochem. Sci.* **11,** 293.

Yeaman, S. J., Danner, D. J., Mutimer, D. J., Fussey, S. P. M., James, O. F. W., and Bassendine, M. F. (1988). *Lancet* **i,** 1067.

Zanger, U. M., Hauri, H. P., Loeper, J., Homberg, J.-C., and Meyer, U. A. (1988). *Proc. Natl. Acad. Sci. U.S.A.* **27,** 8256.

CHAPTER **10**

Autoimmune Diabetes Mellitus

WILLIAM HAGOPIAN
ÅKE LERNMARK
Robert H. Williams Laboratory
Department of Medicine
University of Washington
Seattle, Washington

I. INTRODUCTION AND CLINICAL CHARACTERIZATION

A. Historical Background

Several early documents indicate knowledge of diabetes; the disease was described more than a thousand years ago (Papadopoulos *et al.*, 1984; Bliss, 1982). Of particular interest to this chapter are the early morphological descriptions of pancreatic lesions in diabetes (cf. Gepts, 1965). Already at the beginning of this century, before the discovery of insulin, several authors distinguished between two types of diabetes. The most devastating type, associated with the classic symptoms of insulin-dependent diabetes, showed distinct pancreatic pathology. First, the pancreas was diminished in size in new-onset patients dying of ketoacidosis. Second, the islets of Langerhans were small and showed signs of degeneration. The islet pathology was associated with hydropic degeneration and hyalinosis, and patients had mononuclear cell infiltrates in the islets. Although special fixation and staining techniques were not available, the histopathological descriptions from the pre-insulin era are important since they describe changes that are difficult to document at the present time owing to insulin's lifesaving usefulness. It is of interest that speculations of an inflammatory disease were introduced already at the beginning of this century.

In an early report (Opie, 1901), the author concluded from his histological analysis of pancreas from patients with or without diabetes that "Diabetes mellitus, when the results of a lesion of the pancreas, is caused by destruction of the islands of Langerhans and occurs only when these bodies are in part or wholly destroyed." M. B. Schmidt (cf. Papaspyros, 1964) is likely to have made the first observation of insulitis. In the pancreas of a 10-year-old diabetic boy, he described isolated, acute interstitial inflammation of the islets of Langerhans. This report was followed by numerous similar case reports further documenting severe abnormalities of the endocrine pancreas in children developing diabetes. In these patients, inflammatory cells were observed, and the term insulitis was introduced.

A systematic quantitative study in the postinsulin era did not appear until Gepts (1965) reported on a larger series of newly diagnosed juvenile-onset diabetic patients. In a series of careful investigations, it was documented that there was a major loss of β cells at the time of clinical onset (Gepts, 1965). Other alterations included infiltrates of mononuclear cells in some but not all islets. The frequency of insulitis was, however, reported to be only 9 of 16 (56%) new-onset insulin-dependent diabetes mellitus (IDDM) patients. A critical reevaluation of this early literature indicates that, at the time of clinical onset, the frequency of insulitis may have been slightly exaggerated. In fact, one report failed to detect insulitis (Doniach and Morgan, 1973). Later, reports on new-onset IDDM patients with a young age at onset suggest that the insulitis inflammatory lesion varies not only from patient to patient but also within the individual pancreas (Foulis and Stewart, 1984).

The increased frequency of inflammatory cells in the islets of Langerhans at the time of clinical onset of IDDM stimulated the concept of insulin-dependent diabetes as an autoimmune disease. The original publication by Gepts (1965) inspired a series of investigations to test the hypothesis that the β cells in the pancreatic islets were lost to an autoimmune reaction.

However, the understanding of different forms of diabetes required further work. In 1950, Harris reported evidence to suggest that juvenile- and maturity-onset diabetes have different modes of inheritance (cf. Papaspyros, 1964). The development of the insulin radioimmunoassay provided means by which to estimate the amount of circulating insulin (cf. Rifkin and Porte 1990). Numerous investigations provided evidence for insulinopenia in juvenile-onset, ketosis-prone diabetes, but for hyperinsulinemia associated with maturity onset, non-ketosis-prone diabetes. Since insulinopenic diabetes could, however, occur also in older patients, two forms of diabetes, insulin-dependent (IDDM) and noninsulin-dependent (NIDDM), were suggested (Table I).

The observations that the islets of Langerhans might be affected by immune destruction resulted in a rapid development of our understanding of IDDM. It was reported that IDDM occurs more frequently in patients with autoimmune thyroid disease or in patients with autoimmune Addison's disease (MacCuish *et*

TABLE I
Diagnostic Values for Diabetes Mellitus[a]

	Whole blood		Plasma	
	Venous	Capillary	Venous	Capillary
Diabetes mellitus fasting value	≥6.7 (≥120)	≥6.7 (≥120)	≥7.8 (≥140)	≥7.8 (≥140)
Two hr after glucose load	≥10.0 (≥180)	≥11.1 (≥200)	≥11.1 (≥200)	≥12.2 (≥200)
Impaired glucose tolerance fasting value	<6.7 (<120)	<6.7 (<120)	<7.8 (<140)	<7.8 (<140)
Two hr after glucose load	6.7–10.0 (120–180)	7.8–11.1 (140–200)	7.8–11.1 (140–200)	8.9–12.2 (160–220)

[a]Glucose concentration in mmol/liter (mg/dl). Reprinted from WHO Study Group (1985).

al., 1975). Patients with juvenile-onset diabetes were subsequently found to have an increased frequency of organ-specific autoantibodies (MacCuish *et al.*, 1975). In addition, first-degree relatives of patients with IDDM were found to have an increased frequency of thyroid autoantibodies (Fialkow *et al.*, 1975). The leukocyte migration-inhibition test provided the first evidence for antipancreatic (islet) cellular hypersensitivity in diabetes (Nerup *et al.*, 1971; Nerup *et al.*, 1973). In 1974, islet-cell antibodies (ICA) were first described, suggesting that IDDM represented yet another organ-specific autoimmune disease (MacCuish *et al.*, 1974; Bottazzo *et al.*, 1974). This hypothesis was further substantiated by the demonstration of a close association between diabetes and human leukocyte antigen (HLA) type (Singal *et al.*, 1973; Nerup *et al.*, 1974). Subsequently, patients with IDDM were found also to have antibodies against β-cell plasma membrane antigens (Lernmark *et al.*, 1978). These antibodies mediated complement-dependent cytotoxicity (Dobersen *et al.*, 1980; Eisenbarth *et al.*, 1981) suggesting that they might be of pathogenetic importance. The first islet cell autoantigen, a β-cell specific M_r 64,000 protein, was described in 1981 (Lernmark and Baekkeskov, 1981; Baekkeskov *et al.*, 1982b) and identified in 1990 (Baekkeskov *et al.*, 1990) as glutamic acid decarboxylase (GAD). Insulin autoantibodies, present before exogenous insulin administration, were described in 1983 (Palmer *et al.*, 1983).

Studies in patients as well as in their first-degree relatives showed that markers for IDDM such as ICA may be present years before clinical onset of the disease (Gorsuch *et al.*, 1981). Quantitative analysis of cells in the endocrine pancreas indicated that by the time of clinical diagnosis, the majority of the β-cells have already been lost (Rahier *et al.*, 1983; Rahier, 1988). Taken together, these data suggested that IDDM is not an acute disease, but rather a chronic ailment. The disease has a long prodrome of anti-islet autoimmunity in the patient with young adult or adult age at onset. In very young children, the rate of β-cell destruction appears to be accelerated, and the length of the prodrome may be shortened.

The accumulated evidence of clinical as well as biochemical measures resulted in a set of diagnostic and classification guidelines most recently updated by the World Health Organization (WHO Study Group, 1985).

B. Clinical Definition of IDDM

The WHO diagnostic guidelines of IDDM and other forms of diabetes are summarized in Table I. The untreated disease is characterized by a chronic hyperglycemia. The main diagnostic criterion for diabetes is a fasting blood sugar of ≥ 6.7 mmol/liter glucose. A number of glucose tolerance tests may be used to confirm the diagnosis (WHO Study Group, 1985). These tests are of greater importance in adults than in children, since diabetes in children usually presents with the unequivocal symptoms of hyperglycemia, glycosuria, and ketonuria.

After diagnosis, patients are classified (WHO Study Group, 1985) into either its two major forms, IDDM or NIDDM, or to secondary diabetes (Table II). In the case of IDDM, several studies have already indicated that current guidelines

TABLE II

Classification of Diabetes Mellitus and Other Categories of Glucose Intolerance

Clinical classes
Diabetes mellitus (DM)
Insulin-dependent diabetes mellitus (IDDM)
Non-insulin-dependent diabetes mellitus (NIDDM)
Nonobese
Obese
Malnutrition-related diabetes mellitus (MRDM)
Other types of diabetes associated with certain conditions and syndromes: (1) pancreatic disease; (2) disease of hormonal etiology; (3) drug-induced or chemical-induced conditions; (4) abnormalities of insulin or its receptors; (5) certain genetic syndromes; (6) miscellaneous
Impaired glucose tolerance (IGT)
Nonobese
Obese
Associated with certain conditions and syndromes
Gestational diabetes mellitus (GDM)
Statistical risk classes (subjects with normal glucose tolerance but substantially increased risk of developing diabetes)
Previous abnormality of glucose tolerance
Potential abnormality of glucose tolerance

From WHO Study Group (1985).

of classification may not be sufficient (Wilson *et al.*, 1985). Typically in IDDM (or type 1 diabetes) there is ketoacidosis and hyperglycemia with hyperosmolarity. The body weight is less than or equal to the ideal body weight (IBW). The fasting plasma glucose consistently exceeds 6.7 mmol/liter. In typical NIDDM (type 2 diabetes) there is no history of diabetic ketoacidosis. The body weight of the patient is increased. NIDDM is often asymptomatic and may have been present for years before diagnosis. In fact, sometimes patients are diagnosed because they show signs of diabetic complications. NIDDM in the young, often referred to as MODY (maturity-onset diabetes of the young), is reported as a form of NIDDM inherited in a dominant fashion (Rifkin and Porte, 1990). The presence of such patients indicates that NIDDM may also develop at any age.

Different glucose tolerance tests have been developed to analyze the function of the β-cells and to aid in the classification of diabetes (WHO Study Group, 1985). These tests are, however, not standardized, and interlaboratory comparisons are difficult. Measurements of plasma C-peptide, the connecting peptide that is formed when proinsulin is converted to insulin, and secreted in equimolar concentrations with insulin (cf. Steiner *et al.*, 1989), may be useful as a biochemical measure in the classification of diabetes. It is estimated that NIDDM patients develop IDDM at a rate of 1 to 2% per year. Several investigators have presented data indicating that older patients, usually greater than 20 years of age, are not readily classified into IDDM or NIDDM. For example, ICA have been reported in NIDDM patients with secondary failure to treatment with oral hypoglycemic agents (Irvine *et al.*, 1977; Gleichmann *et al.*, 1984). ICA-positive NIDDM patients followed prospectively are often found to progress to IDDM (Irvine *et al.*, 1977; Groop *et al.*, 1986; Groop *et al.*, 1986). A recent prospective study suggests that the predictive value for insulin dependency is nearly 100% in NIDDM patients who are ICA positive at the time of clinical diagnosis (Landin-Olsson *et al.*, 1990). Interestingly, at the time of diagnosis, these patients showed significantly lower fasting C-peptide than did the ICA-negative patients.

In summary, although IDDM and NIDDM are usually classifiable based on the former being ketosis-prone and with nonelevated IBW, further investigations are necessary to develop diagnostic tests that clearly distinguish IDDM from other forms of diabetes. These tests of differential diagnosis should be made applicable to the subclinical state of IDDM to accurately estimate the residual β-cell function as well as to employ immunological and genetic markers to distinguish between the two major forms of diabetes. More important, however, a diagnosis of IDDM with objective and accurate biochemical tests may permit a diagnosis of IDDM before the β-cell destruction is severe enough to produce glucose intolerance. An early diagnosis will likely be necessary to develop new measures to prevent insulin dependency, perhaps by a specific immune intervention therapy.

C. Clinical Characteristics

A large number of epidemiological studies of IDDM throughout the world suggest that IDDM may develop at any age (Palmer and Lernmark, 1990a; Dahlquist *et al.*, 1989). The incidence rate varies with age and sex. In children, there is an increasing incidence rate until the age of 11 to 14 years, with a decline thereafter. The peak incidence rate occurs slightly earlier in girls than in boys. A sexual dimorphism has been observed in patients with onset as adults, with a significantly higher incidence rate for males (Nyström *et al.*, 1990).

The lifetime risk for IDDM is being quantified based on large population-based studies, primarily in Northern Europe and in England (Dahlquist *et al.*, 1985; Dahlquist *et al.*, 1989; Nyström *et al.*, 1990). It can be estimated from these studies that about 100,000 children are born per year in a population of 10 million inhabitants. Out of these 100,000 newborns, about 1000 will develop IDDM within their lifetimes. It is furthermore estimated that 40% of the patients will develop the disease before 15 years of age; 30%, between 15 and 34 years of age; and the remaining 30% will develop autoimmune diabetes by old age. The use of defined criteria to classify diabetes is therefore critical to our understanding of the role of autoimmunity in IDDM and the detection of this disease before insulin dependency, since the disease may occur at any age (Andres, 1971; Wilson *et al.* 1985; Tattersall, 1986) and is often mistaken for NIDDM (Di Mario *et al.*, 1983; Landin-Olsson *et al.*, 1989; Irvine *et al.*, 1980; Gleichmann *et al.*, 1984; Groop *et al.*, 1986). Second, only 10–13% of new patients have a first-degree relative with the disease (Tillil *et al.*, 1987; Dahlquist *et al.*, 1989; Mason *et al.*, 1987). These and recent phenomena of transient immune markers such as ICA (Gorsuch *et al.*, 1981; Spencer *et al.*, 1984; Landin-Olsson *et al.*, 1989; Karjalainen, 1990) and of subclinical β-cell dysfunction with or without persistent immune markers (McCulloch *et al.*, 1990; Bärmeier *et al.*, 1990) underline the difficulties of ascertaining biochemical and clinical data that clearly identify IDDM.

Genetic inheritance of a disease may often be best understood in studies of monozygotic twins. Most of our information of IDDM among twins is obtained from studies in the United Kingdom (Tattersall *et al.*, 1972; Pyke, 1979). In a first analysis, twins with IDDM who developed their disease before the age of 35 were compared with NIDDM twins who developed their disease after the age of 45. It was found that while 89% of the NIDDM twins were concordant for the disease, this was the case among only 55% of twins with IDDM (Pyke, 1988). The higher the concordance rate, the more likely it is that a disease is attributable to genetic mechanisms, while lower concordance rates suggest that environmental factors predominate. More recent studies in the United Kingdom and other countries with twin registries indicate that the IDDM concordance rate, in fact, may be closer to 30% (Olmos *et al.*, 1988; Rotter *et al.*, 1990). This surprisingly low concordance rate needs to be explained. It is possible that both twins are born susceptible to IDDM. The disease does not develop unless there is an etiological agent in the environment to trigger the pathogenesis that results in β-cell destruction and loss of insulin production. Monozygotic twins, interestingly, show a heterogeneous pattern with respect to the clinical onset of IDDM. Twins who are HLA-DR3/4 positive have a higher concordance rate than twins with only one of these HLA types (Barnett *et al.*, 1981). The data indicate that older twin pairs have less chance of becoming concordant. Similar to siblings, the longer the time from the diagnosis in the first twin, the lesser the possibility of the pairs becoming concordant (Gamble, 1980a). Impaired β-cell function is also reported in nonaffected twins who have failed to develop IDDM during follow-up (Heaton *et al.*, 1987). Several immune abnormalities have been reported, but none of them seems to predict IDDM (Beer *et al.*, 1990; Heaton *et al.*, 1988; Johnston *et al.*, 1989; Millward *et al.*, 1986). It is therefore possible that a previously active diabetogenic process in these individuals has remitted. Immune abnormalities such as ICA have been detected but proven to be transient. It is possible that both twins may have been born with the disease. The pathogenesis of the disorder has progressed differently in the two twins, for example, owing to factors in the environment protecting one of the twins from developing IDDM, rather than inducing the disease in the other twin. This is suggested by animal models of spontaneous IDDM, as well as a study suggesting that families with greater numbers of siblings may be relatively protected from IDDM, perhaps owing to increased exposure to transmitted infectious agents.

Studies in families are the next important approach to uncover patterns of inheritance. Numerous studies on the mode of inheritance of IDDM have been published and reviewed (Köbberling and Tattersall, 1982; Wassmuth *et al.*, 1990; Rotter *et al.*, 1990; Rich, 1990). Despite this effort, it has not yet been possible to clarify the mode of inheritance of IDDM. Nearly every possible model has been proposed, and IDDM has been referred to as the geneticist's nightmare (Köbberling and Tattersall, 1982). A large number of genetic markers or traits have been tested, including markers for blood group types and HLA transplantation antigens. In family studies, none of these markers except HLA has shown linkage to IDDM. Studying IDDM in families is difficult, however, since in patients with onset before age 20 only 10–13% of new patients have a first-degree relative with the disease (Tillil and Köbberling, 1987; Dahlquist *et al.*, 1989; Mason *et al.*, 1987). The familial aggregation has been confirmed in studies comparing the frequency of diabetes among first-degree relatives to that in controls (Rotter *et al.*, 1990). In a recent case-control study, the 13% frequency of IDDM among parents and siblings was confirmed, but familial risk factors were extended to also include NIDDM as well as non-pancreatic diseases of organ-specific autoimmunity (Dahlquist *et al.*, 1989).

The geographic distribution of IDDM varies markedly. In Europe there seems to be a south-to-north gradient of increasing frequency. This is not entirely true, since areas of high incidence rates, such as Sardinia, have recently been documented (Group, 1990). The geographic distribution may therefore rather reflect the distribution of genetic factors. The known incidence rates are highest in Finland and Sweden (Dahlquist *et al.*, 1989; Åkerblom *et al.*, 1988). The incidence rate is higher in American whites than in black or Mexican-Americans. The occurrence of IDDM in these groups may be attributable to transracial admixture of European IDDM susceptibility genes. The lowest recorded incidence rates are obtained from Japan. The role of genetic factors is therefore important to our understanding of IDDM, and will be reviewed briefly below. A more comprehensive review is provided in Chapter 5 by Nepom and Concannon in this volume.

II. GENETIC PREDISPOSITION

Several genes or loci of the human genome have been studied to determine their linkage or association to IDDM. In association studies, the frequency of a marker among patients is compared to that in the control population. In this approach, it is asked whether a gene is distributed with the disease throughout the population. The association with the HLA complex on chromosome 6 was first reported in 1973 for B15 (Singal and Blajchman, 1973) and in 1974 for B8 (Nerup *et al.*, 1974). The availability of HLA as a marker for IDDM generated numerous investigations. Initially HLA typing was carried out by serological techniques. These techniques have to a great extent been replaced by genotyping using cloned probes or oligonucleotides of defined genes (see Chapter 5 by Nepom and Concannon in this volume). A decreased frequency of HLA-DR2 was also observed in IDDM. This haplotype was therefore referred to as protective (conferring resistance to IDDM). This concept is questionable, however, since an increased frequency of an HLA marker in patients compared to its frequency in the controls indicates that other HLA specificities must have a decreased frequency since the number of known HLA specificities or genes is finite.

As indicated above, the first association between HLA and IDDM was with HLA-B15 and B8. The strongest association with the typing sera for the HLA-B class I molecules was with B8/15 heterozygosity (Nerup *et al.*, 1974). The association between HLA-B and IDDM was shortly thereafter shown to be secondary to HLA-Dw3 and Dw4 (Thomsen *et al.*, 1975). In these studies, primed lymphocyte typing was used to identify HLA-D specificities. Using typing sera for HLA-DR (R for related) specificities, DR3 and DR4 were frequent enough to support the conclusion that HLA-B8 and HLA-B15 were associated with IDDM, because these specificities are in strong linkage disequilibrium with HLA-DR3 and DR4, respectively. Subsequently, numerous investigations have confirmed the strong association between HLA-DR3 and/or DR4 and IDDM (for review see Wassmuth and Lernmark, 1990).

About 90 to 95% of patients with IDDM are either DR3 and/or DR4 positive compared to 50 to 60% among the controls. The highest known relative risk is observed for HLA-DR3/4 heterozygosity. The HLA-DR3/4 heterozygosity is particularly prevalent in Northern Europe. In Sweden, 30–40% of patients compared to 3 to 8% among controls are HLA-DR3/4 heterozygous (Wassmuth and Lernmark, 1990). Heterozygosity as such may be important, since the highest risk for Chinese patients with onset of IDDM younger than 11 was observed in HLA-DR3/9 individuals (Hawkins *et al.*, 1987). In Japan the highest risk was in HLA-DR4/9 patients (Kobayashi *et al.*, 1986). Recent data in Swedish, Danish, and Finnish patients and controls suggest that heterozygosity both of HLA-DQw2/8 (Wassmuth *et al.* 1991) and a HLA-DQ β-chain polymorphism (Michelscn *et al.*, 1990; Reijonen *et al.*, 1990) confer higher risks than does HLA-DR3/4.

The discovery of additional genes for HLA class II molecules in the HLA-D region resulted in the demonstration first by analysis of restriction fragment length polymorphism (Owerbach *et al.*, 1983) and later by direct sequence analysis (Todd *et al.*, 1987; Todd *et al.*, 1988) that the DQ region may be closer to IDDM than is DR. Using a similar approach (Platz *et al.*, 1981), it was demonstrated that DR4-positive patients are more often positive for DQw8 than are healthy DR-4 positive controls (Wassmuth *et al.*, 1991). Diabetes risk would therefore be closer to DQ than to DR, yet another example of linkage disequilibrium. These observations illustrate the perils of oversimplification, and teach a lesson that a marker found to be increased in frequency among patients compared to controls does not necessarily represents a *diabetes gene,* nor does the marker necessarily play a role in the pathogenesis of the disease. Further studies on the association between HLA gene markers and IDDM, as well as studies on the linkage between individual HLA markers and IDDM, will be necessary to accurately map the *diabetes susceptibility locus*. Once identified, it is hoped that this locus will contain nucleotide sequences that are found among 100% of the IDDM patients. The frequency among controls is expected to be low since only 0.15–0.3% of the population has IDDM. Future studies on HLA markers in IDDM therefore require a large number of samples from population-based patients and controls. Alternatively (and assuming that this hypothetical locus is the same in ethnic groups other than Caucasians, e.g., Mexican-Americans or U.S. blacks), transracial gene mappings should prove an effective means by which to identify the hypothetical IDDM susceptibility sequences (Jenkins *et al.*, 1990; Todd, 1990).

By sequence comparisons of DQ β-chain genes (Todd *et al.*, 1988) it was concluded that haplotypes associated with IDDM (DR4-DQw8, DR3-DQw2, DR1-DQw5, DR2-DQw1.AZH) were different at amino acid position 57 compared to haplotypes that are negatively associated with IDDM (DR4-DQw7, DR2-DQw1.2, DR2-DQw1.12). Although the crystallographic structures of these HLA-DQ class II molecules is yet to be determined, it has been inferred from analogy to HLA class I molecules (Bjorkman *et al.* 1987) that the position 57 amino acids would be located at one end of the peptide binding groove on the HLA molecule, and therefore accessible to both peptide binding and T cell-receptor recognition (Todd *et al.*, 1988). HLA haplotypes that are associated with IDDM have alanine, serine, or valine in this position, while in nondiabetic haplotypes Asp is present. Numerous studies testing this hypothesis have refuted it, since as many as 2% of Norwegian, 9% of Polish, 22% of Chinese, and 56% of Japanese IDDM patients develop IDDM despite being asp/asp homozygous (see Wassmuth and Lernmark, 1990). Additional observations that do not support the position 57 hypothesis include the findings that HLA-DR7/DQw2 (which has a non-asp in position 57) is negatively associated with diabetes, and that HLA-DQw7, which has an asp in position 57, is positively associated with IDDM in DQw8-positive individuals. It is therefore concluded that genotyping solely for aspartic acid at DQ β position 57 is insufficient to assess disease risk for IDDM.

HLA-DR and -DQ genotyping in Swedish (Wassmuth *et al.*, 1991), American (Baisch *et al.*, 1990), and French IDDM patients and controls has allowed analyses of complete DR–DQ haplotypes. These haplotype analyses represent a way to analyze the degree of linkage disequilibrium between two closely located loci (see Chapter 5, this volume). The common haplotypes with an increased frequency in IDDM are DR3-DQw2 and DR4-DQw8. DR3-DQw2 in DQw8-positive individuals is strongly associated with IDDM. This is also the case for DR1-DQw7 in DQw8-positive individuals. Therefore, some haplotypes may confer risk despite containing a protective DQ type. It is therefore possible that susceptibility to IDDM may require alleles from both the DR and the DQ locus, or a dominant susceptibility may be provided by a gene close to DQw8. However, DQw8 is not always dominant, since DQw1.2 (Baisch *et al.*, 1990) and DQw1.18 (Wassmuth *et al.*, 1991) are negatively associated with IDDM, both alone and when they occur together with HLA-DQw8. In current investigations, it is therefore necessary to perform complete DR–DQ genotyping to accurately assess susceptibility to IDDM. Additional analysis of gene polymorphism associated with the HLA-DR/DQ region (Michelsen and Lernmark, 1987; Reijonen *et al.*, 1990) and new genes in the class II region of the human MHC complex, such as the ATP-binding casette (ABC) genes (Spies *et al.*, 1990; Trowsdale *et al*, 1990) will be of interest. It cannot be excluded that unknown genetic elements in linkage disequilibrium with HLA-DR/DQ represent the true diabetes-susceptibility genes.

In families with IDDM, there will be other family members who carry diabetes-susceptibility genes. Why do not these individuals also develop IDDM? Recent analyses of large numbers of multiplex families suggest that the lifelong risk in first-degree relatives is 3% for parents, 7% for siblings, and 5% for children of parents with IDDM. Several prospective analyses of large numbers of families have confirmed these low conversion rates. The positive predictive value for IDDM in marker-positive (HLA, ICA, or insulin autoantibodies, IAA) first-degree relatives is low. In the Fifth Genetic Analysis Workshop (GAW5), the analysis of affected sib-pair marker sharing confirmed that IDDM is strongly linked to HLA (Risch, 1989). The distribution of HLA markers indicated that the occurrence of IDDM was about 15% if a sibling shared both HLA markers with the proband (HLA-identical), 5% if one (haploidentical), and 1% or less if HLA-nonidentical. In a joint study of Caucasians with IDDM (Thomson *et al.*, 1988), it was found that the susceptibility to IDDM was recessivelike for HLA-DR3 and dominant- or intermediatelike for HLA-DR4. Removing susceptibility effects of HLA-DR3 and HLA-DR4, significant risks were observed for DR1 and DRw8. These residual risk effects are probably explained by linkage to the HLA-DQw-types discussed above. In this multicenter study, the risk estimates for siblings (based on an overall sibling risk of 6%) showed a 13%, 5%, and 2% risk for siblings sharing two, one, and zero HLA haplotypes with the proband, respectively. Again, the highest risk (19%) was observed for HLA-DR3/4 heterozygosity. This analysis, which confirms and extends those of several previous publications (reviewed by Risch, 1987, 1989) therefore suggests that (1) genetic determinants that are not linked to HLA may be more important than HLA, since the lifetime risk for a sibling is five times higher than that predicted by HLA; (2) the mode of inheritance of IDDM is yet to be explained; and (3) a single-locus model is clearly rejected, but there is strong evidence for linkage using maximal-likelihood affected-pair methods (Risch, 1989).

In summary, HLA in IDDM represents factors that are necessary but not sufficient for the disease to develop. This is illustrated by our analysis of HLA-DR/DQ genotypes in Swedish patients, indicating that only 1 of 70 of HLA-DQw2/w8-positive individuals develops IDDM. The HLA gene markers therefore represent merely permissive factors. In animals developing IDDM similar to that of man, such as the NOD mouse and the BB rat, there is evidence for non-MHC genes on chromosomes 1, 3, and 11 that determine susceptibility to IDDM. Family studies rather than association studies may thus better help to become more informative in attempts to detect a second or perhaps third diabetes gene by molecular genetics techniques. Disease linkage may also be obtained by qualified guesses of candidate genes. In the pathogenesis of IDDM, there is no obvious candidate gene (in fact, there are too many of them). Evidence for linkage, using the affected-sib-pair method, was not obtained for the flanking sequences of the insulin gene or for Km nor Gm, all three of which are potential candidate genes as well as genetic markers reported to be associated with IDDM (Risch, 1989). Since it has been calculated that HLA accounts for only 40–80% of the genetic contribution to IDDM (Risch, 1989; Rotter *et al.*, 1990), it will be of interest to explore families with IDDM in several generations as well as to extend the sib-pair analyses with novel techniques of gene mapping using DNA satellite probes and DNA fingerprinting techniques (Hyer *et al.*, 1991) to obtain additional gene markers linked to IDDM.

III. CLINICAL PROGRESSION

A. Triggers of IDDM in Predisposed Individuals

The low concordance rate among monozygotic twins is usually taken to indicate that the environment is of etiological importance in the development of IDDM. Recent studies in the BB rat (Dyrberg *et al.*, 1988) as well as in the NOD mouse (Leiter, 1989) suggest that the environment (including viruses) may confer strong protective effects. Factors in the environment include infectious agents (viruses, bacteria, mycoplasma), environmental chemicals (nitrosamines) or pharmaceutical agents [pentamidine, *N*-3-pyridylmethyl *N′*-*P*-nitrophenylurea (Vacor)] (Palmer and Lernmark, 1990b). It is conceivable that these environmental factors could directly damage the β cells, which may initiate a self-perpetuating β-cell autoreactivity. The alternate hypothesis is that the environmental factors do not represent triggers, but rather potentiators of an inherited immune-system tendency to directly attack the β cells. These two potential mechanisms are most likely to interact with each other, so that lack of tolerance to critical β-cell determinants may result in self-perpetuating autoimmunity initiated by environmental factors. The previous view of viral infection as an acute trigger of IDDM has been modified after the demonstration of the long prodrome of islet autoimmunity in IDDM and the observation that the pancreata from children dying at the acute onset of IDDM in conjunction with viremia have a chronic rather than acute islet inflammation (Foulis *et al.*, 1990). The reader is therefore referred to previous reviews addressing the association between IDDM and viral infections (Notkins and Yoon, 1982; Rayfield and Seto, 1978; Rayfield and Ishimura, 1987; Yoon *et al.*, 1987). It should be kept in mind, however, that several viruses are able to induce diabetes in experimental animals. The mechanisms by which these viruses are able to influence the β cells vary from direct lysis (encephalomyocarditis virus, reo virus), persistent infection (lymphocytic choriomeningitis virus), biochemical lesion (Venezuelan encephalitis virus), to induction of autoimmunity by the possible insertion of neoantigens (rubella).

The evidence for a viral etiology in man is largely circumstantial, and case reports and epidemiological investigations suggest that mumps, Coxsackie, rubella, and cytomegalovirus (CMV) may be involved. The first report of a relationship between mumps and IDDM was published in 1864. Subsequent investigators noted similar associations (Gundersen, 1927), and a lag period of 3 to 4 years between mumps infections and later onset of IDDM was also reported (Sultz *et al.*, 1975). Closer association between mumps infection and later clinical onset of IDDM have also been reported (Gamble, 1980b). ICA was increased in children affected in a mumps epidemic in Germany. However, this was not necessarily associated with subsequent development of IDDM (Helmke *et al.*, 1980; Helmke *et al.*, 1987; Banatvala *et al.*, 1985; Ratzmann *et al.*, 1985). It is not known whether current mumps vaccination practices have influenced association between mumps and IDDM or its study. It is therefore unclear whether mumps is a trigger of ICA or a potentiating agent for already existing ICA. In analyzing the T-cell response to mumps, HLA-DR3 was associated with a decreased number, while HLA-DR4 was associated with an increased number of mumps antigen-reactive T lymphocytes both in controls and in IDDM patients (Bruserud *et al.*, 1985b; Bruserud and Thorsby, 1985c; Bruserud *et al.*, 1985a). The decreased response in HLA-DR3 individuals is of interest since it may indicate a decreased ability of such individuals to clear the virus. Mumps virus was demonstrated to infect cultured human pancreatic β-cells (Prince *et al.*, 1978). It is possible, therefore, that this virus is an etiological agent that potentiates a latent autoimmune process at least in some patients developing IDDM.

Although Coxsackie B virus has also been associated with IDDM, the literature is contradictory. Neutralizing antibodies may (Gamble *et al.*, 1969; Barrett-Connor, 1985; King *et al.*, 1983; Banatvala *et al.*, 1985) or may not (Tuvemo *et al.*, 1989) be found at an increased frequency in new-onset IDDM children. More important, Coxsackie B4 virus was cultured from a child who died in diabetic coma and ketoacidosis. Koch's postulates were fulfilled since it was demonstrated that subsequent *in vitro* virus propagation in isolated islet cells produced a virus diabetogenic to mice (Yoon *et al.*, 1979). Although Coxsackie B viral strains have β-cytopathic effects, IDDM does not always develop, and in more than 100 autopsies of diabetic patients, there was no evidence for the presence of Coxsackie B3 capsid protein (Foulis *et al.*, 1990). Although Coxsackie B virus may confer diabetes in mice, the role of viral tropism in human β-cells remains to be clarified.

Similar to mumps, Coxsackie B4 antigen presented in the context of HLA-DR3 resulted in a low, while HLA-DR4 showed a high T-lymphocyte proliferative response (Bruserud *et al.*, 1985a; Bruserud and Thorsby, 1985c; Bruserud *et al.*, 1985b). It has been suggested that autoimmunity may develop by delayed viral clearance (Southern and Oldstone, 1983), and this hypothesis would be supported by the low response to viral infection in DR3 individuals. A delayed clearance of the virus may either harm the β cells or change the immune system, thereby favoring IDDM. This is consistent with the finding of lower virus antibody titers among IDDM patients who presented during an outbreak of Coxsackie B3 and B4 (Palmer *et al.*, 1982). Future studies are needed to address the question of whether Coxsackie B infections are associated with the appearance of ICA in the general population, and whether a virus infection influences the subclinical progression of IDDM in marker-positive (HLA, ICA, IAA, or 64K antibody) individuals. Recently, a six amino acid homology between a Coxsackie viral protein and one form of glutamic acid decarboxylase (GAD) has been described (Tobin, 1991). A GAD isoform has been identified as the 64K antigen (Baekkeskov *et al.*, 1990) and is relatively specific to beta cells, so this homology raises the possibility that molecular mimicry plays a role in the association of this virus and IDDM.

A strong candidate for virus-induced IDDM is congenital rubella infection (Hay, 1949; Menser *et al.*, 1978; Banatvala *et al.*, 1985; Ginsberg-Fellner *et al.*, 1984). IDDM is an occasional pathologic consequence of congenital rubella, which may also result in both autoimmune thyroid disease and Addison's disease (Rayfield and Ishimura, 1987). The development of IDDM in patients with congenital rubella is HLA-DR restricted, since HLA-DR3 is increased, and HLA-DR2 decreased among the affected (Menser *et al.*, 1978; Ginsberg-Fellner *et al.*, 1984). In congenital rubella patients positive for HLA-DR3 and/or HLA-DR4, the penetrance of IDDM has been estimated to be close to 100% (Rubinstein *et al.*, 1982; Ginsberg-Fellner *et al.*, 1984). Immune markers for IDDM such as ICA, islet cell-surface antibodies (ICSA), and IAA are all reported at increased frequencies in these patients. However, the presence of these markers was not associated with any particular HLA type. It is therefore possible that the congenital rubella infection causes β-cell destruction, resulting in the formation of islet-cell autoantibodies. This response is expected, since autoantibody formation would seem to be a natural response to β-cell lysis or destruction in the context of infection. In HLA-DR3- and/or HLA-DR4-positive individuals, the immune reaction would not be down-regulated but, rather, perpetuated. It will be important to determine to what extent current intensified rubella vaccinations of teenage girls affect IDDM marker frequencies, as well as incidence rates of IDDM.

CMV is only circumstantially associated with IDDM (Rayfield and Ishimura, 1987). CMV inclusion bodies were found in islet cells of a diabetic child with CMV infection (Jansen *et al.*, 1977), but also in 20 of 45 children who died of disseminated CMV infection (Jenson *et al.*, 1980). Additionally, when analyzing blood lymphocytes from newly diagnosed IDDM patients, CMV genome sequences were demonstrated at a significantly increased frequency (Pak *et al.*, 1988). The IDDM patients who were positive for CMV genome showed an increased frequency of ICA and ICSA in their serum. It was therefore speculated that persistent CMV infection may contribute to the pathogenesis of IDDM. In a subsequent report, a mouse monoclonal antibody raised against CMV reacted with a M_r 38,000 human islet-cell antigen (Pak *et al.*, 1990). These cross-reactive antibodies are of interest since they also support the hypothesis of molecular mimicry as a mechanism for development of autoimmunity in IDDM.

The term molecular mimicry, first used in 1964 (Damian, 1988), initially indicated that the sharing of epitopes between parasite and host would have consequences for the nonrecognition of parasite structures. Later the term was adapted to include also the amplification or propagation of autoimmunity in the infected host. A large panel of monoclonal antibodies against virus showed cross-reactivity with many cell types including β-cells (Drell *et al.*, 1987). This pattern of reactivity was observed also when monoclonal antibodies were prepared from both IDDM patients and controls (Prabhakar *et al.*, 1984). These monoclonal antibodies were reactive with multiple organs, and were often of the IgM type. It is still unclear whether these monoclonal IgM antibodies represent an early form of autoantibodies (Casali and Notkins, 1989). It is conceivable that in the presence of an autoantigen, B lymphocytes expressing the IgM receptor (membrane-bound IgM against an islet cell antigen) may further differentiate to stimulate the production of B lymphocytes able to make IgG autoantibodies. It should be noted that at the time of clinical onset, the observed ICA, IAA, 64K antibodies and ICSA are all of the IgG type. In the NOD mouse, it has been reported that IAA show cross-reactivity with antigen p73, which is a group-specific antigen on the intracisternal type A viral particle (Serreze *et al.*, 1988). The reader is referred to Chapter 6 of this volume for a detailed account of the possible role of molecular mimicry in autoimmune diseases.

The role of environmental factors other than viruses is inferred primarily from animal experiments. Alloxan and streptozocin are two well-known β-cytotoxic agents in animals (Palmer and Lernmark, 1990a). Streptozocin is of particular interest since this chemical is a nitrosamine (other nitrosamines are formed in humans after dietary intake of nitrite food preservatives). Streptozocin is occasionally used to treat islet-cell neoplasms. *In vitro,* human but not rat islets are relatively resistant to the toxic effect of streptozocin (Nielsen, 1985). In mice, multiple low-dose injections of streptozocin induce an MHC-dependent inflammatory lesion in the islets of Langerhans, which is associated with a progressive destruction of β-cells (Nedergaard *et al.*, 1983). The diabetes could be prevented by antilymphocyte serum or total body irradiation (Rossini *et al.*, 1978), and it was also possible to passively transfer the disease with lymphocytes (Nedergaard *et al.*, 1983). These experiments provide support for the hypothesis that an environmental trigger may induce a secondary β-cell autoimmunity.

Several compounds related to alloxan and streptozocin have been implicated as possible environmental factors. Vacor (*N*-3-pyridylmethyl *N'*-*p*-nitrophenylurea), a potent rodenticide, is highly diabetogenic in humans (Karam *et al.*, 1980). This drug is toxic to human islets *in vitro* (Nielsen, 1985). Ingestion of Vacor in suicide attempts seems to be associated with direct β-cell cytotoxicity. However, ICSA developed in some of these patients, indicating that β-cell destruction may lead to a secondary β-cell autoimmunity (Karam *et al.*, 1980). It is also possible that the nitrosamine residue present on streptozocin may be diabetogenic when present in other compounds. In a report yet to be confirmed, nitrosamines present in Icelandic cured mutton were not only found to be diabetogenic in mice but also to transfer the disease in germline DNA (Helgason and Jonasson, 1981). Finally, one pharmaceutical agent, pentamidine (4-4′-diamidino-diphenoxy-pentane) is known to be diabetogenic in man (Bouchard *et al.*, 1982). This drug is commonly used to treat acquired immunodeficiency syndrome (AIDS)-related *Pneumocystis carinii,* but despite the escalating use of this drug, the prevalence of diabetes as a side effect is not known. It is possible that the drug has direct β-cytotoxic effects, but studies of autoimmunity are difficult in these patients owing to both their extreme illness and their altered immunologic milieu.

The mechanisms by which drugs, environmental chemicals, or viruses are associated with the pathogenesis of IDDM remain to be elucidated. Are these factors the true etiological agents, with the immune response occurring only in response to cell death, or do they potentiate an underlying autoimmune process? In both the NOD mouse (see Chapter 3) and the BB rat (cf. Mordes *et al.*, 1987), it is possible to influence the frequency and the tempo of clinical onset of IDDM by a variety of dietary manipulations. In humans, although controversial, breast feeding is thought to influence the development of IDDM (Borch-Johnsen *et al.*, 1984; Mayer *et al.*, 1988; Nigro *et al.*, 1985). In this respect, only external factors have been taken into account. Recent studies indicate that cytokines are potent *in vivo* and *in vitro* regulators of β-cell destruction by themselves and by their effects on immune cells (Mandrup-Poulsen *et al.*, 1986; Mandrup-Poulsen *et al.*, 1987; Nerup *et al.*, 1987). Although controlled studies are yet to be performed, it cannot be excluded that increased local levels of interleukin-1β, tumor necrosis factor (TNF), and gamma-interferon alone or in combination would markedly potentiate a subclinical autoimmune reaction against the β cells in susceptible individuals who experience immune reactions toward virus infections in the islet or elsewhere. Daily injections of interleukin-1β to diabetes-prone but not to diabetes-resistant BB rats induced onset at an early age (Wilson *et al.*, 1990).

The association with certain HLA class II molecules is often interpreted to indicate that these molecules are involved in the pathogenesis of IDDM. Class II molecules are known to present peptide antigens. This antigen presentation is the initiator of an immune response and is accomplished by antigen-presenting cells (APC) such as macrophages, monocytes, dendritic cells, but also by B lymphocytes. The peptides, bound to the bimolecular class II HLA molecules, form structures that interact with the T-cell receptor on T (helper) lymphocytes. It has not yet been possible to determine when and where the initial antigen presentation in preclinical IDDM takes place (Table III).

Studies in the BB rat (Dyrberg *et al.*, 1984; Baekkeskov *et al.*, 1984), and the NOD mouse (Atkinson and Maclaren, 1988) suggest that different islet-cell

TABLE III
Hypothetical Staging of Insulin-Dependent Diabetes[a]

	Event	Immunology	Time
Stage 1	Initial β-cell antigen presentations: cell lysis or molecular mimicry	T-cell sensitization, seroconversion, IgM and IgG antibodies.	Weeks
	Autoimmune prodrome		
Stage 2	Islet-cell IgG maintained by varying degree of β-cell lysis; may remit	IgG islet-cell antibodies	Weeks to decades
Stage 3	Persistence of islet-cell and GAD antibodies, progressive β-cell dysfunction; may remit	GAD antibodies, islet macrophage infiltration	Weeks to years
Stage 4	β-cell destruction; insulitis is established; no recovery possible	Mononuclear cell infiltration in islets	Days, weeks, months
	Clinical onset		
Stage 5	β-cell 80–90% destruction. No recovery possible	Insulitis and end-stage islet structures	Days to weeks

[a]Genetics: permissive genes (current HLA-DQw2/ and/or w8); familial hyperautoreactivity; and diabetes gene(s) (including NIDDM, which is a risk factor).

antibodies (ICA, IAA, or 64KA) may be present long before the clinical onset of IDDM. In the BB rat, 64KA were detected at the time of weaning (Baekkeskov *et al.*, 1984) but insulitis, initiated by a macrophage (not T cell) infiltration, did not develop until about 50 to 60 days of age (Logothetopoulos *et al.*, 1984). In humans, the presence of insulitis before the clinical onset of IDDM is not known. Insulitis may be present in children who died from fatal viral infections (Jenson *et al.*, 1980; Foulis *et al.*, 1986). In adults developing IDDM, ICA, IAA, or 64KA have been detected up to 7 to 12 years before clinical diagnosis. The long prodrome and the fact that the different types of islet-cell antibodies are predominantly IgG suggest that the initial antigen presentation (Stage 1, Table III) is an early event occurring before these clinical studies took place, and *therefore* still to be identified. It is also unclear where this early antigen presentation take place. Does it take place in the islets themselves? This would seem unlikely, but the concept of the β cell presenting its own autoantigens by aberrant expression of MHC class II is discussed below. Presentation by islet dendritic cells has also been postulated. Does it take place in lymph nodes? The pancreas is drained to a limited number of lymph nodes. In the case of nonimmune-mediated β-cell destruction, it is conceivable that β-cells debris is brought by the lymphatics to the pancreatic lymph nodes, and is taken up by resident macrophages, processed, and presented. No data are available on such a role for pancreatic lymph nodes. Could autoantibodies be formed by other mechanisms? Polyclonal activation of B lymphocytes (Casali and Notkins, 1989; Papadopoulos *et al.*, 1984; Horita *et al.*, 1982) is a possible mechanism by which autoantibodies may be formed from preexisting B lymphocytes. It has been suggested that *auto*antibodies are formed primarily from CD5-positive B lymphocytes (for a review see Casali and Notkins, 1989).

B. Factors Clinically Associated with Progression

Given our lack of knowledge of the molecular mechanisms of IDDM pathogenesis, it is hard to separate events such as initiation of autoimmunity and its triggers from the progression of β-cell killing. Despite this current arbitrary division, it will be important eventually to stage preclinical IDDM as outlined hypothetically in Table III. Individuals in Stage 1–3 may be treated differently since data are already available showing that such individuals may remit and that the β-cell destructive process can cease. These individuals would remain nondiabetic from a diagnostic point of view, but would shown signs of stable β-cell dysfunction.

Stage 3 (Table III) is of particular interest since it represents the latest stage of the disease, which may either progress to complete destruction of the β cells or to remission. Several studies have addressed this concept. The first controversy arose when it was reported that ICA may fluctuate (Spencer *et al.*, 1984). In reviewing the literature before 1984, it should be noted that the ICA assay had not been standardized. Interlaboratory comparisons may therefore not be possible in these studies. The reports on fluctuating antibodies have, however, been followed by subsequent studies in standardized assays that demonstrate that ICA may be transient (Landin-Olsson *et al.*, 1989; Johnston *et al.*, 1989; Karjalainen, 1990; McCulloch *et al.*, 1990). In some individuals positive for IAA, ICA, or 64KA, alone or in combination, the disease seems to progress to clinical onset (Srikanta *et al.*, 1983; Srikanta *et al.*, 1984; Srikanta *et al.*, 1986; Vardi *et al.*, 1988a). Other more comprehensive studies in first-degree relatives (McCulloch *et al.*, 1990; Riley *et al.*, 1990; Bonifacio *et al.*, 1990; Tarn *et al.*, 1988) have shown that subclinical states of β-cell dysfunction that remain stable can occur among ICA-positive relatives as well as monozygotic twins of IDDM patients without progression to clinical IDDM. ICA are reported among 3–21% of first-degree relatives of IDDM patients (Ginsberg-Fellner *et al.*, 1982; Riley *et al.*, 1990; Bonifacio *et al.*, 1990). ICA are also reported among as many as 2 to 4% of healthy controls (Landin-Olsson *et al.*, 1989; Karjalainen, 1990; Bonifacio *et al.*, 1990), which far outnumbers the prevalence of IDDM (0.15–0.3%). Similarly IAA are also detected at a high frequency among first-degree relatives (Arslanian *et al.*, 1985; McCulloch *et al.*, 1990). This marker, present among 35 to 50% of new-onset patients (Palmer *et al.*, 1983; Atkinson *et al.*, 1986), is of limited predictive value since IAA occur primarily in very young children (Srikanta *et al.*, 1984; Vardi *et al.*, 1988b). It may be advantageous to combine several other markers with ICA and IAA, a strategy that was reported to give an improved prediction (Betterle *et al.*, 1987; Ginsberg-Fellner *et al.*, 1985). In first-degree relatives, a β-cell dysfunction may be stable for years despite the presence of ICA or IAA. In the presence of 64KA, irrespective of ICA or IAA, the β-cell dysfunction was more likely to be unstable, marking individuals at risk for IDDM (Bärmeier *et al.*, 1990).

Factors that determine progression to β-cell destruction and IDDM or remission remain to be identified. It is possible that after some β-cell destruction has taken place and the β-cell mass has decreased, the remaining β cells would therefore have to secrete insulin at an increased rate to maintain homeostasis. This hypersecretion may hasten β cell death through "exhaustion" or by alteration of immune factors such as β cell surface antigen expression.

At the time of clinical onset, nearly all diabetic patients have some residual β-cell function (Fig. 1). Children (Wallensteen *et al.*, 1988; Sochett *et al.*, 1987) have less residual β-cell function than adults, probably owing to their increased insulin sensitivity (Marner *et al.*, 1985). During the first 9–12 months, most patients experience a decrease in insulin requirement associated with an increase in fasting C-peptide (Fig. 1). This period is referred to as thc *honeymoon* period. About 20% of IDDM patients, 15–30 years old at diagnosis, may reach a non-insulin-requiring state during this period (The Canadian–European Randomized Control Trial Group, 1988). However, most undergo continuous decline in β-cell function, and this decline appears to be influenced by the presence of immune markers. First, the rate of loss in β-cell function was greater in ICA-positive children (Wallensteen *et al.*, 1988; Sochett *et al.*, 1987). Second, in young adults and adults developing IDDM whose residual β-cell function was larger, the rate of loss was similarly increased in those patients who were ICA positive (Fig. 1) (Marner *et al.*, 1985; Manna *et al.*, 1988). There is usually no correlation between ICA titer (in JDF units) and residual β-cell function, and the patients have to be followed over time to determine whether the presence of ICA at one time point predicts a lesser endogenous β-cell function at another. It is well known that ICA is evanescent after the clinical onset of IDDM (Irvine *et al.*, 1977; Kolb *et al.*, 1988), and the parallel loss of ICA and C-peptide is taken as an evidence that the ICA is maintained as long as there are β cells left. In contrast (Fig. 2), 64KA (which are as frequent as ICA at the clinical onset) remained positive in a 3-year follow-up study (Christie *et al.*, 1990). The 64KA decreased during the next 3–4 years as the remaining β cells disappeared (Christie *et al.*, 1990). These data indicate that 64KA may be a more sensitive measure of β-cell

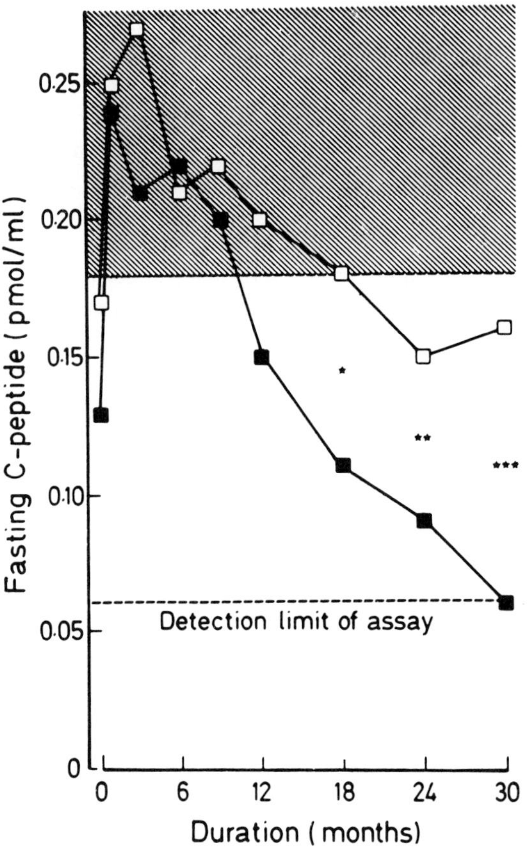

FIG. 1 Fasting C-peptide in insulin-dependent diabetes mellitus patients with newly diagnosed patients without (□) or with (■) persistent islet cell antibodies (ICA). An accelerated loss of fasting C-peptide was observed at 18 ($*p = 0.04$); 24 ($**p = 0.05$) and 30 ($***p = 0.003$) months of follow-up. Reproduced from Marner *et al.* (1985).

specific autoimmunity than are ICA. The fact that the 64K protein has been identified as a GAD isoform supports previous data that this antigen is β-cell specific (Baekkeskov *et al.*, 1982; Christie *et al.*, 1990). Whether the GAD-64 molecule, which is highly hydrophobic (Baekkeskov *et al.*, 1987) and associated with the β-cell membrane fraction (Christie *et al.*, 1990), is expressed on the β-cell surface is not clarified. Future investigations of the β-cell function at the time of clinical onset and during follow-up should therefore include a quantitative analysis of 64KA to determine the possible relationship between preservation of β-cells and levels of this autoimmune marker. For example, intensified insulin therapy at onset improved the β-cell function during the subsequent year (Lud-

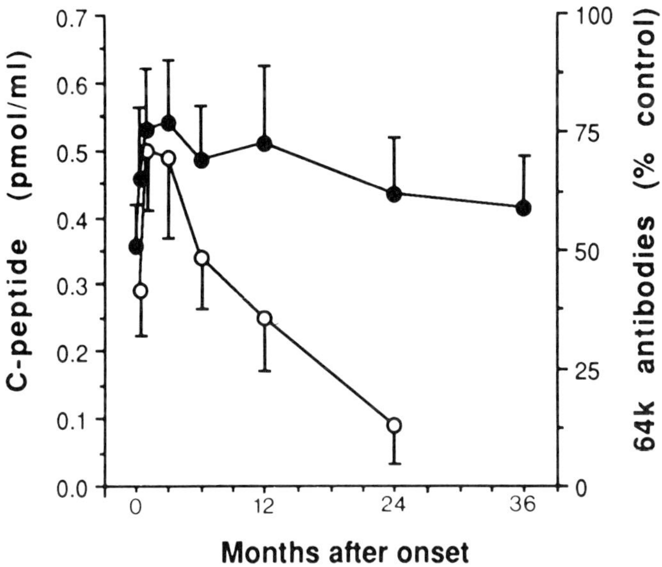

FIG. 2 Residual C-peptide (○) in relation to months after onset in children with insulin-dependent diabetes mellitus. The data illustrate that the frequency of patients positive for antibodies against the 64K protein (●) remains unaffected by increasing duration of the disease. Reproduced from Christie and Delovitch (1990).

vigsson *et al.*, 1977; Shah *et al.*, 1989), and experiments are needed to determine whether a β-cell rest would alter the levels of 64KA and other autoimmune markers. Also, sera from the controlled trials of cyclosporine should be analyzed for 64KA to determine whether non-insulin-requiring patients experienced a decrease in 64K Ab titers.

IV. THE CELLULAR BASIS OF PROGRESSION —INSULITIS

A. Histological Features of Insulitis

What are the histological features of insulitis in IDDM? In man, our knowledge is limited because of the lack of availability of patient material during the various stages of preclinical IDDM as well as after onset (Gepts, 1965; Foulis, 1989). Early studies (Gepts, 1965; Doniach and Morgan, 1973; Foulis and Stewart, 1984) analyzed relatively few patients but demonstrated an overall 32 of 73 (44%) frequency of insulitis. In a subsequent 25-year review of deaths in IDDM patients younger than 20 years in the United Kingdom (Foulis *et al.*, 1986), insulitis was detected in 47 of 60 (78%) of those with recent-onset IDDM. At least three types of islets are reported: (1) unaffected islets containing a normal core of β cells; (2) islets containing β cells and with an inflammatory cell infiltrate; and (3) β cell-deficient islets. Only 1% of type 3 islets showed an inflammatory infiltrate, which supports the view that the cellular infiltrate is associated with the presence of β cell antigens—once the β cells are destroyed, the local islet inflammation resolves. In three patients aged 18 months or younger and with short duration of IDDM, there was no sign of insulitis (Foulis *et al.*, 1986). The difficulty in obtaining a clear histopathological representation of the islet lesion in human IDDM may be because the insulitis is patchy (Gepts, 1965). Further investigations suggested that the disease process in the head of the pancreas is completed sooner than that in the tail (Foulis *et al.*, 1986). Islets of Langerhans were examined in a unique biopsy study in 7 Japanese IDDM patients, 24–49 years of age, who had had diabetes for 2 to 4 months. While all biopsies showed a decrease in β-cells, insulitis was not detected, nor were any of the remaining cells positive for HLA class II molecules (Hanafusa *et al.*, 1990). Provided that Japanese IDDM patients are representative, these studies suggest that insulitis may not always be pathognomonic for IDDM.

B. Role of MHC Molecules in the Islets

The presence of macrophages and T and B lymphocytes has been documented in the few pancreata examined shortly after the time of clinical onset (Bottazzo *et al.*, 1985; Hanafusa *et al.*, 1990; Foulis, 1989). Immunoglobulin deposits within the islets have not been detected. The expression of HLA class I molecules appears to be increased, while the aberrant expression of HLA class II molecules on β cells (Bottazzo *et al.*, 1985) is still controversial (Hanafusa *et al.*, 1990). The concept of aberrant expression is also questioned from the point of view of an artifactual observation, since both normal and insulitis-affected islets contain macrophages. Islet macrophages containing insulin granules have been documented in the BB rat as well as in rats injected with streptozocin (Pipeleers, 1988). Staining with an HLA-DQw8-specific monoclonal antibody showed no staining on endocrine cells but revealed the presence of inflammatory cells in the islets of a 3-year-old boy who died on the day of clinical diagnosis (Fig. 3). On the other hand, the increased HLA class I expression on both endocrine and nonendocrine cells (such as the endothelium) appears to be a reproducible phenomenon. The increased HLA class I levels may reflect an inflammatory state (Foulis *et al.*, 1986), perhaps owing to a viral infection. Immunoreactive α-interferon has been reported in insulin-containing cells in pancreata from IDDM patients (Foulis *et al.*, 1987). Cytokines such as γ-interferon, TNF, and in-

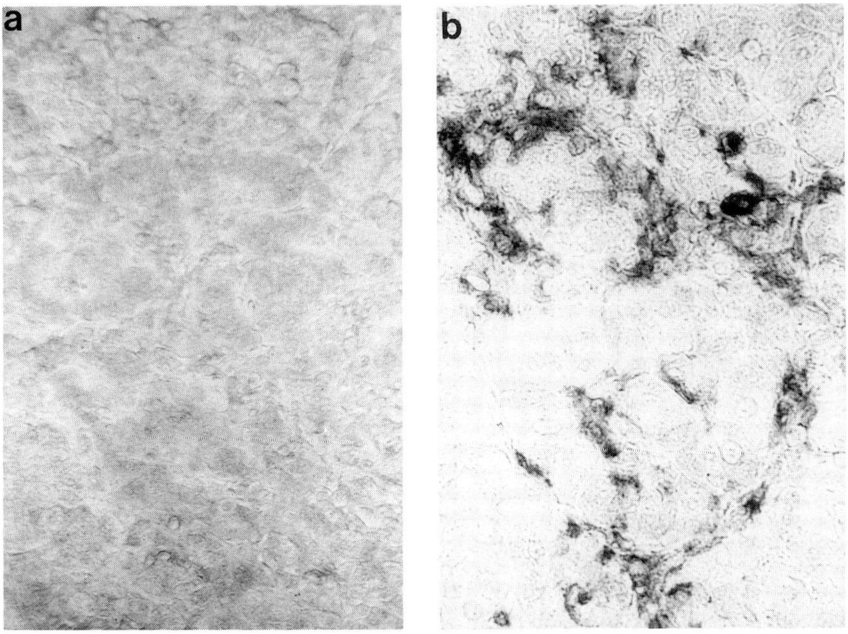

FIG. 3 Presence of HLA-DQw8-positive cells in a 5-year-old nondiabetic child (left panel) and a 3-year-old new-onset diabetic boy (right panel). The diabetic child was HLA-DQw3/w8 positive. The pancreatic sections were stained with a mouse monoclonal antibody specific for HLA-DQw8 (courtesy of Jacob Petersen and Thomas Dyrberg). Whereas the control pancreas showed no reactivity, the islet in the diabetic pancreas revealed the presence of nonendocrine HLA-DQw8-positive cells. Independent experiments show these cells to be macrophages and B lymphocytes, whereas staining for T cells has been negative.

terleukin-1β, alone or in combination, have been found to increase HLA expression in isolated islets (cf. Nerup *et al.*, 1987).

C. Cellular Basis of Toxicity

In the peripheral blood, T-lymphocyte changes in IDDM are most often reported as transient decreases in T-cell suppressor cells (for reviews see Lernmark, 1984; Horita *et al.*, 1982; Drell and Notkins, 1987). In the BB rat and NOD mice, the evidence for a T-cell involvement in the pathogenesis is more substantial. T cells have been used to transfer the disease (Wicker *et al.*, 1986). Spectacular progress has been made, particularly in the NOD mouse, by disease transfer with cloned CD4-positive cells (Mordes *et al.*, 1987; Makino *et al,* 1980). CD8-positive T cells have also been cloned and shown to protect from the development of insulitis and to prevent accelerated onset of diabetes.

As discussed above, macrophages infiltrating the islet seem to be of particular importance (Leiter, 1989). Activated macrophages elaborate cytokines such as interleukin-1. *In vitro* (Mandrup-Poulsen *et al.*, 1986; Spinas *et al.*, 1988) as well as *in vivo* studies in the BB rat (Wilson *et al.*, 1990) show interleukin-1β is an effective modulator of both β-cell function and progression of IDDM. In the BB rat, we demonstrated that daily injections of a high-dose interleukin-1β increase the tempo at which IDDM develops. Low-dose interleukin-1β prevents IDDM and decreases the frequency of diabetes not only in the BB rat but also in the NOD mouse (Jacob *et al.*, 1990). Are these cytokines modulating both the β cells and the immune response? It is important to note that both interleukin-1β and TNF have marked effects on glucose metabolism and seem to enhance the metabolic effects of insulin (DelRay and Besedovsky, 1987).

The protective effects of interleukin-1β in the BB rat and the NOD mouse may also have other explanations. It has been shown that macrophages from autoimmune-prone mice have decreased interleukin-1β production (Donnelly *et al.*, 1990). Autoimmunity in the BB rat, the NOD mouse, and perhaps in humans might therefore be maintained owing to defective interleukin-1β secretion resulting in an inadequate stimulation of suppressor mechanisms. Low-dose interleukin-1β or TNF administration may correct this deficiency. Further investigations are therefore warranted to explore dose-dependent effects *in vivo* of different cytokines tested alone or in combination.

V. THE T-LYMPHOCYTE AND B-LYMPHOCYTE RESPONSES

A. T Lymphocytes

The roles of T lymphocytes in the pathogenesis of IDDM are essentially unknown. It is assumed that T helper-cells will be involved in the initiation of the disease to establish an autoreaction against islet cell antigens (Stage 1, Table III). This early T-cell response may not necessarily take place in the islets themselves. The T helper-cell reaction is expected to induce a B-lymphocyte response, resulting in the production of islet cell autoantibodies (Stage 2, Table III). T cells are likely also involved in β-cell killing in the setting of insulitis, although this may occur late in the pathogenesis of the disease. IDDM can be induced in nonsusceptible NOD mice by passive transfer of CD4 and CD8 cells from diabetic animals (Bendalae, *et al.*, 1987), although it is not known what exact role is played by the transferred T cells.

T cells from new-onset diabetics show specific proliferation to a 38KD membrane protein found on insulin secretory granules (Roep, *et al.* 1990). However, the significance of this finding is not known, since multiple cycles of stimulation in the presence of large amounts of antigen were necessary in order to show a response, and since the time of onset represents a late stage in the process of β-cell destruction.

The wealth of monoclonal antibody markers for lymphocyte subsets has been utilized in numerous studies to test the hypothesis that the onset of IDDM is associated with T-cell abnormalities. HLA class II molecule-positive T lymphocytes were reported at an increased frequency before and at the onset of IDDM (Eisenbarth *et al.*, 1985; Jackson *et al.*, 1982). In particular, measurements have been carried out to test whether there is a suppressor T-cell deficiency associated with β-cell destruction. The results have been far from conclusive (Lernmark, 1984), but the most prevalent effect seems to be a deficit in $CD8^+$ (suppressor/cytotoxic) T lymphocytes (Chatenoud *et al.*, 1989; Horita *et al.*, 1982). However, this deficit is transient, and normalizes after initiation of insulin therapy.

B. Circulating B Lymphocytes

The B lymphocytes comprise only a minor proportion of the blood lymphocytes, and most circulating B lymphocytes are in a resting state. Antibodies are thought to be produced by noncirculating B lymphocytes, because a low percentage of plasma cells are in the peripheral blood. Since a specific β-cell antigen such as GAD (64K protein) has not been available, little is known about the character of B lymphocytes that circulate before the time of clinical onset of IDDM. It has been speculated that an imbalance between helper and suppressor T lymphocytes may affect the ability of blood B lymphocytes to produce antibodies. When *in vitro* antibody production in the Jerne plaque assay was compared between newly diagnosed IDDM patients and controls, it was found that many newly diagnosed patients had increased spontaneous secretion of antibodies (Papadopoulos *et al.*, 1984). Spontaneous antibody secretion was also observed in patients with simultaneous diabetes and Hashimoto's thyroiditis (Horita *et al.*, 1982). These observations are consistent with the presence of polyclonal activation. However, these studies still do not explain the specific loss of pancreatic β cells in IDDM. The availability of a defined antigen such as islet-specific GAD will allow experiments to determine the presence of B lymphocytes able to produce GAD antibodies. Patients with a variety of autoimmune diseases such as rheumatoid arthritis and IDDM (Kidd *et al.*, 1991) have increased levels of CD5+ B lymphocytes, a subpopulation of which normally accounts for up to 10 to 25% of peripheral blood B lymphocytes (Casali and Notkins, 1989). These cells produce mainly IgM, and it has been speculated that they are responsible for the production of *natural* autoantibodies, i.e., IgM antibodies that are polyreactive (Casali and Notkins, 1989) to multiple organs (Prabhakar *et al.*, 1984). It may be speculated that B lymphocytes producing natural autoantibodies may be stimulated by the appearance of autoantigen to differentiate into IgG autoantibody-producing B lymphocytes or plasma cells. This possibility is supported by the observation that patients with Hashimoto's thyroiditis have a high frequency of CD5+ B lymphocytes producing monoreactive thyroglobulin IgG autoantibodies (Casali and Notkins, 1989). Specific islet antigens should be used to find B lymphocytes producing specific autoantibodies, such as to GAD. EBV-transformed human B-lymphocyte clones making GAD-autoantibodies have recently been described (Richter, *et al.*, 1991). This is important, since a recent study demonstrated that the percentage of B lymphocytes expressing CD5 was significantly increased not only in IDDM patients but also in first-degree relatives (Kidd *et al.*, 1991). This observation is reminiscent of several studies demonstrating an increased frequency of organ-specific autoantibodies among healthy first-degree relatives to IDDM patients (Fialkow *et al.*, 1975; Bottazzo *et al.*, 1978; Hägglöf *et al.*, 1986; Nordén *et al.*, 1983). That these organ-specific autoantibodies were detected without association to HLA, suggested that familial hyperautoreactivity (Hägglöf *et al.*, 1986) may be a prerequisite for the development of IDDM and other HLA-associated autoimmune disorders. An *autoimmunity gene* may determine propensity to develop autoantibodies, whereas the HLA type may control the antigen-specific cellular eradication. This is an attractive hypothesis since the response to antigens, both in magnitude and specificity, seems to be controlled by HLA (Strominger, 1986; Bruserud *et al.*, 1985b).

C. Islet Cell Antibodies

Islet-cell antibodies (Table IV) detected in an indirect immunofluorescence assay with frozen sections of human pancreas were first described in 1974 (Bottazzo *et al.*, 1974; MacCuish *et al.*, 1974). Numerous studies were published prior to 1984 using an ICA assay that was neither quantitative nor standardized (for reviews see Lernmark, 1987; Eisenbarth, 1986; Lipton and La Porte, 1989; Drell and Notkins, 1987). A synthesis of these studies suggests that ICA (1) is most common in newly diagnosed IDDM patients, but that the frequency decreases with increasing age of the patient; (2) shows a decrease in frequency and titer with increasing duration of the disease; (3) is increased in frequency among first-degree relatives and patients with other organ-specific autoimmune disease; (4) is associated with a more rapid loss of residual β-cell function when present at a high titer at the time of clinical onset (Fig. 1); (5) precedes the clinical onset of IDDM; (6) is a marker for IDDM in diabetic patients initially classified and treated as NIDDM; and (7) may be evanescent in monozygotic twins discordant for IDDM or in first-degree relatives with stable β-cell dysfunction.

In 1984, the first Immunology of Diabetes Workshop (IDW) on the standardization of islet-cell antibodies indicated poor precision and a large interlaboratory variation in the ICA assay (Bottazzo and Gleichmann, 1986; Gleichmann and

TABLE IV
Assays To Detect Islet-Cell Antibodies

Tissue preparation to detect antibody	Method of detection	Islet-cell antibody
Frozen sections of human pancreas	Indirect immunofluorescence	Islet-cell cytoplasmic antibodies (ICA, ICCA)
Dispersed islet cells	Indirect immunofluorescence Radiobinding	Islet cell-surface antibodies (ICSA)
Purified rat islet β cells	Indirect immunofluorescence	β cell-specific ICSA
Insulin-producing cell lines	Indirect immunofluorescence	ICSA
Monolayers of islet cells or islets	^{51}Cr-release	Islet-cell cytotoxic (C′AMC) antibodies

Bottazzo, 1987). The identification of one serum sample found positive by all participating laboratories allowed the second workshop analysis to demonstrate that the use of a common standard improved the precision of the assay (Bonifacio *et al.*, 1987; Bonifacio *et al.* 1988). The third workshop expressed ICA levels in a common standard (JDF units), which increased concordance among laboratories. Laboratories with poor precision also had poor interlaboratory precision (Boitard *et al.*, 1988). The JDF standard is therefore currently used to express levels of ICA to allow comparisons between laboratories. Several important observations have since been made. First, levels of ICA at the time of clinical onset in large population-based studies have been documented (Landin-Olsson *et al.*, 1989; Karjalainen, 1990). High-titer ICA sera correlate with the presence of IAA (Ludvigsson *et al.*, 1988). The predictive value for IDDM among first-degree relatives is increased with increasing ICA titer (Bonifacio *et al.*, 1990; Riley *et al.*, 1990). Finally, the standardized ICA assay has permitted the frequency of ICA in the background population to be reevaluated, demonstrating a higher frequency (2–4%) (Landin-Olsson *et al.*, 1989; Karjalainen, 1990; Bonifacio *et al.*, 1990) than that (0–0.5%) reported in earlier studies.

D. Islet Cell-Surface Antibodies

Islet cell-surface antibodies (Table IV) are characterized by their ability to bind to antigens expressed on the surface of intact normal β-cells. The assay system used and the detection of β-cell specific ICSA (Van de Winkle *et al.*, 1982; Vercammen *et al.*, 1989) have been reviewed (Lernmark, 1987). In assays using single cells from isolated islets, the cross-species approach necessitates the use of extensive serum absorption to minimize nonspecific reactions. Single, normal human β cells are not yet available. The prevalence of ICSA, 50–70% in new-onset patients, is different from that in first-degree relatives (10–15%) and from that in the background population (2–6%). ICSA are β-cell specific primarily at a young age (Van de Winkle *et al.*, 1982). Insulin-producing cell lines such as RIN (Dobersen and Scharff, 1982) or HIT (Matsuba and Lernmark, 1990) have been found useful to detect ICSA. The ICSA mediate complement-dependent cytotoxicity (Dobersen *et al.*, 1980; Eisenbarth *et al.*, 1981; Rabinovitch *et al.*, 1984) and antibody-dependent cellular cytotoxicity (Charles *et al.*, 1983). Immunoglobulin preparations containing ICSA were reported to inhibit glucose-stimulated insulin release (Kanatsuna *et al.*, 1983; Svenningsen *et al.*, 1983) as well as β-cell glucose transport (Johnson *et al.*, 1990). The mechanisms of these inhibitory effects are unclear, especially since immunoprecipitation analyses have failed to detect glucose transporter (unpublished observations, 1990). Possibly, the surface binding of ICSA interferes with other vital functions of the β cell, thus inhibiting its function. Similar to ICA and IAA, the presence of ICSA may mark an ongoing β-cell destruction. It would therefore be important to correlate ICSA with ICA, IAA, and 64K antibodies. The assays are cumbersome, however, and have not all been subjected to standardization. Further studies are also warranted to determine the ability of ICSA to affect β-cell function *in vivo*.

E. Specific Antigens

1. Insulin

Insulin autoantibodies (IAA) first described by Palmer *et al.* (1983) have been previously reviewed in detail (Palmer *et al.*, 1986; Palmer, 1987). IAA are reported among 28 to 50% of patients with newly diagnosed IDDM and are more frequent among young children (Srikanta *et al.*, 1986; Arslanian *et al.*, 1985; McEvoy *et al.*, 1986). In nondiabetic subjects, IAA tend to occur in individuals with ICA, and the presence of IAA is thought to increase the predictive value for IDDM (Srikanta *et al.*, 1986; Atkinson *et al.*, 1986). The prevalence of IAA was also found to vary between laboratories, and IDW standardization workshops are carried out to evaluate assay reproducibility and precision (Wilkin *et al.*, 1987; Wilkin *et al.*, 1988; Kuglin *et al.*, 1990). These workshop analyses have indicated that the radiobinding assay is reliable, but that enzyme-linked immunosorbent assay (ELISA) generally showed a poor precision and reproducibility. The use of ELISA was questioned in the fourth workshop (Kuglin *et al.*, 1990). ELISA may detect other types of insulin autoantibodies, which are not related to IDDM.

The formation and role of IAA in the pathogenesis of IDDM has not been elucidated. It is speculated that IAA form during the process of active insulitis and β-cell destruction. This possibility is consistent with the presence of proinsulin autoantibodies (Kuglin *et al.*, 1988) (Table V). The reason for higher prevalence of IAA among small children at the time of clinical onset remains

TABLE V
Islet-Cell (Auto)Antigens in Insulin

Antigen	Molecular mass (M_r)	Designation	Prevalence (%) in disease
Insulin	6,000	IAA	35–45
Proinsulin	10,000	PAA	14
Glutamic acid decarboxylase (GAD)(64K)	64,000	64KA or GAD Ab	7–88
38 K	38,000	38K Ab	88
Monoclonal antibody	110,000	1A2	94
1A2 antigens	150,000	Displacement antibodies	
Multiple islet-cell antigens	52,000 84,000 116,000 150,000	Immunoblotting antibodies	71
Monosialoganglioside	GM2 fraction	Tentative ICA antigen	Not reported

obscure. The presence of IAA at onset does not seem to correlate with the subsequent formation of insulin antibodies in response to exogenous insulin. The formation of these latter insulin antibodies is associated with HLA specificities other than those associated with IDDM (Reevers *et al.*, 1984). IAA present before the clinical onset of IDDM had no influence on the first-year clinical course of the disease. The antibodies correlated to ICA but not to mumps virus-specific antibodies or Coxsackie-B4 virus-specific IgA antibodies (Karjalainen *et al.*, 1988). In the NOD mouse, a molecular mimicry has been detected between a retrovirus antigen and IAA (Serreze *et al.*, 1988). In summary, IAA is thought to reflect β-cell destruction in individuals prone to develop IDDM. The IAA are particularly frequent in children younger than 5 to 7 years of age at onset of IDDM. Although the positive predictive value of IAA is low, combining the assay with ICA increases the predictive value by increasing specificity, albeit at the cost of lowered sensitivity.

2. 64K or Glutamic Acid Decarboxylase

The 64K antibodies (Table V) in IDDM were first demonstrated by immunoprecipitation with sera from newly diagnosed IDDM patients (Lernmark and Baekkeskov, 1981; Baekkeskov *et al.*, 1982b) using detergent extracts of metabolically labeled human islets. In addition, an M_r 38,000 component (Table V) was detected in some sera when the donor of the islets was HLA-DR3 positive (Baekkeskov *et al.*, 1982b; Baekkeskov *et al.*, 1987). The initial studies indicated that the 64K protein was (1) present in islet from several species (Baekkeskov and Lernmark, 1982a; Gerling *et al.*, 1986; Christie *et al.*, 1988; (2)

present at very low levels (Baekkeskov *et al.*, 1982b; (3) specific to β cells (Christie *et al.*, 1990); (4) associated with a membrane-enriched subcellular fraction (Christie *et al.*, 1990); but (5) not necessarily expressed on the β-cell surface (Colman *et al.*, 1987) and (6) immunoprecipitated by IDDM sera as two subunits (Baekkeskov *et al.*, 1990). Analysis of sera from newly diagnosed IDDM patients and from first-degree relatives suggested that 64K antibodies were a better marker for the disease than were ICA and IAA (Baekkeskov *et al.*, 1987; Atkinson *et al.*, 1990). The laborious nature of the assay limited the clinical studies that could be performed. In 40 newly diagnosed 0–14-year-old IDDM patients, the frequency of 64KA was 71% in a rat-islet assay (Christie *et al.*, 1988), whereas 17 of 19 (89%) 15- to 32-year-old patients had 64KA in the human and dog-islet assay compared to 15 of 19 (79%) in the rat-islet assay (Bärmeier *et al.*, 1991). The identification of the 64K protein as GAD should permit the development of immunoassays, which would then allow proper estimations of autoantibodies against this antigen, and therefore, the predictive value of these autoantibodies for IDDM.

Multiple attempts were made to identify and characterize the 64K protein from the β cells, initially with little success. The incisive use of sera from patients with stiff man syndrome, which shows an increased frequency of IDDM, led Solinema *et al.* (1990) to demonstrate first that sera from stiff man syndrome patients with GAD antibodies stained β cells in sections of human pancreas. Second, Baekkeskov and coworkers (1990) demonstrated shortly thereafter that stiff man syndrome and IDDM sera each precipitated a 64K islet protein with GAD activity. Figure 4 shows results from our laboratory demonstrating that sera from a diabetic patient and a monoclonal antibody to GAD each immunoprecipitate the same material from a labeled islet extract. The human islet isoform of GAD which likely represents the actual 64K antigen has recently been cloned by our laboratory (Karlsen, A. E., *et al.*, 1991). Decarboxylase activity in the pancreatic β-cells was demonstrated in early experiments with isolated β cells (Lernmark, 1971), and gamma-aminobutyric acid (GABA) and glutamic acid were found to be the most abundant free amino acids in the β cells (Briel *et al.*, 1972). The large quantities of the neurotransmittor GABA in the β cells were puzzling, however, since GABA (in contrast to 5-hydroxytryptamine) did not accumulate in the β-cell granules (Gylfe, 1977), although data in the literature are conflicting (Vincent *et al.*, 1983; Okada, 1986). GABA has been localized to the β cells by immunocytochemistry. GAD was localized by electron-microscope immunocytochemistry to the β-cell cytoplasm, perhaps in association with microvesicles (Garry *et al.*, 1988). It has been suggested that GABA in the β cells does not function as a neurotransmitter but rather as a source of reduced nicotinamide adenine dinucleotide (NADH) and adenosine triphosphate (ATP) (Vincent *et al.*, 1983), a role it is likely to play in spermatozoa. Alternatively, there is evidence supporting a paracrine role for GABA from β cells in modulating

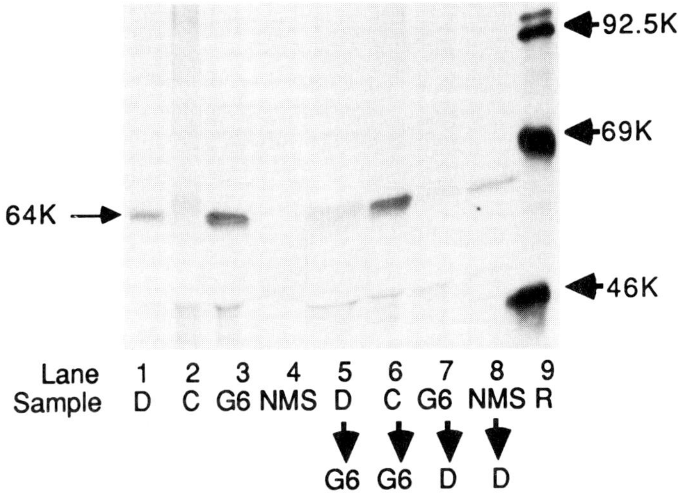

FIG. 4 The islet 64K protein is glutamic acid decarboxylase (GAD). The fluorogram shows the results of polyacrylamide gel electrophoresis of sequential immunoprecipitations of detergent extracts of ^{35}S-methionine-labeled dog islets. The extract was first immunoprecipitated with serum from a patient with IDDM (lane 1, D), serum from a healthy control (lane 2, C), mouse monoclonal antibody to GAD (lane 3, G6), or normal mouse serum control (lane 4, NMS). Following the first immunoprecipitation, the supernatant detergent extract from each immunoprecipitation was separately subjected to a second immunoprecipitation of the material from the diabetic serum with the mouse monoclonal antibody G6 (lane 5), from the control human serum with G6 (lane 6), from G6 with the diabetic serum D (lane 7), and from the normal mouse serum with the diabetic serum D (lane 8). Note that the mouse monoclonal antibody G6 quantitatively immunoprecipitates the 64K protein to leave the supernatant negative for the subsequent diabetic serum immunoprecipitation (lane 7). Similarly, initial diabetic serum immunoprecipitation decreases the amount of 64K immunoprecipitated by the monoclonal antibody to GAD (compare lane 5 with lane 6).

glucagon secretion by alpha cells (Rorsman *et al.*, 1989). Further experiments will be necessary to uncover the role of GAD and GABA in the function of the islet and as an autoantigen in IDDM.

3. Sialoglycoconjugate

The demonstration of GAD as the 64K protein showed that GAD antibody-positive patient sera induced a cytoplasmic staining of β-cells but not of the non-β endocrine cells (Solinema *et al.*, 1990). The ICA reaction, on the other hand, involves all endocrine islet cells. Treatment of human pancreatic sections with proteolytic enzymes or a variety of solvents indicated that the ICA immunofluorescent reaction was sensitive to lipid solvents rather than to proteolysis (Nayak *et al.*, 1985). These initial experiments indicated that a major ICA antigen was a sialic acid-containing glycolipid (Table V). More extensive extraction studies indicated that the islet-cell autoantigen in frozen sections is a glycolipid migrating with a mobility characteristic of a monosialoganglioside (Colman *et al.*, 1988). Binding of human sera to gangliosides was also analyzed by ELISA (Gillard *et al.*, 1989), demonstrating a significantly elevated binding of IDDM sera to the GT3 ganglioside. The limited availability of islet material for lipid extractions and isolation has hampered the possibility of identifying tentative β cell-specific antigens in IDDM. Antibodies against these components may also signify β-cell destruction.

4. Miscellaneous Antigens

A variety of methods are available to detect islet-cell antibodies (Table IV). A multitude of approaches to identify islet cell antigens are also available (Table V). The 64K protein is the major islet-cell antigen detected by immunoprecipiation. Oddly enough, the 64K protein is difficult to detect by immunoblotting (Baekkeskov *et al.*, 1990). It is possible that islet GAD-64 is labile and that the antibody-binding region is destroyed by adsorption to plastic for ELISA or to nitrocellulose for Western blotting. In an extensive Western blotting study (Karounos and Thomas, 1990a; Karounos *et al.*, 1990b), little reactivity was found to a 64K component. However, with different tissue preparations, antigens of M_r 52,000, 84,000, 116,000, and 150,000 were detected by IDDM sera (Table V). Similarly, in an attempt to identify novel β cell-surface antigens, the monoclonal antibody 1A2 (Table V) was used in competition-binding experiments to RIN 5F cells to demonstrate that the binding of this antibody was inhibited by IDDM but not by control sera (Thomas *et al.*, 1990). The nature of the antigen(s) recognized by this β cell-surface IgM monoclonal antibody remains to be identified.

VI. IDENTIFICATION AND TREATMENT OF ONGOING β-CELL DESTRUCTION AND OF DIABETES

Stopping autoimmune β-cell destruction is useful only if enough endocrine mass remains to maintain normoglycemia. Only then would one expect to avoid the neuropathy, nephropathy, retinopathy, and premature mortality that accompany diabetes. Therefore, early and presymptomatic detection of β cell-directed autoimmunity is necessary. Studies of twins and siblings of IDDM patients, as well as of serum immune markers, suggest that the disease process develops over months to years before clinical onset, providing a *window of opportunity* for detection and prevention.

Prediabetics come largely from general populations rather than from identifiable subgroups, such as relatives of diabetics or residents of a certain country, so general populations must be screened.

Provocative tests of β-cell function such as glucose tolerance tests or even i.v. secretogogue infusions can probably detect an estimated 30–50% reduction in insulin-secretory reserve, but are limited from increased sensitivity by large intra- and interindividual variations. These tests are also expensive and laborious, and are unsuited for screening large populations. HLA typing may help define susceptibility and relative risk, but is not of sufficient predictive power to identify prediabetics; current technology is expensive and impractical for population screening, although more rapid PCR-based methods are on the horizon. Therefore, most interest has focused on identification of specific serum markers of β-cell autoimmunity.

As shown in Table IV, tests of serum markers include assays of (1) ICA using immunofluorescence on sections of human pancreas; (2) ICSA using indirect immunofluorescence on viable dispersed islet cells; (3) IAA using soluble-phase immunoassay; (4) antibody-dependent islet cytotoxicity using complement (C′AMC) or immune effector cells; (5) anti-islet monoclonal antibody displacement by serum; and (6) autoantibodies to a 64K islet cell protein (64KA). Of these tests, ICA, ICSA, C′AMC, and the current 64KA assay are all impractical for general screening. Studies analyzing a combination of tests to create an index of risk have improved on the individual test results, but again are impractical as large-scale screening tests. Given the identification of the 64K antigen as islet GAD, a more practical and widely applicable test for serum 64K autoantibodies may soon be available.

Despite the limited power and practicality of the current tests, they can effectively be used on defined high-risk groups (such as first-degree relatives of IDDM patients) to identify prediabetics. However, given the risk of experimental immunotherapy, newly diagnosed IDDM patients themselves have provided the majority of subjects for trials of immunosuppression. Given the strong evidence that early initiation of treatment is critical, beginning therapy after clinical onset may have doomed these studies to partial success at best. The clearest example of early treatment is in living related-donor pancreatic grafts in identical twins discordant for diabetes, in which early immunosuppression is both necessary and sufficient to prevent insulitis and graft failure (Sutherland, 1981). Therefore, the most recent position statement by the American Diabetic Association (ADA), while endorsing the idea of prevention trials given current knowledge, suggests that future trials treat *pre*diabetics selected from limited study groups (Diabetes, 1990). Standardized treatment–response parameters for such trials have also been suggested (Pozzilli and Kolb, 1989), and it appears that islet-secretory function (insulin or C-peptide) and glucose control ($HgbA_{1c}$) are more useful in following study patients than are the aforementioned serum immune markers.

The concept of β-cell rest was introduced early (Ludvigsson *et al.*, 1977) in attempts to preserve the residual β-cell function in new-onset IDDM children. Early insulin therapy in the BB rat decreased the frequency of IDDM (Gotfredsen *et al.*, 1985). One treatment that may offer partial preservation of β-cell secretory function is short-term (1–2 week) intensive insulin therapy, such as that provided by the closed-loop insulin pump (artificial pancreas) (Ludvigsson *et al.*, 1977; Shah *et al.*, 1989). It has been suggested that avoidance of hyperglycemic toxicity or alteration of β-cell antigen expression may be the responsible mechanism. However, it appears that less rigorous, albeit intensive forms of insulin therapy such as open-loop pumps or multiple injections do not have this effect, limiting the practicality of such treatment. However, insulin therapy *preceding* the clinical onset of IDDM in man is yet to be tested.

By far the most widely used immunomodulatory agent has been cyclosporine, an inhibitor of T-lymphocyte function. Several large randomized and placebo-controlled trials have achieved clinical remission in 20 to 30% of treated patients versus 5 to 10% of controls (The Canadian-European Randomized Control Trial Group, 1988; Assan *et al.* 1990; Bougneres *et al.*, 1988), suggesting that cyclosporine treatment preserves β-cell function in those treated early enough. Benefit is lost, however, after the drug is discontinued (Chase *et al.*, 1990). Furthermore, cyclosporine has significant renal toxicity, and can also inhibit islet function (Nielsen, 1985), and these are severe limitations to its use. Other agents tried have included nicotinamide, an enhancer of radical-scavenger activity, which, despite efficacy in the NOD mouse model and in streptozocin models of IDDM, has not consistently preserved islet function in human IDDM (Herskowitz *et al.*, 1989; Chase *et al.*, 1990). Trials of azathioprine and prednisone have shown limited efficacy in previous studies (Cook *et al.*, 1987; Elliott *et al.*, 1981; Harrison *et al.*, 1985), and a multicenter trial using low-dose azathioprine treatment of high-risk first-degree relatives (as defined by ICA and IAA) is currently underway (Silverstein *et al.*, 1988). Finally, while *immune shock therapy* with interperitoneal Freund's complete adjuvant has been shown to block IDDM development in animal models of disease when given early enough (Sadelain *et al.*, 1990), it is difficult to envision a workable human protocol employing this treatment.

Because of the toxicity and tumor risk of general immunosuppression, and the lengthy treatment likely to be necessary in individuals in whom an autoimmune process is already established, specific antigen-guided immunosuppression would be superior treatment. Current rapid progress in general and diabetes immunology makes this goal conceivable, and thus such treatments as T-cell vaccination, antigen–toxin complexes, or antigen-blocking peptides might possibly prevent IDDM with less associated morbidity.

For patients already diabetic, significant effort and progress have been made in whole pancreas or islet transplantation. The first whole pancreas transplants in Minnesota in 1966 were largely unsuccessful, but, since the introduction of cyclosporine in the late 1970s, the number of such transplants worldwide is over 2,000, and the 1-year actuarial graft survival rate has improved dramatically from 5% pre-1977 to 56% in the 1986–1988 interval (Sutherland *et al.*, 1989). Islet transplantation, successful in a syngeneic rat model (Ballinger and Lacy, 1972) and later in canines, has proven much more difficult in allogeneic human transplants, although a few successful patients have recently been demonstrated (Scharp *et al.*, 1990). Interestingly, it appears that autografts of isolated islets in previously nondiabetic patients undergoing elective pancreatectomy for unrelated indications are successful in reversing the surgical diabetes with far fewer islets (fewer than 100,000) than in diabetic patients receiving allografts (more than 500,000 islets), suggesting that immunologic factors due to the host IDDM or the allograft nature of the transplant may play a large role in graft function. Recently, it has been shown that intrathymic islet transplantation tolerizes rats to subsequent islet allografts (Posselt *et al.*, 1990), and it is hoped that this or other maneuvers may someday be clinically useful in islet transplantation. Until then, whole pancreas transplants will be more practical despite the necessity of chronic immunosuppression and the limited availability of donor organs.

VII. CONCLUDING REMARKS—FUTURE PROSPECTS

The clinical onset of IDDM is associated with a number of immune abnormalities. Using islet cell antibodies as a marker for IDDM, it has been established that diabetes exists for extended periods as a subclinical disease. Subclinical or preclinical diabetes may be present for several years before enough β-cell destruction has occurred that clinical IDDM develops. Although IDDM is genetically linked to certain HLA-DR/DQ class II molecules, the role of these molecules in the pathogenesis is unclear. The reviewed evidence of yet another gene necessary for IDDM is important, since studies in both the BB rat (Markholst *et al.*, 1990; Jackson *et al.*, 1984) and the NOD mouse (Leiter, 1989) suggest the presence of a diabetes gene outside the MHC. The availability of a human linkage map and a growing number of polymorphic DNA probes should make it possible to eventually identify the human non-MHC diabetes gene(s).

Since monozygotic twins tend to be discordant for IDDM, a major challenge to our understanding of IDDM is the effect of the environment. HLA class II molecules present foreign antigens or epitopes to the immune system. Are there diabetogenic sequences in the major β-cell autoantigen, glutamic acid decarboxylase (64K antigen)? Is it possible that individuals prone to develop IDDM are poor presentors of this self-antigen during the induction of tolerance? Severe β-cell destruction by virus (rubella, mumps, Coxsackie, etc.) may initiate a disease process that is perpetuated by a genetic propensity to develop autoimmunity. Recent data in spontaneously diabetic BB rats and NOD mice suggest, however, that environmental factors may be protective, since diabetes in these animals reaches 100%, but only in specific pathogen-free environments. Similar phenomena may also occur in man, and research aimed at understanding the preclinical stages of IDDM (Table III) will be necessary to uncover the sequence of events that eventually results in chronic autoimmune islet destruction.

ACKNOWLEDGMENTS

We thank Sue Blaylock for her secretarial assistance. Studies in our laboratory were supported by the National Institutes of Health (DK26190, DK33873, DK41801), the Greenwall Foundation, and by a Howard Hughes Medical Institute Fellowship for Physicians (W.H.).

REFERENCES

Åkerblom, H. K., Ballard, D. J., Bauman, B., *et al.* (1988). *Diabetes* **37,** 1113–1119.

Andres, R. (1971). Aging and diabetes. *Med. Clin. North Am.* **55,** 835–846.

Arslanian, S. A., Becker, D. J., Rabin, B., Atchinson, R., Eberhardt, M., Cavender, D., Dorman, J., and Drash, A. L. (1985). *Diabetes* **34,** 926–930.

Assan, R., Feutren, G., Sirmai, J., Laborie, C., Boitard, C., Vexiau, P., Du Rostu, H., Rodier, M., Figoni, M., Vague, P., Hors, J., and Bach, J.-F. (1990). *Diabetes* **39,** 768–774.

Atkinson, M. A., and Maclaren, N. K. (1988). *Diabetes* **37,** 1587–1590.

Atkinson, M. A., Maclaren, N. K., Riley, W. J., Winter, W. E., Fish, D. D., and Spillar, R. P. (1986). *Diabetes* **35,** 894–898.

Atkinson, M. A., Maclaren, N. K., Scharp, D. W., Lacy, P. E., and Riley, W. J. (1990). *Lancet* **335,** 1357–1360.

Baekkeskov, S., Aanstoot, H. J., Christgau, S., Reetz, A., Solimena, M., Cascalho, M., Folli, F., Richter-Olesen, H., and De Camilli, P. (1990). *Nature* **347,** 151–156.

Baekkeskov, S., Dyrberg, T., and Lernmark, Å. (1984). *Science* **224,** 1348–1350.

Baekkeskov, S., Landin-Olsson, M., Kristensen, J. K., Srikanta, S., Bruining, G. J., Mandrup-Poulsen, T., de Beaufort, C., Soeldner, J. S., Eisenbarth, G., Lindgren, F., Sundkvist, G., and Lernmark, Å. (1987). *J. Clin. Invest.* **79,** 926–934.

Baekkeskov, S., and Lernmark, Å. (1982a). *Acta Biol. Med. Germ.* **41,** 1111–1115.

Baekkeskov, S., Nielsen, J. H., Marner, B., Bilde, T., Ludvigsson, J., and Lernmark, Å. (1982b). *Nature* **298,** 167–169.

Baekkeskov, S., Warnock, G., Christie, M., Rajotte, R. V., Larsen, P. M., and Fey, S. (1990). *Diabetes* **38,** 1133–1141.

Baisch, J. M., Weeks, T., Giles, R., Hoover, M., Stastny, P., and Capra, J. D. (1990). *N. Engl. J. Med.* **322,** 1836–1882.

Ballinger, W. F., and Lacy, P. E. (1972). *Surgery* **72,** 72–175.

Banatvala, J. E., Schernthaner, G., Schober, E., De Silva, L. M., Bryant, J., Borkenstein, M., Brown, D., and Menser, M. A. (1985). *Lancet* **ii,** 1409–1412.

Bärmeier, H., Ahlmen, J., Landin-Olsson, M., Rajotte, R. V., Sundkvist, G., Warnock, G., and Lernmark, Å. (1991). (submitted for publication).

Bärmeier, H., McCulloch, D., Neifing, J., Rajotte, R., Palmer, J., and Lernmark, Å. (1990). *Diabetes* **39** (Suppl. 1), 122A.

Barnett, A. H., Eff, C., Leslie, R. D. G., and Pyke, D. A. (1981). *Diabetologia* **20,** 87–93.

Barrett-Connor, E. (1985). *Rev. Infect. Dis.* **7,** 207–15.

Beer, S. F., Heaton, D. A., Alberti, K. G. M. M., Pyke, D. A., and Leslie, R. D. G. (1990). *Diabetologia* **33,** 497–502.

Bendelae, A., Carnaud, C., Boitard, C., Bach, J. (1987). *J. Exp. Med.* **166,** 823–832.

Betterle, C., Presotto, F., Pedini, B., Moro, L., Slack, R. S., Zanette, F., and Zanchetta, R. (1987). *Diabetologia* **30,** 292–297.

Bjorkman, P. J., Saper, M. A., Samraoui, B., Bennett, W. S., Strominger, J. L., and Wiley, D. C. (1987). *Nature* **329,** 512–518.

Bliss, M. (1982). "The Discovery of Insulin" McClelland and Stewart, Toronto, Canada.

Boitard, C., Bonifacio, E., Bottazzo, G. F., Gleishmann, H., and Molenaar, J. (1988). **31,** 451–452.

Bonifacio, E., Bingley, P. J., Shattock, M., Dean, B. M., Dunger, D., Gale, E. A. M., and Bottazzo, G. F. (1990). *Lancet* **335,** 147–149.

Bonifacio, E., Dawkins, R. L., and Lernmark, A. (1987). *Diabetologia* **30,** 273.

Bonifacio, E., Lernmark, Å., and Dawkins, R. L. (1988). *J. Immunol. Methods* **106,** 83–88.

Borch-Johnsen, K., Mandrup-Poulsen, T., Zachau-Christiansen, B. Z., *et al.* (1984). *Lancet* **ii,** 1083–6.

Bottazzo, G. F., Cudworth, A. G., Moul, D. J., Doniach, D., and Festenstein, H. (1978). *Br. Med. J.* **2,** 1253–1255.

Bottazzo, G. F., Dean, B. M., McNally, J. M., MacKay, E. H., Swift, P. G. F., and Gamble, D. R. (1985). *N. Engl. J. Med.* **313,** 353–360.

Bottazzo, G. F., Florin-Christensen, A., and Doniach, D. (1974). *Lancet* **ii,** 1279–1283.

Bottazzo, G. F., and Gleichmann, H. (1986). *Diabetologia* **29,** 125–126.

Bouchard, P. H., Sai, P., Reach, G., Caubarrère, I., Ganeval, D., and Assan, R. (1982). *Diabetes* **31,** 40–45.

Bougneres, P. F., Carel, J. C., Castano, L., Boitard, C., Gardin, J. P., Landais, P., Hors, J., Mihatsch, M., Paillard, M., Chaussain, J. L., and Bach, J. F. (1988). *N. Engl. J. Med.* **318,** 663–667.

Briel, G., Gylfe, E., Hellman, B., and Neuhoff, V. (1972). *Acta Physiol. Scand.* **84,** 247–253.

Bruserud, Ø., Jervell, J., and Thorsby, E. (1985a). *Diabetologia* **28,** 420–426.

Bruserud, Ø., Stenersen, M., and Thorsby, E. (1985b). *Tissue Antigens* **26,** 179–92.

Bruserud, Ø., and Thorsby, E. (1985c). *Scand. J. Immunol.* **22,** 509–518.

Casali, P., and Notkins, A. B. (1989). *Immunol. Today* **10,** 364–368.

Charles, M. A., Suzuki, M., and Waldeck, N. (1983). *J. Immunol.* **130,** 1189–1194.

Chase, P. H., Butler-Simon, N., Garg, S. K., Hayward, A., Klingensmith, G. J., Hamman, R. F., and O'Brien, D. (1990). *Pediatrics* **85,** 241–245.

Chatenoud, L., Feutren, G., Nelson, D. L., Boitard, C., and Bach, J. F. (1989). *Diabetes* **38,** 249–256.

Christie, M., and Delovitch, T. L. (1990). *Diabetes* **39,** 653–659.

Christie, M., Landin-Olsson, M., Sundkvist, G., Dahlquist, G., Lernmark, Å., and Baekkeskov, S. (1988). *Diabetologia* **31,** 597–602.

Christie, M. R., Pipeleers, D. G., Lernmark, Å., and Baekkeskov, S. (1990). *J. Biol. Chem.* **265,** 376–381.

Colman, P. G., Campbell, I. L., Kay, T. W. H., and Harrison, L. C. (1987). *Diabetes* **36,** 1432–1440.

Colman, P. G., Nayak, R. C., Campbell, I. L., and Eisenbarth, G. S. (1988). *Diabetes* **37,** 645–652.

Cook, J. J., Hudson, I., Harrison, L. C., *et al.* (1987). *Diabetologia* **30,** 509A.

Dahlquist, G., Blom, L., Holmgren, G., Hägglöf, B., Larsson, Y., Sterky, G., and Wall, S. (1985). *Diabetologia* **28,** 802–808.

Dalhquist, G., Blom, L., Tuvemo, T., Nyström, L., Sandström, A., and Wall, S. (1989). *Diabetologia* **32,** 2–6.

Damian, R. T. (1988). Parasites and molecular mimicry. *In* "Molecular Mimicry in Health and Disease" (Å. Lernmark, T. Dyrberg, L. Terenius, and B. Hökfelt, eds.), pp. 211–218. Elsevier Science Publishers, Amsterdam, The Netherlands.

DelRay, A., and Besedovsky, H. (1987). *Am. J. Physiol.* **252,** R794–R798.
Di Mario, U., Irvine, W. J., Borsey, D. Q., Kyner, J. L., Weston, J., and Galfo, C. (1983). *Diabetologia* **25,** 392–395.
Diabetes, C. (1990, September). *Diabetes Care* 1026–1027.
Dobersen, M. J., and Scharff, J. E. (1982). *Diabetes* **31,** 449–462.
Dobersen, M. J., Scharff, J. E., Ginsberg-Fellner, F., and Notkins, A. L. (1980). *N. Engl. J. Med.* **303,** 1493–1498.
Doniach, I., and Morgan, A. G. (1973). *Clin. Endocrinol.* **2,** 233–248.
Donnelly, R. P., Levine, J., Hartwell, D. W., Frendl, G., Fenton, M. J., and Beller, D. I. (1990). *J. Immunol.* **145,** 001–010.
Drell, D. W., and Notkins, A. L. (1987). *Diabetologia* **30,** 132–143.
Dyrberg, T., Poussier, P., Nakhooda, F., Marliss, E. B., and Lernmark, Å. (1984). *Diabetologia* **26,** 159–165.
Dyrberg, T., Schwimmbeck, P. L., and Oldstone, M. B. A. (1988). *J. Clin. Invest.* **81,** 928–931.
Eisenbarth, G. S. (1986). *N. Engl. J. Med.* **314,** 1360–1368.
Eisenbarth, G. S., Morris, M. A., and Scearce, R. M. (1981). *J. Clin. Invest.* **67,** 403–408.
Eisenbarth, G. S., Srikanta, S., Jackson, R., Rabinowe, S., Dolinar, R., Aoki, T., and Morris, M. A. (1985). *Diabetes Res.* **2,** 271–276.
Elliott, R. B., Crossley, J. R., Berryman, C. C., and James, A. G. (1981). *Lancet* **ii,** 119–23.
Fialkow, P. J., Zavala, C., and Nielsen, R. (1975). *Ann. Intern. Med.* **83,** 170–176.
Foulis, A. K. (1989). *Diabetic Med.* **6,** 666–674.
Foulis, A. K., and Farquharson, M. A. (1986). *Diabetes* **35,** 1215–1224.
Foulis, A. K., Farquharson, M. A., Cameron, S. O., McGill, M., Schönke, H., and Kandolff, R. (1990). *Diabetologia* **33,** 290–298.
Foulis, A. K., Farquharson, M. A., and Meager, A. (1987). *Lancet* II: 1423–1427.
Foulis, A. K., Liddle, C. N., Farquharson, M. A., Richmond, J. A., and Weir, S. R. (1986). *Diabetologia* **29,** 267–274.
Foulis, A. K., and Stewart, J. A. (1984). *Diabetologia* **26,** 456–461.
Gamble, D. R. (1980a). *Diabetologia* **19,** 341–344.
Gamble, D. R. (1980b). *Epidemiol. Rev.* **2,** 49–70.
Gamble, D. R., Kinsley, M. L., Fitzgerald, M. G., Bolton, R., and Taylor, K. W. (1969). *Br. Med. J.* **3,** 627–630.
Garry, D. J., Appel, N. M., Garry, M. G., and Sorenson, R. L. (1988). *J. Histochem. Cytochem.* **36,** 573–580.
Gepts, W. (1965). *Diabetes* **14,** 619–633.
Gerling, I., Baekkeskov, S., and Lernmark, Å. (1986). *J. Immunol.* **137,** 3782–3785.
Gillard, A. K., Thomas, J. W., Nell, L. J., and Marcus, D. M. (1989). *J. Immunol.* **142,** 3826–3832.
Ginsberg-Fellner, F., Dobersen, M. J., Witt, M. E., Rayfield, E. J., Rubenstein, P., and Notkins, A. L. (1982). *Diabetes* **31,** 292–297.
Ginsberg-Fellner, F., Witt, M. E., Franklin, B. H., Yagihashi, S., Togushi, Y., Dobersen, M. J., Rubinstein, P., and Notkins, A. L. (1985). *J.A.M.A.* **254,** 1469–1470.
Ginsberg-Fellner, F., Witt, M. E., Yagihashi, S., Dobersen, M. J., Taub, F., Fedun, B., McEvoy, R. C., Roman, S. H., Davies, T. F., Cooper, L. Z., Rubinstein, P., and Notkins, A. L. (1984). *Diabetologia* **27,** 87–89.
Gleichmann, H., and Bottazzo, G. F. (1987). *Diabetes* **36,** 578–584.
Gleichmann, H., Zörcher, B., Greulich, B., *et al.* (1984). *Diabetologia* **27,** 90–92.
Gorsuch, A. N., Spencer, K. M., Lister, J., McNally, J. M., Dean, B. M., Bottazzo, G. F., and Cudworth, A. G. (1981). *Lancet* **ii,** 1363–1365.
Gotfredsen, C. F., Buschard, K., and Frandsen, E. K. (1985). *Diabetologia* **28,** 933–935.
Groop, L. C., Pelkonen, R., Koskimies, S., Bottazzo, G. F., and Doniach, D. (1986). *Diabetes Care* **9,** 129–33.

Group, D. E. R. I. (1990). *Diabetes* **39,** 858–864.
Gundersen, E. (1927). *J. Infect. Dis.* **41,** 197–202.
Gylfe, E. (1977). *Acta Physiol. Scand.* **452,** 125–128.
Hägglöf, B., Rabinovitch, A., Mackay, P., Huen, A., Rubenstein, A. H., Marner, B., Nerup, J., and Lernmark, Å. (1986). *Acta Pœdiatr. Scand.* **75,** 611–618.
Hanafusa, T., Miyazaki, A., Miyagawa, J., *et al.* (1990). *Diabetologia* **33,** 105–111.
Harrison, L. C., Colman, P. G., Dean, B., Baxter, R., and Martin, F. I. R. (1985). *Diabetes* **34,** 1306–1308.
Hawkins, B. R., Lam, K. S. L., Ma, J. T. C., Low, L. C. K., Cheung, P. T., Serjeantson, S. W., and Yeung, R. T. T. (1987). *Diabetes* **36,** 1297–1300.
Hay, D. R. (1949). *N.Z. Med. J.* **48,** 604–608.
Heaton, D. A., Millward, B. A., Gray, I. P., Tun, Y., Hales, C. N., Pyke, D. A., and Leslie, R. D. G. (1988). *Diabetologia* **31,** 182–184.
Heaton, D. A., Millward, B. A., Gray, P., Tun, Y., Hales, C. N., Pyke, D. A., and Leslie, R. D. G. (1987). *Br. Med. J.* **294,** 145–146.
Helgason, T., and Jonasson, M. R. (1981). *Lancet* **ii,** 716–720.
Helmke, K., Otten, A., Mäser, E., Wolf, H., and Federlin, K. (1987). *Horm. Metab. Res.* **19,** 312–315.
Helmke, K., Otten, A., and Willems, W. (1980). *Lancet* **ii,** 211–212.
Herskowitz, R. D., Jackson, R. A., Soeldner, J. S., and Eisenbarth, G. S. (1989). *J. Autoimmunol.* **2,** 733–737.
Horita, M., Suzuki, H., Onodera, T., Ginsberg-Fellner, F., Fauci, A. S., and Notkins, A. L. (1982). *J. Immunol.* **129,** 1426–1429.
Hyer, R. N., Julier, C., Buckley, J. D., Trucco, M., Rotter, J., Spielman, R., Barnett, A., Bain, S., Boitard, C., Deschamps, I., Todd, J. A., Bell, J. I., and Lathrop, G. M. (1991). *Am. Soc. Hum. Genet.* (in press).
Irvine, W. J., Gray, R. S., and Steel, J. M. (1980). *In* "Immunology of Diabetes" Irvine, W. J. (Ed.), pp. 117–154. Teviot Scientific Publications, Edinburgh, Scotland.
Irvine, W. J., McCallum, C. J., Gray, R. S., Campbell, C. J., Duncan, L. J. P., Farquhar, J. W., Vaughan, H., and Morris, P. J. (1977). *Diabetes* **26,** 138–147.
Jackson, R., Buse, J. B., Rifai, R., Pelletier, D., Milford, E. L., Carpenter, C. B., Eisenbarth, G. S., and Williams, R. M. (1984). *J. Exp. Med.* **159,** 1629–1636.
Jackson, R. A., Morris, M. A., Haynes, B. F., and Eisenbarth, G. S. (1982). *N. Engl. J. Med.* **306,** 785–788.
Jacob, C. O., Aiso, S., Michie, S. A., McDevitt, H. O., and Acha-Orbea, H. (1990). *In* "Tumor Necrosis Factor: Structure, Mechanism of Action, Role in Disease and Therapy" pp. 222–227. Benjamin Bonavida, Gale Granger (Eds) Publ. Basel; New York; Karger
Jansen, F. K., Münterfering, H., and Schmidt, W. A. K. (1977). *Diabetologia* **13,** 545–549.
Jenkins, D., Mijovic, C., Fletcher, J., Jacobs, K. H., Bradwell, A. R., and Barnett, A. H. (1990). *Diabetologia* **33,** 387–395.
Jenson, A. B., Rosenberg, H. S., and Notkins, A. L. (1980). *Lancet* **ii,** 354–358.
Johnson, J. H., Crider, B. P., McCorkle, K., Alford, M., and Unger, R. H. (1990). *N. Engl. J. Med.* **322,** 653–659.
Johnston, C., Millward, B. A., Hoskins, P., Leslie, R. D. G., Bottazzo, G. F., and Pyke, D. A. (1989). *Diabetologia* **32,** 382–386.
Kanatsuna, T., Baekkeskov, S., Lernmark, Å., and Ludvigsson, J. (1983). *Diabetes* **32,** 520–524.
Karam, J. H., Lewitt, P. A., Young, C. W., Nowlain, R. E., Frankel, B. J., Fujiya, H., Freedman, Z. R., and Grodsky, G. M. (1980). *Diabetes* **29,** 971–978.
Karjalainen, J. (1990). *Diabetes* **39,** 1144–1150.
Karjalainen, J., Knip, M., Hyöty, P., Leinikki, P., Ilonen, J., Käär, M.-L., and Åkerblom, H. K. (1988). *Diabetologia* **31,** 146–152.

Karlsen, A. E., Hagopian, W. A., Grubin, C. E., *et al.* (1991). *Proc. Nat. Acad. Sci.* **88:** 8337–8341.

Karounos, D., and Thomas, J. W. (1990a). *Diabetes* **39,** 1085–1090.

Karounos, D. G., Nell, L. J., and Thomas, J. W. (1990b). *Autoimmunity* **6,** 79–91.

Kidd, P. G., McLaren, T., McCulloch, D. K., Neifing, J., and Palmer, J. P. (1991). *Diabetes* (in press).

King, M. L., Bidwell, D., Shaikh, A., Voller, A., and Banatvala, J. E. (1983). *Lancet* **i,** 1397–1399.

Kobayashi, T., Sugimoto, T., Itoh, T., Kosaka, K., Tanaka, T., Suwa, S., Sato, K., and Tsuji, K. (1986). *Diabetologia* **35,** 335–340.

Köbberling, J., and Tattersall, B. (Ed.). (1982). "The Genetics of Diabetes Mellitus. Academic Press, London, England.

Kolb, H., Dannehl, K., Grüneklee, D., Zielasek, J., Bertrams, J., Hübinger, A., and Gries, F. A. (1988). *Diabetologia* **31,** 189–194.

Kuglin, B., Gries, F. A., and Kolb, H. (1988). *Diabetes* **37,** 130–132.

Kuglin, B., Kolb, H., Greenbaum, C., Maclaren, N. K., Lernmark, Å., and Palmer, J. P. (1990). *Diabetologia* **33,** 638–639.

Landin-Olsson, M., Karlsson, A., Dahlquist, G., Blom, L., Lernmark, Å., and Sundkvist, G. (1989). *Diabetologia* **32,** 387–395.

Landin-Olsson, M., Nilsson, K. O., Lernmark, Å., and Sundkvist, G. (1990). *Diabetologia* **33,** 561–568.

Leiter, E. (1989). *FASEB J.* **3,** 2231–2241.

Lernmark, Å. (1971). *Horm. Metab. Res.* **3,** 305–309.

Lernmark, Å. (1984). *In* "Immunology in Diabetes" D. Andreani, U. Di Mario, K. F. Federlin, and L. G. Heding (eds.), pp. 121–131. Kimpton Medical Publications, London, England.

Lernmark, Å. (1987). *Diabetic Med.* **4,** 285–292.

Lernmark, Å., and Baekkeskov, S. (1981). *Diabetologia,* **212,** 431–435.

Lernmark, Å., Freedman, Z. R., Hofmann, C., Rubenstein, A. H., Steiner, D. F., Jackson, R. L., Winter, R. J., and Traisman, H. S. (1978). *N. Engl. J. Med.* **299,** 375–380.

Lipton, R., and LaPorte, R. E. (1989). *Epidemologic Reviews,* **11,** 182–203.

Logothetopoulos, J., Valiquette, N., Madura, E., and Cvet, D. (1984). *Diabetes* **33,** 33–36.

Ludvigsson, J., Binder, C., and Mandrup-Poulsen, T. (1988). *Diabetologia* **31,** 647–651.

Ludvigsson, J., Heding, L. G., Larsson, Y., and Leander, E. (1977). *Acta Pædiatr. Scand.* **66,** 177–184.

MacCuish, A. C., Barnes, E. W., Irvine, W. J., and Duncan, L. J. P. (1974). *Lancet* **ii,** 1529–1531.

MacCuish, A. C., and Irvine, W. J. (1975). *Clin. Endocrinol. Metab.* **4,** 435–471.

Makino, S., Kunimoto, K., Muraoka, Y., Mizushima, Y., Katagiri, K., and Tochima, Y. (1980). *Exp. Anim.* **29,** 1–13.

Mandrup-Poulsen, T., Bendtzen, K., Dinarello, C. A., and Nerup, J. (1987). *J. Immunol.* **139,** 4077–4082.

Mandrup-Poulsen, T., Bendtzen, K., Nerup, J., Dinarello, C. A., Svenson, M., and Nielsen, J. H. (1986). *Diabetologia* **29,** 63–67.

Manna, R., Salvatore, M., Scuderi, F., Papa, G., Marietti, G., Greco, A. V., and Ghirlanda, G. (1988). *Diabetes Res.* **9,** 101–103.

Markholst, H., Andreasen, B., Eastman, S., and Lernmark, Å. (1990). *J. Exp. Med.* (in press).

Marner, B., Agner, T., and Binder, C. (1985). *Diabetologia* **28,** 875–880.

Mason, D. R., Scott, R. S., and Darlow, B. A. (1987). *Diabetic Res. Clin. Prac.* **3,** 21–29.

Matsuba, I., and Lernmark, Å. (1990). *Reg. Immunol.* **3,** 23–28.

Mayer, E. J., Hamman, R. F., Gay, E. C., Lezotte, D. C., Savitz, D. A., and Klingensmith, G. J. (1988). *Diabetes* **37,** 1625–1631.

McCulloch, D. K., Klaff, L. J., Kahn, S. E., Schoenfeld, S. L., Greenbaum, C. J., Mauset, R. S., Benson, E. A., Nepom, G. T., Shewey, L., and Palmer, J. P. (1990). *Diabetes* **39,** 549–556.

McEvoy, R. C., Witt, M. E., Ginsberg-Fellner, F., and Rubenstein, P. (1986). *Diabetes* **35,** 634–641.

Menser, M. A., Forrest, J. M., and Bransby, R. D. (1978). *Lancet* **i,** 57–60.

Michelsen, B., and Lernmark, Å. (1987). *J. Clin. Invest.* **79,** 1144–1152.

Michelsen, B., Wassmuth, R., Ludvigsson, J., Lernmark, Å., Nepom, G. T., and Fisher, L. (1990). *Scand. J. Immunol.* **31,** 405–413.

Millward, B. A., Alviggi, L., Hoskins, P. J., Johnston, C., Heaton, D., Bottazzo, G. F., Vergani, D., Leslie, R. D., and Pyke, D. A. (1986). *Br. Med. J.* **292,** 793–796.

Mordes, P. P., Desemone, J., and Rossini, A. A. (1987). *Diabetes Metab. Rev.* **3,** 725–750.

Nayak, R. C., Omar, M. A. K., Rabizadeh, A., Srikanta, S., and Eisenbarth, G. S. (1985). *Diabetes* **34,** 617–619.

Nedergaard, M., Egeberg, J., and Kromann, H. (1983). *Diabetologia* **24,** 392–396.

Nerup, J., Andersen, O. O., Bendixen, G., *et al.* (1973). *Acta Endocrinol. (Copenh)* **28,** 231–249.

Nerup, J., Andersen, O. O., Bendixen, G., Egeberg, J., and Poulsen, J. E. (1971). *Diabetes* **20,** 424–427.

Nerup, J., Mandrup-Poulsen, T., and Molvig, J. (1987). *Diabetes Metab. Rev.* **3,** 779–802.

Nerup, J., Platz, P., and Anderssen, O. O. (1974). *Lancet* **ii,** 864–866.

Nielsen, J. H. (1985). *Acta Endocrinol.* **108,** 1–39.

Nigro, G., Campea, L., De Novellis, A., and Orsini, M. (1985). *Lancet* **i,** 467.

Nordén, G., Jensen, E., Stilbo, I., Bottazzo, G. F., and Lernmark, Å. (1983). *Acta Med. Scand.* **213,** 199–203.

Notkins, A. L., and Yoon, J.-W. (1982). *N. Engl. J. Med.* **306,** 486.

Nystrom, L., Dahlquist, G., Östman, J., Wall, S., Arnqvist, H. J., Blohme, G., Lithner, F., Littorin, B., Schersten, B., and Wibell, L. (1990). (Submitted for publication.

Okada, Y. (1986). "Localization and Function of GABA in the Pancreatic Islets." Raven Press, New York.

Olmos, P., Aherne, R., Heaton, D. A., Millward, B. A., Risley, D., and Pyke, D. A. (1988). *Diabetologia* **31,** 747–750.

Opie, E. (1901). *J. Exp. Med.* **5,** 393.

Owerbach, D., Lernmark, Å., Platz, P., Ryder, L. P., Rask, L., Peterson, P. A., and Ludvigsson, J. (1983). *Nature* **303,** 815–817.

Pak, C., McArthur, R. G., Eun, H.-M., and Yoon, J.-W. (1988). *Lancet* **i,** 1–4.

Pak, C. Y., Cha, C. Y., Rajotte, R. V., McArthur, R. G., and Yoon, J. W. (1990). *Diabetologia* **33,** 569–572.

Palmer, J. P. (1987). *Diabetes Metab. Rev.* **3,** 1005–1015.

Palmer, J. P., Asplin, C. M., Clemons, P., Lyen, K., Tatpati, O., Raghu, P. K., and Paguette, T. L. (1983). *Science* **222,** 1337–1339.

Palmer, J. P., Asplin, C. M., Raghu, P. K., Clemons, P., Lyen, K., Tatpati, O., McKnight, B., Paquette, T. L., Sperling, M., Baker, L., and Guthrie, R. (1986). *Pediatr. Adolescent Endocrinol.* **15,** 111–116.

Palmer, J. P., Cooney, M. K., Ward, R. H., Hansen, J. A., Brodsky, J. B., Ray, C. G., Crossley, J. R., Asplin, C. M., and Williams, R. H. (1982). *Diabetologia* **22,** 426–429.

Palmer, J. P., and Lernmark, Å. (1990a). "Diabetes Mellitus" In Rifkin, H. and Porte, D. (Eds), pp. 414–435. Elsevier, New York.

Palmer, J. P., and Lernmark, Å. (1990b). "Diabetes Mellitus" In Rifkin, H. and Porte, D. (Eds), pp. 414–435. Elsevier, New York.

Papadopoulos, G., Petersen, J., and Andersen, V. (1984). *Acta Endocrinol.* **105,** 521–527.

Papaspyros, N. S. (1964). "The History of Diabetes Mellitus" (2nd Ed.). Stuttgart: Georg Thieme Verlag

Pipeleers, D. G. (1988). *J. Clin. Invest.* **82,** 1123–1128.

Platz, P., Jakobsen, B. K., and Morling, M. (1981). *Diabetologia* **21,** 108–115.

Posselt, A. M., Barker, C. F., Tomaszewski, J. E., Markmann, J. F., Choti, M. A., and Naji, A. (1990). *Science* **249,** 1293–1295.

Pozzilli, P., and Kolb, H. (1989). *Immunol. Today* **10,** 321–322.

Prabhakar, B. S., Saegusa, J., Onodera, T., and Notkins, A. L. (1984). *J. Immunol.* **133,** 2815–2817.

Prince, G. A., Jenson, A. B., Billups, L. C., and Notkins, A. L. (1978). *Nature* **271,** 158–161.

Pyke, D. A. (1979). *Diabetologia* **17,** 333–343.

Pyke, D. A. (1988). *Adv. Exp. Med. Biol.* **246,** 255–258.

Rabinovitch, A., MacKay, P., Ludvigsson, J., and Lernmark, Å. (1984). *Diabetes* **33,** 224–228.

Rahier, J. (1988). *In* "The Pathology of the Endocrine Pancreas" (P. Lefebvre and D. Pipeleers, eds.), pp. 17–40. Springer-Verlag, Berlin/Heidelberg.

Rahier, J., Goebbels, R. M., and Henquin, J. C. (1983). *Diabetologia* **24,** 366–371.

Ratzmann, K. P., Strese, J., Witt, S., Berling, H., Keilacker, H., and Michaelis, D. (1985). *Diabetes Care* **7,** 170–173.

Rayfield, E. J., and Ishimura, K. (1987). *Diabetes Metab. Rev.* **3,** 925–957.

Rayfield, E. J., and Seto, Y. (1978). *Diabetes* **27,** 1126–1140.

Reevers, W. G., Gelsthorpe, K., Van der Minne, P., Torensma, R., and Tattersall, R. B. (1984). *Clin. Exp. Immunol.* **57,** 443–448.

Reijonen, H., Ilonen, J., Knip, M., Michelsen, B., and Åkerblom, H. K. (1990). *Diabetologia* **33,** 357–362.

Rich, S. S. (1990). *Diabetes* **39,** 1315–1319.

Richter, W., Eierman, T., Enell, J., *et al.* (1991). *Diabetologia* **34** (Suppl. 2), A57, 1991.

Rifkin, H., and Porte, J., D. (Ed.). (1990). "Ellenberg and Rifkin's Diabetes Mellitus (4th Ed.). Elsevier, New York.

Riley, W. J., Maclaren, N. K., Krischer, J., Spillar, R. P., Silverstein, J. H., Schatz, D. A., Schwartz, S., Malone, J., Shah, S., Vadheim, C., and Rotter, J. I. (1990). *N. Engl. J. Med.* **323,** 1167–1172.

Risch, N. (1987). *Am. J. Hum. Genet.* **40,** 1–14.

Risch, N. (1989). *Genet. Epidemiol.* **6,** 143–148.

Roep, B., Arden, S., De Vries, R., Hutton, J. (1990). *Nature* **345,** 632–634.

Rorsman, P., Berggren, P-O., Bokvist, K., Ericson, H., Möhler, H., Ostenson, C-G., Smith, P. (1989). *Nature* **341,** 233–236.

Rossini, A. A., Williams, R. M., Appel, M. C., and Like, A. A. (1978). *Nature* **276,** 182–184.

Rotter, J. I., Vadheim, C. M., and Rimoin, D. L. (1990). "Genetics of Diabetes Mellitus" (4th Ed.). Elsevier, New York.

Rubinstein, P., Walker, M. E., Fedun, B., Witt, M. E., Cooper, L. Z., and Ginsburg-Fellner, F. (1982). *Diabetes* **31,** 1088–1091.

Sadelain, M. W. J., Oin, H. Y., Lauzon, J., and Singh, B. (1990). *Diabetes* **39,** c583–589.

Scharp, D. W., Lacy, P. E., Santiago, J. V., McCullogh, C. S., Weide, L. G., Falqui, L., Marchetti, P., Gingerich, R. L., Jaffe, A. S., Cryer, P. E., Anderson, C. B., and Glye, M. W. (1990). *Diabetes* **39,** 515–518.

Serreze, D. V., Leiter, E. H., Kuff, E. L., Jardieu, P., and Ishizaka, K. (1988). *Diabetes* **37,** 351–358.

Shah, S. C., Malone, J. I., and Simpson, N. E. (1989). *N. Engl. J. Med.* **320,** 550–554.

Silverstein, J., MacLaren, N., Riley, W., Spillar, R., Radjenovic, D., and Johnson, S. (1988). *N. Engl. J. Med.* **319,** 599–604.

Singal, D. P., and Blajchman, M. A. (1973). *Diabetes* **22,** 429–432.

Sochett, E. B., Daneman, D., Clarson, C., and Ehrlich, R. M. (1987). *Diabetologia* **30,** 453–459.

Solinema, M., Folli, F., Aparisi, R., Pozza, G., and Pietro, D. C. (1990). *N. Engl. J. Med.* **322,** 1555–1560.

Southern, P., and Oldstone, M. B. A. (1983). *N. Engl. J. Med.* **314,** 359–367.

Spencer, K. M., Tarn, A., Dean, B. M., Lister, J., and Bottazzo, G. F. (1984). *Lancet* **i,** 764–766.

Spies, T., Bresnahan, M., Bahram, S., Arnold, D., Blanck, G., Mellins, E., Pious, D., and DeMars, R. (1990). *Nature* **348,** 744–747.

Spinas, G. A., Palmer, J. P., Mandrup-Poulsen, T., Andersen, H., Nielsen, J. H., and Nerup, J. (1988). *Acta Endocrinol. (Copenh)* **119,** 307–311.

Srikanta, S., Ganda, O. P., Eisenbarth, G. S., and Soeldner, J. S. (1983). *N. Engl. J. Med.* **308,** 321–325.

Srikanta, S., Ganda, O. P., Gleason, R. E., Jackson, R. A., Soeldner, J. S., and Eisenbarth, G. S. (1984). *Diabetes* **33,** 717–720.

Srikanta, S., Ricker, A. T., McCulloch, D. K., Soeldner, J. S., Eisenbarth, G. S., and Palmer, J. P. (1986). *Diabetes* **35,** 139–142.

Steiner, D. F., Bell, G. I., and Tager, H. S. (Ed.). (1989). "Chemistry and Biosynthesis of Pancreatic Protein Hormones (2nd Ed.). W.B. Saunders, Philadelphia, Pennsylvania.

Strominger, J. L. (1986). *J. Clin. Invest.* **77,** 1411–1415.

Sultz, H. A., Hart, B. A., Zielezny, M., and Schlesinger, E. R. (1975). *J. Pediatr.* **86,** 654–656.

Sutherland, D. E., Moudry, K. C., Goetz, F. C., and Najarian, J. S. (1989). *Transplant. Proc.* **21,** 2845–2849.

Sutherland, D. E. R. (1981). *Diabetologia* **20,** 161–185.

Svenningsen, A., Dyrberg, T., Gerling, I., Lernmark, Å., Mackay, P., and Rabinovitch, A. (1983). *J. Clin. Endocrinol. Metab.* **57,** 1301–1304.

Tarn, A. C., Thomas, J. N., Dean, B. M., Ingram, D., Schwarz, G., Bottazzo, G. F., and Gale, E. A. M. (1988). *Lancet* **i,** 845–850.

Tattersall, R. B. (1986). *Diabetologia* **27,** 167–173.

Tattersall, R. B., and Pyke, D. A. (1972). *Lancet* **ii,** 1120–1125.

The Canadian-European Randomized Control Trial Group (1988). *Diabetes* **37,** 1574–1582.

Thomas, N. M., Ginsberg-Fellner, F., and McEvoy, R. C. (1990). *Diabetes* **39,** 1203–1211.

Thomsen, M., Platz, P., Andersen, O. O., Christy, M., Lyngsoe, J., Nerup, J., Rasmussen, K., Ryder, L. P., Staub-Nielsen, L., and Svejgaard, A. (1975). *Transplant. Proc.* **22,** 125–147.

Thomson, G., Robinson, W. P., Kuhner, M. K., Joe, S., MacDonald, M. J., Gottschall, J. L., Barbosa, J., Rich, S. S., Bertrams, J., Baur, M. P., Partanen, J., Tait, B. D., Schober, E., Mayr, W. R., Ludvigsson, J., Lindblom, B., Farid, N. R., Thompson, C., and Deschamps, I. (1988). *Am. J. Hum. Genet.* **43,** 799–816.

Tillil, H., and Köbberling, J. (1987). *Diabetes* **36,** 93–99.

Tobin, A. (1991). Autoimmunity to two forms of glutamic acid decarboxylase in IDDM. Symposium presentation, 14th International Diabetes Federation Congress, 26 June 1991, Washington, D.C.

Todd, J. A. (1990). *Immunol. Today* **11,** 122–129.

Todd, J. A., Acha-Orbea, H., Bell, J. L., *et al.* (1988). *Science* **240,** 1003–1009.

Todd, J. A., Bell, J. I., and McDevitt, H. O. (1987). *Nature* **329,** 599–604.

Trowsdale, J., Hanson, I., Mockridge, I., Beck, S., Townsend, A., and Kelly, A. (1990). *Nature* **348,** 741–744.

Tuvemo, T., Dahlquist, G., Frisk, G., Blom, L., Friman, G., Landin-Olsson, M., and Diderholm, H. (1989). *Diabetologia* **32,** 745–747.

Van de Winkle, M., Smets, G., Gepts, W., and Pipeleers, D. G. (1982). *J. Clin. Invest.* **70,** 41–49.

Vardi, P., Keller, R., Dib, S., Eisenbarth, G. S., and Soeldner, J. S. (1988a). *Diabetes* **37,** 28A.

Vardi, P., Ziegler, A. G., and Mathews, J. H. (1988b). *Diabetes* **9,** 736–739.

Vercammen, M., Gorus, F., Foriers, A., Segers, O., Somers, G., Van de Winkel, M., and Pipeleers, D. (1989). *Diabetologia* **32,** 611–617.

Vincent, S. T., Hökfelt, T., Wu, J.-Y., Eide, R. P., Morgan, L. M., and Kimmel, J. R. (1983). *Neuroendocrinology* **36,** 197–204.

Wallensteen, M., Dahlquist, G., Persson, B., Landin-Olsson, M., Lernmark, Å., Sundkvist, G., and Thalme, B. (1988). *Diabetologia* **31,** 664–669.

Wassmuth, R., Kockum, I., Nepom, G. T., Holmberg, E., Ludvigsson, J., and Lernmark, Å. (1991). (Submitted for publication).

Wassmuth, R., and Lernmark, Å. (1990). *Clin. Immunol. Immunopathol.* **53,** 358–399.

WHO Study Group (1985). "Diabetes Mellitus." *WHO Technical Report Series,* 727.

Wicker, L. S., Miller, B. J., and Mullen, Y. (1986). *Diabetes* **35,** 855–860.

Wilkin, T., Palmer, J., Bonifacio, E., Diaz, J.-L., and Kruse, V. (1987). *Diabetologia* **30,** 676–677.

Wilkin, T., Palmer, J., Kurtz, A., Bonifacio, E., and Diaz, J.-L. (1988). *Diabetologia* **31,** 449–450.

Wilson, C. A., Jacobs, C., Baker, P., Baskin, D. G., Dower, S., Lernmark, Å., Toivola, B., Vertrees, S., and Wilson, D. (1990). *J. Immunol.* **144,** 3784–3788.

Wilson, R. M., Van der Minne, P., Deverill, I., Heller, S. R., Gelsthorpe, K., Reeves, W. G., and Tattersall, R. B. (1985). *Diabetic Med.* **2,** 167–172.

Yoon, J.-W., Kim, C. J., Pak, C. Y., and McArthur, R. G. (1987). *Clin. Invest. Med.* **10,** 457–469.

Yoon, J. W., Austin, M., Onodera, T., and Notkins, A. L. (1979). *N. Engl. J. Med.* **300,** 1173–1179.

CHAPTER **11**

Autoimmune Vasculitis

J. CHARLES JENNETTE
Department of Pathology
University of North Carolina
School of Medicine
Chapel Hill, North Carolina

DREW A. JONES
Department of Medicine
University of Iowa
Iowa City, Iowa

RONALD J. FALK
Division of Nephrology
Department of Medicine
University of North Carolina
School of Medicine
Chapel Hill, North Carolina

I. INTRODUCTION

Vasculitis is induced by a variety of etiologies and pathogenic mechanisms, all of which mediate vascular inflammatory injury. The two most common mechanisms are direct injury to vessels by infectious pathogens, and immune-mediated inflammation. For example, the systemic vasculitis of the spotted fever rickettsial diseases, such as Rocky Mountain spotted fever, results from the proliferation of pathogens in vessel walls, resulting in vascular necrosis and influx of inflammatory cells. The inflammatory response in infectious vasculitides involves both nonimmune and immune mechanisms, but the former predominate, especially during the initial phases of vascular injury. In those vasculitides in which immune-mediated injury is the primary pathogenic process, infectious pathogens may play an indirect role, but the vascular injury is not produced by direct invasion of vessels by the pathogens. For example, hepatitis B virus infection of the liver can be associated with systemic necrotizing arteritis that is mediated by the deposition in vessel walls of immune complexes containing viral antigens and antibodies against viral antigens (Duffy *et al.*, 1976; Sergent, 1980). However, most immune-mediated vasculitides, including most immune complex-mediated vasculitides, do not have evidence for participation of pathogen-derived antigens. In fact, there is increasing evidence that many, if not most, systemic vasculitides are induced by a variety of autoimmune mechanisms. This chapter will focus on the vasculitides for which there is evidence of autoimmune pathogenesis.

A. Nomenclature of Systemic Vasculitides

There is no universally accepted classification system for the systemic vasculitides, or even an agreement as to what diseases should be considered in the general category of systemic vasculitis (e.g., is the vascular injury of malignant hypertension a vasculitis or a thrombotic microangiopathy?). Classification systems categorize the vasculitides on the basis of pathologic features, clinical syndromes, or pathogenetic mechanism, or most often, a combination of these characteristics. The pathologic features that are usually taken into consideration are type of vessel involved (e.g., large, medium, or small arteries, arterioles, venules, capillaries), and pattern of inflammation (e.g., neutrophil predominance, mononuclear leukocyte predominance, or granulomatous with giant cells). The clinical feature that is most often used in classification is the organ distribution of disease. Categorization of vasculitides based on different patho-

TABLE I
Classification of Immune-Mediated Systemic Vasculitides

Pathogenic mechanism	Clinicopathologic syndrome
Immune Complex mediated	
Immune	Leukocytoclastic angiitis, e.g., secondary to serum sickness
	Polyarteritis nodosa, e.g., secondary to hepatitis B
Autoimmune	Leukocytoclastic angiitis, e.g., cryoglobulinemic
	Polyarteritis nodosa, e.g., secondary to lupus
Direct Antibody Attack	
Anti-basement membrane	Pulmonary-renal syndrome, i.e., Goodpasture's syndrome
Anti-endothelial cell	Kawasaki disease
	Polyarteritis nodosa
Antineutrophil cytoplasmic Autoantibody associated	Wegener's granulomatosis
	Polyarteritis nodosa
	Pulmonary-renal syndrome, with capillaritis
	Churg-Strauss syndrome
Cell mediated	Allograft rejection vasculitis
	Giant-cell arteritis

genic mechanisms is more problematic, because the exact pathogenesis for most vasculitides is presumptive, if not unknown. Nevertheless, Table I attempts to categorize immune-mediated systemic vasculitides based on a combination of pathogenic, clinical, and pathologic features. This categorization demonstrates that autoimmune processes are considered to be a major cause of systemic vasculitis.

B. Autoimmune Pathogenic Mechanisms Causing Vasculitis

Both humoral and cellular autoimmune mechanisms have been implicated in the pathogenesis of vasculitis. In some instances, this is based only on the identification of autoreactive antibodies or lymphocytes with specificity for antigens in vessel walls or for antigens in immune complexes within vessel walls. In other instances, autoimmune pathogenesis is further supported by *in vivo* and *in vitro* experimental data demonstrating pathogenic effects caused by these autoantibodies and autoreactive lymphocytes.

1. Immune Complex Mediation

Although some investigators have concluded that most systemic vasculitides are caused by vascular immune complex deposition (Fauci *et al.*, 1978), others have reported observations that suggest that only a minority of systemic vasculitides are immune complex mediated (Ronco *et al.*, 1983). Rich was one of the earliest proponents of immunologic mediation of vasculitis. This was based both on the clinical observation of polyarteritis nodosa developing in patients who had hypersensitivity responses to horse serum and sulfonamide drugs (Rich, 1942), and on the experimental observation that rabbits injected with horse serum developed necrotizing vasculitis (Rich and Gregory, 1943). Germuth (1953) and Dixon *et al.* (1958) demonstrated that the vascular injury of serum sickness in rabbits was associated with antigen-excess immune complexes in the blood and the presence of immune complexes in vessel walls. The latter was documented by identifying immune complex constituents in vessel walls using immunofluorescence microscopy, which continues to be a standard technique for implicating immune complexes in the pathogenesis of vasculitis (Fig. 1). Whether these immune complexes accrue in vessel walls by deposition from the circulation, by *in situ* formation, or by a combination of these mechanisms has not been completely elucidated (Christian and Sergent, 1976); the pathogenic effects of their presence in vessel walls would be the same no matter which accumulation mechanism took place.

Mural immune complexes cause vascular inflammation by activating the many interconnected humoral and cellular inflammatory mediator systems; for example, the complement, kinin, plasmin, and coagulation humoral systems, and the

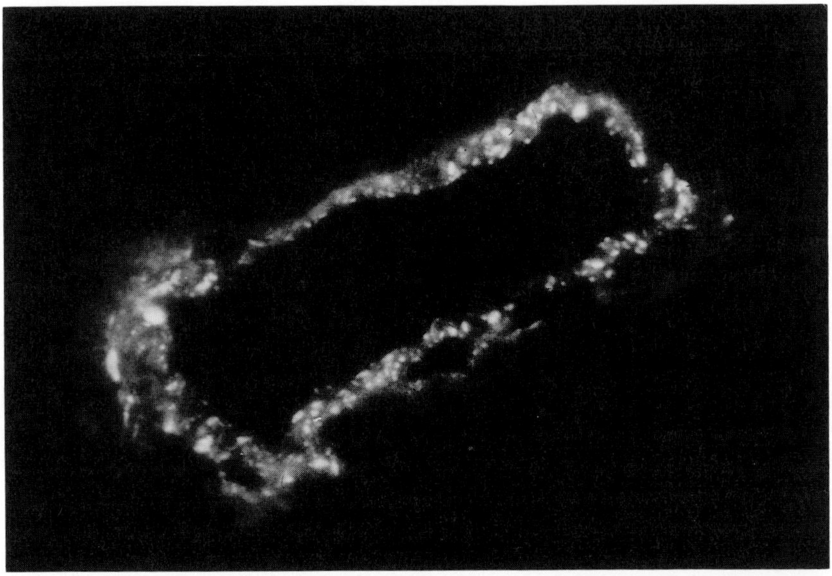

FIG. 1 Direct immunofluorescence micrograph demonstrating granular IgG deposits in an artery from a patient with immune complex-mediated vasculitis.

neutrophil, mononuclear phagocyte, and platelet cellular systems. Endothelial cells and mural smooth muscle cells are capable of modulating vascular inflammation, for example, by producing lipid metabolites with cytokine activity, and, in the case of endothelial cells, by up-regulating leukocyte adhesion molecule and altering surface thrombogenicity (Pober, 1988). This complex interplay of humoral and cellular events results in the pathologic changes that characterize immune complex-mediated necrotizing vasculitis, i.e., influx of inflammatory cells (especially neutrophils), necrosis, and sometimes thrombosis (Fig. 2). It must be realized, however, that this same pathologic phenotype of vascular injury can be produced by other mechanisms that do not involve vascular immune complexes. The pathologic features of immune complex-mediated vascular injury are no different if the constituent antigen is an autoantigen or a heterologous antigen. Autoimmune immune complex-mediated injury can affect vessels ranging in size from capillaries (e.g., lupus glomerulonephritis), to postcapillary venules (e.g., cryoglobulinemic cutaneous leukocytoclastic angiitis), to arteries (e.g., necrotizing arteritis in patients with systemic lupus erythematosus).

2. Direct Autoantibody Attack

Autoantibodies directed against constituents of vessel walls (e.g., endothelial cells and basement membrane) can also mediate vascular injury. The interaction

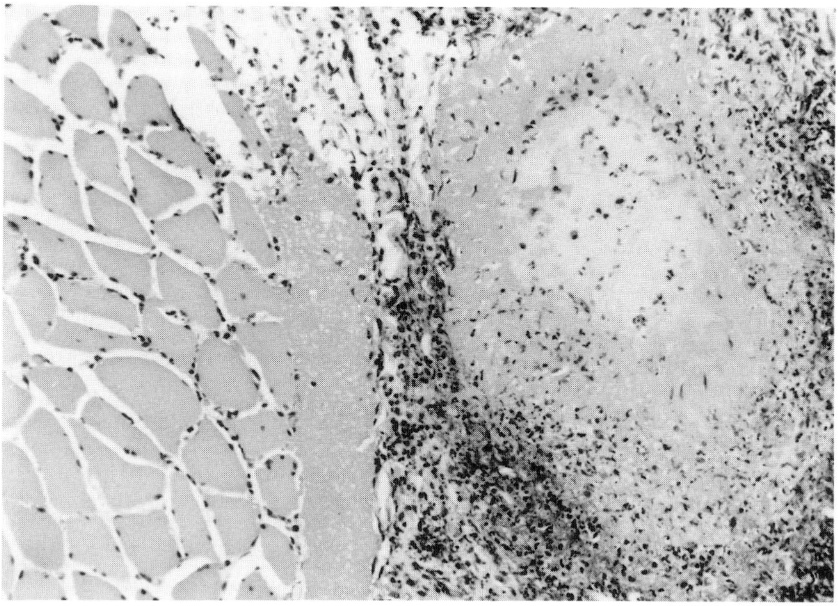

FIG. 2 Artery in a skeletal muscle biopsy from a patient with hepatitis B-associated polyarteritis nodosa demonstrating mural fibrinoid necrosis, leukocyte infiltration, and leukocytoclasia (hemotoxylin and eosin stain).

of an autoantibody with vascular autoantigens may require synergistic events, such as endothelial alterations to expose basement membrane antigens, and induction of expression of surface membrane antigens in endothelial cells. Once autoantibodies are able to bind to antigens in vessel walls, the effect is, in essence, *in situ* immune complex formation. Therefore, the resultant pathogenic events share a common pathway with injury induced by immune complexes that arrive in vessel walls by deposition from the circulation; i.e., activation of humoral and cellular mediators leading to vascular inflammation.

If the autoantigens are of high density in the vessel wall, and adequate autoantibodies are bound, immunofluorescence microscopy will detect the bound autoantibodies. For example, in anti-basement membrane antibody-mediated Goodpasture's syndrome, immunofluorescence microscopy demonstrates linear deposition of immunoglobulin along the basement membranes of glomerular and pulmonary alveolar capillaries (Lerner *et al.*, 1967), which is quite different from the granular vascular staining indicative of immune complex deposits containing nonconstitutive antigens. However, in a number of human and experimental vasculitides in which autoantibodies against vascular antigens (e.g., antiendothelial-cell antibodies) are thought to be of pathogenic importance, no vascular immunoglobulin binding can be detected by immunofluorescence microscopy.

This may be because pathogenic levels of autoantibody binding are below the sensitivity of this detection method.

3. Autoantibody-Induced Leukocyte Activation

A recently postulated mechanism of autoimmune vasculitis proposes that autoantibodies specific for proteins within neutrophil cytoplasmic granules and monocyte lysosomes (e.g., myeloperoxidase and proteinase 3) can cause vascular inflammation (Falk *et al.*, 1990a; Ewert *et al.*, 1991). According to this hypothesis, these antineutrophil cytoplasmic autoantibodies (ANCA) interact with granule and lysosome proteins that are released at the surface of neutrophils and monocytes during synergistic inflammatory processes (such as a viral respiratory tract infection), resulting in intravascular activation of neutrophils and monocytes. These activated leukocytes would in turn activate the interconnected humoral and cellular inflammatory mediators discussed above, causing vasculitis. The patterns of systemic vasculitis in which ANCA have been observed most frequently are Wegener's granulomatosis and microscopic polyarteritis nodosa.

Because all three types of autoantibody-mediated vascular inflammation share a common final pathogenic pathway, it is not surprising that a particular clinical and pathologic phenotype of vasculitis can be produced by entirely different autoimmune pathogenic processes. For example, pulmonary–renal syndrome (i.e., severe pulmonary hemorrhage and glomerulonephritis) can be caused by vascular immune complex deposits (e.g., in mixed cryoglobulinemia and lupus), direct attack by anti-basement membrane autoantibodies (i.e., Goodpasture's syndrome), and putatively by ANCA-induced leukocyte activation (e.g., Wegener's granulomatosis and Churg-Strauss syndrome). Similarly, there is evidence that pathologically indistinguishable systemic necrotizing arteritis can be caused by a variety of humoral mechanisms (e.g., polyarteritis nodosa with demonstrable mural immune complex deposits caused by immune complexes, and polyarteritis nodosa without demonstrable immune complex deposits caused by direct attack by antiendothelial autoantibodies or by leukocytes activated by ANCA).

4. Autoimmune Cell-Mediated Vasculitis

There is less evidence for the participation of autoreactive T lymphocytes in the pathogenesis of vasculitis than there is for autoantibodies. The pathologic features of some vasculitides, for example, the giant cell arteritides and lymphocyte-predominant cutaneous vasculitis, suggest the possibility of a cell-mediated immune pathogenesis, but this has not been confirmed. Because of the granulomatous nature of the inflammation, and the absence of detectable antibodies in the lesions, some investigators have proposed that Wegener's granulomatosis is a form of cell-mediated vasculitis; but there is no compelling evidence to support this.

The best documented example of cell-mediated vasculitis is the T cell-mediated vascular injury that occurs as one form of acute allograft rejection. This lesion is characterized by T lymphocytes adhering to vascular endothelium and penetrating into the intima, and ultimately the muscularis, to produce a vasculitis in which mononuclear leukocytes are the predominant inflammatory cell. This pattern of cell-mediated vasculitis is not well reproduced in any setting that might be considered an autoimmune process.

As will be discussed later in this chapter, there are experimental models of vasculitis in which there is some evidence that autoreactive T lymphocytes are primary pathogenic effectors.

II. VASCULITIS CAUSED BY IMMUNE COMPLEXES CONTAINING AUTOANTIGENS AND AUTOANTIBODIES

A. Human Diseases

1. Lupus Vasculitis

Systemic lupus erythematosus is the archtypical immune complex-mediated autoimmune human disease. Localization of immune complexes in tissues, either by deposition from the circulation or *in situ* formation, is the major pathogenic event in much of the tissue inflammation in lupus patients. Except for glomerular inflammation, which is one of the most frequent lesions in lupus patients, overt vasculitis, especially arteritis, is relatively uncommon. For example, the estimated frequency for cutaneous vasculitis in systemic lupus erythematosus patients is only 10–30% (Watson, 1989).

Those lupus patients who do develop vasculitis can manifest a broad range of pathologic and clinical presentations that are similar to those in patients with nonlupus vasculitides [e.g., small and medium artery necrotizing arteritis morphologically identical to polyarteritis nodosa (Korbet *et al.*, 1984), cutaneous leukocytoclastic angitis (Watson, 1989; Tan and Kunkel, 1966), and pulmonary alveolar capillaritis (Eagen *et al.*, 1978; Myers and Katzenstein, 1986)]. Deposits of immunoglobulin and complement can be demonstrated by immunofluorescence microscopy in the walls of vessels in patients with systemic lupus erythematosus. The vascular immune complexes are presumably the cause of vasculitis; however, in lupus patients, immune complexes can often be demonstrated in the walls of vessels that are not involved with vasculitis.

The classic explanation for vascular injury in systemic lupus erythematosus posited that circulating immune complexes containing autoantigens and autoantibodies (especially DNA and anti-DNA) deposited from the circulation into vessel walls, where they induced inflammatory injury. There is still strong support for this being an important mechanism of injury in lupus, but there is mounting support for vessel wall *in situ* immune-complex formation as a cause for vascular injury. One proposed mechanism suggests that DNA, because of its strong affinity for basement membrane collagen, becomes a planted antigen in vessel walls and acts as a nidus for *in situ* immune-complex formation with anti-DNA autoantibodies (Izui *et al.*, 1976). Another proposed mechanism involves cross-reactivity of anti-DNA autoantibodies with non-DNA vessel wall antigens, such as glycosaminoglycans (Winfield *et al.*, 1975; Maddison and Reichlin, 1979).

There is evidence that lupus sera contain immune complexes and antiendothelial cell autoantibodies that can bind directly to endothelial cells (Cines *et al.*, 1984). This leads to complement activation and endothelial damage, which *in vitro* is manifested by loss of cell adhesion, secretion of PGI_2, and adherence of platelets.

A role for immune complexes in the pathogenesis of vasculitis in other connective tissue diseases has been proposed, for example, in rheumatoid arthritis (Breedveld *et al.*, 1988) and Sjögren's syndrome (Molina *et al.*, 1985; Tsokos *et al.*, 1987).

2. Cryoglobulinemic Vasculitis

Cryoglobulins can be divided into three major types: (1) monoclonal, (2) mixed monoclonal–polyclonal, and (3) polyclonal. Cryoglobulins often contain anti-immunoglobulin autoantibodies (Grey and Kohler, 1973). Mixed cryoglobulins are more pathogenic than are monoclonal or polyclonal cryoglobulins. Monoclonal cryoglobulins usually occur in patients with plasma cell dyscrasias or B-cell lymphomas, and cause morbidity primarily by precipitating within vessels and producing occlusion. Monoclonal cryoglobulins are not effective activators of inflammatory mediator systems, and therefore rarely cause overt vasculitis. Mixed cryoglobulins, however, are immune complexes that are capable of activating inflammatory mediators, including the complement system, and therefore characteristically cause systemic vasculitis.

Mixed cryoglobulinemic vasculitis can affect vessels of many types, including small and medium-sized arteries, postcapillary venules (e.g., in the skin), and glomerular and pulmonary alveolar capillaries (Gorevic *et al.*, 1980). Immunofluorescence microscopy reveals granular deposits of immunoglobulins and complement in vessel walls, and sometimes lumenal aggregates of cryoglobulins and complement. The clinical and pathologic manifestations of cryoglobulinemic vasculitis overlap with those of other systemic vasculitides, and include purpura with leukocytoclastic angiitis, glomerulonephritis, and, in severe cases, pulmonary hemorrhage with alveolar capillaritis. As with many systemic vasculitides, arthralgias and arthritis caused by synovitis are a common feature.

Antiimmunoglobulin autoantibodies may participate in pathogenic immune complex formation other than that of mixed cryoglobulinemia. Both anti-Fc rheumatoid factorlike autoantibodies and anti-Fab antiidiotypic antibodies may accrete onto immune complexes containing other antigen–antibody systems. This antiimmunoglobulin binding could then enhance the pathogenicity of the immune complexes.

B. Animal Models

The best animal models of immune complex-mediated vasculitis are induced by injection of heterologous proteins, e.g., serum sickness in rabbits (Rich and Gregory, 1943; Germuth, 1953; Dixon *et al.*, 1958). Such models have shed a great deal of light on the characteristics of immune complexes, vessel walls, and inflammatory mediator systems that influence vascular injury by immune complexes (Cochrane and Koffler, 1973). Vascular-wall immune complexes may play a role in virus-induced vasculitis, such as that in Aleutian mink virus disease and murine lymphocytic choriomeningitis virus disease (Gunby, 1984). However, there is no evidence that these animal models of vasculitis involve autoimmune events.

Because vasculitis in patients with systemic lupus erythematosus is thought to be an example of immune complex-mediated autoimmune vasculitis, a reasonable place to look for an animal model of immune complex-mediated autoimmune vasculitis would be in mice with lupus-like diseases, such as NZB/W, BXSB, and MRL/lpr mice. Of these strains, MRL/lpr have the highest frequency of vasculitis; but, as will be discussed later in this chapter, there is no strong evidence that it is immune complex-mediated, and considerable evidence that it is not.

Although NZB/W and BXSB mice have a very high incidence of immune complex-mediated glomerulonephritis (in fact, much more so than MRL/lpr mice), they rarely have true vasculitis elsewhere. This is reminiscent of lupus patients who also have high-frequency glomerulonephritis but low-frequency extraglomerular vasculitis. When arteritis does occur in NZB/W and BXSB mice (for example, coronary arteritis), immunoglobulins and complement often are demonstrable in vessel walls; however, some of the vasculitis in lupus mice has pathologic features that do not suggest immune-complex pathogenesis (Staszak and Harbeck, 1985).

Gyotoku *et al.* (1987) have described an experimental model of cryoglobulinemic vasculitis. They established monoclonal IgG rheumatoid factor-secreting hybridomas from MRL/lpr mice. These monoclonal rheumatoid factor antibodies were capable of forming cryoglobulins, and, when injected into normal mice, caused peripheral vasculitis and glomerulonephritis resembling that seen in patients with mixed cryoglobulinemia.

III. VASCULITIS CAUSED BY AUTOANTIBODIES SPECIFIC FOR VESSEL-WALL AUTOANTIGENS

A. Human Diseases

Until recently, the only example of vascular injury caused by direct binding of an autoantibody to constitutive vessel-wall molecules was anti-basement membrane disease. The presence of these autoantibodies can be demonstrated by the relatively insensitive techniques of direct and indirect immunofluorescence microscopy. The advent of better cell-culture techniques and more sensitive immunochemical assays has allowed a more careful search for autoantibodies that react with vessel-wall antigens. Antiendothelial autoantibodies have been detected using these more sensitive techniques. In the future, additional pathogenic autoantibodies may come to light via this approach.

1. Anti-Basement Membrane Autoantibodies

The first human vascular disease in which autoantibodies against vessel-wall constituents were shown to be pathogenic was Goodpasture's syndrome. Lerner *et al.* (1967) established the pathogenic role of anti-basement membrane autoantibodies in patients with pulmonary hemorrhage and glomerulonephritis (i.e., Goodpasture's syndrome). They demonstrated the presence of anti-basement membrane autoantibodies in the walls of injured vessels and in the circulation, and transferred the disease to monkeys using patient serum and tissue eluates.

The vascular injury caused by anti-basement membrane autoantibodies is almost totally confined to glomerular and pulmonary alveolar capillaries; however, rare patients also will have vasculitis affecting arterioles and small arteries (Ming-Jiang *et al.*, 1980). We have seen three patients with anti-basement membrane autoantibodies who had typical pulmonary and glomerular changes of Goodpasture's syndrome along with the presence of necrotizing arteritis; but all three patients also had antineutrophil cytoplasmic autoantibodies, which are frequently associated with arteritis. Therefore, these patients could represent concurrent expression of both anti-basement membrane autoantibody and antineutrophil cytoplasmic autoantibody disease.

2. Antiendothelial Autoantibodies

As mentioned previously, antiendothelial antibodies have been incriminated as a pathogenic factor in vascular injury in patients with systemic lupus erythematosus (Cines *et al.*, 1984). Antiendothelial autoantibodies also have been identified in patients with other forms of vascular injury (Cines, 1989), including Kawasaki disease (Leung *et al.*, 1986a), rheumatoid vasculitis (Heurkens *et al.*, 1989), IgA nephropathy (Yap *et al.*, 1988), hemolytic uremic syndrome (Leung *et al.*, 1988), Wegener's granulomatosis (Frampton *et al.*, 1990), and polyarteritis nodosa (Framptom *et al.*, 1990).

The pathogenic potential of antiendothelial autoantibodies has been studied most extensively in Kawasaki disease. Kawasaki disease is a systemic necrotizing arteritis that affects children predominantly. It was first described in Japan (Kawasaki, 1967), but occurs worldwide, and is a major cause of childhood cardiac disease. Clinical manifestations include fever, polymorphous erythematous rash, diffuse mucosal inflammation, nonsuppurative lymphadenopathy, indurative edema of extremities, and, in some patients, cardiac failure secondary to coronary arteritis (Kawasaki *et al.*, 1974; Rauch and Hurwitz, 1985). Pathologically, a necrotizing vasculitis affects small and medium-sized arteries, arterioles, and venules throughout the body, with frequent involvement of the coronary arteries. Because of these clinical and pathologic features, alternative names for Kawasaki disease are mucocutaneous lymph node syndrome (Kawasaki *et al.*, 1974), and infantile polyarteritis nodosa (Magilavy *et al.*, 1977).

Leung and associates (1986a, 1986b) have studied autoimmune events in Kawasaki disease that appear to be involved in the pathogenesis of vasculitis. They have observed that patients with Kawasaki disease have circulating autoantibodies that react with cytokine-inducible non-major histocompatibility complex (MHC) molecules on endothelial cells, resulting in endothelial cell lysis *in vitro*. Specifically, they detected IgG and IgM antiendothelial autoantibodies that caused complement-mediated lysis of human umbilical and saphenous vein endothelial cells that had been pretreated with gamma interferon, interleukin-1, or tumor necrosis factor. From these observations, a pathogenic mechanism for vasculitis in Kawasaki disease would entail two events; production of antiendothelial autoantibodies (possibly related to the polyclonal B-cell activation that occurs in Kawasaki disease patients), and increased cytokine production (possibly related to the increased activity of CD4 T lymphocytes and monocytes that also occurs in Kawasaki disease patients). The antiendothelial autoantibodies would bind to up-regulated endothelial antigens, and cause endothelial death and vascular inflammation.

High-dose intravenous gamma globulin has therapeutic benefits in patients with Kawasaki disease (Furusho *et al.*, 1984; Nagashima *et al.*, 1987; Rowley *et al.*, 1988). If the interaction of antiendothelial autoantibodies with cytokine-activated endothelial cells is the major pathogenic mechanism in Kawasaki disease, intravenous gamma globulin could be acting by reducing (e.g., through negative feedback control) or neutralizing (e.g., by antiidiotypic binding) antiendothelial autoantibodies, or by preventing cytokine stimulation of endothelial cells. Leung *et al.* (1989) have studied these possibilities, and have concluded that the beneficial effects of intravenous gamma globulin result from reduced circulating cytokines and reduced endothelial cell activation, and not from reduced antiendothelial autoantibody activity.

Antiendothelial autoantibodies have recently been described in adults with polyarteritis nodosa and Wegener's granulomatosis (Frampton *et al.*, 1990). As will be discussed later, these patients also have circulating antineutrophil cytoplasmic autoantibodies. Frampton *et al.* (1990) suggest that the antiendothelial autoantibodies and antineutrophil cytoplasmic autoantibodies in these patients may in fact react with molecules that are shared by endothelial cell and neutrophils.

B. Animal Models

Although experimental antiendothelial autoantibody-mediated vascular injury has been reported (Hart *et al.*, 1981), the only extensively studied animal models of vascular injury induced by direct autoantibody attack involve anti-basement membrane antibodies.

Experimental anti-basement membrane autoantibody-mediated disease can be induced either by active immunization of an animal with basement membrane antigens (Steblay, 1962), or by passive administration of anti-basement membrane antibodies (Hammer and Dixon, 1963). As with the analogous human disease, vascular injury is essentially confined to glomerular capillaries and pulmonary alveolar capillaries. This indicates that anti-basement membrane autoantibodies have a limited pathogenic potential for inducing vascular inflammation, probably because of the inaccessibility of basement membrane antigens in most vessels to circulating antibodies.

IV. VASCULITIS ASSOCIATED WITH ANTINEUTROPHIL CYTOPLASMIC AUTOANTIBODIES

Two of the most common forms of systemic vasculitis are polyarteritis nodosa and Wegener's granulomatosis. Although these diseases have long been thought to be mediated by immune mechanisms, until recently, there has been little evidence for immunopathogenic processes in most patients with polyarteritis nodosa and Wegener's granulomatosis. For example, Ronco *et al.* (1983) studied 43 patients with polyarteritis nodosa and Wegener's granulomatosis looking for evidence of immune-complex mediation. They observed that only a minority of patients had vascular immunoglobulin deposits or detectable circulating immune complexes, and none had hypocomplementemia. They suggested the possibility that most polyarteritis nodosa and Wegener's granulomatosis is not mediated by immune complexes, which was contrary to some of the conventional wisdom at the time.

The discovery of a specific class of autoantibodies in the circulation of most patients with polyarteritis nodosa and virtually all patients with Wegener's granulomatosis has suggested a new mechanism of autoimmune injury that involves autoantibody-mediated leukocyte activation (Falk *et al.*, 1990a; Ewert *et al.*, 1991). These autoantibodies react with proteins in the cytoplasmic granules of neutrophils and lysosomes of monocytes, and are called antineutrophil cytoplasmic autoantibodies (ANCA) (reviewed by Jennette and Falk, 1990a).

A. Human Diseases

ANCA were first reported in the serum of patients with systemic vasculitis and necrotizing glomerulonephritis, most of whom also had inflammatory pulmonary disease (Davies *et al.*, 1982; Hall *et al.*, 1984). In 1985, a collaborative study from The Netherlands and Denmark documented a strong association between ANCA and active Wegener's granulomatosis (van der Woude *et al.*, 1985). Subsequent studies have revealed the presence of ANCA in patients with polyarteritis nodosa, Churg-Strauss syndrome, and "idiopathic" crescentic glomerulonephritis (Savage *et al.*, 1987; Venning *et al.*, 1987; Wathen and Harrison, 1987; Falk and Jennette, 1988; Jennette *et al.*, 1989; Cohen Tervaert *et al.*, 1990).

Although ANCA-associated diseases have varied clinical expressions, primarily because of different organ distributions of vasculitis, there is a basic pathologic vascular lesion that is shared among patients with different syndromes and among different types of vessels in a given patient (Jennette *et al.*, 1989; Jennette, 1991). This lesion is characterized by mural fibrinoid necrosis with karyorrhexis and infiltrating leukocytes. Neutrophils predominate in early lesions, and mononuclear leukocytes in later lesions. The only pathologic change that is relatively segregated into a specific syndrome is granulomatous inflammation, which is found in patients with Wegener's granulomatosis. Wegener's granulomatosis patients, however, also have other nongranulomatous vascular lesions identical to those in patients with other ANCA-associated clinical syndromes. A common vascular lesion in patients with ANCA-associated diseases is a necrotizing and crescentic glomerulonephritis, which can occur as the only vascular lesion in some patients. By immunofluorescence microscopy, all the vascular lesions of ANCA-associated diseases are characterized by the absence or paucity of immunoglobulin deposits in vessel walls.

As is true for antinuclear antibodies, there are ANCA with different specificities. When detected by indirect immunofluorescence microscopy using alcohol-fixed neutrophils as substrate, this diverse specificity is reflected in two staining patterns: cytoplasmic (C-ANCA) and perinuclear (P-ANCA) (Fig. 3).

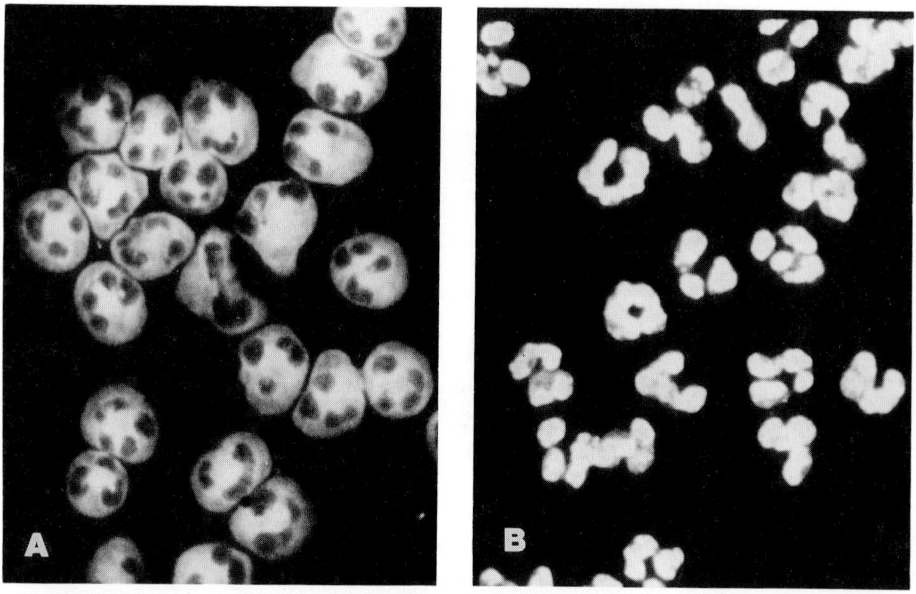

FIG. 3 Indirect immunofluorescence staining of alcohol-fixed normal human neutrophils caused by C-ANCA (A) and P-ANCA (B). Alcohol-fixed neutrophils were first incubated with human serum, followed by fluorescein-conjugated antihuman IgG.

The perinuclear distribution of antigen is an artifact of substrate preparation. The antigens that react with P-ANCA are in the cytoplasm *in vivo,* but become solubilized during substrate preparation, and diffuse to and bind to the nuclei (Charles *et al.*, 1989). When analyzed by specific immunoassays, the most frequent C-ANCA specificity is for proteinase 3 (PR3) (Jennette *et al.*, 1990b; Ludemann *et al.*, 1990), and the most frequent P-ANCA specificity is for myeloperoxidase (MPO) (Falk and Jennette, 1988). A less frequent C-ANCA specificity is for 57-kDa cationic protein (Falk *et al.*, 1990c), and a less frequent P-ANCA specificity is for elastase (Goldschmeding *et al.*, 1989).

Although there is a great deal of overlap, the specificity of ANCA does correlate to a degree with the clinical expression of vasculitis (Fig. 4) (Jennette and Falk, 1990a; Jennette 1991). For example, patients with active Wegener's granulomatosis in whom granulomatous inflammation has been documented pathologically have a greater than 90% frequency of C-ANCA, whereas patients with ANCA-associated vascular injury confined to the renal glomeruli most often have P-ANCA.

In patients with polyarteritis nodosa and Wegener's granulomatosis, the high frequency of ANCA in the circulation, the correlation of ANCA titers with

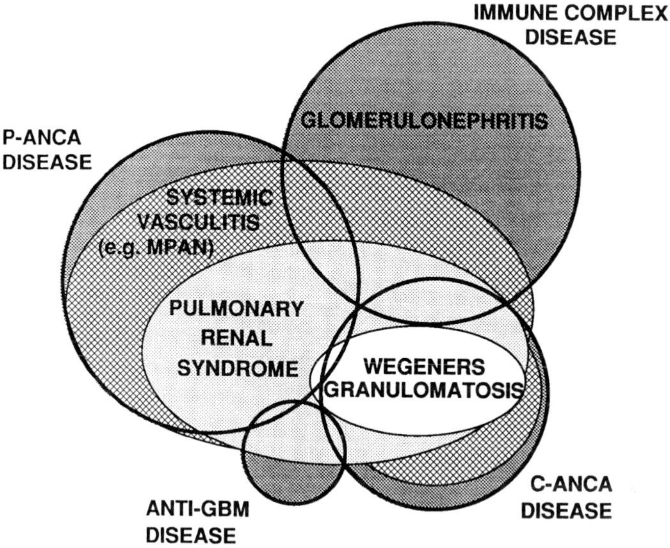

FIG. 4 Diagram representing the distribution of different types of vasculitis and glomerulonephritis with respect to the four major immunopathologic categories (i.e., immune complex disease, anti-GBM disease, C-ANCA disease, and P-ANCA disease) represented by the four circles. Note that a given type of vasculitis, e.g., microscopic polyarteritis nodosa (MPAN) can be caused by more than one immunopathogenic mechanism. Modified from Jennette (1991) with permission.

disease activity (Nolle *et al.*, 1989), and the absence of strong evidence for an alternative pathogenic mechanism, raise the possibility that ANCA have a role in disease induction. Falk *et al.* (1990a) have proposed that ANCA are able to interact with cytokine-primed neutrophils to cause total neutrophil activation. This is supported by the *in vitro* observations that ANCA incubated with primed neutrophils induce the release of toxic reactive oxygen species and the release of lytic granule enzymes (Fig. 5). Neutrophil priming, as occurs with exposure to certain cytokines, results in the expression of small amounts of ANCA-antigens at the surface of neutrophils where they can interact with ANCA, resulting in neutrophil activation.

Ewert *et al.* (1991) have demonstrated that ANCA-activated neutrophils can injure endothelial cells *in vitro*. If this process occurs *in vivo*, it would cause vasculitis.

According to the hypothesis of Falk *et al.*, ANCA-associated diseases occur in patients with circulating ANCA who develop some synergistic inflammatory process (such as a viral respiratory tract disease) that primes neutrophils and monocytes so that they can be activated with vessels by ANCA.

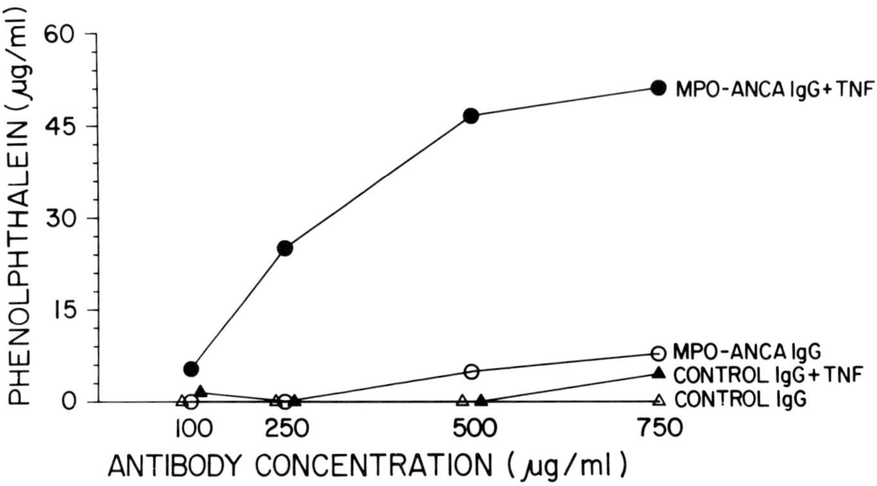

FIG. 5 Degranulation of neutrophils after priming with tumor necrosis factor (TNF) and incubation with myeloperoxidase (MPO)-specific ANCA as measured by the cleavage of phenolphthalein from phenolphthalein glucuronic acid by beta glucuronidase. Note that synergism between ANCA and the cytokine is required for activation. From Falk *et al.* (1990a) with permission.

1. Wegener's Granulomatosis

As mentioned above, active Wegener's granulomatosis has a very high frequency of ANCA. As defined by Godman and Churg (1954), Wegener's granulomatosis is characterized by necrotizing granulomatous inflammation of the upper or lower respiratory tract, necrotizing arteritis, and necrotizing glomerulonephritis. The term limited Wegener's granulomatosis has been used for patients who do not express all three components of the syndrome, especially whose with exclusively respiratory tract disease (Carrington and Liebow, 1966). There is some uncertainty about the absolute requirement for granulomatous inflammation to make a diagnosis of Wegener's granulomatosis, because some patients with the syndrome of severe respiratory vascular inflammation, systemic arteritis, and necrotizing glomerulonephritis will have pulmonary capillaritis rather than granulomatous inflammation (Yoshikawa and Watanabe, 1986).

The definition of Wegener's granulomatosis being used has a bearing on the sensitivity and specificity of C-ANCA for Wegener's granulomatosis. As depicted in Fig. 4, when a strict Godman and Churg definition of Wegener's granulomatosis is used, C-ANCA are very sensitive (but not very specific) for Wegener's granulomatosis, but when all cases of pulmonary–renal–sinus syndrome are considered to be Wegener's granulomatosis, C-ANCA are less sensitive, since many patients will have P-ANCA rather than C-ANCA.

2. Polyarteritis Nodosa

As discussed earlier and reflected in Table I, the pathologic phenotype called polyarteritis nodosa can apparently be caused by multiple pathogenic mechanisms (Fig. 4). In our experience, most patients with polyarteritis nodosa have ANCA, with an almost equal frequency of C-ANCA and P-ANCA (Jennette and Falk, 1990a).

The earliest detailed description of polyarteritis nodosa was by Kussmaul and Maier (1866). They reported a patient with fever, muscle weakness, gastrointestinal symptoms, and renal disease who was found at autopsy to have vascular inflammation of medium and small arteries, arterioles, and glomeruli. A workable clinical and pathologic definition of polyarteritis nodosa is somewhat elusive, but a reasonably practical one is systemic necrotizing arteritis with no evidence for a more specific vasculitic syndrome (e.g., no evidence for Wegener's granulomatosis, Churg–Strauss syndrome, or Kawasaki disease) (Rosen *et al.*, 1991).

Although medium-sized artery-necrotizing arteritis is the classic lesion of polyarteritis nodosa, patients with polyarteritis nodosa typically have vasculitis affecting many different types of vessels, including small arteries (Fig. 6),

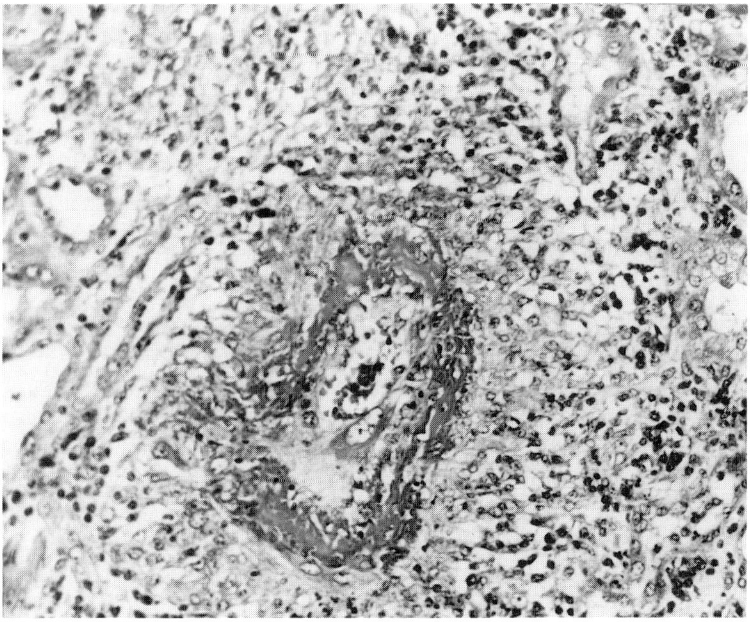

FIG. 6 ANCA-associated necrotizing arteritis in an artery demonstrating fibrinoid necrosis and inflammatory cell infiltration (Masson trichrome stain).

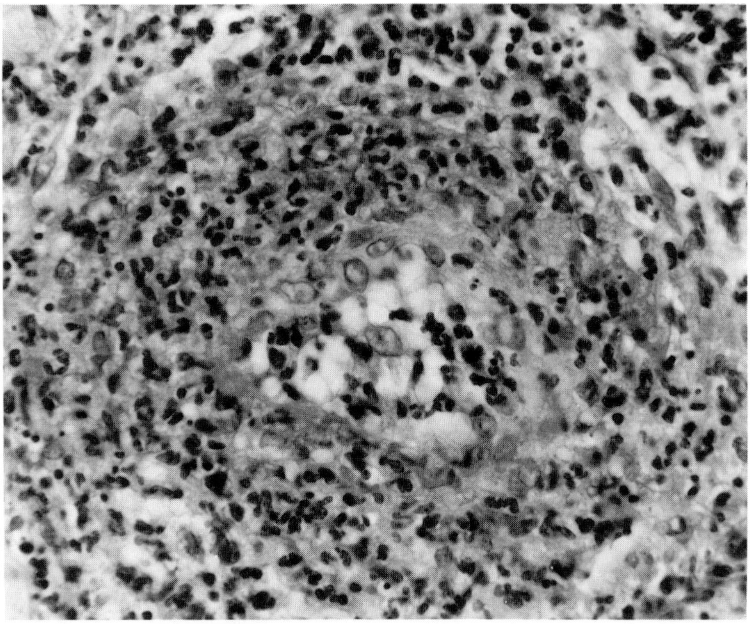

FIG. 7 ANCA-associated dermal angiitis demonstrating intense neutrophilic infiltration and leukocytoclasia (hematoxylin and eosin stain).

arterioles, postcapillary venules (Fig. 7), and glomerular capillaries. In addition to affecting many different types of vessels, many different organs can be involved, including muscle, nerves, gut, heart, and kidneys. Therefore, the clinical features of polyarteritis nodosa are protean, and the disease is often a differential consideration in a patient with an undiagnosed multisystem disease. In such patients, an ANCA test can be useful for supporting a diagnosis of polyarteritis nodosa.

In patients with polyarteritis nodosa affecting vessels no smaller than main visceral arteries (i.e., no involvement of arterioles or glomeruli) ANCA are rarely if ever present; but this variant of polyarteritis nodosa is uncommon. Most patients with polyarteritis nodosa have vascular inflammation involving not only arteries, but also arterioles and glomeruli; and these patients often have ANCA.

The usual treatment for polyarteritis nodosa, and other ANCA-associated diseases, such as Wegener's granulomatosis and severe crescentic glomerulonephritis, is aggressive immunosuppression. This most often entails steroid (e.g., pulse methylprednisolone), cytotoxic drug (e.g., oral or intravenous cyclophosphamide), or combined steroid and cytotoxic drug treatment (Falk *et al.*, 1990b). Plasmapheresis and high-dose intravenous gammaglobulin are advocated by some, but their efficacy has not been well documented.

B. Animal Models

To date, no animal models of ANCA-associated disease have been published. Proof that ANCA are in fact capable of causing vasculitis, rather than being a serologic epiphenomenon, will probably await experiments in *in vivo* models. We have several potential *in vivo* models under development, but the data are too preliminary to report at this time. One problem in the design of animal models is the lack of reactivity of human ANCA with neutrophils from animals other than primates.

V. Vasculitis Caused by Cell-Mediated Vascular Damage

A. Human Diseases

As was stated earlier, the evidence that any forms of human vasculitis are caused by cell-mediated autoimmune mechanisms is circumstantial and weak. Observations that are used to incriminate a cell-mediated pathogenesis include a predominance of mononuclear leukocytes in the inflammatory infiltrates, and absence of substantial immunoglobulin and complement in vessel walls. Obviously, such evidence does not prove cell-mediated immune pathogenesis.

Vasculitides that have most often been considered candidates for cell-mediated pathogenesis are the giant-cell arteritides (e.g., Takayasu's aortitis and giant-cell temporal arteritis) (Hamilton *et al.*, 1971), and Wegener's granulomatosis. As noted earlier, there are now data that raise the possibility that Wegener's granulomatosis is mediated by autoantibody-induced leukocyte activation rather than by a T cell-mediated inflammatory process.

The only form of human vasculitis for which there is a clear-cut, cell-mediated immune pathogenesis is acute cellular vascular rejection occurring in an allograft. Cell-mediated vascular rejection is most likely directed against endothelial cell MHC antigens. Autoimmune responses directed at MHC antigens are uncommon. Therefore, it may be that autoimmune cell-mediated vasculitis is uncommon because of this infrequency of T-cell autoimmunity against MHC antigens.

B. Animal Models

1. MRL/lpr Mice

Vasculitis in MRL/lpr mice has been proposed as a model of cell-mediated autoimmune vasculitis (Moyer *et al.*, 1987; Moyer and Reinisch, 1989).

MRL/lpr mice spontaneously develop a lymphoproliferative disease characterized morphologically by lymphoid hyperplasia in many tissues; and immunologically by increased numbers of helper/inducer T cells, polyclonal B-cell activation, and production of autoantibodies (e.g., antinuclear antibodies and rheumatoid factor), and autoreactive T cells. Presumably as a result of these immunologic abnormalities, MRL/lpr mice develop autoimmune diseases that resemble a number of human diseases, including systemic lupus erythematosus, rheumatoid arthritis, Sjögren's syndrome, graft-versus-host syndrome, glomerulonephritis, and vasculitis (Fig. 8) (Moyer *et al.*, 1987).

MRL vasculitis has varied morphologic appearances, with some lesions having a predominance of neutrophils and others, a predominance of mononuclear leukocytes (sometimes with a granulomatous character). The appearance of the former lesions suggests an antibody-mediated process and that of the latter, a cell-mediated process thus suggesting that more than one pathogenic mechanism might be operational in MRL mice. Alexander (1986), however, concludes that the mononuclear leukocyte-predominant vasculitis can evolve into neutrophil-predominant vasculitis. When examined by immunofluorescence microscopy, the vasculitic lesions in MRL/lpr mice contain no or very little immunoglobulin and complement; therefore, an immune complex-mediated pathogenesis is unlikely.

Moyer and Reinisch (1984, 1989) have reported data that support the hypoth-

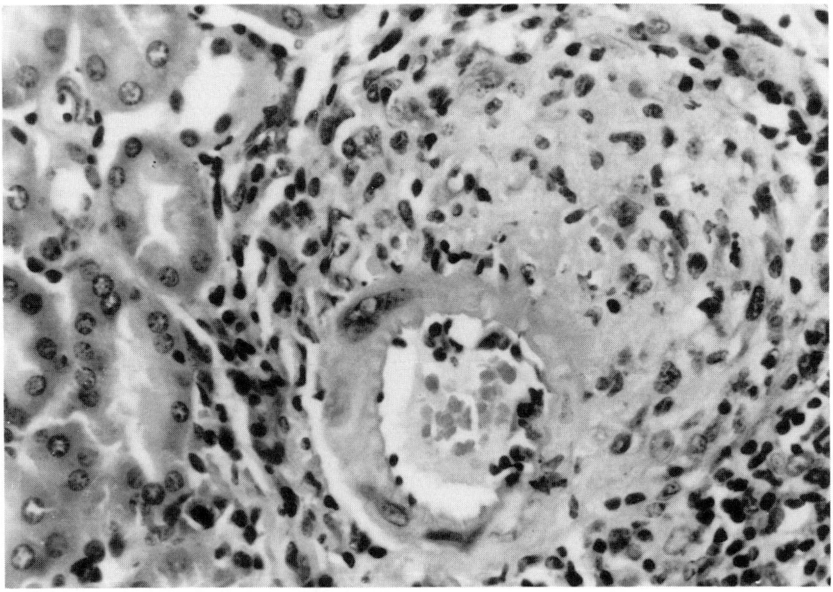

FIG. 8 Vasculitis affecting a small renal artery in an MRL/lpr mouse (hemoatoxylin and eosin stain).

esis that MRL/lpr vasculitis, at least the mononuclear leukocyte-rich form, is induced by cell-mediated attack against vascular smooth muscle cells. When they cocultured MRL/lpr vascular smooth muscle cells with MRL/lpr (autoimmune) or H-2 histocompatible C3H (normal) splenocytes, massive mononuclear leukocyte clusters enveloped the smooth muscle cells and caused detachment from the tissue culture plates. This event did not occur when C3H vascular smooth muscle cells were cocultured with MRL/lpr or C3H splenocytes. Moyer and Reinisch (1989) postulate that "vascular smooth muscle cells derived from autoimmune, but not normal, mice stimulate a mononuclear inflammatory response which culminates in autoimmune vascular smooth muscle destruction." They further propose that the targets of this autoimmune response are aberrantly expressed Ia-d antigens on vascular smooth muscle cells.

In support of more than one pathogenic mechanism of vascular injury in MRL mice are the observations of Nose *et al.* (1989). They used genetic manipulations to demonstrate that the development of the autoimmune glomerulonephritis and vasculitis could be dissociated, thus suggesting independent pathogenic mechanisms for glomerular and extraglomerular vascular injury.

2. Murine Vasculitis Caused by Lymphocytes Sensitized against Vessel Wall Cells

Hart and associates (1983, 1985) developed experimental models of vasculitis that are induced by first coculturing murine lymphocytes with endothelial cells or vascular smooth muscle cells, and then injected the lymphocytes into syngeneic mice.

Mice injected with endothelium-activated lymphocytes developed vasculitis in small and medium-sized veins and in arterioles (Hart *et al.*, 1983). The vasculitis was observed in many organs, including lungs and brain. The vascular lesions were characterized by mural and perivascular mononuclear leukocyte infiltration, sometimes accompanied by eosinophils and neutrophils.

Mice injected with smooth muscle cell-activated lymphocytes also developed a mononuclear leukocyte-predominant vasculitis (Hart *et al.*, 1985). Unlike the previous model, in approximately 20% of animals, the vascular inflammation was granulomatous and displayed substantial medial involvement.

The mechanism by which lymphocytes that have been cocultured with vascular cells cause vasculitis is unknown. One hypothesis is that subpopulations of lymphocytes with autospecificity are activated, undergo clonal expansion, and are then capable of mediating autoimmune vasculitis.

VI. SUMMARY

A variety of autoimmune pathogenic mechanisms mediate vasculitis. Clinically, and even pathologically, identical disease can be produced by distinctly different mechanisms; and a given pathogenic mechanism can produce more than one clinical and pathologic pattern of vasculitic disease. In addition, because different organs can be affected in different patients, the clinical manifestations of even relatively specific types of vasculitis are protean. Therefore, the classification (i.e., diagnosis) of systemic vasculitis, including autoimmune vasculitis, is problematic, and requires the integration of clinical, pathologic, and laboratory data.

REFERENCES

Alexander, E. L. (1986). *Scand. J. Rheumatol. (Suppl.)* **61,** 280–285.

Breedveld, F. C., Heurkens, A. H., Lafeber, G. J., van-Hinsbergh, V. W., and Cats, A. (1988). *Clin. Immunol. Immunopathol.* **48,** 202–213.

Carrington, C. B., and Liebow, A. A. (1966). *Am. J. Med.* **41,** 497–527.

Charles, L. A., Falk, R. J., and Jennette, J. C. (1989). *Clin. Immunol. Immunopathol.* **53,** 243–253.

Christian, C. L., and Sergent, J. S. (1976). *Am. J. Med.* **61,** 385–392.

Cines, D. B. (1989). *Rev. Infect. Dis.* **11,** 705–711.

Cines, D. B., Lyss, A. P., Reeber, M., Bina, M., and DeHoratius, R. J. (1984). *J. Clin. Invest.* **73,** 611–625.

Cochrane, C. G., and Koffler, D. (1973). *Adv. Immunol.* **16,** 185–264.

Cohen Tervaert, J. W., Goldschmeding, R., Elema, J. D., van der Giessen, M., Huitema, M. G., van der Hem, G. K., The, T. H., von dem Borne, A. E. G., Jr., and Kallenberg, C. G. M. (1990). *Kidney Int.* **37,** 799–806.

Davies, D. J., Moran, J. E., Niall, J. F., and Ryan, G. B. (1982). *Br. Med. J.* **285,** 606.

Dixon, F. J., Wazuez, J. J., and Weigle, W. O. (1958). *Arch. Pathol.* **65,** 18–28.

Duffy, J., Lidsky, M. D., Sharp, J. T., Davis, J. S., Person, D. A., Hollinger, F. B., and Min, K.-W. (1976). *Medicine* **5,** 19–37.

Eagen, J. W., Memoli, V. A., Robert, J. L., Matthew, G. R., Schwartz, M. M., and Lewis, E. J. L. (1978). *Medicine* **57,** 545–560.

Ewert, B. H., Jennette, J. C., and Falk, R. J. (1991). *Am. J. Kidney Dis.* **18,** 188–193.

Falk, R. J., and Jennette, J. C. (1988). *N. Engl. J. Med.* **318,** 1651–1657.

Falk, R. J., Terrell, R. S., Charles, L. A., and Jennette, J. C. (1990a). *Proc. Natl. Acad. Sci. U.S.A.* **87,** 4115–4119.

Falk, R. J., Hogan S., Carey, T. S., and Jennette, J. C. (1990b). *Ann. Intern. Med.* **113,** 656–663.

Falk, R. J., Becker, M., Pereia, H. A., Spitznagel, J. K., Hoidal, J., and Jennette, J. C. (1990c). *Blood* submitted.

Fauci, A. S., Haynes, B. F., and Katz, P. (1978). *Ann. Intern. Med.* **89,** 660–676.

Frampton, G., Perry, G. J., Jayne, D., Lockwood, C. M., and Cameron, J. S. (1990). *Proceedings of the XIth International Congress of Nephrology (Tokyo, Japan)* 340A.

Fursusho, K., Nakano, H., Shinomiya, K., *et al.* (1984). *Lancet* **2,** 1055–1061.

Germuth, F. G. (1953). *J. Exp. Med.* **97,** 257–282.

Godman, G. C. and Churg, J. (1954). *Arch. Pathol.* **58,** 533–553.

Goldschmeding, R., van der Schoot, C. E., ten Bokkel Huinink, D., Hack, C. E., van den Ende, M. E., Kallenberg, C. G. M., and von dem Borne, A. E. G., Jr. (1989). *J. Clin. Invest.* **84,** 1577–1587.

Gorevic, P. D., Kasab, H. J., Levo, Y., Kohn, R., Meltzer, M., Prose, P., and Franklin, E. C. (1980). *Am. J. Med.* **69,** 287–308.

Grey, H. M., and Kohler, P. F. (1973). *Semin. Hematol.* **10,** 87–112.

Gunby, P. (1984). *J.A.M.A.* **251,** 1131–1132.

Gyotoku, Y., Abdelmoula, M., Spertini, F. Izui, S., and Lambert, P. H. (1987). *J. Immunol.* **138,** 3785–3792.
Hall, J. B., Wadham, B. McN., Wood, C. J., Ashton, V., and Adam, W. R. (1984). *Aust. N. Z. J. Med.* **14,** 277–278.
Hamilton, C. R., Shelley, W. M., and Tumulty, P. A. (1971). *Medicine* **50,** 1–27.
Hammer, D. K., and Dixon, F. J. (1963). *J. Exp. Med.* **117,** 1019–1034.
Hart, M. N., Debault, L. E., Sadewasser, K. L., Cancilla, P. A., and Henriquez, P. A. (1981). *J. Neuropathol. Exp. Neurol.* **40,** 84–91.
Hart, M. N., Sadewasser, K. L., Cancilla, P. A., and DeBault, L. E. (1983). *Lab. Invest.* **48,** 419–427.
Hart, M. N., Tassell, S. K., Sadewasser, K. L., Schelper, R. L., and Moore, S. A. (1985). *Am. J. Pathol.* **119,** 448–455.
Heurkens, A. H., Hiemstra, P. S., Lafeber, G. J., Daha, M. R., and Breedveld, F. C. (1989). *Clin. Exp. Immunol.* **78,** 7–12.
Izui, S., Lambert, P. H., and Miescher, P. A. (1976). *J. Exp. Med.* **144,** 428–443.
Jennette, J. C. (1991). *Am. J. Kidney Dis.* **18,** 164–170.
Jennette, J. C., and Falk, R. J. (1990a). *Am. J. Kidney Dis.* **15,** 517–529.
Jennette, J. C., Hoidal, J. H., and Falk, R. J. (1990b). *Blood* **75,** 2263–2264.
Jennette, J. C., Wilkman, A. S., and Falk, R. J. (1989). *Am. J. Pathol.* **135,** 921–930.
Kawasaki, T. (1967). *Jpn. J. Allergol.* **16,** 178–222.
Kawasaki, T., Kosaki, F., Okawa, S., Shigematsu, I., and Yanagawa, H. (1974). *Pediatrics* **54,** 271–276.
Korbet, S. M., Schwartz, M., and Lewis, E. J. (1984). *Am. J. Med.* **77,** 141–146.
Kussmaul, A., and Maier, R. (1866). *Dtsch. Arch. Klin. Med.* **1,** 484–518.
Lerner, R. A., Glassock, R. J., and Dixon, F. J. (1967). *J. Exp. Med.* **126,** 989–1004.
Leung, D. Y. M., Collins, T., Lapierre, L. A., Geha, R. S., and Pober, J. S. (1986a). *J. Clin. Invest.* **77,** 1428–1435.
Leung, D. Y. M., Geha, R. S., Newburger, J. W., Burns, J. C., Fiers, W., Lapierre, L. A., and Pober, J. S. (1986b). *J. Exp. Med.* **164,** 1958–1972.
Leung, D. Y. M., Cotran, R. S., Kurt-Jones, E., Burns, J. C., Newburger, J. W., and Pober, J. S. (1989). *Lancet* **2,** 1298–1302.
Leung, D. Y. M., Moake, J. L., Havens, P. L., Kim, M., and Pober, J. S. (1988). *Lancet* **2,** 183–186.
Ludemann, J., Utecht, B., and Gross, W. L. (1990). *J. Exp. Med.* **171,** 357–362.
Maddison, P. J., and Reichlin, M. (1979). *Arthritis Rheum.* **22,** 858–863.
Magilavy, D. B., Petty, R. E., Cassidy, J. T., and Sullivan D. C. (1977). *J. Pediatr.* **91,** 25–30.
Ming-Jiang, W., Rajaram, R., Shelp, W. D., Beirne, G. J., and Burkholder, P. M. (1980). *Arch. Pathol. Lab. Med.* **104,** 300–302.
Molina, R., Provost, T. T., and Alexander, E. L. (1985). *Arthritis Rheum.* **28,** 1251–1258.
Moyer, C. F., and Reinisch, C. L. (1984). *Am. J. Pathol.* **117,** 380–390.
Moyer, C. F., and Reinisch, C. L. (1989). *Toxicol. Pathol.* **17,** 122–128.
Moyer, C. F., Strandberg, J. D., and Reinisch, C. L. (1987). *Am J. Pathol.* **127,** 229–242.
Myers, J. L., and Katzenstein, A. A. (1986). *Am. J. Clin. Pathol.* **85,** 552–556.
Nagashima, M., Matsushima, M., Matsuoka, H. *et al.* (1987). *J. Pediatr.* **110,** 710–712.
Nolle, B., Specks, U., Ludemann, J., Rohrbach, M. S., DeRemee, R. A., and Gross, W. L. (1989). *Ann. Intern. Med.* **111,** 28–40.
Nose, M., Nishimura, M., and Kyogoku, M. (1989). *Am. J. Pathol.* **135,** 271–280.
Pober, J. S. (1988). *Am. J. Pathol.* **133,** 426–433.
Rauch, A., and Hurwitz, E. (1985). *Pediatr. Infect. Dis.* **4,** 702–703.
Rich, A. R. (1942). *Bull. Johns Hopkins Hosp.* **71,** 123–140.
Rich, A. R., and Gregory, J. E. (1943). *Bull. Johns Hopkins Hosp.* **72,** 65–88.

Ronco, P., Verroust, P., Mignon, F., Kourilsky, O., Vanhille, Ph., Meyrier, A., Mery, J. Ph., and Morel-Maroger, L. (1983). *Q. J. Med.* **52,** 212–223.
Rosen, S., Falk, R. J., and Jennette, J. C. (1991). *In* "Systemic Vasculitides" (A. Churg and J. Churg, eds.), Chapter 5, pp. 57–78. Igaku-Shoin, New York.
Rowley, A. H., Duffy, C. E., and Shulman, S. T. (1988). *J. Pediatr.* **113,** 290–294.
Savage, C. O. S., Winearlsk C. G., Jones, S., Marshall, P. D., and Lockwood, C. M. (1987). *Lancet* **1,** 1389–1393.
Sergent, J. S. (1980). *Clin. Rheum. Dis.* **6,** 339–356.
Staszak, C., and Harbeck, R. J. (1985). *Am. J. Pathol.* **120,** 99–105.
Steblay, R. W. (1962). *J. Exp. Med.* **116,** 253–272.
Tan, E. M., and Kunkel, J. G. (1966). *Arthritis Rheum.* **9,** 37–46.
Tsokos, M., Lazarou, S. A., and Moutsopoulos, H. M. (1987). *Am. J. Clin. Pathol.* **88,** 26–31.
van der Woude, F. J., Rasmussen, N., Lobatto, S. Wiik, A., Permin, H., van Es, L. A., van der Giessen, M., van der Hem, G. K., and The, T. H. (1985). *Lancet* **1,** 425–429.
Venning, M. C., Arfeen, S., and Bird, A. G. (1987). *Lancet* **2,** 850.
Wathen, C. W., and Harrison, D. J. (1987). *Lancet* **1,** 1037.
Watson, R. (1989). *Med. Clin. North Am.* **73,** 1091–1111.
Winfield, J. B., Koffler, D., and Kunkel, H. G. (1975). *J. Clin. Invest.* **56,** 563–570.
Yap, H. K., Sakai, R. S., Bahn, L., Rappaport, V., Woo, K. T., Ananthuraman, V., Lim, C. H., Chiang, G. S. C., and Jordan, S. C. (1988). *Clin. Immunol. Immunopathol.* **46,** 450–462.
Yoshikawa, Y., and Watanabe, T. (1986). *Hum. Pathol.* **17,** 401–410.

CHAPTER **12**

Autoimmune Heart Disease

NOEL R. ROSE[1,2]
DAVID A. NEUMANN[1]
C. LYNNE BUREK[1]
AHVIE HERSKOWITZ[2]
Departments of [1]Immunology and Infectious Diseases and [2]Medicine
The Johns Hopkins Medical Institutions
Baltimore, Maryland

I. INTRODUCTION

In the first edition of this book, M. A. Vadas (1985) commented: "There are few areas of clinical medicine that have been so little influenced by immunological considerations as that of cardiovascular disease" (p. 429). This comment is particularly striking when one recalls the years of research effort devoted to establishing a link between streptococcal infection and rheumatic heart disease on the basis of an autoimmune response. The presence of heart-reactive antibodies in patients with acute rheumatic fever is cited as a classic example of molecular mimicry wherein the Group A streptococcal membrane shares antigens with the myocyte (Zabriskie *et al.*, 1970). Only slightly less investigative energy was invested in elucidating the possible autoimmune origin of chronic Chagas' disease based on a cross-reaction of antibodies to *Trypanosoma cruzi* with the myocardium or cardiac-conductive tissue (Sadigursky *et al.*, 1982). Finally, postpericardiotomy syndrome and postmyocardial infarction syndrome are often cited as instances of an autoimmune response instigated by damaged or necrotic tissue (Van der Geld, 1964).

The comment of Vadas that these immunological studies had so little influence on clinical medicine is based not so much on a failure to recognize that autoantibodies frequently accompany several important forms of heart disease, as on a deficit of information that autoimmunity plays a causative role in these diseases. For that reason, we undertook the task of analyzing in depth one prevalent form of heart disease, Coxsackievirus-induced myocarditis, to see whether a causative link could be established between the virus and the heart disease based on an autoimmune response (Rose *et al.*, 1987). If a pathogenetic role of autoimmunity can be established, new, more rational modes of treatment become possible.

This chapter will describe the newer investigations by our group and other groups designed to establish the role of autoimmunity in heart disease and to associate a particular viral infection with the initiation of that autoimmune response.

II. CLINICAL AND PATHOLOGICAL MANIFESTATIONS OF MYOCARDITIS AND DILATED CARDIOMYOPATHY

A. Myocarditis

The classic clinical signs of individuals with acute myocarditis are fever, malaise, persistent tachycardia, and rapid onset of ventricular failure. These findings can be supported by electrocardiographic changes such as nonspecific ST-T wave abnormalities, conduction and voltage disturbances, and Q-wave abnormalities, mimicking myocardial infarction. Sometimes, a pericardial rub indicates pericarditis. Unfortunately, the majority of cases of myocarditis cannot be traced back to an obvious febrile illness, and most patients with biopsy-proven myocarditis present with unexplained congestive heart failure or arrhythmias as their only signs. Focal or diffuse myocardial inflammation is seen in 3 to 4% of routine autopsy cases and in 10 to 20% of cases of sudden death.

The introduction of the endomyocardial biopsy by Sakakibara and Konno in 1962 dramatically altered the clinical diagnosis of myocarditis by permitting direct histological confirmation. The so-called Dallas criteria, the consensus of a group of cardiovascular pathologists (Aretz *et al.*, 1986), has led to better standardization of the histopathologic examination. These criteria require both lymphocytic cell infiltration and evidence of myocyte necrosis. Yet, a large number of patients with signs and symptoms of myocarditis do not fulfill both of these requirements on biopsy. For example, inflammatory cell infiltration may be found in the heart without evidence of muscle cell injury. Part of the problem may be related to the limited sample size of biopsies, but the finding may also result from a dynamic process of injury and healing. To further investigate heart muscle damage, radioisotopic scans of the heart, using radioisotope-labeled monoclonal antibodies to myosin, have sometimes proved valuable.

Laboratory tests can be used to establish the diagnosis of virus-induced myocarditis. First, an increasing antibody titer to a particular virus should be documented, using the patient's serum. Usually, a fourfold rise in neutralizing antibody titer between acute and convalescent stages is acceptable evidence of a recent virus infection. Second, it may be possible to isolate the virus from biopsy tissues or pericardial fluid, using appropriate cell cultures or experimental animals. Finally, specific nucleic acid probes can be applied to sections of biopsied tissue. The polymerase chain reaction greatly increases the sensitivity of *in situ* nucleic acid hybridization. Although these methods are useful in clinical investigation, they are rarely applied in routine diagnosis of myocarditis.

B. Idiopathic Dilated Cardiomyopathy

Dilated cardiomyopathy is a chronic form of heart disease characterized by left and right ventricular dilatation and impaired contraction, which usually results in clinically evident congestive heart failure. The diagnosis requires exclusion of heart failure associated with valvular or coronary vessel disease or with systemic or pulmonary vascular disease.

The number of etiological agents associated with dilated cardiomyopathy is large (Abelmann, 1988) and includes infections; granulomata; hematologic, metabolic, endocrine, and nutritional diseases; neoplasms and neuromuscular diseases; as well as toxins and drugs. However, in well over 90% of patients, no specific etiology can be identified. Most likely, the same condition is the result of a number of different pathological processes.

The incidence of dilated cardiomyopathy in Great Britain is estimated at 0.7–7.5/100,000 population per year with a prevalence of 8.3 cases per 100,000 (Williams and Olsen, 1985). Since a number of these patients eventually require cardiac transplantation, there is a great need for early and definitive diagnosis. It is still uncertain how many cases represent progression from acute myocarditis to chronic myocarditis and dilated cardiomyopathy, since in most patients the symptoms of the acute disease are nonspecific and mild. For that reason, the link between these diseases is based mostly on relatively small case series and anecdotal case reports. For example, Kline and Saphir (1960) documented progressive myocardial failure and death in 29 patients within months to years after acute myocarditis. Miklozek *et al.* (1986) found that 12 of 16 patients diagnosed as having viral myocarditis had continued cardiac functional abnormalities. Abelman (1984) reported that 45% of patients had cardiac symptoms, and 63% had physical evidence of persistent cardiac dysfunction after recovery from acute myocarditis. In 50 infants and children with dilated cardiomyopathy, Ayuthya *et al.* (1974) found significantly increased titers of neutralizing antibody to Coxsackieviruses. More recently, Bowles *et al.* (1986) and Kandolf *et al.* (1987) demonstrated Coxsackie B-specific nucleic acid sequences in the heart tissue of a small number of patients with dilated cardiomyopathy.

III. VIRAL MYOCARDITIS

A. COXSACKIEVIRUSES

Acute myocarditis is associated with infections of many types, including bacterial, rickettsial, viral, mycotic, protozoal, and helminthic (Weinstein and Fenoglio, 1987). In Europe and North America, however, the most common agents are the Coxsackieviruses of Group B. The association is based on a rising titer of viral antibodies in approximately 50% of cases, as well as the occasional detection of virus in blood or other tissue fluids and the demonstration of virus antigen or nucleic acid sequences in heart muscle.

Coxsackieviruses are members of the Picornavirus family, which comprises four genera: enteroviruses, cardioviruses, rhinoviruses, and polio viruses (Wolfgram and Rose, 1989). Among the enteroviruses that infect humans are the Coxsackie Group A and Group B. In addition to myocarditis and pericarditis, the Group B Coxsackieviruses have been implicated in pleurodynia, aseptic meningitis, postviral fatigue syndrome, and insulin-dependent diabetes, but they are most often responsible for undifferentiated febrile illness. As their name implies, picornaviruses are small (*pico*) RNA viruses. The single-stranded RNA genome composes approximately 30% of the molecular mass and is enclosed by an icosahedral protein capsid. The capsid consists of 60 protomers, comprising 4 proteins designated VP-1 through VP-4.

Like other enteroviruses, Coxsackieviruses enter the alimentary tract and are acid stable (Wolfgram and Rose, 1989). They multiply in the small intestine. Following replication, viremia develops, seeding the infectious agents in selected tissues. Some variants of Coxsackie Group B have a predilection for cardiac or pancreatic tissue.

These tissue tropisms are determined mainly by the distribution of specific cellular receptors. A receptor protein for Coxsackievirus B has been extensively studied by Crowell and his associates (1988). They have hypothesized the diverse manifestations of Coxsackie B infection are owing to polymorphism of the cellular receptors and to variable affinity of individual virus strains for different host-cell receptors. They have, for example, shown that the receptor protein found on HeLa cells differs from that found on a human rhabdomyosarcoma cell line. Receptor variation among genetically dissimilar persons selects virus variants that are more or less virulent than parental virus.

Cell receptors serve both to bind virus and to initiate virus disassembly (Crowell *et al.*, 1987). Entry of the virus into the cell is mediated by receptor endocytosis. Binding of virus to the cellular receptor is through a protein referred to as virion attachment protein. Capsid protein VP-2 of Coxsackievirus B3 (CB3), which induces neutralizing antibody, may serve as the virion attachment protein. Viral protein synthesis occurs in the rough endoplasmic reticulum, while

RNA synthesis takes place at the smooth endoplasmic reticulum. The positive-stranded RNA assembles with capsid proteins at the cytoplasmic membrane, and the newly synthesized virus is probably released into the culture medium following cell lysis.

Infection produces significant alterations in the host cell (Jen and Thach, 1982). The virus inhibits host-cell protein synthesis, turning the cell to manufacturing viral protein. Host-cell RNA synthesis is also inhibited. The cytopathic effects of the virus are probably mediated through alterations in the membrane composition, resulting in increases in plasma-membrane permeability. Intracellular components leak into the surrounding medium, and the cell disintegrates, allowing virus to escape. In addition to producing overt cell necrosis, the virus may persist in the host cell for prolonged periods, as evident by the presence of viral RNA in apparently healthy cells.

B. Genetics of Susceptibility to Viral Myocarditis

Although infections by Group B Coxsackieviruses are relatively common, the development of clinically significant myocardial disease is uncommon, suggesting that differences in host response play a role in disease susceptibility. These differences are likely to be genetically determined and may relate to the virus-specific receptor or to the immune response of the host. Because of the difficulty in diagnosing Coxsackie-induced myocarditis, it is difficult to examine the role that genetic polymorphisms play in humans. Therefore, investigators have developed models of Coxsackievirus-induced myocarditis in mice, in which a large number of genetically defined strains are available. An investigation undertaken by Wolfgram *et al.* (1986) examined the genetic role of the immune response of the host in influencing susceptibility to Coxsackie-induced myocarditis.

Based on the pioneering studies of Lerner (1969), Rose *et al.* (1986) developed a murine model of CB3-induced myocarditis by infecting 14-day-old mice of a variety of inbred strains with a standard myocardiogenic strain of virus. The mouse strains were chosen to reveal both major histocompatability complex (MHC)-linked and non-MHC-linked traits that influenced the course of disease.

All animals had infectious CB3 virus in the bloodstream 2 days after infection. There was, however, a significant difference among strains on day 3, since some inbred strains had high levels of viremia at that time, whereas other strains were virtually negative. At that time, neutralizing antibody could be demonstrated in serum of all of the strains free of circulating virus and none of the viremic mice. This finding suggests that neutralizing antibody is the major mechanism for clearing virus from the bloodstream. There was, furthermore, a direct correlation between the susceptibility of the mouse strain to virus infection as determined by the level and duration of viremia and the extent of cardiac pathology. By comparing genetically different inbred strains, it became apparent that both MHC and non-MHC determinants influence susceptibility to viral myocarditis.

C. Myocarditis as an Autoimmune Sequela

Further studies reveal that it is possible to separate CB3-induced myocarditis into two distinct phases (Rose *et al.*, 1986). The first phase usually occurs during the first week after infection and is characterized by focal necrosis of myocytes and an accompanying acute inflammatory response. The second phase of CB3-induced myocarditis became evident about 9 days after infection and was fully manifested by 15 to 21 days after infection. Histologically, the inflammatory process was diffuse and consisted mainly of a mononuclear interstitial infiltrate. The two phases overlapped between days 9 and 15. Infectious virus could be isolated only during the first phase of disease; no virus was isolated after day 9. Heart-specific autoantibodies were present in all strains that developed the second phase of virus-induced myocarditis. This finding suggested that the second phase represents an autoimmune response initiated by the initial virus infection. It should be emphasized that only certain inbred strains of mice developed this secondary autoimmune myocarditis. Susceptibility was determined by non-H-2-background genes, although H-2-encoded differences accounted for the vigor of the autoimmune response. Susceptibility to the autoimmune sequela, however, clearly differed from genetic susceptibility to the early phase of viral myocarditis.

The demonstration of autoantibodies in the late phase of CB3-induced myocarditis led to evaluating the significance of the autoimmune response, namely, the characterization and isolation of the target antigen. The studies of Alvarez *et al.* (1987) showed that myosin heavy chain is the major antigen. Absorption studies further showed that heart-specific determinants are present on the myosin molecule.

Using purified mouse cardiac myosin incorporated in complete Freund's adjuvant, Neu *et al.* (1987) were able to produce cardiac lesions that resembled the late phase of CB3-induced myocarditis. Moreover, the inbred strains of mice that were genetically susceptible to late-phase disease were also susceptible to myosin-induced myocarditis, whereas the strains resistant to the autoimmune phase of viral myocarditis were also resistant to myosin-induced myocarditis. Taken together, these investigations suggested that the late phase of CB3-induced myocarditis, which occurs in a few genetically susceptible strains of mice, results from an autoimmune response to cardiac-specific determinants on the myosin heavy chain molecule.

Coincident with the humoral autoimmune response to myosin among both CB3-infected and cardiac myosin-immunized mice, there is evidence that pathogenesis is associated with the induction of autoreactive T cells. Huber and Job

(1983) demonstrated that CB3 infection of BALB/c mice results in the induction of two populations of autocytotoxic T cells, one which is specific for CB3-infected myocytes and one which is specific for uninfected myocytes. Although the antigen specificity of the latter population has not been determined, Huber *et al.* (1988) suggested that the reactivity was directed against myocyte 'neo-antigens' which were expressed on myocyte surfaces as a consequence of altered myocyte metabolism. Our own experiments (Neumann *et al.*, 1991) indicate that spleen cells from CB3-infected mice respond to in vitro stimulation with myosin. Among mice immunized with cardiac myosin, Smith and Allen (1991) were able to demonstrate the presence of myosin-specific spleen cells by in vitro stimulation of cellular proliferation. Mice depleted of either $CD4^+$ or $CD8^+$ T cells failed to develop myocarditis when immunized with cardiac myosin (Neu *et al.*, 1991). The pathological significance of these results is unclear since one would expect antigen-specific T cells to engage cell surface antigens leading to target cell lysis. Myosin is not generally considered to be expressed on myocyte surfaces, hence the role of myosin-specific T cells in pathogenesis remains to be determined. It is likely that both humoral and cellular immune processes contribute to the continuing pathology in susceptible strains of mice.

IV. IMMUNOLOGIC ASPECTS OF HUMAN MYOCARDITIS AND IDIOPATHIC DILATED CARDIOMYOPATHY

A. Circulating Antibodies

The ambiguities in diagnosing inflammatory disease of the heart muscle have been described. Although the availability of endomyocardial biopsy has helped to clarify the situation, many cases are still inconclusive. There is, in addition, need for a noninvasive, inexpensive diagnostic procedure. The evidence related in the previous section points to a significant role of autoimmunity in some cases of heart muscle disease. It is logical, therefore, to propose that a serological test, based on the demonstration of circulating autoantibodies, might be useful in the identification of autoimmune forms of myocarditis and dilated cardiomyopathy.

Three levels of testing have been applied in the search for practical diagnostic tests of autoimmune heart disease. Screening tests utilize indirect immunofluorescence or cytotoxicity to detect antibodies in patient serum to cardiac tissue. The Western immunoblot is valuable because it separates the soluble components of heart tissue based on their molecular mass and permits the identification of antibodies to individual components. Finally, it has been possible to set up immunoassays using well-defined constituents of cardiac tissue to measure quantitatively the antibody content of patient serum.

1. Immunofluorescence and Cytotoxicity

Immunofluorescent tests utilize cardiac tissue of rat or human origin. Both frozen sections and isolated myocytes have been employed. Antibody generally localizes at the surface of the myocyte, the so-called sarcolemmal or myolemmal pattern, or on the striations, producing the so-called fibrillar pattern. Whether these two immunofluorescent patterns represent different populations of antibodies has not yet been determined. It is interesting that both patterns are produced by sera from mice immunized with purified cardiac myosin. A major problem in the application of indirect immunofluorescence is the high prevalence of reactions obtained with sera from healthy control subjects. Maisch (1987) found that 91% of patients with Coxsackie B influenza or mumps myocarditis gave positive reactions with human or rat cardiocytes, whereas 31–35% of healthy controls showed similar reactions. In our own studies (Neumann *et al.*, 1990), more conservative criteria have been used, so that 40% of patients with biopsy-proven myocarditis were positive, as were 20% of dilated cardiomyopathy patients. In contrast, none of the healthy controls and only 4% of patients with ischemic heart disease were positive in this test.

Maisch (1986) found that sera of patients with Coxsackie myocarditis demonstrated complement-dependent cytotoxicity with isolated cardiomyocytes. The cytotoxicity could be eliminated by absorption with Coxsackievirus preparations and with enriched sarcolemmal proteins, indicating that the antibody is both complement-fixing and cross-reactive.

2. Western Immunoblots

The Western immunoblot is potentially more sensitive as well as capable of identifying particular antigens recognized by heart-reactive antibodies. In our laboratory (Neumann *et al.*, 1990), for example, heart antibodies were detected in 48 of 103 samples by immunofluorescence, whereas 97 of the 103 samples exhibited reactivity by Western immunostaining. No single pattern of antigen reactivity was unique to patients with myocarditis or dilated cardiomyopathy. Myocarditis sera showed an elevated prevalence of antibody against proteins in the 190- to 199-kDa class, whereas cardiomyopathy sera exhibited a greater prevalence of reactivity against 40- to 49-kDa and 100- to 109-kDa antigens. Although the identity of the reactive antigens is not known, it is possible that the 190- to 199-kDa class includes the heavy chain of cardiac myosin and the 40- to 49-kDa class includes actin.

It seems to be a common experience that multiple components are evident when patient sera are tested with tissue extracts using Western immunoblots. Similar findings have been described for autoimmune hepatitis (Swanson *et al.*, 1989).

3. Immunoassays with Defined Antigens

Among the well-characterized antigens used for the study of antibodies in sera of patients with myocarditis and dilated cardiomyopathy are myosin (Neumann *et al.*, 1990), laminin (Wolff *et al.*, 1989), beta-adrenergic receptors (Limas *et al.*, 1989), and the mitochondrial components, adenine nucleotide translocator (ANT) protein (Schultheiss *et al.*, 1986) and branched-chain ketoacid dehydrogenase (BCKD) (Ahmed-Ansari *et al.*, 1988). It is curious that the mitochondrial enzyme, BCKD, is also an autoantigen in primary biliary cirrhosis.

ANT facilitates the transport of adenosine triphosphate (ATP) into the cytosol and the return of adenosine diphosphate (ADP) to the inner mitochondrial space. Therefore, it plays a significant role in the energy metabolism of the myocardiocyte. Using a sensitive enzyme-linked immunosorbent assay (ELISA), Schultheiss *et al.* (1986) found that autoantibodies directed to this ADP–ATP carrier protein (ANT) were significantly elevated in 24 of 32 patients with dilated cardiomyopathy. Controls with coronary heart disease, alcoholic cardiomyopathy, and heterotrophic obstructive cardiomyopathy were all within normal limits. Since there was less binding of the autoantibodies to the analogous protein from the liver, there was a suggestion of organ specificity. Therefore, absorption experiments were carried out, which demonstrated that ADP–ATP carrier from heart absorbed most of the autoantibodies, whereas the residual activity of antiserum after absorption with the liver protein was significantly higher.

Purified IgG fractions of serum were found to inhibit nucleotide exchange in myocytes. Preabsorption of the antisera by isolated heart mitochondria prevented the inhibition of the ADP–ATP functional activity. In addition to showing that these antibodies are physiologically effective, these experiments suggest that some determinants of the ANT protein are accessible on the surface of the myocardiocyte, possibly as epitopes shared with connexon or calcium channel molecules embedded in the membrane (Morad *et al.*, 1988; Schultheiss *et al.*, 1988). Ansari *et al.* (1991) recently reported that both ANT and BCKD were aberrantly expressed on the surface of cardiac myocytes isolated from myocarditis and cardiomyopathy patients. All three of the myocarditis patients presented evidence of CB3 infection, suggesting that virus-associated changes in myocyte metabolism may contribute to the expression of intracellular molecules on the myocyte surface.

In our own studies, autoantibodies to ANT were found in 79% of 14 patients with acute myocarditis and in 90% of 41 patients with idiopathic dilated cardiomyopathy. Almost all patients who possessed antibody to ANT also had antibody to BCKD. Sera from the following groups were used as controls: lupus patients (n = 52); rheumatoid arthritis patients (n = 35); normal adults (n = 42). None of these samples reacted with ANT or BCKD. By ELISA, the titers of circulating antibodies to ANT served as useful indicators of therapeutic response, since the majority of patients with improved ejection fractions showed a drop in ANT titers early in the course of immunosuppressive treatment with oral prednisone and azathioprine.

Antibodies to laminin are also prominent in patients with dilated cardiomyopathy and myocarditis. By ELISA, 78% of 41 dilated cardiomyopathy cases were found to be positive by Wolff *et al.* (1989) as were 75% of myocarditis patients; only 5% of 65 controls were positive.

A decrease in the density of beta-1 adrenergic receptors has been described in patients with clinical heart failure. Based on this finding, Limas and Limas (1988) evaluated the possible role of anti-beta receptor antibodies in dilated cardiomyopathy. Antibodies were measured by detecting inhibition of radiolabeled dihydro-L-prenalol binding to rat cardiac membranes. Of 48 patients with idiopathic dilated cardiomyopathy, 32% gave positive reactions. In contrast, 7% of 36 patients with ischemic or valvular heart disease and none of 25 controls were positive.

Based on the experimental studies in mice described previously, our laboratory has carried out tests for antibody to myosin. Using a sensitive enzyme immunoassay, 40% of patients with cardiomyopathy and 60% of myocarditis patients were positive in contrast to 7% of patients with ischemic heart disease.

These results show that patients with myocarditis and, to a lesser extent, with idiopathic dilated cardiomyopathy develop autoantibodies to a number of cardiac constituents. Further large-scale evaluation is necessary before one can conclude that detection of any single antibody or group of antibodies is sufficiently sensitive and specific to replace the endomyocardial biopsy as a primary diagnostic tool. It does seem, even at this early stage of investigation, that a decline in some antibody titers during treatment may predict a favorable therapeutic response.

The presence of multiple autoantibodies in diseases of autoimmune origin is quite expected. There are, for example, several antibodies to thyroid in patients with chronic thyroiditis and to pancreatic islets in patients with insulin-dependent diabetes. None of these investigations, as yet, has been able to establish that antibodies to cardiac antigens play a pathogenetic role in the disease. The presence of antibodies to beta-adrenergic receptors is highly suggestive, since the antigen is available on the surface of the myocardiocyte, and the blocking of this receptor is likely to produce functional effects. Similar receptor-specific antibodies are known to have functional consequences in myasthenia gravis and Graves' disease. Antibodies to beta-adrenergic receptors have been described in patients with intractable asthma, where they are reputed to have functional consequences. Antibodies to the mitochondrial antigens, ANT and BCKD, may also have adverse consequences on cardiac function. It is not clear, however, whether these antibodies have access to their target antigens *in vivo*. Morad *et al.* (1988) have provided evidence that ANT antibodies interfere with calcium flux in the isolated myocardial cell, perhaps because a related antigen is available at the cell surface.

The pathogenetic importance of antibodies to laminin and to myosin is still problematic. The finding that purified myosin can induce a florid myocarditis in susceptible strains of mice is a strong indication that this antigen has pathological importance. Investigations in mice have not yet resolved the relative roles of cell-mediated and humoral immunity in producing the myocardial lesions.

B. Immunologic Assessment of Biopsies

In addition to studies of circulating antibody, immunological methods can contribute to the diagnosis of heart disease by the identification of immunoglobulin and complement in biopsy specimens. Hammond *et al.* (1988) found that 55% of 18 patients with active myocarditis have deposits of IgG and C3 in their biopsies. Of 13 borderline myocarditis (inflammation without necrosis) cases, 39% were positive, as were 6% of dilated cardiomyopathy cases. Patients with other autoimmune diseases, such as systemic lupus erythematosus and scleroderma, sometimes showed deposits of IgG and C3 in their hearts, but these usually were coarse, granular deposits in the interstitial spaces, probably representing immune complexes.

Immunofluorescence with defined antisera has been used to identify infiltrating cells in cardiac biopsies. Hammond *et al.* (1988) found that approximately half of the infiltrating cells in all patients with myocarditis were macrophages. The majority of infiltrating lymphocytes in patients with myocarditis was T lymphocytes. These cells were equally divided between CD4 and CD8 subsets.

The expression of MHC class I and class II antigens in biopsy specimens was evaluated by Herskowitz *et al.* (1990). In control samples, only low levels of MHC class I antigens were expressed on interstitial cells and vascular epithelium, while MHC class II could not be demonstrated immunohistologically. Increased myocardial expression of MHC class I and *de novo* expression of class II antigens were found in 85% of the myocarditis patients and 33% of the dilated cardiomyopathy patients.

V. SUMMARY AND CONCLUSIONS

The study of autoimmunity in inflammatory disease of the heart muscle has undergone a recent renaissance. This renewed interest is attributable to a number of factors, including the demonstration of autoantibodies with defined specificities in many cases of myocarditis, the availability of specific nucleic acid probes to demonstrate the presence of virus in cardiac tissue, and the still controversial introduction of immunosuppressive treatment. The progression of myocarditis to dilated cardiomyopathy and persistent cardiac dysfunction has also spurred the need for clinical and basic research on the involvement of immunological factors.

The presence of autoantibodies in the sera of many myocarditis patients has raised the possibility that autoimmunity may be responsible for progression of the disease from an acute, self-limited virus infection of the heart muscle to a chronic inflammatory, degenerative disease. A cause-and-effect relationship between the autoimmune response and ongoing myocardial disease has been difficult to establish. For that purpose, an animal model of CB3-induced myocarditis has proved to be useful. By testing a large number of strains of inbred mice, we have shown that the same strain of virus induces severe or mild myocarditis depending on the genetic constitution of the host. There was close correspondence between disease severity and time of appearance of neutralizing antibody.

In most mouse strains, CB3 induced a self-limited myocardial inflammation followed by complete resolution. A few strains developed ongoing disease characterized by diffuse monocytic infiltration of the myocardium. Heart-specific autoantibodies were present only in the strains of mice susceptible to this ongoing form of myocarditis. The corresponding antigen was determined to be the heavy chain of cardiac myosin. Immunization of the susceptible strains of mice with purified cardiac myosin, but not skeletal myosin, reproduced the major histological features of interstitial myocarditis.

Human subjects with myocarditis frequently evince elevated titers of antibody to myosin as well as to a number of other cardiac antigens, especially ANT and BCKD. Their myocytes may also show increased expression of MHC products. These immunological indicators may prove to be of great value in improving the diagnosis of myocarditis, in distinguishing the autoimmune form of disease from that produced directly by the infecting virus, and in providing a rational basis for therapy. When the underlying mechanisms of sensitization and pathogenesis have been defined, it may become possible to identify individuals at great risk of developing the ongoing, autoimmune form of myocarditis and to institute preventive measures.

Finally, it should be emphasized that autoimmune myocarditis may be one of several causes of *idiopathic* cardiomyopathy. The clinical problem is to separate the different etiological types of this disease.

REFERENCES

Abelmann, W. H. (1984). *Prog. Cardiovasc. Dis.* **27,** 73–94.

Abelmann, W. H. (1988). *In* "New Concepts in Viral Heart Disease" (H.-P. Schultheiss, ed.), pp. 3–21. Springer-Verlag, Berlin.

Ahmed-Ansari, A., Herskowitz, A., Danner, D. J., Necklemann, N., Gershwin, M. E., Gravanis, M. B., and Sell, K. W. (1988). *Circulation* **11,** 457.

Alvarez, F. L., Neu, N., Rose, N. R., Craig, S. W., and Beisel, K. W. (1987). *Clin. Immunol. Immunopathol.* **43,** 129–139.

Ansari, A. A., Wang, Y.-C., Danner, D. J., Gravanis, M. B., Mayne, A., Neckelmann, N., Sell, K. W., and Herskowitz, A. (1991). *Am. J. Pathol.* **139,** 337–354.

Aretz, H. T., Billingham, M. E., Edwards, W. D., Factor, S. M., Fallon, J. T., Fenoglio, J. J., Olsen, E. G. J., and Schaen, F. J. (1986). *Am. J. Cardiovasc. Pathol.* **1,** 3–14.

Ayuthya, P. S. N., Jayavasu, V. J., and Pongpenich, B. (1974). *Am. Heart J.* **88,** 311–314.

Bowles, N. E., Richardson, P. J., Olsen, E. G. J., and Archard, L. C. (1986). *Lancet* **i,** 1120–1122.

Crowell, R. L., Hsu, K.-H.L., Schultz, M., and Landau, B. J. (1987). *In* "Positive Strand RNA Viruses" (M. A. Brinton and R. R. Rueckert, eds.), pp. 453–466. Liss, New York.

Crowell, R. L., Finkelstein, S. D., Hsu, K.-H.L., Landau, B. J., Stalhandske, P., and Whittier, P. S. (1988). *In* "New Concepts in Viral Heart Disease" (H.-P. Schultheiss, ed.), pp. 79–92. Springer-Verlag, Berlin.

Hammond, E. H., Menlove, R. L., and Anderson, J. L. (1988). *In* "New Concepts in Viral Heart Disease" (H.-P. Schultheiss, ed.), pp. 303–311. Springer-Verlag, Berlin.

Herskowitz, A., Ahmed-Ansari, A., Neumann, D. A., Beschorner, W. E., Rose, N. R., Soule, L. M., Burek, C. L., Sell, K. W., and Baughman, K. L. (1990). *J. Am Coll. Cardiol.* **15,** 624–632.

Huber, S. A., and Job, L. P. (1983). *Adv. Exp. Med. Biol.* **161,** 491–508.

Huber, S. A., Heintz, N., and Tracy R. (1988). *J. Immunol. 141:*3214–3219.

Jen, G., and Thach, R. C. (1982). *J. Virol.* **43,** 250–261.

Kandolf, R., Ameis, D., Kirschner, P., Canue, A., and Hofschneider, P. H. (1987). *Proc. Natl. Acad. Sci. U.S.A.* **84,** 6272–6276.

Kline, I. K., and Saphir, O. (1960). *Am. Heart J.* **59,** 681–697.

Lerner, A. M. (1969). *J. Infect. Dis.* **120,** 496.

Limas, C. J., and Limas, C. (1988). *In* "New Concepts in Viral Heart Disease" (H.-P. Schultheiss, ed.), pp. 217–224. Springer-Verlag, Berlin.

Limas, C. J., Goldenberg, I. F., and Limas, C. (1989). *Circ. Res.* **64,** 97.

Maisch, B. (1986). *Basic Res. Cardiol.* **81,** 217–242.

Maisch, B. (1987). *In* "Pathogenesis of Myocarditis and Cardiomyopathy" (C. Kawai and W. H. Abelmann, eds.), pp. 245–267. University of Tokyo Press, Tokyo.

Miklozek, C. L., Kingsley, E. M., Crumpaker, C. S., Modlin, J. F., Royal, H. D., Come, P. C., Mark, R., and Abelmann, W. H. (1986). *Postgrad. Med. J.* **62,** 577–579.

Morad, M., Näbauer, M., and Schultheiss, H.-P. (1988). *In* "New Concepts in Viral Heart Disease" (H.-P. Schultheiss, ed.), pp. 236–242. Springer-Verlag, Berlin.

Neu, N., Rose, N. R., Beisel, K. W., Herskowitz, A., Gurri-Glass, G., and Craig, S. W. (1987). *J. Immunol.* **139,** 3630–3636.

Neu, N., Pummerer, C., Rieker, T., and Berger, P. (1991). 2nd Internatl. Symp. on Myocarditis, Airlie, VA, 5–8 May.

Neumann, D. A., Burek, C. L., Baughman, K. L., Rose, N. R., and Herskowitz, A. (1990). *J. Am. Coll. Cardiol.* **16,** 839–846.

Neumann, D. A., Wulff, S. M., Frondoza, C., Herskowitz, A., and Rose, N. R. (1991). *J. Cell. Biochem. 15A:*273 (Abst.).

Rose, N. R., Wolfgram, L. J., Herskowitz, A., and Beisel, K. W. (1986). *Ann. N. Y. Acad. Sci.* **475,** 146–156.

Rose, N. R., Beisel, K. W., Herskowitz, A., Neu, N., Wolfgram, L. J., Alvarez, F. L., Traystman, M. D., and Craig, S. W. (1987). *In* "Autoimmunity and Autoimmune Disease" (D. Evered and J. Whelan, eds.), pp. 3–24. John Wiley, Chichester, United Kingdom.

Sadigursky, M., Acosta, A. M., and Santos-Buch, C. A. (1982). *Am. J. Trop. Med. Hyg.* **31,** 934.

Sakakibara, S., and Konno, S. (1962). *Jpn. Heart J.* **3,** 537–543.

Schultheiss, H.-P., Schulze, K., Kühl, U., Ulrich, G., and Klingenberg, M. (1986). *Ann. N. Y. Acad. Sci.* **488,** 44.

Schultheiss, H.-P., Kühl, U., Schauer, R., Schulze, K., Kemkes, B., and Becker, B. F. (1988). *In* "New Concepts in Viral Heart Disease" (H.-P. Schultheiss, ed.), pp. 243–258. Springer-Verlag, Berlin.

Smith, S. C., and Allen, P. M. (1991). 2nd Internatl. Symp. on Myocarditis, Airlie, VA, 5–8 May.

Swanson, N. R., Reed, W. D., Yarred, L. J., Bartholomaeus, W. N., Shilkin, K. B., and Joske, R. A. (1989). *Clin. Immunol. Immunopathol.* **52,** 291–304.

Vadas, M. A. (1985). *In* "The Autoimmune Diseases" (N. R. Rose and I. R. Mackay, eds.), pp. 429–441. Academic Press, Orlando, Florida.

Van der Geld, A. (1964). *Lancet* **i,** 617.

Weinstein, C., and Fenoglio, J. J. (1987). *Hum. Pathol.* **18,** 613–618.

Williams, D. G., and Olsen, E. G. L. (1985). *Br. Heart J.* **54,** 153.

Wolff, P., Kühl, U., and Schultheiss, H.-P. (1989). *Am. Heart J.* **117,** 1303.

Wolfgram, L. J., Beisel, K. W., Herskowitz, A., and Rose, N. R. (1986). *J. Immunol.* **136,** 1846–1852.

Wolfgram, L. J., and Rose, N. R. (1989). *Immunol. Res.* **8,** 61–80.

Zabriskie, J. B., Hsu, K. C., and Seegal, B. C. (1970). *Clin. Exp. Immunol.* **7,** 147–159.

CHAPTER **13**

Autoimmune Diseases of Muscle

PETER N. HOLLINGSWORTH
ROGER L. DAWKINS

Department of Clinical Immunology
Royal Perth Hospital
Perth, Western Australia

RANJENY THOMAS

Department of Rheumatology
University of Texas
Southwestern Medical Center
Dallas, Texas

I. INTRODUCTION

Symptomatic involvement of skeletal muscle is common in several quite different autoimmune diseases. In diseases such as rheumatoid arthritis and systemic lupus erythematosus, myalgia and even weakness are often dismissed as being secondary to inflammation of joints and tendons; specific investigation and treatment of any associated myositis are often unnecessary. In this chapter we shall restrict ourselves to those autoimmune diseases associated with profound weakness due to immunologically mediated injury to the myofiber itself. Autoimmune diseases principally affecting the neuromuscular junction are considered elsewhere.

The terms polymyositis and idiopathic inflammatory myopathy are often used interchangeably to describe apparently noninfectious but inflammatory disorders that can result in essentially symmetrical weakness of multiple muscle groups. Undoubtedly the mechanisms of the injury are heterogeneous, but several clinical entities can be distinguished. The validity of the distinctions between these diseases remains unclear with respect to the pathogenesis of the muscle injury, but there do appear to be correlations between some pathological and immunological characteristics on the one hand and the response to treatment on the other. For example, adult polymyositis (PM) and dermatomyositis (DM) are often steroid responsive, whereas inclusion body myositis appears to be rather less so. DM and mixed connective tissue disease (MCTD) can often be distinguished by their autoantibody profiles and perhaps their human leukocyte antigen (HLA) associations.

Unfortunately, relevant etiological agents have not been identified and specific immunotherapy is not yet possible. For the time being, clinical approaches must be largely empirical, but recent discoveries have suggested that some generalizations may be possible in the near future. We shall argue that several etiological agents including drugs such as D-penicillamine and perhaps certain viruses can lead to an immune response, which will vary depending on the immunogenetics of the host. Cytotoxic T cells may be generated, and these are capable of destroying myofibers. Capillaries may also be destroyed, especially in juvenile DM, possibly by immune complex-mediated reactions. Various autoantibodies also develop, many of these having specificity for intracellular proteins involved in transcription and translations of genetic code to protein. Particular autoantibodies correlate with particular syndromes, such as PM associated with interstitial lung disease, PM associated with progressive systemic sclerosis, DM, and MCTD.

II. CLASSIFICATION

For the present purposes, we shall make a distinction between polymyositis as a descriptive term for necrotizing myositis and polymyositis (PM) and dermatomyositis (DM) as clinical entities. The clinical syndrome of PM/DM has been variously subclassified according to age of onset, skin involvement, and associated features such as C2 deficiency (Bohan and Peter, 1975; Mastaglia and Walton, 1982; Dawkins *et al.*, 1982) (Table I). Further classification according to histopathological details, type of associated connective tissue disease, autoantibodies, and immunogenetic associations, will be argued here (Table I). Drug-induced polymyositis, particularly D-penicillamine-induced polymyositis (Carroll *et al.*, 1987) is pathologically similar to PM but separated from PM on the basis of etiological and immunogenetic features (Table I). Inclusion body myositis is now recognized as a disease entity (Lotz et al., 1989). It is not associated with polymyositis specific autoantibodies and responds poorly to prednisolone. It will be discussed here, with the autoimmune diseases of muscle, because the histological changes (Bertolini, 1988; Carpenter, 1988; Sawchak, 1988), cellular infiltrates (Arahata and Engel, 1990), changes in blood lymphocytes (Miller *et al.*, 1990) and prevalence of associated autoimmune diseases (Lotz *et al.*, 1989) are so similar to PM. The diseases that should be considered in the differential diagnosis of PM/DM are shown in Table II. Inflammatory changes in muscle (polymyositis) may occur in several of these conditions but are usually mild and

TABLE I

Clinicopathological Classification of Inflammatory Myopathies

Infective
Viral
Bacterial
Parasitic
Idiopathic
Polymyositis
Dermatomyositis
Polymyositis and dermatomyositis associated with malignancy
Myositis associated with connective tissue diseases
Mixed connective tissue disease
Systemic lupus erythematosus
Progressive systemic sclerosis
Interstitial lung disease
D-penicillamine-induced polymyositis
Juvenile dermatomyositis
Myositis associated with vasculitis
Inclusion-body myositis
Eosinophilic polymyositis, hypereosinophilic syndrome
Granulomatous myositis
Sarcoidosis
Connective tissue diseases

TABLE II

Differential Diagnosis of Inflammatory Myopathy

Rheumatoid arthritis
Polymyalgia rheumatica
Myasthenia gravis and myasthenic myopathy
Neurogenic atrophy, Guillain-Barré syndrome
Motor neuron disease
Muscular dystrophy
Endocrine myopathy
Metabolic myopathy
Periodic paralysis
Electrolyte disturbances–hypokalemia, hypercalcemia
Enzyme deficiency
Drug and toxic myopathies
Carcinomatous myopathy (paraneoplastic)
Amyloidosis

focal, may not be symptomatic and should not necessarily justify the diagnosis of PM/DM.

III. EXPERIMENTAL MODELS

Generalized myositis can be induced in experimental animals by immunization with skeletal muscle or fractions of skeletal muscle in Freund's complete adjuvant (Dawkins, 1975). These animals develop uniphasic disease characterized by segmental necrosis of skeletal muscle. Lymphocyte-mediated cytotoxicity to cultured muscle has been demonstrated and is thought to be the major pathogenic mechanism in experimental autoallergic myositis. Antibodies reactive with contractile proteins of skeletal muscle (e.g., actomyosin) are also demonstrable in sera (Dawkins, 1975). These antibodies resemble those found in patients with MG and a thymoma. Interestingly, they are not found in patients with PM/DM.

Inflammatory muscle disease may also be induced experimentally by means of a number of viruses including Semliki Forest virus, encephalomyocarditis virus, Ross River virus, and Coxsackievirus (Whitaker, 1982). Polymyositis induced by Coxsackie B1 virus in mice is strain dependent (Ray *et al.*, 1979) and may provide a model with which to explore the immunogenetic basis of some forms of polymyositis.

The breadth and complexity of autoimmune muscle disease is illustrated by the spontaneous disease that occurs in the African Mastomys. These animals appear to be predisposed to several autoimmune diseases and thymoma. In some respects their muscle disease resembles myasthenia gravis plus polymyositis, and in this regard, they may be similar to the occasional patient with coexistent thymoma, MG, and polymyositis.

IV. CLINICAL FEATURES

Previous extensive reviews are provided in Mastaglia and Walton (1982) and Bohan (1988). The incidence of polymyositis is approximately 5 per million per year, with a peak in the fifth and sixth decades, and a smaller peak in childhood. It is more frequent in blacks than whites and in females than males.

As with other forms of myopathy, the presenting feature of autoimmune muscle disease will generally be weakness. The nature of the weakness will largely determine the clinician's approach. If there is excessive fatiguability, that is, reversible weakness that improves after rest, the differential diagnosis will include disorders of the neuromuscular junction such as MG. Clinical testing is generally sufficient to demonstrate deterioration with exercise and improvement after rest, but it is often useful to show that the patient improves after anticholinesterase therapy. Electromyography may also assist in that it may be possible to demonstrate a decremental response and to distinguish this change from that which occurs in the Eaton–Lambert syndrome and other disorders associated with myasthenia.

In other patients, the weakness may be "fixed" in that it remains relatively constant throughout the day and from day to day. In such patients one can generally assume that there is an abnormality of the muscle fiber per se rather than of the neuromuscular junction. Other possibilities, such as denervation, need to be excluded. Evidence in favor of myofiber necrosis might be provided by demonstration of elevated serum creatine kinase activity and by biopsy.

The distribution of weakness is also very useful. In generalized myasthenia gravis, extraocular, facial, bulbar, and proximal musculature is generally involved. In PM/DM, extraocular muscles are spared, but proximal and truncal muscles are usually affected.

Other symptoms and signs of autoimmune muscle disease depend on the nature of the lesion. If there is major inflammatory component, or acute rhabdomyolysis, the patient may complain of muscle pain and tenderness, but these features are generally more pronounced in the presence of synovitis, tenosynovitis, or interstitial inflammation.

The tempo of polymyositis varies. A minority of patients will have acute very severe myositis and necrosis, developing in a few days. They may be systemically ill with fever, malaise, dysphagia, joint pains, and edema and with very high plasma concentrations of muscle enzymes, myoglobinuria, and renal failure. Some of these will have PM and some, DM, with associated cancer. This syndrome must be distinguished from rhabdomyolysis due to drugs, toxins, metabolic disease, and viral infection. Most have a subacute illness, developing over weeks to months. There is symmetrical weakness of pelvic and shoulder girdle muscles, particularly affecting neck flexors, with sparing of distal muscles and of facial and extraocular muscles. Weakness is disproportionate to apparent wasting, muscles are rarely tender, and reflexes are preserved. DM skin involvement, associated connective tissue disease, or cancer may be present. Some will have a chronic disease, evolving gradually over several years, often involving distal as well as proximal muscles, without skin involvement, associated connective tissue disease, or cancer. This presentation is typical of inclusion-body myositis.

Associated features are important. The characteristic dermal involvement of DM is almost pathognomonic. This comprises an erythematous rash in the "butterfly" distribution of sun-exposed skin on the cheeks, nose, and forehead, with heliotrope discoloration of eyelids, a scaling erythematous rash on the dorsal aspects of the knuckles of the metacarpophalangeal and interphalangeal joints (Gottron's sign), periungual erythema, and telangiectasis. There may also be acrosclerosis: shiny, thin, inelastic skin in the hands. In juvenile DM, calcinosis of skin may occur, especially over the elbows, knuckles, and heels. Dysphagia,

Raynaud's phenomenon, and joint pain occur particularly in those with acute rhabdomyolysis, and those with associated connective tissue disease. MCTD, scleroderma, and systemic lupus erythematosus (SLE) are discussed elsewhere in this book, and diagnostic criteria for myasthenia gravis, polymyositis, and MCTD have been discussed elsewhere (Dawkins *et al.*, 1982).

Cancer has been associated in 7 to 24% of PM/DM, with the average from combined studies of adults being 13% (Hochberg, 1986). Patients with cancer tend to be older, and cancer is not associated with JDM (Pachmann and Maryjowski, 1984). Lakhanpal *et al.* (1986) have asserted that any increase in malignancy is not clinically significant, mainly reflecting referral bias, and that there is no increased risk of malignancy after the diagnosis of PM/DM.

The case fatality rate was 17.1% in a study by Hochberg *et al.* (1986). Mortality is higher in older patients, those with cardiac involvement, higher white cell count, and pneumonia, but not with malignancy (Hochberg *et al.*, 1986; Benbassat, 1985).

V. PATHOLOGY

A. Histopathology and Electron Microscopy

Examination of muscle biopsies is useful, not only to confirm and classify polymyositis, but also to assess response to treatment in problem cases, to confirm or exclude other forms of myopathy, and to assess vascular changes. Needle biopsy gives sufficient tissue in many cases and should lead to more frequent use of muscle biopsy. The pathology of polymyositis (inflammatory myopathy) has been reviewed in Mastaglia and Walton (1982), and in Dalakas (1988), by Bertorini (1988), Carpenter (1988), and briefly by Plotz *et al.* (1989).

Muscle tissue exhibits only a limited range of changes in response to injury. While myofiber necrosis, regeneration, and mononuclear inflammatory infiltrate are the key features, none of these is of itself specific to primary inflammatory disease of muscle (Mastaglia and Walton, 1982).

The key features of polymyositis are segmental myofiber necrosis and regeneration occurring *pari passu,* and associated inflammatory infiltration (Fig. 1). The extent of these changes varies from patient to patient. In those with acute rhabdomyolysis, extensive necrosis will be apparent, often with minimal inflammatory infiltrate. In those with subacute polymyositis, there may be necrosis of scattered or even single fibers. Necrotic fibers show hyalinization, loss of staining, and invasion by macrophages. Regenerating fibers can be recognized by the appearance of myotubes containing myoblasts with enlarged, central nuclei with prominent nucleoli, and cytoplasmic basophilia due to increased RNA. Lymphocytes, plasma cells, and macrophages predominate in the inflammatory infiltrate, occurring focally within fascicles and fibers, in perimyseal connective tissue and within or surrounding small blood vessels (Fig. 1). However, differences are now recognized between inclusion-body myositis and PM on the one hand, and DM and juvenile DM on the other (Bertolini, 1987; Carpenter, 1987).

In adult PM, necrosis is apparently confined to the muscle fibers, with no necrosis or loss of capillaries. The inflammatory cells occur within the fascicles rather than in perimyseal or perivascular areas (Carpenter, 1988). Close contact, partial invasion, and invasion of non-necrotic fibers by lymphocytes is characteristic (Fig. 2), (Mastaglia and Walton, 1982; Engel *et al.*, 1990).

In JDM, and commonly in DM, vascular damage, particularly necrosis and loss of capillaries precedes muscle necrosis and infiltration by inflammatory cells (Engel *et al.*, 1990). Atrophic and necrotic fibers are concentrated around the edge of the fascicle (perifascicular atrophy), farthest from the supplying arteriole that penetrates to the center of the fascicle before branching (Carpenter, 1988). Electron microscopy studies show endothelial swelling in capillaries, with protrusion into the lumen causing occlusion. Endothelial necrosis, degeneration, and regeneration occur *pari passu,* and replication of the basal lamina results from repeated cycles of degeneration and regeneration (Fenichel, 1988). Platelet thrombi occlude larger vessels (Fenichel, 1988). Portions of fascicles, or whole fascicles and adjacent connective tissue, may be necrotic. Inflammatory infiltrates are less conspicuous, and mainly in fibrous septa adjacent to lymphatics and larger vessels. These findings in juvenile DM and DM are similar to those in necrotizing vasculitis (Wegener's granulomatosis, polyarteritis, and some cases of SLE) and imply that the muscle fibers are damaged by ischemia (Carpenter, 1988; Fenichel, 1988). JDM may be considered a systemic angiopathy in which vascular occlusion accounts for the observed changes in muscle as well as ischemic lesions of skin and gut (Fenichel, 1988).

Inclusion-body myositis, according to Lotz *et al.* (1989), can now be recognized as a disease entity in which a set of pathologic features is consistently associated with a constellation of clinical findings. Light microscopy demonstrates eosinophilic granules and vacuoles with basophilic granules at their rim in the cytoplasm of muscle fibers. The basophilic granules are phospholipid containing membranous whorls, which may dissolve during processing for routine H and E sections, but are demonstrable on frozen section. Electron microscopy shows abnormal tubular filaments associated with and adjacent to the vacuoles in cytoplasm and in the nucleus of muscle fibers (Mastaglia and Walton, 1982; Sawchak and Kula, 1988). Neither the vacuoles nor the filaments alone are specific for inclusion-body myositis, but the filaments are not seen in PM or DM (Lotz *et al.*, 1989). Pathological features essential for the diagnosis were defined by Lotz *et al.* (1989) in a study of 48 cases of suspected IBM in a series of 170 consecutive cases of polymyositis. They are (1) more than one rimmed vacuole per high-power field (100%); (2) more than one group of atrophic fibers per

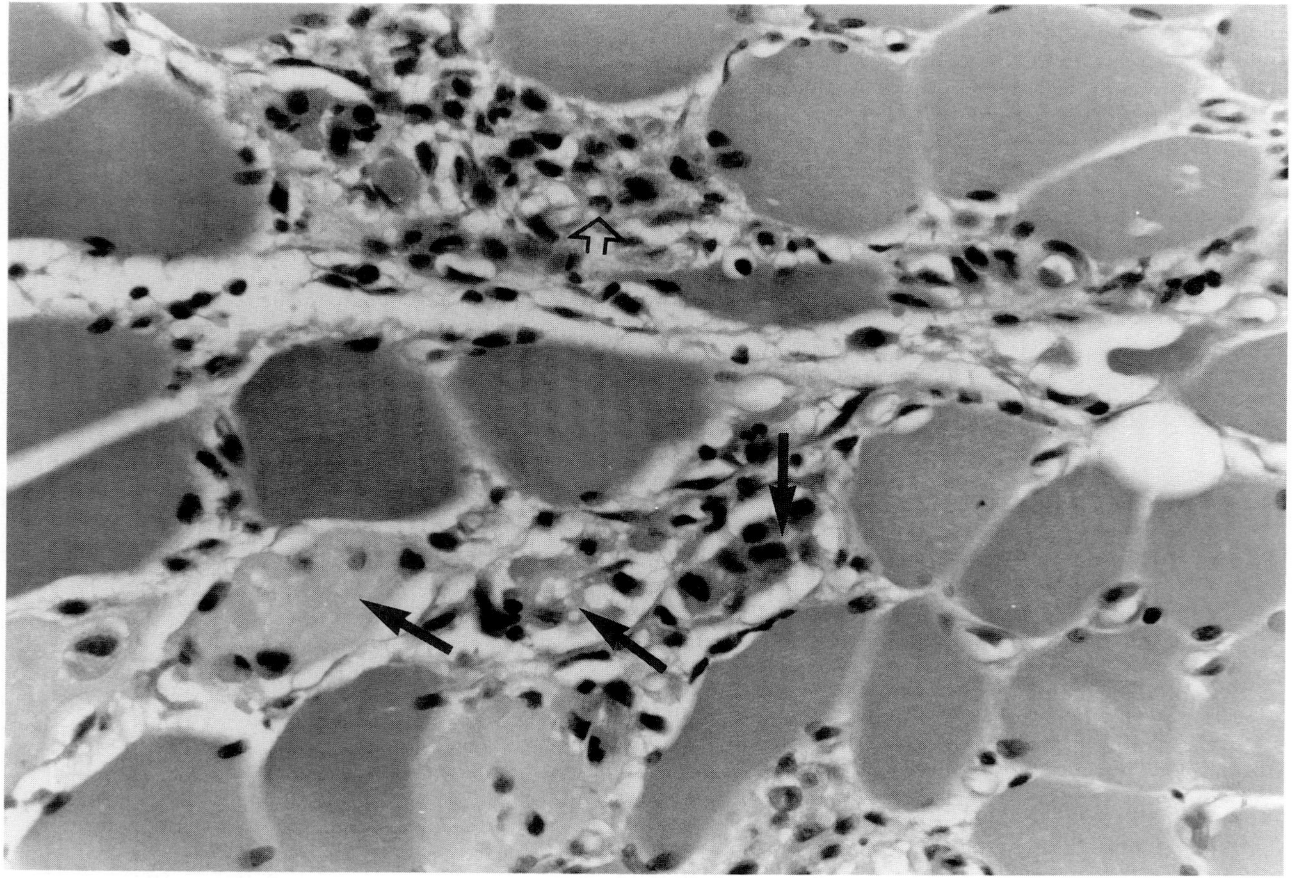

FIG. 1a Polymyositis. Mononuclear phagocytic cells are seen invading several myofibers which are undergoing necrosis (arrows). A scant lymphohistiocytic infiltrate permeates the endomysium (arrowhead). Haematoxylin and eosin (530 ×).

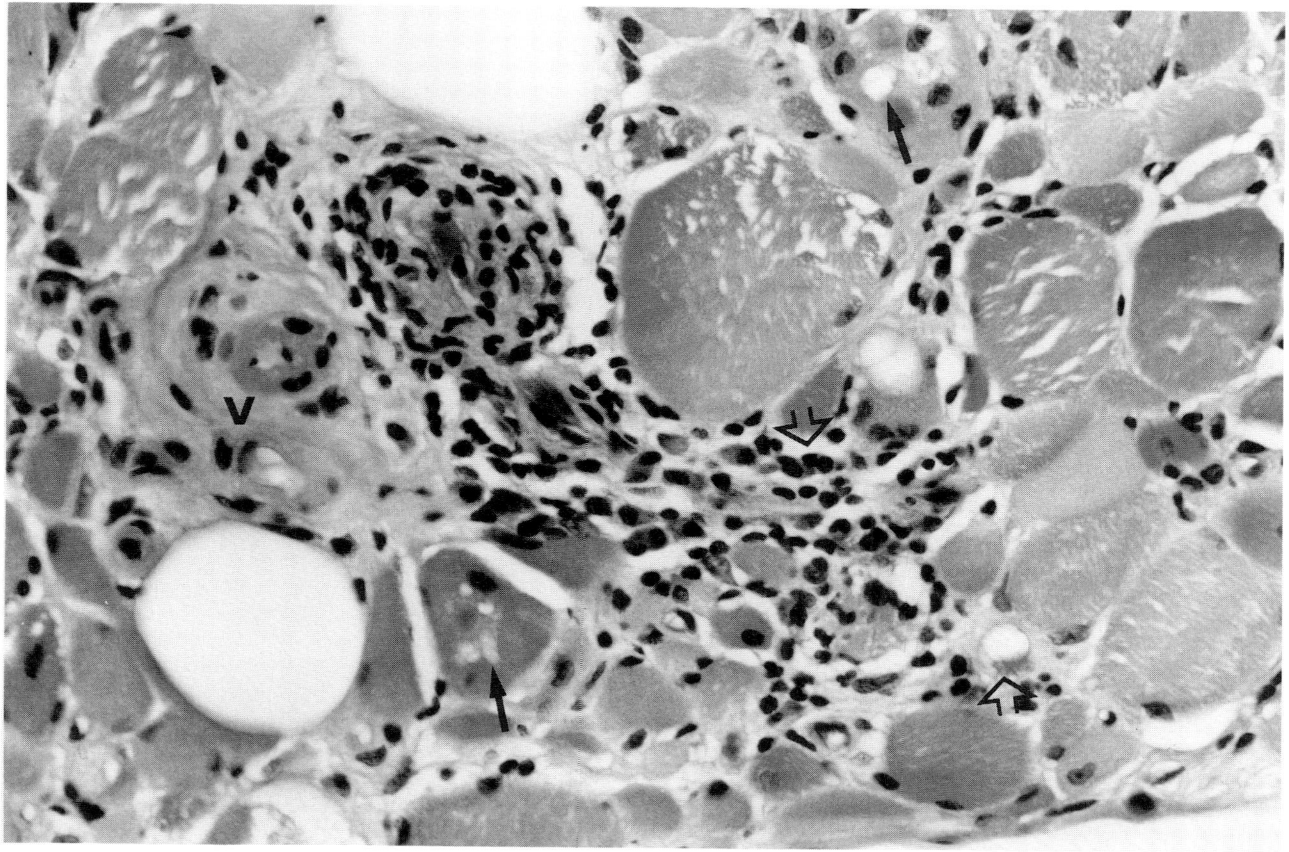

FIG. 1b Polymyositis. A heavy mononuclear inflammatory infiltrate is present in the perivascular (V) and interfascicular connective tissues and extending into the fascicle (arrowheads). Several necrotic fibers show vacuolar change and phagocytic invasion (arrows). Perifascicular atrophy is apparent. Haematoxylin and eosin (530×). (Figures provided by Dr. J. Harvey).

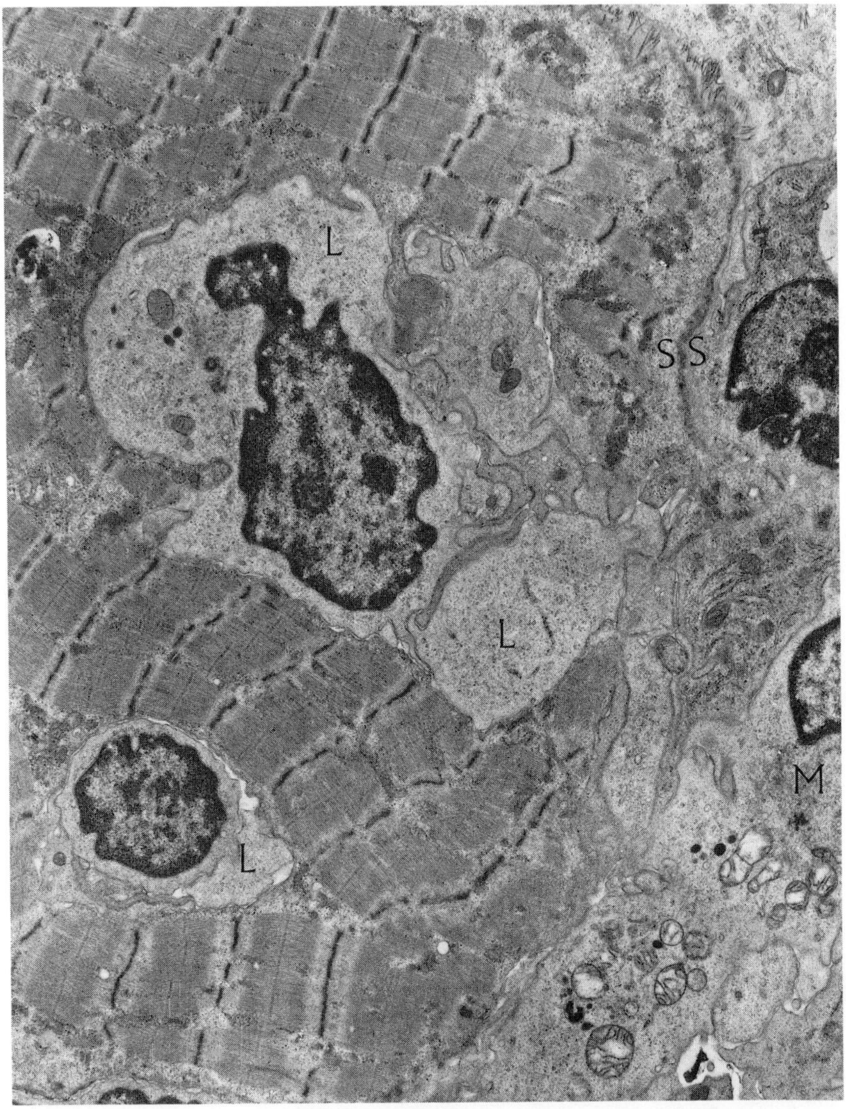

FIG. 2 Polymyositis. Electron micrograph showing inflammatory cells including lymphocytes (L), and macrophages (M) penetrating a striated muscle fiber via a defect in the sarcolemmal sheath (SS). Cytoplasmic spikes from the lymphocytes are invading the sarcoplasm. Magnification × 22,000. Figure provided by Professor J. M. Papadimitriou.

low-power field (96%); (3) an endomyseal (intrafascicular) and autoaggressive inflammatory exudate (92%); and (4) typical filamentous inclusions shown by electron microscopy (93%). There is no loss of capillaries, and inflammatory cells are sparse in perifascicular and perivascular areas.

In a series of 177 consecutive cases of polymyositis, the frequency of pathological diagnoses was PM, 31.2%; inclusion-body myositis, 28.2%; DM, 18.2%; perivascular inflammation, 8.3%; MCTD, 4.7%; eosinophilic fasciitis, 2.9%; necrotizing vasculitis, 2.3%; scleroderma with polymyositis, 2.3%; granulomatous myositis, 1.2%; and focal myositis, 0.6% (Lotz *et al.*, 1989).

VI. IMMUNOLOGY

A. Autoantibodies

In polymyositis, the most notable serological feature is the presence of antibodies to one or more nuclear or cytoplasmic antigens. Antinuclear antibodies as detected by immunofluorescence on rodent tissue are relatively infrequent (16–35%), and of low titer. However, 89% of a series of 114 patients studied by Reichlin and Arnett (1984) had antibodies detectable by immunofluorescence on Hep-2 cells and/or immunoprecipitation with thymus extract. Some of these antibodies have high specificity and predictive value for myositis syndromes (Table IV). The majority of myositis patients have at least one such antibody. The antigens are summarized in Table III, and have certain remarkable features in common (Tan, 1989; Plotz *et al.*, 1989). They are usually combinations of RNA and protein, highly conserved, and functioning in transcription and translation of genetic code to protein. The antigenic epitopes are on functional sites of the protein, and the autoantibodies inhibit their function (Matthews and Bernstein, 1983; Dang *et al.*, 1988). The antibodies to aminoacyl tRNA synthetases are of particular interest, and the best studied is anti-Jo-1 or anti-histidyl-t-RNA synthetase (Matthews and Bernstein, 1983; Plotz *et al.*, 1989; Cronin *et al.*, 1988). This enzyme binds histidine and t-RNA, and attaches the histidine to the tail of the RNA. It may also bind the genomic RNA of picornaviruses such as Coxsackie, and attach histidine to it (Plotz, 1983). Indeed, picornaviruses would be expected to exploit such enzymes during their replication. Anti-Jo-1 is predominantly IgG1, persists but fluctuates with disease activity, and its titer is independent of total IgG1 (Plotz *et al.*, 1989). These findings suggest that it is a T cell-dependent, antigen-driven response, as originally suggested by Tan and reviewed by Tan (1989). The antibody may then be a *reporter* of the original event that initiated the disease. Several explanations of the origin of the antibodies are suggested: (1) They may be directed against a viral product and cross-react with the autoantigen (Matthews and Bernstein, 1983); (2) They may be an antiidiotype

TABLE III

Biochemical Characteristics of Antigens Recognized by Myositis-Related Autoantibodies

Antigen	Location	Immunofluorescence pattern	Properties or function	Reference
nRNP	Nucleus	Speckled	mRNA splicing	Tan (1989)
Ku	Nucleus	Reticular[a]	Binds free ends of dsDNA	Mimori *et al.* (1985)
Mi_1	Nucleus	Rim Particulate[b]	Unknown	Targoff *et al.* (1983)
Mi_2	Nucleus	Homogeneous[c]	Unknown	Targoff and Reichlin (1985)
56-kDa protein	Nucleus	Speckled	RNA processing	Arad-Dann *et al.* (1989)
PM-Scl	Nucleolus	Nucleolar	Related to preribosomes	Reimer (1986)
Jo-1	Cytoplasm	Variable	Histidyl tRNA synthetase	Hochberg *et al.* (1984)
PL-7	Cytoplasm	Homogeneous	Threonyl tRNA synthetase	Targoff *et al.* (1988)
PL-12	Cytoplasm	Homogeneous	Alanyl tRNA synthetase and alanyl tRNA	Targoff and Arnett (1990) Bunn and Mathews (1987)
Isoleucyl tRNA synthetase	Cytoplasm	?	Isoleucyl tRNA synthetase	Targoff *et al.* (1988)
Glycyl tRNA synthetase	Cytoplasm	?	Glycyl tRNA synthetase	Targoff *et al.* (1988)
K-J	Cytoplasm	Homogeneous	Protein associated with ribosomal translation	Targoff *et al.* (1989)
SRP	Cytoplasm	?	Ribonuclear protein: translocates nascent polypeptides across ER	Plotz *et al.* (1989)

[a]On human liver substrate.
[b]On mouse liver substrate.
[c]On mouse spleen substrate.

TABLE IV

Approximate Prevalence of Certain Autoantibodies in Patients with Myositis

	PM	PM or DM	DM	PM + ILD	PM + PSS	MCTD	Reference
Antibodies to t-RNA synthetases							
Histidyl	30		<10	50–100	<5	<5	Nishikai and Reichlin (1980), Hochberg *et al.* (1984)
Threonyl		3–5		H[b]	NA[a]	NA	Mathews *et al.* (1984), Targoff *et al.* (1988)
Alanyl		<5		H	NA	NA	Bunn and Mathews (1987), Targoff (1990)
Isoleucyl		<5		H	NA	NA	Targoff *et al.* (1988)
Glycyl		<5		H	NA	NA	Targoff *et al.* (1988)
Antibodies to other intracellular antigens							
Mi_1	0		3	0	<5	<5	Targoff *et al.* (1983)
Mi_2	<5		20	<5	NA	<5	Targoff and Reichlin (1985)
56 kDa		85		NA	NA	NA	Arad-Dann *et al.* (1989)
nRNP		4–15		<5	5–10	85–100	Arnett *et al.* (1981), Reichlin *et al.* (1984)
Ku	<5		NA	NA	50	<5	Mimori *et al.* (1985), Nakamura and Arnett (1985)
Pm-Scl	8		NA	NA	50	NA	Reichlin and Arnett (1984)
KJ		<5		NA	NA	NA	Targoff *et al.* (1989)
+SRP	<5		0	NA	NA	NA	Plotz *et al.* (1989)

[a]NA, data not available.
[b]H, few cases, but highly associated with PM + ILD.

to viral antibody (Plotz, 1983). The coincidence of antibody to alanyl tRNA synthetase and to alanyl tRNA (Bunn and Mathews, 1987) in the serum of the same patient has been quoted as evidence for idiotype networks; (3) They may be a response to viral protein bound to self-protein, with peptides from degraded viral protein being presented to T helper cells, thereby providing help for B cells reactive with epitopes on the self-protein; or (4) They may be a response to the self-protein that has been presented in an aberrant way to the immune system.

Anti Jo-1 is associated with the combination of myositis, interstitial lung disease, Raynaud's phenomenon, joint pains, and with HLA-DR3 or -DR6 (Plotz *et al.*, 1989; Arnett *et al.*, 1981). It is not associated with interstitial lung disease without myositis (Wasicek *et al.*, 1990). The other antibodies to tRNA synthetases are apparently specific for the combination of myositis and interstitial lung disease, but relatively few cases have been reported. Anti-Mi_1 and anti-Mi_2 are associated with DM, but anti-Mi_1 was found also in 5% of SLE patients, including 7% of those with anti-RNP and 9% of those with anti-Sm

(Targoff and Reichlin, 1985; Targoff *et al.*, 1983). Anti-Ku and anti-PM-Scl identify the combination of polymyositis and progressive systemic sclerosis (Mimori *et al.*, 1981). High titers of antibodies to ribonucleoprotein (RNP) have been used as part of the definition of MCTD (Chapter 8), but there is little doubt that high-titer anti-RNP is associated with inflammatory muscle disease occurring in diverse clinical situations. Other autoantibodies including anti-SSA(Ro), antithyroid microsome, and rheumatoid factor have been detected, but are not specific for polymyositis syndromes (Cronin *et al.*, 1988).

Nishikai and Homma (1977) detected antibodies to myoglobin in 70% of patients with PM, but also found them with high frequency in other diseases (e.g., MG). Wada *et al.*, (1983) reported the detection of antibodies to skeletal muscle myosin in 90% of patients with PM as well as in a smaller percentage of patients with other diseases of muscle (e.g., MG, muscular dystrophy). Detection of these antibodies bore no relationship to the presence of AStr antibodies. By contrast, Carrano *et al.* (1983) were unable to demonstrate reactivity of PM sera with crude actomyosin by enzyme-linked immunosorbent assay (ELISA), although reactivity with this antigen correlated with the presence of AStr antibodies in sera from patients with MG. We conclude that antibodies to contractile proteins and certainly anti-Str are rarely detectable in PM, and in this respect the human disease contrasts with EAM.

Despite the presence of several autoantibodies in polymyositis, none seems to play a direct role in producing the damage to skeletal muscle. Serum from PM and DM patients has not been shown to be cytotoxic to cultured muscle cells (Dawkins and Mastaglia, 1973). The presence of immunoglobulin and complement in the necrotic fibers seems to be a consequence of the damage rather than its cause (Fig. 3). IgG can occasionally be demonstrated in apparently intact myofibers in the absence of complement components or fibrinogen (Dawkins *et al.*, 1982), but the significance of this apparent *in vivo* binding of IgG is unclear. Controversy also exists as to the significance of apparent *in vivo* binding of speckled antinuclear antibody seen in skin and muscle biopsies of patients with MCTD, and occasionally, DM. Some suggest that this is an artefact of high-titer circulating antinuclear antibody, which binds to the nuclei during processing of the biopsy. Others (Alarcon-Segovia *et al.*, 1978) have demonstrated entry of anti-RNP into human monocytes via Fc receptors and speculated that the entry of autoantibody into viable cells in this way may be of pathogenetic importance.

B. Immunoglobulin and Complement

Reduced complement concentrations are not a usual feature of PM (Cumming *et al.*, 1977). If C3 and C4 concentrations are normal but hemolytic activity is low, then C2 deficiency might be suspected, particularly given a family history of

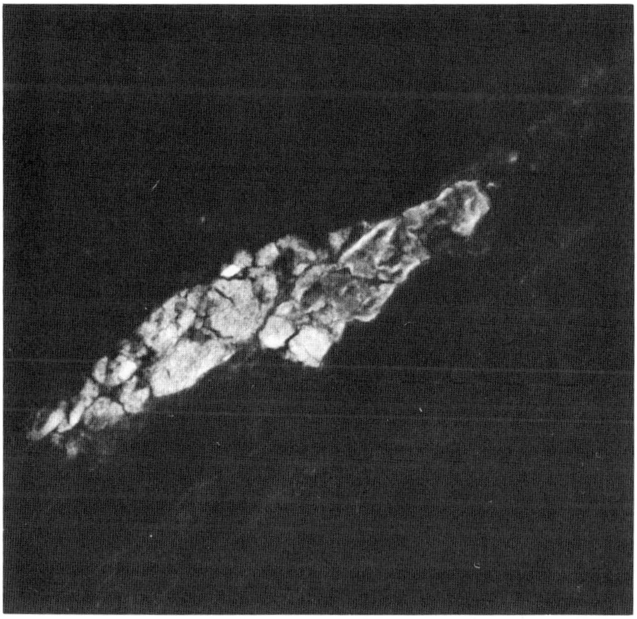

FIG. 3 Indirect immunofluorescent staining of immunoglobulin in a biopsy of skeletal muscle from a patient with polymyositis. Similar intrafiber staining was seen using antifibrinogen and anticomplement reagents (originally × 160). Reproduced from Garlepp and Dawkins (1984), with permission from the editor of *Clinics in Rheumatic Disease*.

relevant diseases (Dawkins *et al.*, 1982). In MCTD, serum-complement activity is reduced in some cases, particularly those with cryoglobulinemia. If serum C4 is decreased and anti-DNA antibodies are elevated, then the possibility of coincident SLE should be considered.

Circulating immune complexes, and deposition of IgG, IgM, and C3 and of the late complement components or membrane attack complex (MAC) in blood vessel walls are demonstrable in JDM and in some cases of DM (Whittaker and Engel, 1972; Behan and Behan, 1977; Engel *et al.*, 1990).

By examining biopsies from clinically unaffected and histologically normal muscles from patients with DM, Engel *et al.* (1990) demonstrated that capillary depletion precedes muscle-fiber necrosis and that MAC components are deposited on remaining capillaries.

PM/DM can occur in the presence of agammaglobulinemia and hypogammaglobulinemia, and some patients do have low or borderline low serum-IgG concentrations and respond poorly to tetanus immunization. By contrast, patients classified as MCTD tend to have elevated serum-IgG concentration.

C. Mononuclear Cells

There is good evidence for cell-mediated immunity and cellular cytotoxicity in some but not necessarily all cases of polymyositis. Intimate contact and invasion of nonnecrotic muscle fibers by lymphocytes (Mastaglia and Walton, 1982 and Fig. 2) occur particularly in PM and inclusion body myositis. Lymphocyte-mediated cytotoxicity to cultured muscle has been demonstrated in some cases of PM/DM and in experimental autoallergic myositis (Dawkins *et al.*, 1975). Lymphocyte transformation in response to the patient's own skeletal muscle (syngeneic) and to muscle from other patients (allogeneic) has been demonstrated in over 50% of cases of active untreated PM/DM (Kalovidoris *et al.*, 1989). This carefully controlled study did address the shortcomings of previous such studies by including syngeneic as well as allogeneic muscle and by including healthy subjects, patients with neuromuscular diseases, with connective tissue diseases, and with treated polymyositis as comparison groups.

Detailed analysis of the distribution and subsets of mononuclear cells in muscle biopsies of patients with polymyositis has been undertaken by Engel, Arahata and colleagues and reviewed by Engel *et al.*, (1990). In DM and juvenile DM, the location of the inflammatory cells is predominantly perivascular and perimysial (around fascicles) and to a lesser extent, endomysial (within fascicles). In contrast, in PM and inclusion-body myositis the exudate is predominantly focal and endomysial. In PM the exudate is also perivascular and perimysial (Arahata and Engel, 1984).

The proportion of macrophages is similar at each site, but the proportion of lymphocyte subsets differs at these sites and differs between DM, PM, and inclusion body myositis. In DM and juvenile DM, B cells are increased in the perivascular region. Here they are close to T helper (CD4) cells and macrophages, as would be expected in a local response with antibody production. T cells predominate in perimysial and endomysial areas. Invasion of nonnecrotic fibers (by CD8-bearing cytotoxic T cells, not NK cells) was observed in only a few fibers, in fewer than half of the cases.

In PM and inclusion body myositis approximately 70% of endomysial cells are T cells and 80% of these are CD8-bearing cytotoxic T cells. Most of the remainder are macrophages, with 2% or fewer B cells or mature NK cells. The CD8 T cells invade nonnecrotic fibers. Many of these cells, and the fibers they attack, bear increased HLA class I molecules (Karpati *et al.*, 1988). These findings imply that MHC-restricted cytotoxic T cells rather than non-MHC-restricted NK cells injure muscle fibers in PM and inclusion-body myositis. In addition, fibers with segmental necrosis, invaded mainly by macrophages and having components of the membrane attack complex of complement on their surface, occur in PM and less frequently in inclusion-body myositis. It is possible, therefore, that a second cytotoxic mechanism, probably antibody and complement, operates in PM (Engel and Arahata, 1986; Engel *et al.*, 1990).

In summary, the findings of these studies imply a spectrum of pathogenetic mechanisms in polymyositis. In juvenile DM, and DM, antibody and complement mediated vascular and muscle fiber injury predominate. In PM both antibody and complement and cytotoxic T cells injure muscle fibers. In inclusion body myositis T cell cytotoxicity predominates.

D. Immunogenetics

Immunogenetic analysis of PM requires consideration of various clinical subgroups. Most studies have shown that HLA-B8 and -DR3 are increased in adult PM and DM, but Hirsch *et al.* (1981) showed no increase in a small group of patients with adult DM. In juvenile DM it seems clear that B8 and DR3 are increased in frequency, most probably by virtue of the A1,B8,DR3 (8.1) ancestral haplotype (Table V).

Comprehensive MHC typing of our patients with PM, DM, MCTD, and D-P PM (Table VI, VII) yields several conclusions. First, the data confirm an association between PM/DM and the 8.1 ancestral haplotype, which is also associated with MG, SLE, and many other autoimmune diseases. The present results lead us to the conclusion that PM, DM, and JDM are similar at least with respect to the immunogenetic association with the 8.1 ancestral haplotype. Presently undefined are differences in the relative importance of the HLA genes themselves (e.g., DR, DQ, and the central, non-HLA genes of the MHC). The complete 8.1 haplotype HLA-A1, B8, BfS, C4AQ0, C4B1, DR3, DQ2 is not always present, and the central part containing the haplospecific complotype BfS, C4AQ0, C4B1 is the most frequent association (Table VIIA,B). If confirmed by further studies, this finding suggests that the HLA associations may reflect gene(s) present within the central MHC. It is interesting that some of these (e.g., C4, C2, TNF) are potentially immunoregulatory products of macrophages and are polymorphic in structure and/or gene copy number (French and Dawkins, 1990). The 8.1 ancestral haplotype appears to predispose to hyperreactivity so that other factors must determine the nature of the clinical syndrome (French and Dawkins, 1990).

The immunogenetic associations of the myositis of MCTD are different (Table VIIC). There is a very clear increase in DR4 and particularly in DQ3. In contrast to another DR4-DQ3-associated disease [insulin-dependent diabetes mellitus (IDDM)] the increment appears to reflect the DQw7 split of DQ3.

In D-Penicillamine PM/DM there is also an increase in DR4. This could reflect the underlying disease, rheumatoid arthritis (RA), for which D-Penicillamine was prescribed. However, D-Penicillamine-induced MG is associated with DR1 and/or DR7 (Garlepp *et al.*, 1983), and, therefore, differs from RA and from idiopathic MG, which is associated with A1,B8,DR3 and D-Penicillamine myositis associated with DR4. We may speculate that D-Penicillamine binds to and alters the peptide-binding groove of the MHC class II molecule, thereby altering presentation of antigen and inducing autoimmunity.

TABLE V
Polymyositis and Dermatomyositis Have Been Associated with HLA-B8 and -DR3

			Antigen frequency (%)		
Condition	n	Antigen	Disease	Healthy controls	References
PM	37	B8	44	28	Cumming *et al.* (1978)
PM	14	B8	61	NS[b]	Behan *et al.* (1978)
PM	13	B8	54	21	Hirsch *et al.* (1981)
PM	33	B8	18	30	Walker *et al.* (1982)
PM	12	DR3	67	24	Hirsch *et al.* (1981)
PM, Jo-1	11	DR3	64	22	Arnett *et al.* (1981)
PM, Jo-1	11	DRw6	45	31	Arnett *et al.* (1981)
PM, Jo-1	11	DR3 or DRw6	100	50	Arnett *et al.* (1981)
PM	25	DR3	71	23	Goldstein *et al.* (1988)
Jo-1 (White)	25	DRw52	88	62	Goldstein *et al.* (1988)
PM	24	DR3	45	31	Goldstein *et al.* (1988)
Jo-1 (Black)	24	DRw52	96	76	Goldstein *et al.* (1988)
PM, Jo-1		B8, DR3	80	NS	Plotz *et al.* (1989)
PM/DM	27	B8	48	25	McDonald (1981)
PM		B14	40	8	Cumming *et al.* (1978)
PM/DM (White)	52	DR3	48	NS	Plotz *et al.* (1989)
DM	7	B8	0	21	Hirsch *et al.* (1981)
DM	23	B8	35	20	Mellins *et al.* (1982)
DM	23	DR3	43	23	Mellins *et al.* (1982)
DM	14	A1, B8, DR3	21	5	Mandel *et al.* (1982)
DM	14	A1, B8, Cw7	28	10	Mandel *et al.* (1982)
JDM	67	B8	37	17.5	Friedman *et al.* (1983a)
JDM	36	DR3	53	23	Friedman *et al.* (1983b)
IBM	12	DR1	50	15	Plotz *et al.* (1989)
SRP[a]	NS	DR5	67	NS	Plotz *et al.* (1989)

[a]Signal-recognition protein.
[b]NS Not stated.

Adult DM has been reported in association with C2 deficiency (Leddy *et al.*, 1975; Dawkins *et al.*, 1982). In both cases the ancestral haplotype carrying the C2 null allele was A25,B18,DR2,BfS. The role of C2 deficiency in the induction of autoimmune disease is unknown, but an explanation in terms of immunoregulation (see previous sections), as in the case of systemic lupus erythematosus, is favored.

E. Laboratory Diagnosis

The essential first step is to establish the diagnosis of polymyositis. In terms of the criteria of Bohan and Peter (1975), this requires demonstration of proximal

TABLE VI
Certain HLA Antigen and Ancestral Haplotype Frequencies Differ in MCTD, PM, and DM, and D-Pen Polymyositis

		MCTD (6)	DM (16)	PM (9)	D-Pen (8)	Health (78)
HLA	B7	14	25	45	0	30
	B8	14	27	55	25	29
	B18	0	0	18	25	7
	B12[a]	43	13	0	12	29
	B40[b]	57	7	9	12	7
	B15	0	13	9	25	7
HLA	DR3	14	33	45	0	32
	DR4[c]	71	25	9	100	34
AH	7.1	0	17	9	0	20
	8.1	14	33	27	25	22
	18.2	0	0	18	0	1

[a] $p < 0.05$ MCTD versus other myositis; $p < 0.04$ PM versus healthy.

[b] $p < 0.05$ MCTD versus other myositis; $p < 0.003$ anti-RNP versus healthy.

[c] $p < 0.03$ MCTD versus DM; $p < 0.02$ MCTD versus other myositis; $p < 0.001$ D-Pen versus PM and DM. Only 11 of 16 DM cases had DR as well as B-locus typing.

myopathy and any two of: raised muscle enzymes in the serum; a biopsy showing muscle fiber necrosis and regeneration with inflammatory cells; and typical EMG changes. Laboratory testing to exclude the potentially confounding conditions (listed in Table II) may also be required, but will not be discussed here.

Identification of polymyositis-specific and polymyositis-associated autoantibodies by the immunology laboratory may then assist in the subclassification of polymyositis, and in prognosis. Indirect immunofluorescence to detect serum antibodies reactive with cells such as HEp-2 remains a useful first step. This was positive in 78% of 114 polymyositis patients reported by Reichlin and Arnett (1984). The most prevalent patterns were speckled nuclear (59%), homogenous cytoplasmic (19%), nucleolar (10%), centromere (3%), and bright speckles (3%). Immunofluorescence detected 100% of sera with precipitating antibody to RNP, PM-Scl and Ro + La (SSA + SSB); and 60–70% of sera with precipitating antibody to Jo-1, Ro (SSA), and other unidentified antigens.

Immunodiffusion in gels is a well-established, simple, and robust technique for detection and identification of particular antibody specificities. In Reichlin and Arnett's (1984) study 18% of polymyositis patients had precipitating antibody to

TABLE VIIA

MHC Phenotypes and Probable Haplotypes in Patients with Polymyositis

CODE	A	B	Bf	C4A	C4B	DR	DQ
C0325569	1	8	S	0	1	3	2
	9	7	S	3	1	4	3
A0138699	1	8	S	0	1	3	
		15	S	5	2	10	
B4257078	2	18	F_1	3	0	3	2
		7	S	3	1	2	1
C0691561	3	18	F_1	3	Y[a]	5	7
		7	S	X	1		
J0406282	1,2	40	SS	3,X	2,Y	1	1
G6040920	11,28	8	SS				
A0315117	1	8					
E2086715	2,26	8, 35					
G4156169	2	7,35	3,3	1,0			

[a]X,Y = Homozygous of type allele or null allele. The loci HLA A, HLA B, Factor Bf, C4A, C4B, HLA DR and HLA DQ are listed in the order in which they occur on the short arm of chromosome 6. Patients are listed by a code number. Phenotypes are displayed, and where possible, we have deduced probable haplotypes. These are shown above and below the central line for each case. The ancestral haplotype (AH) 8.1 (A1, B8 BFs, C4AO, C4B1, DR3, DQ2), or recombinant fragments thereof, is boxed. DR4 and DQ3 or DQ7 are also boxed. For a discussion of ancestral haplotypes, see Dawkins (1987).

Jo-1, 13% to RNP, 8% to PM-Scl, 7% to Ro (SSA), 5% to unidentified antigens, and 4% to Mi. By immunofluorescence anti-RNP, La (SSB), and Mi gave a speckled nuclear pattern. Anti-PM-Scl was nucleolar with added nucleoplasmic staining. Anti-Jo-1 and anti-SSA were negative in 30–40% and nuclear, cytoplasmic, or both in the remainder. Nishikai (1990) has also shown that affinity-purified anti-Jo-1 binds to an antigen in the cytoplasm. Heterogeneity of reported patterns probably reflects presence or absence of additional autoantibodies.

TABLE VIIB

MHC Phenotypes and Probable Haplotypes in Patients with Dermatomyositis

CODE	A		B	Bf	C4A	C4B	DR		DQ	
			38	S	2	1	4			
K0225322	2,	24							1,	3
			62	S	4	4	6			
		1	8	S	0	1	3		2	
H0318182										
		28	15	S	3	Y	2		1	
		1	8			1	3			
K0070420					3					
		24	15			Y	1			
		1	8	S	0	1	3		2	
F2087640										
		1	8	S	0	1	3		2	
		2	8	S	0	1	3			
E4155298										
		3	7	S	3	1	2			
				F	3	0	1			
G0344702	1,	2	7						1,	3
				S	6	1	7			
				S	X	1	6			
D066636	3,	11	7,14						1	
				F	3	Y	1			
			7	S	3	1	2			
H0393103	3,	11								
			22	F	2 + 3	0	4			
				S	0	1	6			
L6183209	2,	3	35,41							7
				S	3	1	4			
				S	X	1				
J6121288	11,	26	5,62				4,	5		3
				S	3	Y				

(*continued*)

TABLE VIIB
(Continued)

CODE	A		B	Bf	C4A	C4B	DR	DQ	
				S	X	1	6		
K4174025	2		5					1	
				F	3	Y	2		
				F	3	Y			
D0312315	2,	10					6	1	
				F	X	1			
H2074926	9,	11	41	SS	4,X	2,Y			7
				S	X	1	6	2	
F0406466	11		5,44						
				F	3	Y		1	
K4189436	29,	32	44,61	SF	3	1			
K0673825	2,	9	35,40	SS	3,4	1,2	12		3

TABLE VIIC
MHC Phenotypes and Probable Haplotypes in Patients with Myositis and Mixed Connective Tissue Disease

CODE	A	B	Bf	C4A	C4B		DR		DQ
L0279157	2,11	22,40	SF	2,3	0,0		4		7
L6137163	2,3	40	SS	3,3	1,0		1,5		1
		44	S	3	Y				
D3145574	2						4		7
		27	S	X	1				
			F	0	1				7
K4214824	2,9	44					4		
			F	3	1				1
C6119951	2	40		4,4	2,1		4	1,	3
K0447577	2	12,40	SS	3,3	1,0	5,	6	1,	7

Western immunoblotting can be used to detect these antibodies, with the exception of anti-PM-Scl. Analytical sensitivity is higher than that of immunodiffusion, and additional reactivity, such as anti-56kd described by Arad-Dann (1987), may be identified if special antigen extracts are used. Affinity-purified and cloned antigens can be used in ELISA assays, which are sensitive, convenient and readily automated. These techniques are not yet widely available in routine diagnostic laboratories.

Although clinical–serological subgroups are recognizable, it must be said that the polymyositis syndromes associated with particular autoantibodies are not absolutely homogenous. The exception appears to be the complete association of anti-Mi_2 with DM. A majority of those with anti-Jo-1 will have PM (Nishikai and Reichlin, 1980; Nishikai, 1990) and over half of these will have joint pain, Raynaud's phenomenon, and interstitial lung disease (Hochberg *et al.*, 1984; Yoshida *et al.*, 1983; Plotz *et al.*, 1989). The majority of those with anti-RNP have other features of mixed connective tissue disease but others have PM or DM (Reichlin and Arnett, 1984). Only 2 out of 9 with anti-PM-Scl had overlapping PM and scleroderma, the remainder having PM or DM (Reichlin and Arnett, 1984).

The diagnostic *sensitivity* of these antibodies individually for *polymyositis* is low. They can not therefore be used as excluding tests. The diagnostic specificity is high, so they do have potential as confirmatory tests. For *particular* syndromes, for example, PM and interstitial lung disease or PM plus scleroderma, both diagnostic sensitivity and specificity appear to be high. The anti-tRNA synthetases, including anti-Jo-1, predict associated interstitial lung disease (Bernstein *et al.*, 1984; Targoff *et al.*, 1988; Wasicek, 1989; Targoff and Arnett, 1990) and anti-PM-Scl and anti-Ku predict associated progressive systemic sclerosis (Treadwell *et al.*, 1984; Mimori *et al.*, 1981). Anti-RNP predicts the overlapping features typical of mixed connective tissue disease and a relatively quick response to relatively low doses of prednisolone.

Immunogenetic markers, including HLA typing, do not usually provide diagnostic benefit to individual patients. Nevertheless, continuing attempts to subclassify polymyositis in terms of immunogenetic as well as serological, clinical, and pathological features should continue.

VII. TREATMENT

Before planning therapy, it is crucial to consider the differential diagnosis and to exclude certain conditions that require a different approach. For example, hypothyroidism can mimic PM, but clearly requires different therapy. SLE can present as an inflammatory myopathy and may respond to standard therapy, but it is preferable to determine the extent of involvement and especially the extent of glomerulonephritis before commencing corticosteroid therapy. If

D-Penicillamine appears to be the trigger factor, it may be possible to discontinue the drug and to observe in the hope that there may be spontaneous recovery.

Corticosteroid therapy is the mainstay of treatment for inflammatory myopathy leading to weakness. It is usual to commence therapy with 40 to 80 mg prednisone each day. A sustained remission can be induced, but this may require at least months of therapy and relatively high doses. In those who fail to respond, methotrexate and other forms of immunosuppression may be useful (Bunch, 1988; Hughes, 1987). We use intravenous methotrexate initially, but the oral form may also be effective.

Patients have been reported to respond to plasmapheresis (Clark, 1986) and gammaglobulin (Roifman, 1987), suggesting that alteration of a humoral factor may be beneficial. This approach to therapy may be particularly valuable in active but steroid-resistant disease. An alternative approach may be irradiation (Hughes, 1987).

VIII. CONCLUDING REMARKS

In this chapter we have taken the view that autoimmune muscle disease is heterogeneous, but that some mechanisms of injury can be identified. Clinical, histological, ultrastructural, serological, and immunogenetic clusters are emerging and will lead to further subclassification.

There are already suggestions that this approach has practical value in relation to diagnosis and therapy, and further progress can be anticipated. It seems highly likely that most forms of autoimmune muscle disease can be considered to be the consequence of aberrant immunoregulation in the genetically predisposed subject. Various inducing factors appear important, and it should be possible to identify at least some of these. Further study of the drug-induced syndromes should be particularly useful in this regard.

ACKNOWLEDGMENTS

The authors gratefully acknowledge the contributions of Dr. J. B. Peter, the secretarial assistance given by J. Wakefield, J. Key, and B. Harvey, and reviews of the manuscript by J. Papadimitriou, M. A. H. French, and F. Mastaglia.

REFERENCES

Alarcon-Sergovia, D., Ruiz-Arguelles, A. and Fishbein, E. (1978). *Nature* 58, 83–91.

Arad-Dann, H., Isenberg, D., Ovadia, E., Shoenfeld, Y., Sperling, J., and Sperling, R. (1989). *J. Autoimmun.* **2,** 877–888.

Arahata, K., and Engel, A. G. (1988). *Ann. Neurol.* **23**(2), 168–173.

Arnett, F. C., Hirsch, T. H., Bias, W. B., Nishikai, M., and Reichlin, M. (1981). *J. Rheumatol.* **8,** 925–930.

Arnett, F. C., Goldstein, R., Duvic, M., and Reveille, J. D. (1988). *Am. J. Med.* **85** (Suppl.6A), 38–41.

Behan, W. M. H., and Behan, P. O. (1977). *J. Neurol. Sci.* **34,** 241–246.

Behan, W. M. H., Behan, P. O. and Dick, H. A. (1978). *N. Engl. J. Med.* **298**(22), 1260–1261.

Benbassat, J., Gefel, D., Larholt, K., Sukenik, S., Morgenstern, V., and Zlotnick, A. (1985). *Arthritis Rheum.* **28**(3), 249–255.

Bernstein, R. M., Morgan, S. H., and Chapman, J. (1984). *B. Med. J.* **289,** 151–152.

Bertorini, T. E. (1988). *In* "Polymyositis and Dermatomyositis" (M. C. Dalakas, ed.), pp. 157–194. Butterworth, Boston, Massachusetts.

Bohan, A. (1988). *In* "Polymyositis and Dermatomyositis" (M. C. Dalakas, ed.), pp. 19–36. Butterworth, Boston, Massachusetts.

Bohan, A., and Peter, J. B. (1975). *N. Engl. J. Med.* **292**(7), 344–347.

Bunch, T. W. (1988). *Mount Sinai J. Med.* **55**(6), 483–493.

Bunch, T. W., Worthington, J. W., Combs, J. J., Ilstrup, D. M., and Engel, A. G. (1980). *Ann. Int. Med.* **92**(3), 365–369.

Bunn, C. C., Bernstein, R. M., and Mathews, M. B. (1986). *J. Exp. Med.* **163,** 1281–1291.

Bunn, C. C., and Mathews, M. B. (1987). *Science* **238,** 1116–1119.

Carpenter, S. (1988). *In* "Polymyositis and Dermatomyositis" (M. C. Dalakas, ed.), pp. 195–216. Butterworth, Boston, Massachusetts.

Carrano, J. A., Swanson, N. R., and Dawkins, R. L. (1983). *J. Immunol. Methods* **59,** 301–314.

Carroll, G. J., Will, R. K., Peter, J. B., Garlepp, M. J., and Dawkins, R. L. (1987). *J. Rheumatol.* **14**(5), 995–1001.

Clarke, C. R., Dyall-Smith, D. J., Mackay, I. R., Emery, P., Jennings, I.D., and Becker, G. (1988). *J. Clin. Lab. Immunol.* **27,** 149–152.

Cronin, M. E., Plotz, P. H., and Miller, F. W. (1988). *In Vivo* **2,** 25–30.

Cumming, W. J. K., Hudgson, P., Lattimer, D., Sussman, M., and Wilcox, C. B. (1977). *Lancet* **2,** 978–979.

Cumming, W. J. K., Hudgson, P., and Wilcox, C. B. (1978). *N. Engl. J. Med.* **299,** 1365–1365.

Dalakas, M. C. (Ed.). (1988). "Polymyositis and Dermatomyositis" 1st Ed. Butterworth, Stoneham, Massachusetts.

Dang, C. V., Tan, E. M., and Traugh, J. A. (1988). *FASEB.* **2,** 2376–2379.

Dawkins, R. L. (1975). *Clin. Exp. Immunol.* **21,** 185–201.

Dawkins, R. L., and Mastaglia, F. L. (1973). *N. Engl. J. Med.* **288,** 434–438.

Dawkins, R. L., Garlepp, M., and McDonald, B. (1982). *In* "Skeletal Muscle Pathology" (F. L. Mastaglia and J. Walton, eds.), pp. 461–482. Churchill Livingstone, Edinburgh, Scotland.

Dawkins, R. L., Kay, P. H., Martin, E., and Christiansen, F. T. (1989). *In* "Immunology of HLA: Histocompatibility Testing 1987" (B. Dupont, ed.), pp. 893–895. Springer-Verlag, New York.

Engel, A. G., and Arahata, K. (1986). *Hum. Pathol.* **17**(7), 704–721.

Engel, A., Arahata, K., and Emslie-Smith, A. (1990). *Nerv. Ment. Dis.* **68,** 141–157.

Fenichel, G. M. (1988). *In* "Polymyositis and Dermatomyositis" (M. C. Dalakas, ed.), pp. 71–84. Butterworth, Boston, Massachusetts.

French, M. A. H., and Dawkins, R. L. (1990). *Immunol. Today* **11,** 271–274.

Friedman, J. M., Pachman, L. M., Maryjowski, M. L., Jonasson, O., Battles, N. D., Crowe, W. E., Fink, C. W., Hanson, V., Levinson, J. E., Spencer, C. H., and Sullivan, D. B. (1983a). *Tissue Antigens* **21,** 45–49.

Friedman, J. M., Pachman, L. M., Maryjowski, M. L., Radvany, R. M., Crowe, W. E., Hanson, V., Levinson, J. E., and Spencer, C. H. (1983b). *Arthritis Rheum.* **26,** 214–216.

Garlepp, M. J., Dawkins, R. L., and Christiansen, F. T. (1983). *B. Med. J.* **286,** 338–340.

Goldstein, R., Duvic, M., Targoff, I. N., Reichlin, M., Warner, W. B., Pollack, M. C., and Arnett, F. C. (1988). *Arthritis Rheum.* **31,** S33.

Hirsch, T. J., Enlow, R. W., Bias, W. B., and Arnett, F. C. (1981). *Hum. Immunol.* **3,** 181–186.

Hochberg, M. C., Feldman, D., Stevens, M. B., Arnett, F. C., and Reichlin, M. (1984). *J. Rheumatol.* **11,** 663–665.

Hochberg, M. C., Feldman, D., and Stevens, M. B. (1986). *Semin. Arthritis Rheum.* **15**(3), 168–178.

Hughes, G. R. V. (1987). Polymyositis and dermatomyositis. *In* "Connective Tissue Diseases," pp. 172–184. Blackwell Scientific, Oxford, England.

Kalovidouris, A. E., Pourmand, R., Passo, M. H., and Plotkin, Z. (1989). *Arthritis Rheum.* **32**(4), 446–453.

Karpati, G., Pouliot, Y., and Carpenter, S. (1988). *Ann. Neurol.* **23,** 64–72.

Lakhanpal, S., Bunch, T. W., and Melton, L. J., III. (1986). *Mayo Clin. Proc.* **61,** 645–653.

Leddy, J. P., Griggs, R. C., Klemperer, M. R., and Frank, M. M. (1975). *Am. J. Med.* **58,** 83–91.

Lotz, B. P., Engel, A. G., Nishino, H., Stevens, J. C., and Litchy, W. J. (1989). *Brain* **112,** 727–747.

Mandel, D., Segal, A., and Mayes, M. (1982). *Arthritis Rheum.* **25,** S151.

Mastaglia, F. L., and Walton, J. N. (1982). *In* "Skeletal Muscle Pathology" (F. L. Mastaglia and J. N. Walton, eds.), pp. 360–392. Churchill Livingstone, Edinburgh, Scotland.

Mathews, M. B., and Bernstein, R. M. (1983). *Nature* **304,** 17–19.

Mathews, M. B., Reichlin, M., Hughes, G. R. V., and Bernstein, R. M. (1984). *J. Exp. Med.* **160,** 420–434.

McDonald, B. L. (1981). "Anti-Muscle Antibodies and Inflammatory Muscle Disease." Ph.D. Thesis, University of Western Australia.

Mellins, E., Malleson, P., Schaller, J., and Hansen, J. (1982). *Arthritis Rheum.* **25,** 5151.

Miller, F. W., Love, L. A., Barbieri, S. A., Balow, J. E., and Plotz, P. H. (1990). *Clin. Exp. Immunol.* **81,** 373–379.

Mimori, T., Akizuki, M., Yamagata, H., Inada, S., and Homma, M. (1981). *J. Clin. Invest.* **68,** 611–620.

Mimori, T., Hardin, J. A., and Steitz, J. A. (1985). *Arthritis Rheum.* **28,** S74.

Nakamura, M., Mimori, T., and Hardin, J. (1985). *Arthritis Rheum.* **28,** S96.

Nishikai, M., Homma, M. (1977). *J.A.M.A.* **237,** 1842–1844.

Nishikai, M., Aoyagi, S., Kanazawa, N., and Sato, A. (1990). *J. Rheumatol.* **2,** 245–250.

Pachman, L. M., and Maryjowski, M. C. (1984). *Clin. Rheum. Dis.* **10,** No 1, 95–111.

Plotz, P. H. (1983). *Lancet* **11,** 824–826.

Plotz, P. H., Dalakas, M., Leff, R. L., Love, L. A., Miller, F. W., and Cronin, M. E. (1989). *Ann. Int. Med.* **111,** 143–157.

Ray, C. G., Minnich, L. L., and Johnson, P. C. (1979). *J. Infec. Dis.* **140**(2), 239–243.

Reichlin, M., and Arnett, F. C. (1984). *Arthritis Rheum.* **27,** 1150–1156.

Reichlin, M., Maddison, P. J., Targoff, I. N., Bunch, T., Arnett, F. C., Sharp, G. C., Treadwell, E. and Tan, E. M. (1984). *J. Clin. Immunol.* **4,** 40–44.

Reimer, G., Scheer, U., Peters, J.-M., and Tan, E. M. (1986). *J. Immunol.* **137**(12), 3802–3808.

Roifman, C. M., Schaffer, F. M., Wachsmuth, S. E., Murphy, G., and Gelfand, E. W. (1987). *J.A.M.A.* **258**(4), 513–515.

Sawchak, J. A., and Kula, R. W. (1988). *In* "Polymyositis and Dermatomyositis" (M. C. Dalakas, ed.), pp. 121–132. Butterworths, Boston, Massachusetts.

Tan, E. M. (1989). *Adv. Immunol.* **44,** 93–151.

Targoff, I. N., and Arnett, F. C. (1990). *Am. J. Med.* **88,** 241–251.

Targoff, I. N., and Reichlin, M. (1985). *Arthritis Rheum.* **28,** 796–803.

Targoff, I. N., and Reichlin, M. (1987). *J. Immunol.* **138,** 2874–2882.

Targoff, I. N., Raghu, G., and Reichlin, M. (1983). *Clin. Exp. Immunol.* **53,** 76–82.
Targoff, I. N., Arnett, F. C., and Reichlin, M. (1988). *Arthritis Rheum.* **31**(4), 515.
Targoff, I. N., Arnett, F. C., Berman, L., O'Brien, C., and Reichlin, M. (1989). *J. Clin. Invest.* **84,** 162–172.
Wada, K., Ueno, S., Hazama, T., Ogasahara, S., Kang, J., Takahashi, M., and Tarui, S. (1983). *Clin. Exp. Immunol.* **52,** 297–304.
Walker, G. L., Mastaglia, F. L., and Roberts D. F. (1982). *Acta Neurol. Scand.* **66,** 432–443.
Wasicek, C. A., Reichlin, M., Montes, M., and Raghu, G. (1990). *Am. J. Med.* **76,** 538–544.
Whitaker, J. N. (1982). *Muscle Nerve* **5,** 573–592.
Whitaker, J. N., and Engel, W. K. (1972). *N. Engl. J. Med.* **286**(7), 333–338.

CHAPTER **14**

Autoimmune Aspects of Ocular Disease

BARBARA DETRICK
Vaccine Research & Development Branch
Division of AIDS
National Institute of Allergy and Infectious Diseases
National Institutes of Health
Bethesda, Maryland

JOHN J. HOOKS
Immunology & Virology Section
Laboratory of Immunology
National Eye Institute
National Institutes of Health
Bethesda, Maryland

I. AUTOIMMUNE INFLAMMATORY DISEASES OF THE EYE

Autoimmune phenomena can occur throughout the body. The eye is no exception. In fact, the ocular microenvironment may be a unique location in which to study and identify etiologies, mechanisms of pathogenesis, and modes of interventive therapy.

This chapter gives a brief overview of some of the autoimmune inflammatory diseases of the eye, both in man and in animal models. This will be followed by an evaluation of recent developments that may aid in a better understanding of immunopathologic mechanisms. Finally, approaches to therapy and intervention of ocular immunopathogenic processes will be addressed.

The term uveitis is used to identify intraocular inflammatory disease in man and animals (Nussenblatt, 1988). The etiology of these disorders may be ascribed to exogenous infectious agents, such as toxoplasmosis or cytomegalovirus, or it may be the result of endogenous, autoimmune phenomena. These inflammatory disorders are also identified by the anatomic site of the inflammation. Thus, the uveitis may be referred to as anterior, intermediate, or posterior.

A. Animal Models

Animal models exist for both antibody-mediated and T cell-mediated ocular autoimmune diseases. The standard model system for antibody-mediated disease is referred to as lens-induced uveitis, whereas the T cell-mediated disease in a variety of animals is referred to as experimental autoimmune uveoretinitis (EAU).

Hyperimmunization of rats with lens antigens and the subsequent disruption of the lens capsule results in intraocular inflammation (Marak *et al.*, 1974, 1976a,b, 1977; Gery *et al.*, 1981). This disease can be passively transferred using immune serum. Deposition of immunoglobulin and complement can be identified in the injured lens. This model mimics a human disease, phacoantigenic uveitis, which can be triggered by trauma to the lens.

Experimental autoimmune uveoretinitis in animals is an acute disease that can reproduce many of the pathological changes present in human diseases (Wacker *et al.*, 1977). In fact, this disease is frequently regarded as a prototype of sympathetic ophthalmia. The disease is initiated by a variety of retinal proteins, such as S-antigen, opsin, rhodopsin, and interphotoreceptor retinoid-binding protein (IRBP) (Schalken *et al.*, 1989; Sanui *et al.*, 1989; Shinohara *et al.* 1990). S-antigen is a protein found in photoreceptor cells and in the pineal gland. It has also been referred to as *48-kDa protein* or *arrestin*. This protein has been shown to play an important role in visual transduction. A major soluble protein in the interphotoreceptor matrix, IRBP is synthesized by the photoreceptors and is believed to act by transporting retinoids between the photoreceptors and the retinal pigment epithelium.

Induction of EAU is achieved by injecting specific retinal antigens formulated in complete Freund's adjuvant into the footpad of a susceptible host. Rabbits, guinea pigs, rats, and subhuman primates are all susceptible to this disease. The ability to induce the disease is greatly enhanced by the addition of *Bordetella pertussis* or pertussis toxin. The disease may also be adoptively transferred to syngeneic hosts with immune T cells and T-cell lines (Mochizuki *et al.*, 1985; Hu *et al.*, 1989). Recent studies also show that the induction of EAU in response to retinal proteins is mediated by T helper/inducer cells ($CD4^+$), which recognize antigen expressed or presented via major histocompatibility complex (MHC) class II (Ia) interaction. EAU is an acute and dramatic inflammatory disease of short duration (Wacker *et al.*, 1977). Eleven to 14 days after immunization, animals develop both clinical and histopathological ocular inflammation. This response is characterized by inflammation of the anterior chamber, vitreous, uveal tissue, and retina. Often a serous retinal detachment can be observed. The inflammatory cell infiltrate persists for approximately 2 weeks and is followed by a more or less complete destruction of the photoreceptor cell layer (Chan *et al.*, 1986a; Wetzig *et al.*, 1988). The usefulness of this model in understanding immunopathologic mechanisms and in designing interventive treatments is described below.

A modification of the immunization procedure that allows for the development of EAU in mice has been identified (Caspi *et al.*, 1990; Chan *et al.*, 1990). Initial studies showed that when mice are pretreated with cyclophosphamide, and then administered two doses of *Bordetella pertussis* and two doses of IRBP in complete Freund's adjuvant, EAU is induced. This schedule can be further modified to a single immunization of IRBP formulated in complete Freund's adjuvant if pertussis toxin is substituted for the bacterium. This model system may potentially be useful in evaluating chronic uveitis.

A general description of models of autoimmunity, including examples of ocular autoimmunity, is further explored in Chapter 3.

B. Human Diseases

In man autoimmune diseases of the eye may be primary or secondary to various systemic autoimmune diseases (Table I). These have been extensively reviewed (Nussenblatt and Silverstein, 1985; Kraus-Mackiw and O'Connor, 1986; Friedlaender and O'Connor, 1987). However, it may be important to highlight some of these disorders in order to illustrate their relationships to immunopathologic mechanisms.

Numerous human eye disorders may be considered as primary ocular disorders associated with autoimmune phenomena (Table I). These disorders may be primarily associated with autoantibody production, activated cytotoxic T cells, or a combination of these. The human disorder associated with autoantibody production is lens-induced uveitis or phacoantigenic uveitis. In this disorder the disease process has been correlated with antibody responses to lens material. In 1903 Uhlerhuth demonstrated that lens-induced uveitis was associated with organ-specific antibodies. Fifty years later, Witmer determined that the antibody to lens tissue was produced by lymphoid cells in the ciliary body (Witmer, 1964). This is a relatively rare disorder, which can be observed in individuals whose lens capsules are permeable as a result of trauma or other diseases. It is of interest to note that up to 50% of normal individuals can have antibodies to lens antigens or lens alpha crystallins (Hackett and Thompson, 1964; Sandburg and Closs, 1979). This disease clearly requires a series of events, two of which probably involve preexisting antilens antibody and damage to the lens through trauma or surgery.

On the other hand, sympathetic ophthalmia and Vogt-Kayanagi-Harada syndrome (VKH) have been associated with cell-mediated immune responses.

TABLE I
Eye Diseases Associated with Alterations in Immune Function

Human	
Primary Eye Involvement	Sympathetic ophthalmia
	Vogt-Koyanagi-Harada syndrome
	Lens-induced uveitis
	Birdshot choroidopathy
	Pars planitis
Systemic disorders with ocular involvement	Behcet's syndrome
	Sjögren's syndrome
	Rheumatoid arthritis
	Ankylosing spondylitis
	Reiter's syndrome
	Ulcerative colitis
	Juvenile rheumatoid arthritis
	Systemic lupus erythematosus
	Sarcoidosis
	Wegener's granulomatosis
	Ocular cicatrical pemphigoid
Animal models	Experimental autoimmune uveitis
	Lens-induced uveitis

Sympathetic ophthalmia is a fascinating and devastating disease (Kraus-Mackiw and O'Connor, 1986). This ocular inflammatory (autoimmune) disease is associated with a perforating injury. The hallmark of this disease is that the injured eye undergoes a massive lymphocytic infiltration and at any time from the second week to several years following the trauma, a spontaneous lymphocytic infiltrate occurs in the "sympathizing" eye. Recent studies have shown that the lymphocytic infiltrate in the sympathizing eye consists predominantly of T cells, and that the infiltrating cells and the resident ocular cells, namely the retinal pigment epithelial cells, are activated to express MHC class II determinants (Jacobiec *et al.*, 1983; Muller-Hermelink *et al.*, 1984; Chan *et al.*, 1986b). Moreover, the infiltrating T cells are actively producing interferon-gamma (IFN-gamma) and interleukin-2 (IL-2) (Hooks *et al.*, 1988). How these findings relate to immunologic pathogenesis of sympathetic ophthalmia will be touched upon later.

Systemic diseases of presumed autoimmune etiology can be associated with ocular manifestations (Table I) (Nussenblatt and Silverstein, 1985; Friedlander and O'Connor, 1987). For example, juvenile rheumatoid arthritis and rheumatoid arthritis can be associated with scleritis and uveitis. Likewise, iridocyclitis is seen in patients with ankylosing spondylitis, papillary conjunctivitis has been noted in patients with Reiter's disease, and vasculitis of the retinal nerve fiber can be observed in patients with systemic lupus erythematosus. Other examples include intraepithelial bullae of the conjunctiva, which have been described in patients with pemphigus vulgaris; panuveitis, which has been noted in sarcoidosis patients; and recurrent iridocyclitis with hypopyon and occlusive vasculitis, which has been observed in patients with Behcet's syndrome.

II. RECENT DEVELOPMENTS IN UNDERSTANDING IMMUNOPATHOLOGIC MECHANISMS

The key challenge is to determine the multiple ways in which ocular autoimmune phenomena or processes are initiated and perpetuated. Fortified with this knowledge, investigators may identify effective ways to modify these pathologic processes in the ocular microenvironment. New information on factors that participate in this process will first be explored and then new therapeutic approaches to modify these autoimmune events will be reviewed.

Many of the recent developments in understanding immunopathologic mechanisms concentrate on the activation of resident ocular cells, cytokine production, MHC class II antigen expression, and antigen presentation (Hanafusa *et al.*, 1983; Babbit *et al.*, 1985; Matsunga *et al.*, 1986; Touraine *et al.*, 1989). Numerous studies indicate that a variety of autoimmune diseases are associated with the IFN-gamma-induced tissue-specific expression of MHC class II molecules (Hanafusa *et al.*, 1983; Bottazo *et al.*, 1983; Hickley *et al.*, 1985; Dalavanga *et al.*, 1987; Frohman *et al.*, 1991). This series of events may elicit a T-cell response against tissue-specific antigen (Frohman *et al.*, 1991). These interrelated phenomena will be addressed in this section.

A. Cytokines

Cytokines are a group of specialized, hormone-like proteins, which can exert profound influences on cellular development and on a variety of cellular functions. The efficient functioning of the immune response requires a series of interactions among a variety of cell types, which can be facilitated by cytokines. For example, IL-2, which is produced by T cells, can activate T cells and natural killer (NK) cells in cytotoxic processes. IFN-gamma, a major immunoregulatory protein, induces the synthesis and expression of MHC class II antigens on a variety of cell types (Basham and Merigan, 1983; Hooks and Detrick, 1987; Pober, 1988). MHC class II antigens are membrane-associated glycoproteins that are encoded by genes in the major histocompatibility complex. Unlike class I antigens that can be detected on most nucleated cells, the class II antigens are limited to select populations of cells, such as B cells, activated T cells, macrophages, and other cell types termed accessory cells. These molecules play an important role in the cellular interactions that initiate and sustain immune responses. For example, T helper cells recognize exogenous antigen in association with class II molecules on the antigen-presenting cell (Babbitt *et al.*, 1985).

B. Augmentation of MHC Expression

Determining how this immunologic network relates to the microenvironment of the eye has been a formidable challenge to ocular immunologists for many years. We shall highlight recent data demonstrating how this network may act in the posterior pole of the eye. The retinal pigment epithelium consists of a single layer of cells situated at a crucial interface between the choroidal blood supply and the photoreceptor cell layer of the neural retina (Fig. 1). The retinal pigment epithelial (RPE) cell has long been considered an important regulating cell, maintaining physiological and structural balance within the retina (Clark, 1986). The RPE cells influence the transport of metabolites between the blood and neural retina, play a role in the rhodopsin cycle, consistently absorb excess light energy, and phagocytize the photoreceptor outer segments. This phagocytic ability of the RPE cells is reminiscent of macrophage phagocytic capabilities. RPE cells manifest all of the classical properties of phagocytic cells, including discrimination between particles of different types, ingestion of particulate matter into vacuoles bounded by a plasma membrane, production of a large variety of hydrolytic enzymes, and the capacity to digest engulfed particles. Recent studies indicate that the RPE cell may also be important in autoimmunity and transplantation (Detrick *et al.*, 1985; Li and Turner, 1988; Lopez *et al.*, 1989; Percopo *et al.*, 1990).

The fact that human RPE cells *in vitro* could express MHC class II antigens (HLA-DR), and that this expression can be modulated by human recombinant IFN-gamma was first reported in 1985 (Detrick *et al.*, 1985). These studies have recently been confirmed and extended. Human RPE cells maintained *in vitro* can be induced by IFN-gamma to express both HLA-DR and HLD-DQ antigens (Baudouin *et al.*, 1989). Furthermore, RPE cells from two additional species, rats and guinea pigs, also express MHC class II antigens in response to IFN-gamma (Fujikawa *et al.*, 1987; Liversidge *et al.*, 1988).

Subsequent studies have described the inappropriate or deviant expression of HLA-DR antigen on RPE cells in inflammatory diseases (uveitis and sympathetic ophthalmia), in a degenerative disease (retinitis pigmentosa) and in progressive diabetic retinopathy (Detrick *et al.*, 1986; Chan *et al.*, 1986b; Baudouin *et al.*, 1988). In each of these examples, the cells do not express HLA-DR antigen under normal physiologic conditions but are activated to express the antigen during a degenerative or an immunologically mediated disease. In these disorders, it is postulated that IFN-gamma is the inducer of class II antigen expression. Using immunocytochemistry, we were able to show that both lymphokines, IL-2 and IFN-gamma, are present in the human eye during inflammatory (uveitis) and autoimmune diseases (sympathetic ophthalmia) (Hooks *et al.*, 1988). Furthermore, the presence of these lymphokines was correlated with a lymphocyte infiltrate, predominantly of T-cell origin, and with the expression of MHC class

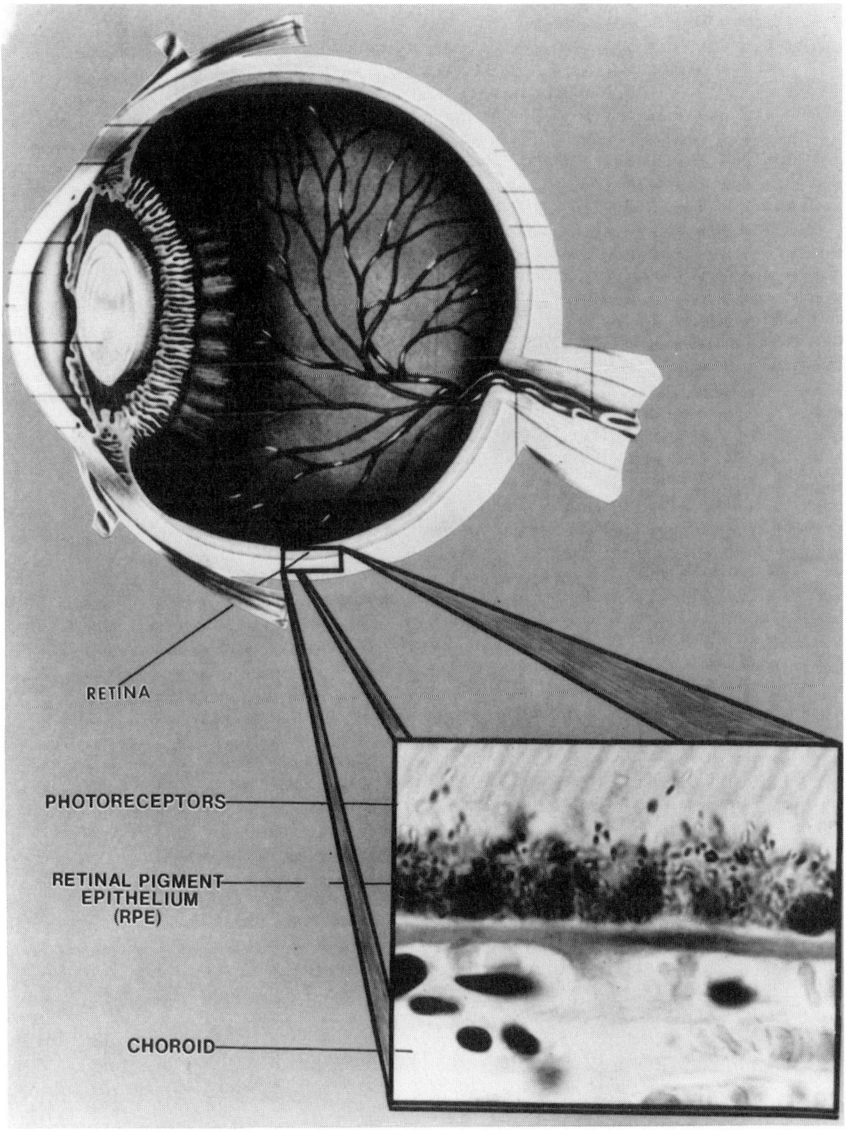

FIG. 1 Diagram of the eye. The retina is highlighted. The RPE cells are arranged as a single layer of cells situated at a crucial interface between the choroidal blood supply and the photoreceptor cell layer. This cell is activated by IFN-gamma to express MHC class II antigens and to process and present retinal antigens to T helper cells.

II antigens on both infiltrating cells and ocular resident cells, that is, RPE cells and retinal vascular endothelial cells. Similar findings have been generated when patients with anterior uveitis were examined (Abi-Hanna *et al.*, 1989). Both class I and class II antigens were identified in iris biopsy specimens, and the level of expression correlated with the concentration of IFN-gamma detected in the aqueous humor.

In order to more clearly delineate the sequence of events in ocular inflammation, we also compared the development of Ia antigen on RPE cells to the clinical and histopathologic processes in EAU (Chan *et al.*, 1986a). EAU was induced in Lewis rats by immunization against retinal S-antigen. Rat RPE cells were activated to express Ia antigen during the course of EAU. In contrast, these antigens were not detected on RPE cells from unimmunized (normal) rats. Interestingly, the presence of these antigens was identified 4 days before clinical and 2 days before histopathological evidence of EAU. This observation shows that RPE cells express class II antigens before observable ocular inflammation and suggests that the expression of MHC class II antigens on RPE cells may be functionally important for the initiation and perpetuation of certain forms of ocular autoimmune disease.

The Lewis rat was also used to further evaluate the direct effect of IFN-gamma on ocular tissue (Hamel *et al.*, 1990). Eyes evaluated 24 hr after inoculation of recombinant IFN-gamma revealed Ia expression on a variety of ocular cells. These cells were localized to the conjunctiva and anterior segment, and included conjunctival epithelial, keratocytes, iris epithelial, ciliary epithelial, and choroidal cells. In the retina, the RPE cells were also Ia positive. These studies clearly show that IFN-gamma can regulate class II antigen expression in the ocular microenvironment.

C. Critical Role of the RPE Cell as an Antigen-Presenting Cell

The most recent piece of experimental evidence implicating a role for cytokine-activated RPE cells in autoimmune phenomena demonstrates that the RPE cell is capable of presenting antigens *in vitro* (Percopo *et al.*, 1990). RPE cell cultures were established from 12-day-old rats. The isolated rat RPE cells alone do not express Ia antigens. However, these cells can be induced to express Ia antigen following incubation with rat recombinant IFN-gamma. T-cell proliferative responses and IL-2 production were used as a measure of antigen presentation. RPE cells (Ia positive and Ia negative) were incubated with T helper cells (retinal protein specific) in the presence of retinal proteins. The retinal proteins used were S-antigen and interphotoreceptor-binding protein. Significant thymidine uptake and IL-2 production were observed when Ia-positive RPE cells were incubated with T helper cells in the presence of specific retinal proteins (Fig. 2).

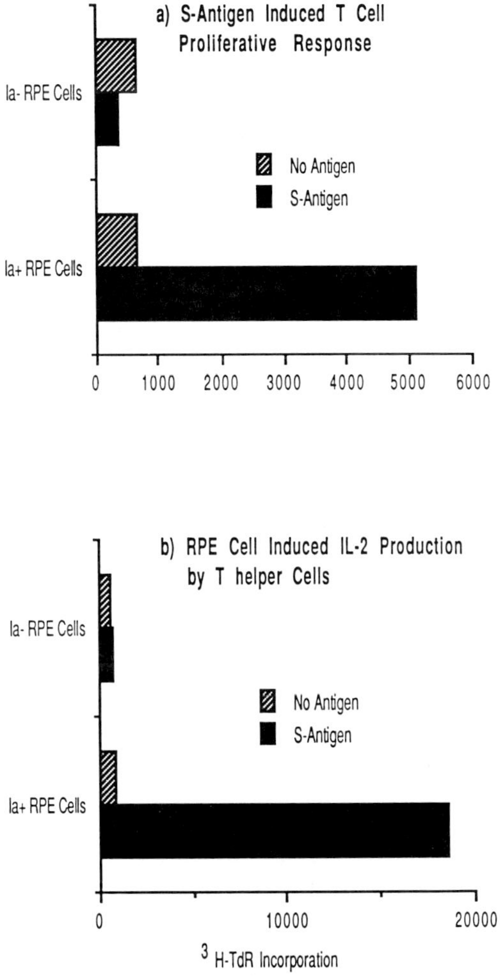

FIG. 2 Antigen presentation by RPE cells. T-cell proliferative responses (a) and IL-2 production (b) were used to measure the ability of rat RPE cells to present retinal S-antigen to specifically sensitized T helper cells.

However, minimal thymidine uptake and IL-2 production were noted when Ia-positive RPE cells were incubated without T helper cells either in the absence or in the presence of specific retinal proteins. Moreover, Ia-negative RPE cells failed to incorporate significant amounts of thymidine or produce IL-2, even when they were incubated with T helper cells in the presence of retinal proteins. These data clearly demonstrate that RPE cells, which express Ia antigens, are capable of presenting a retina-specific protein to T helper cells.

In order to determine whether RPE cells process antigen before presenting it to T cells, RPE cells and thymocytes were incubated with chloroquine. Chloroquine is a potent inhibitor of lysosomal activity, which can block the ability of cells to properly process antigen. Treatment of Ia-positive RPE cells with chloroquine results in an 87% inhibition of thymidine incorporation. These data suggest that RPE cells are indeed capable of processing antigen before presenting it to T cells. These studies further substantiate the concept that cytokine-mediated activation of RPE cells may be a basic component of ocular immunity and may have major immunological consequences for RPE cell transplantation studies (Li and Turner, 1988; Lopez *et al.*, 1989).

Based on these studies, it is now possible to propose the following hypothesis on pathogenic mechanisms in the eye during autoimmune disease. An initiating event, such as trauma or a virus infection, may sufficiently traumatize the posterior pole of the eye to induce the release of mediators. One notable consequence of mediator production is increased vascular permeability. This breach in the endothelial cell barrier of the microvasculature, coupled with the migration of cells into the damaged tissue, are of prime importance in the development of an inflammatory reaction. Once mononuclear cells invade the retina, the release of cytokines can help to sustain the inflammatory reaction. For example, sensitized T cells can interact with retinal antigens in the context of MHC class II antigens on monocytes, endothelial cells, and RPE cells. Moreover, IFN-gamma can enhance the killing ability of cytotoxic T cells and augment antibody synthesis by B cells. Finally, the presence of these mediators can result in the coincident generation of other cytokines at the inflammatory site. Once set into motion, this cyclic pattern of cytokine production and cell activation leads to destruction of ocular tissue.

Numerous additional cytokines and alternative processes may participate in various aspects of ocular autoimmune phenomena. A number of investigators are beginning to probe the effects of interleukins and neuropeptides in the eye (Unger and Butler, 1988). This approach will be an exciting avenue to follow in the future.

D. IFN-gamma Enhancement of Neuronal Cell Protein

Recent studies have described a novel effect of IFN-gamma on a retinal and pineal protein. As a pluripotent lymphokine, IFN-gamma modulates a variety of cellular processes, such as inhibition of viral replication, cell growth and differentiation, and gene regulation (Hooks and Detrick, 1987; Detrick *et al.* 1988, 1991). One of the mechanisms involved in these processes is the ability of IFN-gamma to alter the regulation and expression of cellular proteins (Korber *et al.*, 1988). Using analytical flow cytometry, recombinant human IFN-gamma was shown to enhance the expression of retinal S-antigen in retinoblastoma cells (Hooks *et al.*, 1990; Detrick *et al.*, 1991). This enhancement was selective since other retinal cell proteins were not affected by IFN-gamma treatment. Retinal S-antigen plays an important role in vision and is one of the retinal proteins capable of inducing EAU. These studies therefore demonstrate yet another important role for this lymphokine, that is, the enhanced expression of a neuronal cell protein. In this case, IFN-gamma may be acting as a differentiation agent. Studies such as this may help to identify additional mechanisms by which IFN-gamma may participate in immunopathologic events in nervous tissue.

E. Molecular Mimicry

Autoimmune responses may be generated by a variety of different known or proposed mechanisms. A number of investigators have suggested molecular mimicry as one of these mechanisms (Fujinami and Oldstone, 1985). In this process, epitopes may be shared between a microbial agent (virus, bacteria, yeast) and a host protein. These homologous but not identical determinants, differing in one or more amino acids, may be foreign enough to elicit an immune response. The immune response initiated against a foreign epitope may also react with a closely homologous *self* host protein. In this way, antibody or cytotoxic lymphocytes generated against a microbial agent may cross-react with a self protein resulting in cellular injury and disease. A more detailed discussion on molecular mimicry can be found in Chapter 6 by Dr. Fujinami.

Shinorhara and associates have presented evidence that molecular mimicry may occur in the ocular microenvironment (Shinohara *et al.*, 1990). These studies have identified sequence homology between the uveitopathogenic site of S-antigen and selected viral proteins, i.e., *Escherichia coli* protein and yeast histone H-3 protein (Singh *et al.*, 1989a,b, 1989a, 1990). Sequence homology with S-antigen was identified in the following viruses: hepatitis B virus DNA polymerase, gag-pol polyprotein of baboon endogenous virus, and gag-polyprotein of AKV murine leukemia virus. Inoculation of Lewis rats with these different synthetic peptides triggered the process of EAU. Moreover, native histone H-3 alone was demonstrated to induce EAU (Singh *et al.*, 1989a).

Many autoimmune diseases have been associated with preceding infections and thus, infectious agents have been implicated in these diseases. The data presented in these studies provide evidence that ocular inflammatory conditions may be triggered by an antigenically similar, cross-reacting environmental biological agent.

Until now cellular actions and cytokine activation have been the main focus discussed with respect to immune mechanisms. However, the production of antibodies directed against ocular cells and associated antigen–antibody complex formation as well as complement activation probably also play a role in selected forms of ocular diseases. In fact, Kaplan and co-workers (1986) have identified examples of human posterior uveitis that may be associated with B-cell activation and immunoglobulin production. Much remains to be done in order to better define the role of B cells in these disorders. Development and exploration of animal models to address some of these questions may be a fruitful area of investigation.

III. EXPERIMENTAL INTERVENTION OF IMMUNOPATHOGENIC PROCESSES

EAU is a widely used model system for the study of immune-mediated destruction of the posterior pole of the eye. Manipulation of the induction of this experimental disease continues to provide valuable information on pathogenesis and potential modes of therapy.

Studies during the past few years have clearly shown that the induction of EAU in response to retinal proteins is mediated by T-helper/inducer cells ($CD4^+$), which recognize antigen expressed or presented by means of MHC class II (Ia) interaction. Knowledge of this sequence of events has allowed researchers to attempt some innovative approaches to modulate this process. *In vivo* administration of anti-Ia monoclonal antibodies (at the time of S-antigen sensitization) results in a diminution of the disease process and protection from disease (Fig. 3) (Wetzig *et al.*, 1988). Furthermore, immunocytochemical evaluation demonstrated that tissue obtained from animals receiving anti-Ia therapy contained fewer Ia-positive cells, and fewer infiltrating T cells. These data show that anti-Ia treatment significantly modifies the course of EAU in the rat. In subsequent studies, the MHC Ia region was divided into its components I-A and I-E determinants (Rao *et al.*, 1989). The anti-I-A antibodies appeared to be more effective in inhibiting disease activity. These studies underscore the critical role that is played by the expression of MHC class II antigens in inflammatory eye diseases.

Another avenue that has been used to modify the disease process is to present the initiating protein, S-antigen, so that tolerance or suppression of the immune response is the end product. Mizuno *et al.* (1989) found that pretreatment of rats with injections of S-antigen into the anterior chamber markedly reduces the incidence and expression of EAU. These authors speculate that S-antigen released from the diseased retina could gain access to the anterior chamber. The resultant induction of S-antigen specific anterior chamber-associated immune deviation (ACAID) would then actively prevent or down-regulate autoimmune retinitis. Nussenblatt and co-workers (1990) have shown that pretreatment with S-antigen or fragments of S-antigen by the oral route induces tolerance and inhibits S-antigen-induced EAU. In this case, as was observed with the experimental allergic encephalomyelitis model, the tolerant state is associated with the

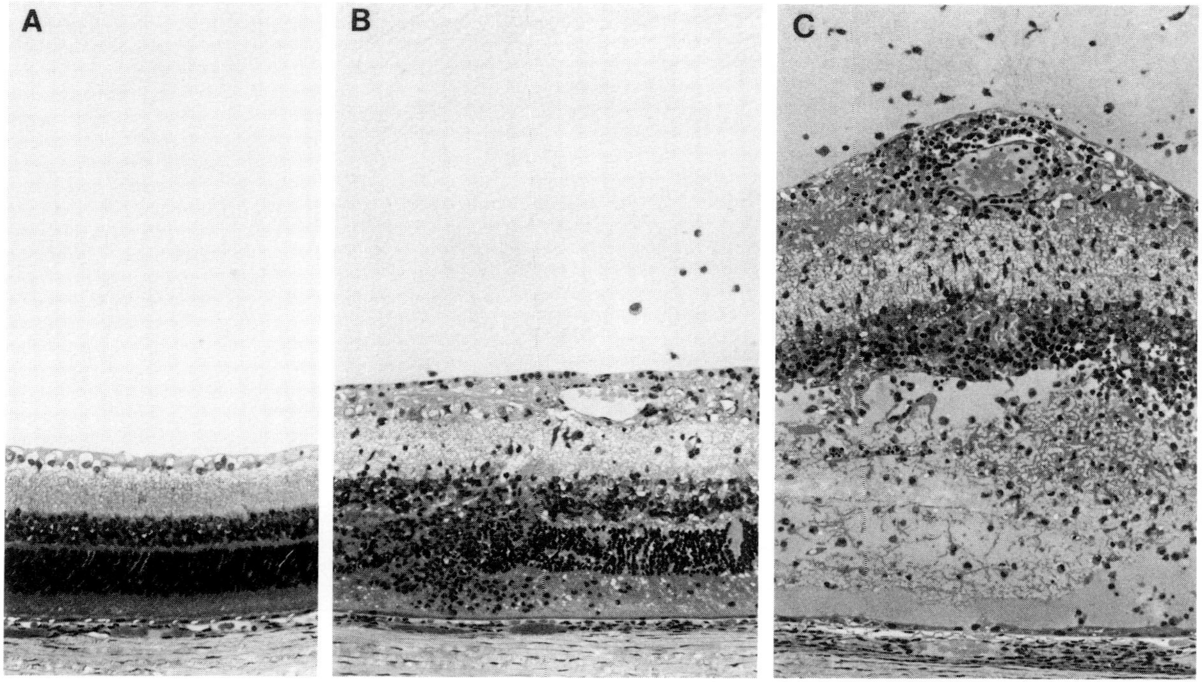

FIG. 3 Histopathology of the posterior pole of the eye. (A) normal rat tissue, (B) rat tissue obtained from EAU rat treated with anti-Ia antibodies, and (C) EAU rat tissue. Anti-Ia antibody treatment diminishes ocular inflammation in EAU. Reprinted with permission from Wetzig *et al*. (1988).

generation of $CD8^+$ T cells. These suppressor cells may then help to suppress the retinal responses of T-helper cells.

Treatment and intervention in autoimmune diseases is described in detail by Dr. Wekerle in Chapter 16 of this volume. The mode of treatment of autoimmune intraocular diseases in humans has been reviewed by Nussenblatt (1988). Immunosuppressive therapy has been achieved with corticosteroids, cytotoxic agents, particularly alkylating agents, and cyclosporine.

IV. IMMUNODIAGNOSTIC TECHNIQUES

Inflammatory diseases of the eye may have an infectious or autoimmune etiology. In addition, infectious agents such as bacteria or viruses may trigger autoimmune phenomena. Differentiation of these initiating and/or perpetuating events, especially in the posterior pole of the eye, is extremely difficult. Routine serologic diagnostic markers are presently not available for identifying the subset of uveitis that has an autoimmune etiology.

The rapid and accurate diagnosis of immunologic and/or infectious diseases may be critical to the management of ocular disorders. Since the eye provides us with a window to evaluate the pathogenic situation, we should try to exploit this fact. Scheiffarth and associates (1990) have imaginatively used their knowledge of immunology and ophthalmology to develop a new noninvasive technique that permits staining of specific structures in the living eye. These investigators have combined the specificity of immunofluorescence with the *in vivo* practicability of fluorescein angiography. The technique is based on intravenous application of specific antibodies, labeled with fluorescein. The antibody staining within the eye can be directly recorded as low-contrast fluorescence on high-speed film, which can then be combined with digital image processing. With the advent of monoclonal antibodies directed against ocular structures and specific infectious agents, this technique may prove to be a revolutionary and very effective means of differential diagnosis in immunological uveitis.

V. CONCLUDING REMARKS

Advances in our knowledge of ocular autoimmune diseases have progressed steadily during the past 2 decades. These advances have paralleled the development of an appreciation of the complex nature of immune responses and autoimmune phenomena. The studies described herein highlighted the fact that the release of cytokines, such as IFN-gamma, within the ocular microenvironment, and the subsequent induction of MHC class II antigen expression on resident and infiltrating cells may be critical elements in a cascading effect leading to ocular cell destruction. The RPE cell within the retina may play a critical role in autoimmune uveitis. This cell expresses MHC class II molecules during ocular autoimmune diseases in humans and animals. Moreover, *in vitro* IFN-gamma treated RPE cells express MHC class II molecules and subsequently process and present retinal antigen to T-cell clones. These studies suggest that some autoimmune eye disorders may result from a localized or chronic infection that elicits the release of IFN-gamma. IFN-gamma-induced expression of MHC class II molecules on RPE cells may then lead to T cell-dependent autoimmune disease in the ocular microenvironment.

The exact stimuli that initiate the autoimmune responses in ocular diseases are not known. Genetic and environmental factors, such as viruses, other infectious agents, and chemicals, may contribute in the presentation of retinal proteins to the immune system. There is a need for continued studies on the etiology and pathogenic mechanisms involved in ocular autoimmune disorders. We have presented some of the new avenues of treatment that have been identified using EAU model systems. With a better understanding of the varied etiologies and pathogenic mechanisms, new advances in our knowledge of managing these diseases may be possible.

REFERENCES

Abi-Hanna, D., McCluskey, P., and Wakefield, D. (1989). *Invest. Ophthalmol. Vis. Sci.* **30,** 990–994.

Babbitt, B. P., Allen, P. M., Matsueda, G., Haber, E., and Unanue, E. R. (1985). *Nature* **317,** 359–361.

Basham, T. Y., and Merigan, T. C. (1983). *J. Immunol.* **130,** 1492–1495.

Baudouin, C., Fred-Reygrobellet, D., Jambou, D., Gastaud, P., and Lapalus, P. (1989). *Graef's Arch. Clin. Exp. Ophthalmol.* **228,** 86–88.

Baudouin, C., Fredj-Reygrobellet, D., Lapalus, P., and Gastaud, P. (1988). *Am. J. Ophthalmol.* **105,** 383–388.

Bottazo, G. R., Pujol-Borrel, R., Hanafusa, T., and Feldman, M. (1983). *Lancet* **2,** 1115–1116.

Caspi, R. R., Chan, C. C., Leake, W. C., Higuchi, M., Wiggert, B., and Chader, G. J. (1990). *J. Autoimmunity* **3,** 237–246.

Chan, C. C., Hooks, J. J., Nussenblatt, R. B., and Detrick, B. (1986a). *Curr. Eye Res.* **5,** 325–330.

Chan, C. C., Detrick, B., Nussenblatt, R., Palestine, A., Fujikawa, L. S., and Hooks, J. J. (1986b). *Arch. Ophthalmol.* **104,** 725–729.

Chan, C. C., Caspi, R. R., Ni, M., Leake, W. C., Wiggert, B., Chader, G. J., and Nussenblatt, R. B. (1990). *J. Autoimmunity* **3,** 247–255.

Clark, V. M. (1986). *In* "The Retina: A Model for Cell Biology Studies" (R. Adler and D. Farber, eds.), pp. 129–168. Academic Press, Orlando, Florida.

Dalavanga, Y. A., Detrick, B., Hooks, J. J., Drosos, A. A., and Moutsopoulos, H. M. (1987). *Ann. Rheum. Dis.* **46,** 89–92.

Detrick, B., Newsome, D. A., Percopo, C., and Hooks, J. J. (1985). *Clin. Immunol. Immunopathol.* **36,** 201–211.

Detrick, B., Rodrigues, M., Chan, C. C., Tso, M. O. M., and Hooks, J. J. (1986). *Am. J. Ophthalmol.* **101,** 584–590.

Detrick, B., and Hooks, J. J. (1987). *Adv. Biosci.* **62,** 479–488.

Detrick, B., Chan, C. C., Rodrigues, M., Kyritsis, A., Chader, G. J., and Hooks, J. J. (1988). *Cancer Res.* **48,** 1633–1641.

Detrick, B., Evans, C. H., Chader, G. J., Percopo, C. M., and Hooks, J. J. (1991). *Invest. Ophthalmol. Vis. Sci.* **32,** 1714–1722.

Friedlaender, M. H., and O'Connor, G. R. (1987). *In* "Basic & Clinical Immunology" (D. P. Stites, J. D. Stobo, and J. V. Wells, eds.), pp. 610–618. Appleton & Lange, Norwalk, Connecticut.

Frohman, M., Francfort, J. W., and Cowing, C. (1991). *J. Immunol.* **146,** 2227–2234.

Fujikawa, L. S., Chan, C. C., McAllister, C., Gery, I., Hooks, J. J., Detrick, B., and Nussenblatt, R. B. (1987). *Cell. Immunol.* **98,** 139–150.

Fujinami, R. S., and Oldstone, M. B. A. (1985). *Science* **230,** 1043–1045.

Gery, I., Nussenblatt, R., and BenEzra, D. (1981). *Invest. Ophthalmol. Vis. Sci.* **20,** 32–39.

Hackett, E., and Thompson, A. (1964). *Lancet* **2,** 663–666.

Hamel, C. P., Detrick, B., and Hooks, J. J. (1990). *Exp. Eye Res.* **50,** 173–182.

Hanafusa, T. R., Fujoi-Borrell, L., Chiovato, R. G. G., Coniach, D., and Bottazo, G. F. (1983). *Lancet* **2,** 1111.

Hickley, W. F., Osborn, J. P., and Kirby, W. M. (1985). *Cell. Immunol.* **91,** 528–533.

Hooks, J. J., and Detrick, B. (1987). *In* "The Interferon System: A Current Review to 1987" (S. Baron, F. Dianzani, F. J. Stanton, and W. R. Fleischman, Jr., eds.), pp. 319–325. The Univ. of Texas Press, Austin, Texas.

Hooks, J. J., Chan, C. C., and Detrick, B. (1988). *Invest. Ophthalmol. Vis. Sci.* **29,** 1444–1451.

Hooks, J. J., Detrick, B., Percopo, C., Hamel, C., and Siraganian, R. (1989). *Invest. Ophthalmol. Vis. Sci.* **30,** 2106–2113.

Hooks, J. J., Chader, G., Evans, C. H., and Detrick, B. (1990). *J. Neuroimmunol.* **26,** 245–250.

Hu, L. H., Redmond, T. M., Sanui, H., Kuwabara, T., McAllister, C. G., Wiggert, B., Chader, G. J., and Gery, I. (1989). *Cell. Immunol.* **122,** 251–261.

Jacobiec, F. A., Marboe, C. C., and Knowles, D. M. (1983). *Ophthalmology* **90,** 76–95.

Kaplan, A., Waldrep, J. C., Chan, W. C., Nicholson, J. K., Wright, and J. D. (1986). *Arch. Ophthalmol.* **104,** 240–244.

Korber, B., Mermod, N., Hook, L., and Stroynowski, I. (1988). *Science* **239,** 1302–1303.

Kraus-Mackiw, E., and O'Connor, G. R. (1986). "Uveitis, Pathophysiology, and Therapy." Thieme Medical, New York.

Li, L., and Turner, J. (1988). *Exp. Eye Res.* **47,** 911–917.

Liversidge, H. F. S., Thomson, A. W., and Forrester, J. V. (1988). *Immunology* **63,** 313–317.

Lopez, R. P., Gouras, H., Kjeldbye, B., Sullivan, M., Reppucci, R., Wapner, F., and Goluboff, E. (1989). *Invest. Ophthalmol. Vis. Sci.* **30,** 586–588.

Marak, G. E., Jr., Font, R. L., Czawlytko, L. N., and Alepa, F. P. (1974). *Exp. Eye Res.* **19,** 311–316.

Marak, G. E., Jr., Font, R. L., and Alepa, F. P. (1976a). *Mod. Probl. Ophthalmol.* **16,** 75–79.

Marak, G. E., Jr., Font, R. L., and Alepa, F. P. (1976b). *Ophthalmic Res.* **8,** 117–120.

Marak, G. E., Jr., Font, R. L., and Alepa, F. P. (1977). *Ophthalmic Res.* **9,** 162–170.

Matsunga, A., Katsumi, E., Fukuda, T., Hurata, K., Tezuka, H., Shimoumura, C., Otsubo, O., Ishikaqa, S., Ito, K., and Nagataki, H. (1986). *J. Clin. Endocrinol. Metab.* **62,** 723–728.

Mizuno, K., Clark, A. F., and Streilein, J. W. (1989). *Invest. Ophthalmol. Vis. Sci.* **30,** 772–774.

Mochizuki, M., Kuwabara, T., McAllister, C., Nussenblatt, R. B., and Gery, I. (1985). *Invest. Ophthalmol. Vis. Sci.* **26,** 1–9.

Muller-Hermelink, H. K., Kraus-Mackiw, E., and Daus, W. (1984). *Arch. Ophthalmol.* **102,** 1353–1357.

Nussenblatt, R. B., and Silverstein, A. M. (1985). *In* "The Autoimmune Diseases" (N. R. Rose and I. R. Mackay, eds.), pp. 371–398. Academic Press, New York.

Nussenblatt, R. B. (1988). *J. Autoimmunity* **1,** 615–621.

Nussenblatt, R. B., Caspi, R. R., Mahdi, R., Chan, C. C., Roberge, F., Lider, O., and Weiner, H. L. (1990). *J. Immunol.* **144,** 1689–1695.

Percopo, C. M., Hooks, J. J., Shinohara, T., Caspi, R., and Detrick, B. (1990). *J. Immunol.* **145,** 4101–4107.

Pober, J. S. (1988). *Am. J. Pathol.* **133,** 426–433.

Rao, N. A., Atalla, L., Linker-Israeli, M., Chen, F. Y., George, F. W., IV, Martin, W. J., and Steinman, L. (1989). *Invest. Ophthalmol. Vis. Sci.* **30,** 2348–2355.

Sandberg, H. O., and Closs, O. (1979). *In* "Immunology and Immunopathology of the Eye" (A. M. Silverstein and G. R. O'Connor, eds.), pp. 325–330. Masson, New York.

Sanui, H., Redmond, T. M., Kotake, B., Wiggert, B., Hu, L. H., Margalit, H., Berzofsky, J. A., Chader, G. J., and Gery, I. (1989). *J. Exp. Med.* **169,** 1947–1960.

Schalken, J. J., Winkens, H. J., Van Vust, A. H. M., De Grip, W. J., and Broekhuyse, R. M. (1989). *B. J. Ophthalmol.* **73,** 168–172.

Scheiffarth, O. F., Zrenner, E., Disko, R., Stefani, F. H., and Brabander, B. (1990). *Invest. Ophthalmol. Vis. Sci.* **31,** 272–276.

Shinohara, T., Singh, V. K., Tsuda, M., Yamaki, K., Abe, T., and Suzuki, S. (1990). *Exp. Eye Res.* **50,** 751–757.

Singh, V. K., Yamaki, I., Abe, T., and Shinohara, T. (1989a). *Cell. Immunol.* **122,** 262–273.

Singh, V. K., Yamaki, K., Donoso, L. A., and Shinohara, T. (1989b). *J. Immunol.* **142,** 1511–1517.

Singh, V. K., Kalra, H. K., Yamaki, K., Abe, T. Donoso, L. A., and Shinohara, T. (1990). *J. Immunol.* **144,** 1282–1287.

Touraine, J. L., Betuel, H., Pouteil-Noble, C., and Royo, C. (1989). *Adv. Nephrol.* **18,** 325–334.

Uhlenhuth, L. (1903). *In* "Festschrift zum Sechzigsten Geburtstage von Robert Koch." pp. 49–74.

Unger, W. G., and Butler, J. M. (1988). *Eye* **2,** (Suppl. S) 202–212.

Wacker, W. B., Donoso, L. A., Kalsow, C. M., Yankeelov, J. J., and Organisciak, D. J. (1977). *J. Immunol.* **119,** 1949–1950.

Wetzig, R., Hooks, J. J., Percopo, C. M., Nussenblatt, R., Chan, C. C., and Detrick, B. (1988). *Curr. Eye Res.* **7,** 809–818.

Witmer, R. (1964). *In* "Immunopathology of Uveitis" (A. E. Maumenee and A. M. Silverstein, eds.), pp. 111–128. Williams & Wilkins, Baltimore, Maryland.

CHAPTER **15**

Autoimmune Arthropathy: Rheumatoid Synovitis

GARY S. FIRESTEIN
NATHAN J. ZVAIFLER
Division of Rheumatology
University of California, San Diego Medical Center
San Diego, California

I. INTRODUCTION—HISTORICAL BACKGROUND

Rheumatoid arthritis (RA) is a common systemic inflammatory disorder of unknown etiology, characterized largely by the manner in which it involves joints. It is distributed worldwide, affecting approximately 1% of adult populations and involves all racial and ethnic groups. Articular inflammation, the hallmark of the disease, may be remitting but, if continuous, results in characteristic deformities. Thus, it is surprising that victims of RA cannot be clearly identified in ancient art or literature, unlike for instance, victims of gouty arthritis, known since the time of Hippocrates (fourth century B.C.) (Short, 1974). Nor is RA one of the rheumatic diseases definitely identified in ancient skeletons. Based on the evidence from paleopathology, RA of the severity seen today must have been uncommon in previous millenia, if present at all. Exceptions are reports from the United States and Mexico that pre-Columbian skeletons show joint erosions that might represent RA, suggesting that RA, like syphilis, was a New World disease that subsequently spread to Europe (Rothschild, 1989).

In medieval times, joint afflictions were usually ascribed to gout, a term used as nonspecifically as *arthritis* is used today. It was not until the early seventeenth century that Sydenham attempted to distinguish specific diseases from the admixture of rheumatism. Gout was clearly recognized, and there were descriptions compatible with rheumatic fever. Sydenham also noted a chronic phase of arthritis in which the patient "became a cripple until the day of his death and wholly lose the use of his limbs while the knuckles of his fingers shall become knotty and protuberant." By the early 1800s, RA was well described in both the French and English literature, and in 1858, A. B. Garrod coined the term rheumatoid arthritis (Garrod, 1892).

Intensive investigation into the immunologic aspects of RA began after World War II, prompted by the discovery that the addition of RA serum to sheep red blood cells coated or sensitized with rabbit antibodies produced marked agglutination. Waaler, from Oslo, published his initial observations in 1940, and termed the serum material *agglutination activating factor* (Waaler, 1940). In parallel studies, Rose *et al.* (1948) identified a similar activity. Shortly thereafter, it was determined that the activity under study was a serum globulin and a member of the newly recognized antibody family. Because of the frequent disease association, it was termed the rheumatoid factor. The true significance of these observations and their relevance to the pathogenesis of RA awaited the incisive studies of H. G. Kunkel and his associates (Franklin *et al.*, 1957; Kunkel *et al.*, 1959; Kunkel *et al.*, 1961). In a series of landmark publications between 1957 and 1960, they determined that RA serum contained a unique high-molecular-weight protein complex (sedimentation rate in an ultracentrifuge of 22 Svedberg units). This complex could be further dissociated into 19S and 7S components. The 19S component was identified as a high-molecular-weight antibody (now known as the IgM class of immunoglobulin). Subsequently they showed that the high-molecular-weight material was present in both the blood and synovial fluid of patients with RA and defined the gamma globulin–antigammaglobulin nature of the immune complex.

In the next 3 decades, investigations of RA paralleled the advances in our understanding of both humoral and cellular immunity. This information forms the basis of much of this chapter. Currently, these insights are beginning to modify the heretofore empirical nature of RA treatment, and we hope they will be translated into effective, rational treatment for this chronic disabling disorder.

II. GENERAL DESCRIPTION—ANIMAL MODELS

Numerous manipulations can produce chronic inflammatory arthritis in laboratory animals. Most have in common a genetic component and an immune pathogenesis and thus may serve as surrogates for human rheumatic diseases. While no one model accurately recapitulates both the clinical and pathologic features of RA, nevertheless, some valuable lessons have been learned. We shall briefly describe three forms of experimental arthritis that have particular relevance to RA.

A. Collagen-Induced Arthritis

Immunization of certain strains of mice and rats with native type II collagen (the predominant form of collagen in cartilage), results in a symmetrical synovitis reminiscent of RA (Courtenay *et al.*, 1980). Disease susceptibility is closely linked to specific class II MHC genes (Wooley *et al.*, 1981). Some experiments suggest that circulating antibodies to type II collagen play a role, since antibody titers increase dramatically after immunization (Holmdahl *et al.*, 1986), and transient disease can be transferred with serum from affected animals (Stuart and Dixon, 1983). IgG2a and IgG2b antibodies (both of which activate complement) are present in high titer and might contribute to local complement activation. Other soluble factors produced by T cells (e.g., *arthritogenic* factor) have also been implicated (Helfgott *et al.*, 1985). The rolc of T cells is not so well defined, and transfer of disease with splenocytes is inconsistent. However, depletion of T helper populations inhibits anticollagen antibody production and disease expression (Ranges *et al.*, 1985).

The relevance of type II collagen immunity to RA is not established. Early studies demonstrated circulating anticollagen antibodies in RA and other forms of inflammatory arthritis. Cell-mediated responses to type II collagen were also increased. A recent study demonstrated active synthesis of antibodies to type II collagen by RA synovial tissue cells (Tarkowski *et al.*, 1989). Failure to detect the antibody in the circulation could be owing to absorption by antiidiotype antibodies or rheumatoid factors. Although immunity to collagen is probably not a primary event in RA, it is likely that synovial antibody production contributes to cartilage damage, either directly or via local complement activation.

B. Adjuvant Arthritis

Adjuvant arthritis (AA) is induced in Lewis rats after immunization with complete Freund's adjuvant (CFA) (Pearson, 1964). Over the ensuing weeks, the animals develop a self-limited polyarticular arthritis that shares some histopathologic features of RA, including mononuclear cell infiltration of the synovium, pannus formation, destruction of cartilage, and erosion of bone. T cells are thought to play an important role in both the aggressive phases of the disease; some T-cell clones that can induce the disease have been isolated from rats immunized with CFA, while others are protective (Holoshitz *et al.*, 1984; Cohen *et al.*, 1985). The critical antigens in CFA might be mycobacterial heat-shock proteins (van Eden *et al.*, 1985). Some evidence suggests that the link between the joint disease and heat-shock proteins is a shared epitope between a 65-kDa heat-shock protein and a fraction of cartilage proteoglycan (van Eden *et al.*, 1985). It is also intriguing that synovial fluid mononuclear cells from patients with inflammatory arthritis proliferate in response to the 65-kDa protein (Gaston *et al.*, 1989).

C. Streptococcal Cell Wall Arthritis

Lewis rats developed a T cell-dependent, erosive arthritis after intraperitoneal injection with cell wall fragments isolated from streptococci. Control strains (e.g., Fischer rats) are resistant to this disease. Interestingly, the resistant strain develops a rapid increase in corticotropin-releasing factor (CRF), adrenocorticotropic hormone (ACTH), and corticosteroids after injection, while the Lewis rats have a blunted hypothalamic-pituitary-adrenal response (Sternberg *et al.*, 1989). Steroid replacement in the Lewis rats decreases the inflammatory arthritis, while pharmacologic inhibition of the axis dramatically increases the incidence of arthritis in the Fischer rats. These intriguing data support the notion of a neuroendocrine role in immune-mediated diseases.

III. CLINICAL PRESENTATION—JOINT DISEASE

Rheumatoid arthritis is a highly variable disease, ranging from a mild pauciarticular form of brief duration to a relentless, progressive, destructive polyarthritis associated with systemic features (Weisman, 1990). Frequently RA is heralded by prodromal symptoms, such as fatigue, anorexia, weakness, and generalized aching and stiffness that is not clearly localized to articular structures. Joint symptoms usually appear gradually and insidiously over a period of weeks to months. Occasionally there are brief remittent episodes of articular involvement before the development of more persistent arthritis; approximately 20% of patients have an abrupt onset, with the rapid development of polyarthritis, often accompanied by fever, prostration, and severe constitutional symptoms.

Articular involvement is manifested clinically by joint pain, stiffness, limitation of motion, and the signs of inflammation (Zvaifler, 1990). Morning stiffness lasting more than 30 min (and frequently several hours) is highly characteristic. Joint swelling results from a combination of synovial hypertrophy, angiogenesis, infiltration with inflammatory cells, and increase in the volume of synovial fluid (joint effusions). Although RA can affect any diarthrodial joint, symmetrical involvement of the small joints of the hands, the wrists, knees, and feet is the most common distribution. As the disease becomes established, the arthritis spreads to the elbows, shoulders, hips, ankles, subtalar, and sternoclavicular joints.

Examination of the joints generally reveals characteristic abnormalities. Swelling of the proximal interphalangeal finger joints produces a fusiform or spindle-shaped appearance. Bilateral and symmetrical soft-tissue swelling of the metacarpal phalangeal joints, particularly the second and third, is a hallmark of rheumatoid arthritis. By contrast, the distal interphalangeal finger joints are usually spared. As the disease progresses, laxity of tissues increases, and under the pressure of regular use, characteristic hand changes develop, including ulnar deviation of the digits and hyperextension ("swan neck") or flexion ("boutonniere") deformities. Wrist disease is an almost invariable accompaniment of RA, often complicated by carpal tunnel syndrome due to compression of the median nerve by hypertrophied synovium. Flexion contractures of the elbows are frequent, even at an early stage of the disease, and shoulder involvement is common.

In the lower extremities, RA can affect the hip joints, but usually late in the illness. The knee, one of the most commonly involved joints, develops contractures, deformities, and commonly all degrees of ligamentous instability. Pain and limitation of flexion and extension of the foot results from disease of the ankle joint proper, whereas subtalar joint involvement causes pain and limitation of eversion and inversion. In the foot proper, synovitis of the metatarsal phalangeal joints is particularly common, resulting in subluxation of the metatarsal heads, and lateral deviation and clawing of the toes.

A. Extra-Articular Manifestations

Low-grade fever, mild lymphadenopathy, anorexia, and weight loss are all evidence of the systemic nature of RA. Muscle atrophy is common and may be remarkable in its degree and rapidity of development.

Subcutaneous nodules (rheumatoid granuloma) occur at some time in 20 to 25% of RA patients, almost always associated with rheumatoid factor in the blood (Zvaifler, 1990). Nodules usually appear in areas subjected to mechanical pressure, especially the olecranon, extensor surface of the forearms, and the Achilles' tendon periarticular structures. Unusual locations include the pleura, meninges, back of the head, pinna of the ears, and bridge of the nose. As a rule, the nodules are firm, nontender, oval or round masses in the subcutaneous or deeper tissues.

A spectrum of vascular lesions accompany RA. Inflamed capillaries and small venules participate in the development of rheumatoid nodules and synovitis. Other lesions include a bland intimal proliferation, commonly affecting digital and mesenteric vessels; subacute lesions of arterioles and venules; and occasionally a widespread necrotizing arteritis of small and medium-sized arteries, possibly indistinguishable from polyarteritis nodosa. This form of rheumatoid vasculitis characteristically produces polyneuropathy, skin necrosis and ulceration, digital gangrene, perforation of the nasal septum, and visceral infarction. The prognosis in this fulminant vasculitis was exceedingly poor before the advent of immunosuppressive (cyclophosphamide) treatment. Much evidence (see the following sections) suggests a role for immune complexes in the pathogenesis of most vascular lesions.

Involvement of viscera, such as the eyes, heart, lungs, and peripheral nervous system, is a well-recognized complication of RA (Zvaifler, 1990). The basic lesion in most is an admixture of a granulomatous response (analogous to the rheumatoid nodule) and some form of vascular injury. For instance, inflammatory microvascular lesions can be found throughout the myocardium in almost 40% of autopsied RA patients. Less common are granulomatous lesions involving the epicardium, myocardium, and valves. Interstitial pulmonary disease is likely to result from immune complex-mediated vascular abnormalities, whereas intrapulmonary nodules reflect granulomatous responses. Dryness of mucous membranes, particularly dry eyes (xerophthalmia) and dry mouth (xerostomia) due to chronic inflammation of exocrine glands also occurs in about 15% of patients.

IV. HISTOPATHOLOGY

The lining of a normal joint (synovium) is a delicate structure consisting of an intimal lining and a sublining layer. The former is usually one or two layers deep; the latter comprises occasional small blood vessels, loose stroma, fibroblasts, and fat cells. The lining cells (synoviocytes) can be divided into two separate populations based on conventional morphologic studies, histochemical staining, and functional capacities. Type A cells (macrophagelike) synoviocytes possess phagocytic vacuoles, macrophage surface markers, surface HLA-DR, and Fc receptors, while type B cells (fibroblastlike) have features of secretory fibroblasts, including prominent, rough endoplasmic reticulum and regular arrays of ribosomes.

Histopathologic changes in RA vary considerably. Early on, sublining edema and proliferation of blood vessels is prominent. Fibrin deposits onto the surface of the lining facing the joint cavity, and there is a scant interstitial infiltrate with either neutrophils or lymphocytes. As the disease progresses, the lining becomes hyperplastic, and the sublining is infiltrated with mononuclear cells and lymphoid aggregates. The synoviocytes display high levels of HLA-DR (particularly on macrophagelike cells), and large amounts of class II MHC mRNA are demonstrable in this region (Firestein, *et al.*, in press). The lining layer is usually 5 to 10 cells deep as a result of an increase in both type A and type B synoviocytes. Whether the increase is the result of local proliferation or increased migration of new cells into the joint is not clear, although the relative absence of mitotic figures, low expression of cell cycle-specific antigens, and minimal *in situ* incorporation of tritiated thymidine favor the latter explanation (Konttinen *et al.*, 1981; Nykanen *et al.*, 1986; Lalor *et al.*, 1987).

The sublining is often densely infiltrated with lymphocytes. These may be evenly dispersed throughout the tissue or collected in aggregates. T lymphocytes predominate in RA tissue, representing about 40 to 50% of the total number of synovial cells, along with immunoglobulin-producing B cells and plasma cells. Most are CD4-positive T-helper cells, with a CD4:CD8 ratio ranging from 4:1 to

14:1. (in synovial fluid, CD8-positive T cells equal or outnumber helper cells) (Forre *et al.*, 1982; Klareskog *et al.*, 1982; Konttinen *et al.*, 1981; Malone *et al.*, 1984; Young *et al.*, 1984). The CD8 infiltrate in the tissue is scanty and usually located at the periphery of the lymphoid aggregates, suggesting that within the aggregate, macrophages and/or dendritic cells are presenting antigen to the helper T cells and B cells; and the relative absence of a CD8 population results in unopposed activation (Janossy *et al.*, 1981; Preble *et al.*, 1982).

However, this model is somewhat simplistic and not without problems. For instance, synovial biopsies from some RA patients show equal numbers of CD4- and CD8-positive T cells (Lindblad *et al.*, 1983; Young *et al.*, 1984; Malone *et al.*, 1984). In another study, lymphoid aggregates were identified in only a minority of patients, and occasionally the synovium displayed a stromal pattern made up almost exclusively of fibroblasts with only rare T cells. The peripheral blood cells of these RA patients tended to respond briskly to soluble recall antigens (e.g., PPD), while blood mononuclear cells from those with intense lymphocytic infiltrates failed to respond (Malone *et al.*, 1984). This reciprocal relationship between blood anergy and the degree of inflammatory infiltrate implies a different immunopathogenic mechanism in each subset. Finally, the classic histopathologic picture is not unique to RA but is seen in a number of other forms of arthritis, including crystal-induced disease and even osteoarthritis, which are not likely to be antigen-driven processes.

V. IMMUNOLOGIC FEATURES AND MODELS FOR RHEUMATOID ARTHRITIS

The notion that disordered cellular immunity is central to the pathogenesis of RA derives from the histopathologic findings in the joint, but the ontogeny of immunology began in the humoral arm of the immune system with the discovery of rheumatoid factor (RF) in the blood of 80% of RA patients. This antibody, which binds to the Fc portion of human IgG, was initially recognized through its ability to agglutinate sheep red blood cells (RBC) coated with anti-sheep RBC antibodies; this provided evidence for autoimmunity in RA. Later studies demonstrated that, although most RF are IgM, IgG RF is also produced (Pope *et al.*, 1974).

The importance of RF in the pathogenesis of RA was inferred from the fact that circulating B cells in RA spontaneously produce the antibody (Peterson *et al.*, 1983), and RF-producing plasma cells abound in the rheumatoid synovium (Munthe and Natvig, 1972). Also, RF is a major constituent of immune complexes in the blood and synovial fluid (SF) of RA patients, suggesting that local immune-complex formation and complement fixation is involved in rheumatoid synovitis. Chemotactic complement fragments (like C5a) recruit neutrophils, which ingest the complexes and release degradative enzymes and toxic O_2 products into the SF (Ward and Zvaifler, 1971). This model is supported by the observation that serum RF levels correlate positively with complement consumption in RA (Kaplan *et al.*, 1980). A consequence of the intra-articular inflammation is cartilage damage and the release of additional antigens (such as type II collagen) that can contribute to local autoantibody production, complement fixation, and direct tissue injury.

Although RF undoubtedly contributes to synovitis, recent studies have focused on the importance of cellular immunity in RA. Three separate paradigms could explain the histologic findings of chronic rheumatoid synovitis.

A. T Cell-Driven Immune Response

RA is thought to begin when an *arthrotropic* pathogen enters the joint. The etiologic agent is not known, but might be a virus or a nonbiodegradable product of bacteria (as in streptococcal cell-wall arthritis). Persistence in the synovial tissue would presumably result in a specific T cell-mediated immune response. Much evidence has been advanced to support this sequence of events (Cush and Lipsky, 1987). For instance, the joint lesions of Lyme arthritis, in which spirochetal antigens are likely to be pathogenic, are similar to those of RA (Steere *et al.*, 1988). The T cells from RA synovial effusions and subintimal tissues appear "activated" and express cell-surface markers, such as class II MHC antigens, transferrin receptors, and IL-2 receptors (Klareskog *et al.*, 1982; Konttinen, 1981; Burmester *et al.*, 1984). Synovial lining cells and interdigitating macrophages also display large amounts of class II antigens. Lymphocytes intimately associated with Ia-rich accessory cells should produce a variety of lymphokines that, along with macrophage-derived factors, can induce class II MHC expression, and promote synoviocyte proliferation and the growth and differentiation of B lymphocytes. Finally, T cell-specific therapies, such as thoracic duct drainage, total nodal irradiation, and cyclosporine A, are modestly effective in RA.

Thus, the notion that RA synovitis results from a T cell-driven immune response could explain a number of features of RA but, as will be noted below, not all of the data are consistent with this hypothesis. In particular, the surprising finding is that the soluble mediators (i.e., cytokines) produced in the joint are primarily of non-T cell origin (Firestein and Zvaifler, 1990a; Firestein *et al.*, 1990b). Also, the small amount of T-cell proliferation that does occur in the synovium ($<$ 1% of T cells are dividing) is limited to the CD8 population, not the putative CD4 responder cells. Finally, as mentioned earlier, the classic histologic features of RA are not always present, and some patients have an acellular fibrotic synovium.

B. Autoreactive T-Cell Model

Although it is usually assumed that the initiating agent in RA is responsible for both the early changes and the perpetuation of chronic synovitis, this need not be the case. The chronic rheumatoid lesion might be attributable to a response to antigens quite distinct from those responsible for starting the process. Such a scenario has been used to explain other chronic inflammatory lesions, like chronic thyroiditis, in which an appropriate response to a presumed viral insult results in the local elaboration of IFN-gamma (Feldmann, 1987). This cytokine can induce HLA-DR expression on the surface of thyrocytes, rendering them targets for immune attack. This reaction between HLA-DR-bearing stimulator cells and autologous T lymphocytes is termed the autologous mixed-leukocyte reaction (AMLR). The evidence that RA synovitis represents a localized AMLR is largely circumstantial. First, the cytokine profile of synovitis is similar to that of an AMLR in that only small amounts of T cell-derived factors, like IL-2 and IFN-gamma, are present (Firestein and Zvaifler, 1987b; Firestein *et al.*, 1988; Firestein *et al.*, 1990b; Suzuki *et al.*, 1986). In contrast, allogeneic mixed-leukocyte reactions contain a high level of these lymphokines. Also, the cytotoxic T cells present in RA joint effusions are similar to the natural killer (NK)-like cells produced in the AMLR (Goto and Zvaifler, 1983, 1985). Finally, the articular cavity and synovium contain a variety of Ia-rich potential stimulator cells including type A synoviocytes and dendritic cells (Zvaifler *et al.*, 1985).

Autologous stimulation can also occur through other mechanisms. According to theories of molecular mimicry, a foreign antigen can closely resemble a self-antigen, and innocent bystanders can become a target. This is one of the proposed mechanisms implicating Epstein–Barr virus (EBV) in the pathogenesis of RA. B lymphocytes are the primary target; once infected, the cells carry the viral genome for life. Normal B cells that have been superinfected *in vitro* spontaneously proliferate and secrete immunoglobulin (including rheumatoid factors) (Slaughter *et al.*, 1978). In addition, rheumatoids are defective in controlling *in vitro* EBV infection (Hasler *et al.*, 1983), in part owing to deficient IFN-γ secretion by RA T cells (Hasler *et al.*, 1983) and a monocyte-derived IL-1 inhibitor (Lotz *et al.*, 1986). Recent analysis of EBV-encoded proteins revealed sequence homology between the EBV glycoprotein gp110 and human HLA-DW4/DW14/DR1 (Roudier *et al.*, 1989). Disease susceptibility to RA has been mapped to a five-amino-acid sequence in the third hypervariable region of the DR beta 1 chain; this is precisely the epitope shared by gp110 and the RA-associated HLA-DR haplotypes. Hence, immunity directed against the gp110 could inadvertently damage normal cells in hosts expressing these surface MHC molecules and result in perpetuation of synovitis if high levels of Ia were maintained in the joint. In a sense, EBV might initiate an AMLR-like reaction in genetically susceptible individuals, with HLA-DR as the target.

Other self-molecules have been proposed as targets for immune attack in arthritis. For instance, type II collagen can cause arthritis in susceptible animals and might contribute to chronic RA, but is probably not etiologic. Autoantibodies to proteoglycan, a macromolecule with a protein backbone and large glycosaminoglycan side chains, develops in the course of immune synovitis in rabbits, and the affected joints show a loss of cartilage proteoglycan. The relevance of this model to human disease is not yet defined, but as with type II collagen, if immunity to proteoglycan contributes to cartilage damage, it is likely to be a secondary phenomenon.

Mycobacteria cause chronic inflammatory lesions and have long been implicated in the pathogenesis of RA (see preceding discussion on adjuvant arthritis). Interest in mycobacterium as a cross-reactive autoantigen comes from the recent recognition that an immunodominant antigen of the mycobacterium is a 65-kDa protein with sequence homology to an intracellular stress protein present in all eukaryotic cells (Young *et al.*, 1987). A massive increase in stress proteins was first demonstrated after cells were exposed to heat. Thus, heat-shock proteins (HSP) and stress proteins are interchangeable terms. Because of the ubiquitous nature of these highly conserved proteins, the immune system is likely to be tolerant to them. Repeated presentation of cross-reactive bacterial HSP or surface expression of these proteins on T cells or macrophages might result in loss of tolerance and an autoimmune reaction. Another intriguing mechanism for the role of HSP in RA, reminiscent of EBV molecular mimicry, is suggested by the discovery that the QKRAA epitope on the HLA-DR4 beta chain, the putative susceptibility marker for RA, has complete homology with a sequence in a 70-kDa stress protein (Sargent *et al.*, 1989). Finally, another link to arthritis is that an acetone-precipitable fraction of mycobacterium has antigens that cross-react with antibodies to cartilage proteoglycan (van Eden *et al.*, 1985; Holoshitz *et al.*, 1986).

C. Paracrine/Autocrine Model

In the two previous models, T lymphocytes are assigned the major role for the perpetuation of rheumatoid synovitis. Products of these cells theoretically diffuse through the tissues, altering postcapillary venules, inducing the proliferation and differentiation of B cells, and directly influencing macrophages and synoviocytes in the lining. Unfortunately, this picture is not consistent with much of the data about T-cell activation in the joint. For instance, important T-cell cytokines, like IL-2, IL-3, IL-4, IFN-gamma, and TNF-beta, are barely detectable in RA tissue or SF (Firestein and Zvaifler, 1987b; Firestein *et al.*, 1988; Firestein *et al.*, 1990b; Miossec *et al.*, 1990; Saxne *et al.*, 1988), whereas *in vivo* production of these same lymphokines is easily demonstrated in a human T cell-mediated response, such as that in tuberculous pleuritis (Barnes *et al.*, 1990).

In RA, most synovial lymphocytes are small and quiescent in appearance. Little DNA synthesis is demonstrable, and the majority of dividing synovial T cells are $CD8^+$ rather than $CD4^+$. Also, IL-2 receptor expression is actually similar to that of resting peripheral blood cells. Even infiltration of the synovium with HLA-DR-positive T cells is nonspecific, since it also occurs in T cell-

TABLE I
Cytokine Profile of Rheumatoid Synovitis

	T Cell	Macrophage/Fibroblast
IL-2	–	
IL-3	–	
IL-4	–	
IFN-gamma	–	
TNF-beta	–	
IL-6	–	+
GM-CSF	–	+
TNF-alpha	–	+
IL-1		+
M-CSF		+
TGF-beta		+

independent forms of arthritis (like gout) (Laffon *et al.,* 1989). Finally, studies of synovial tissue and synovial fluid T cell-receptor rearrangements have not consistently demonstrated the oligoclonal expansion expected in an antigen-driven response (Stamenkovic *et al.,* 1988; Duby *et al.,* 1989; Brennan *et al.,* 1988; Savill *et al.,* 1987; Keystone *et al.,* 1988; Sakkas *et al.,* 1987).

In contrast, synovial macrophagelike and fibroblastlike cells appear highly activated based on their morphology, surface HLA-DR expression, and elaboration of cytokines (see Table I for a comparison of cytokine production by various synovial cells). Products of these cells, like IL-1 (Fontana *et al.,* 1982; Wood *et al.,* 1983; Nouri *et al.,* 1984; Miossec *et al.,* 1986), TNF-alpha (Saxne *et al.,* 1988), IL-6 (Guerne *et al.,* 1989; Hirano *et al.,* 1988), GM-CSF (Xu *et al.,* 1989), M-CSF (CSF-1) (Firestein *et al.,* 1988), prostaglandins, and collagenase are abundant in synovial fluids and synovial tissues. Recent studies using *in situ* hybridization to quantify cytokine production at the level of gene expression confirm experiments that detected high levels of secreted cytokines in culture supernatants of synovial tissue cells and in synovial effusions (Firestein *et al.,* 1990b). For instance, IL-1 beta and TNF-alpha genes were expressed by large numbers of synovial macrophages. IL-6 probes also hybridized to a high percentage of RA synovial cells. Although T cells can produce IL-6 under some circumstances, *in situ* hybridization experiments show most of the IL-6 gene expression in the nonmacrophage, non-T cell population; these cells are located mainly in the intimal lining of the joint. GM-CSF and TGF-beta gene expression was observed in a lesser number of cells. As predicted from earlier studies on synovial IFN-gamma production (Firestein and Zvaifler, 1987b), the IFN-gamma probe did not bind to synovial tissue cells. Interestingly, the failure to detect cytokine mRNA (including IL-1, TNF-alpha, and IL-6) in mononuclear cells

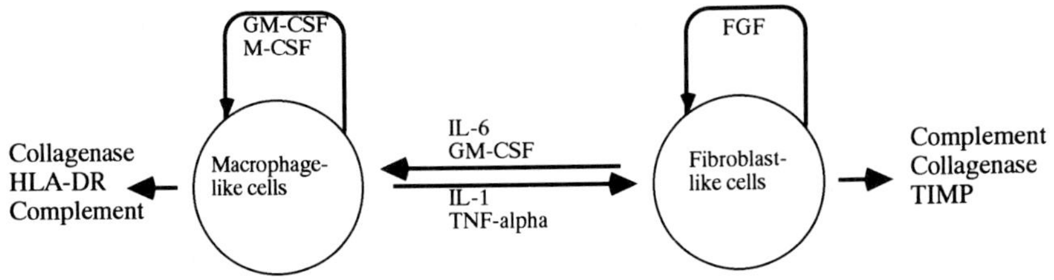

FIG. 1 Paracrine and autocrine cytokine loops in rheumatoid arthritis synovium.

isolated from synovial effusions indicates that the synovium is the source of most articular cytokines.

The cytokine profile of the rheumatoid synovium suggests that chronic articular inflammation might be sustained by factors produced by neighboring macrophages and synovial fibroblasts in a paracrine or autocrine model. This non-T cell-driven pathogenesis of synovitis has support in some animal models. For instance, synoviocytes from rats injected with complete Freund's adjuvant show evidence of activation (surface class II MHC antigen) before the onset of arthritis or the appearance of mononuclear cells in the synovial membrane. Also, T cell-dependent autoantibody production directed against type II collagen in the MRL/l mouse arthritis model is probably triggered by cartilage destruction and is, therefore, a secondary phenomenon (Gay *et al.*, 1987). Many factors already identified in the joint could explain lining-cell hyperplasia, Ia induction, and synovial angiogenesis. Figure 1 shows a simplified scheme of the complex cytokine circuits that exist between synovial cells. For instance, IL-1 and TNF-alpha (synovial macrophage products) stimulate fibroblast proliferation and increase secretion of IL-6, GM-CSF, and collagenase (Guerne *et al.*, 1989; Kaushansky *et al.*, 1988; Dayer *et al.*, 1986; Dayer *et al.*, 1985). GM-CSF, produced by synovial macrophages, can stimulate fibroblastlike synoviocytes, is a potent inducer of IL-1 secretion, and increases Ia expression on macrophages (Morrissey *et al.*, 1987; Alvaro-Gracia *et al.*, 1989). TNF-alpha can synergize with GM-CSF and probably also contributes to macrophage HLA-DR expression (Alvaro-Garcia *et al.*, 1989). The local production of cytokines by macrophages and fibroblasts could also affect T cells and contribute to the modest degree of T-cell activation observed. B-cell activation and RF production might result through T-cell independent mechanisms or as yet undefined cell products.

A prediction of this alternative (paracrine) model is that T cells are not necessarily sequestered in the joint in response to a specific antigen; rather they accumulate under the influence of factors made in the lining. The RA synovium has an overrepresentation of mature memory helper cells ($CD4^+$, $4B4^+$, or UCHL-1^+ subset) while naive 2H4-bearing cells (the suppressor–inducer subset) are conspicuously absent (Kidd *et al.*, 1989). This could be explained by the fact that the movement of lymphocytes from the circulation into the joint is not a random process. Their site of egress is the postcapillary venules, notably those with "high" endothelium (HEV) that express adhesion molecules, like ICAM-1 and/or LFA-3 (Streeter *et al.*, 1988; Cavender *et al.*, 1987). A recent immunofluorescence study of RA synovium demonstrated large amounts of these molecules on the surface of synovial fibroblasts and endothelial cells (Hale *et al.*, 1989). The ligands for ICAM-1 and LFA-3 (LFA-1 and CD2, respectively) are expressed on all T cells, but in significantly greater amounts on mature $4B4^+$ cells (Sanders *et al.*, 1988). A consequence might be the preferential accumulation of cells with this phenotype in inflamed synovium. The expression of other integrins, such as very late activation (VLA) markers (recognized by the 4B4 antibody) on T cells could also be important for T-cell retention, since these heterodimers are receptors for matrix proteins that are abundant in the synovium. The implications of the nonspecific accumulation of T cells in synovitis are profound: No one can argue with the fact that memory T cells are present in the rheumatoid synovium. The germane question is whether they have been activated by antigen and how they express this. To date, there is little functional data to support this occurrence in RA.

D. Immunogenetics

Some of the genes responsible for susceptibility to RA and other autoimmune disorders (see Chapter 4 of this volume) reside on the short arm of chromosome 6 in man. This region contains the histocompatibility loci (HLA class I and HLA class II), and between them, a large number of loci that include genes for complement components and tumor necrosis factor. Classic genetic techniques such as comparisons between monozygotic and dizygotic twins, HLA haplotype sharing in siblings affected by the disease in multicase families, and an analysis of the estimate of the risk of RA in siblings that do not share an HLA haplotype all support the conclusion that perhaps 25–50% of the disease susceptibility is linked to HLA and the remainder comes from non-MHC genes (Wordsworth, 1990). In most populations the relevant HLA gene is associated with DR4 specificity. Prominent exceptions in Israelis, Yakima American Indians, and some other ethnic groups have been revealing. In the Israeli study, for instance, only DR1 is associated with an increased relative risk for the development of RA. Taking advantage of the information that different DR and Dw specificities originate from variations in the DR beta chain, Gregersen *et al.*, demonstrated that amino acid sequences in the third allelic hypervariable region of the DR beta chain from RA susceptible haplotypes (i.e., DR1; DR4, Dw4; DR4, Dw14; DR4, Dw15) were essentially the same and differed from non-RA-susceptible haplotypes (like DR4, Dw10). Thus, it appears that different haplotypes can share common epitopes and confer disease susceptibility (Gregerson *et al.*,

1989). This concept was subsequently confirmed employing T-cell clones, oligonucleotide probes, and Southern blotting. The shared amino acid sequences appear to reside in the third diversity region of the alpha-helical segment of the DR beta chain between position 67 and 74. This region is a critical binding site for foreign antigens and supports the notion that associations between class II antigens and specific diseases are likely to involve discrete disease-related epitopes that are immunologically relevant in terms of T-cell recognition. A search of computer-based data banks for peptides analogous to the RA susceptibility QKRAA amino acid sequence revealed homology with a 110-kDa glycoprotein from the capsular antigen of the Epstein–Barr virus (Roudier *et al.*, 1989) and a sequence in the 70-kDa HSP (Sargent *et al.*, 1989). It is probably not coincidental that both EBV and HSP have independently been implicated in the pathogenesis of RA.

While DQ haplotypes have not been incriminated in an overall susceptibility to RA, some are strongly associated with Felty's syndrome (DQ w4), vasculitis, and other extra-articular manifestations of the disease (Sansom *et al.*, 1989).

E. Laboratory Diagnosis

RA is a clinical diagnosis, but laboratory tests are useful to support the clinical assessment and to monitor disease activity (Bull *et al.*, 1989). Acute-phase reactants such as the erythrocyte sedimentation rate, serum orosomucoid, CRP, alpha-2 macroglobulins, and fibrinogen are all increased, probably reflecting the release from inflamed articular tissues of cytokines, particularly IL-1 and IL-6 (Scott *et al.*, 1989). Anemia, usually associated with low serum iron, may be explained by similar factors.

Rheumatoid factors (antigammaglobulins) are detected in the serum of approximately 70% of RA patients. Very high titers of IgM rheumatoid factor are usually associated with more aggressive, destructive arthritis and more extra-articular features, including vasculitis. Titers of rheumatoid factor fluctuate very little in the course of the disease, and only occasionally do they fall in response to treatment. However, IgM rheumatoid factors are not specific for rheumatic diseases but are found in a variety of chronic and inflammatory conditions. Rheumatoid factors of the IgG class, while probably important pathogenetically, particularly in the synovial space, are not measured in the conventional clinical laboratory tests because they are poor agglutinators.

Much information about the immunopathogenesis of RA comes from studies of cellular immunity in synovial tissues and fluids, but they are of limited clinical utility (Firestein *et al.*, 1987a). Determinations of circulating lymphocyte numbers, subclasses, and surface markers have been disappointing (Cush *et al.*, 1990). Recently, however, some new methods have been developed for assessing disease activity. For instance, serum levels of soluble IL-2 receptor appear to correlate with increased disease activity in RA (Wood *et al.*, 1988). Likewise, soluble CD8 molecules, presumably shed from subsets of lymphocytes during activation, correlate inversely with IL-2 receptor levels. Small amounts of IL-1β can be detected in the plasma of normal and RA subjects. Although there is a considerable overlap, half of the RA patients have markedly elevated levels that seem to correlate with disease activity.

Inflammatory joint disease is associated with an accelerated metabolism of bone and cartilage matrix constituents. Connective tissue turnover can be quantified by measurements of proteoglycans, type III procollagen peptides, hyaluronic acid in blood, and hydroxyproline in urine. Unfortunately, these determinations are of little value in assessing clinical status, apart from proteoglycans, whose levels appear to be increased during acute inflammation (Ratcliff *et al.*, 1988).

Synovial fluid (SF) analysis confirms that RA is an inflammatory joint disease. The increased protein content is characteristic of an exudate. White blood cells range from 5 to 20,000 per mm^3, and counts in excess of 50,000 mm^3 are occasionally encountered. Approximately two thirds of the cells are polymorphonuclear leukocytes, except in very early disease (Firestein *et al.*, 1987a). Total hemolytic complement activity is reduced to less than one third of the serum values, especially in patients with seropositive RA. Early classic pathway components (C2 and C4) are most profoundly depressed. This is distinctly different in other inflammatory forms of joint disease and supports a role for intra-articular immune complexes in the pathogenesis of RA (Pekin and Zvaifler, 1964). Mononuclear cell-surface antigens, cytokines, and constituents of the inflammatory reaction have all been measured in SF but are of limited utility. A possible exception is neopterin, a product of activated macrophages, whose concentration in SF appears to correlate directly with disease activity measurements (Krause *et al.*, 1989).

Roentgenograms, particularly of the hands and feet, remain the standard for assessing joint damage and progression in RA (Sharp, 1989). Erosions of articular cartilage and bone predict a poorer outcome and are used as an indication for aggressive drug treatment.

VI. TREATMENT OUTCOME (PROGNOSIS)

The course that RA will follow in any individual seen at the inception of the disease cannot be reliably predicted, but there are several recognized patterns of outcome (Short, 1968). Approximately 10% of patients have a short-lived joint disease that remits without significant residua. In another 15 to 25%, arthritis persists for some time and then leaves with only mild to moderate damage to the joints. Fifty percent of patients have persistent activity of arthritis, punctuated by exacerbations and remissions, but invariably leading to progressive deformity and disability. The remaining 10% have a relentless disease that is unresponsive to treatment and, before the availability of joint replacement, resulted in complete disability with the patient restricted to a bed or wheelchair existence.

Features that portend either a favorable or a dismal outcome for RA have been identified. In general, remissions are most likely to occur during the first year of disease, especially after an acute onset with systemic manifestations. Factors that presage a less-favorable disease course are an insidious onset; older age (> 45 years); gender (female is worse); persistence beyond 1 year without remission; early appearance of bone erosions on radiologic examination of the joints; development of nodules and the presence of serum RF, particularly in high titers (Short, 1968; Feigenbaum *et al.*, 1979). Rheumatoid patients may succumb to overwhelming sepsis or complications of drug or surgical therapy, but the majority generally die of the same diseases as age-matched cohorts, except 5 to 10 years sooner. In fact the life expectancy for RA patients with advanced (Stage IV) joint disease is similar to that of Hodgkin's disease patients (Mitchell *et al.*, 1986). The dim outlook in these patients has been used to justify trials with toxic compounds or experimental modalities.

The natural course of RA is characterized by spontaneous remissions and exacerbation; therefore, the evaluation of therapy is difficult. In this review, the discussion will be limited to drug therapies, with an emphasis on classes of drugs. A total management program for RA, however, requires the participation of various medical and paramedical personnel: physiatrists, orthopedic surgeons, rheumatologists, visiting nurses, and when indicated, other medical specialists. Successful treatment also depends on an empathetic doctor–patient relationship.

Nonsteroidal anti-inflammatory drugs (NSAID) are mainstays of RA therapy. All have the capacity to inhibit prostaglandin and thromboxane synthesis by interfering with the cyclooxygenase enzyme. However, the fact that nonacetylated salicylates are poor inhibitors of prostaglandin synthesis and that the anti-inflammatory effect of NSAIDs requires doses that are in excess of those needed to inhibit prostaglandin synthesis suggests that these agents must have anti-inflammatory effects independent of arachidonic acid metabolism (Hochberg, 1989). Indeed, they can influence neutrophil function and activation, interfere with the guanosine triphosphate-binding regulatory protein (G protein), and probably have other effects through their ability to associate with the plasma membrane of certain cells. Many of these same pharmacologic properties may account for important toxicities that develop in the course of NSAID use. Upper gastrointestinal injury occurs in many patients who take these compounds, and although infrequent (1–2% per annum), massive upper gastrointestinal bleeding or perforation are recognized as significant public health problems. Likewise, prostaglandins play an important role in renal blood flow, and NSAID use introduces a significant risk for the development of renal impairment and congestive heart failure, particularly in elderly patients and/or those with decreased blood volume.

Glucocorticosteroids are used in RA to modify both inflammation and immune function. Their effects are multiple and complex (Harrison and Lippman, 1989). Glucocorticoids alter leukocyte trafficking and recruitment of cells to sites of inflammation. By interfering with the conversion of phospholipase A2 to arachidonic acid, they inhibit both the 5-lipoxygenase and cyclooxygenase pathways. Cellular responses to cytokine and cytokine production are reduced by steroids. Glucocorticoids are potent suppressors of collagenase production by cultured synoviocytes, in part by their ability to block the expression of c-jun, an important transcriptional regulator of the procollagenase gene. Higher concentrations diminish or block lymphocyte proliferation *in vitro*. Clinically, however, glucocorticoids are usually employed at small daily doses (prednisone 5–7.5 mg) in an attempt to reduce the side effects associated with their chronic use (Weiss, 1989). They are seldom the exclusive therapeutic agent in RA; rather they are used in combination with NSAIDs or other slower-acting drugs.

A second class of drugs used to treat RA have in common a slow onset of action (hence the acronym SARD). The members of the group have similar structural or pharmacological properties, but have serendipitously been observed to act as disease-modifying antirheumatic drugs (DMARD) (Weiss, 1989). They include intramuscular gold, oral gold (auranofin), penicillamine, sulfasalazine, and a number of amino-quinoline compounds such as chloroquine and hydroxychloroquine. In contrast to NSAID, which act rapidly (often within hours or days) and lose their effects just as quickly, the second-line antirheumatic drugs often need to be taken for months before improvement is recognized, and their benefits may persist long after the drug is discontinued. Their exact mode of action is unknown (Paulus, 1990a). Gold compounds appear to influence cells of the monocyte/macrophage lineage by interfering with lysosomal enzyme activity, antigen processing, or cytokine production. Penicillamine, on the other hand, seems to exert its effect on T-cell proliferation. Anti-malarials have actions in both the nucleus and cytoplasm of cells. Their ability to interrupt the appearance of HLA class II molecules on the surfaces of monocytes theoretically could interfere with antigen presentation or T-cell activation.

Second-line drugs are considered in patients with persistent synovitis or progressive disability despite NSAID therapy. The appearance of periarticular erosions on radiographic evaluation or development of extra-articular disease are additional indications.

In the past few years there has been increasing skepticism about the long-term benefits of treatment with second-line drugs (Weisman, 1990). Most studies enforce the notion that RA is a relentlessly progressive disease. Conventional interventions appear to benefit a limited number of patients (one third to one half) in the short term (18–30 months), but at the end of 5 to 7 years, there is little evidence for alteration in the natural history of the disease. This has evoked a number of responses, including use of combination therapies employing several second-line agents together, based on the notion that there are multiple pathways in the pathogenesis of chronic synovitis, and intervention at several points might improve effectiveness. An alternative approach is to introduce second-line agents earlier in the disease, when a theoretical window of opportunity exists between the inception of RA and its subsequent perpetuation by autoimmune or chronic inflammatory processes. The evidence that either of these strategies improves outcome is yet to be shown (Paulus, 1990b).

Immunosuppressive treatment has been used in RA for more than 25 years. Initial enthusiasm for alkylating agents such as nitrogen mustard, chlorambucil, and cyclophosphamide was tempered by a high rate of toxicity and the development of skin and hematologic malignancies. Alkylating agents are usually reserved for patients with systemic, life-threatening complications such as necrotizing vasculitis. In contrast, azathioprine has a low incidence of side effects that are easily managed with appropriate attention to hematologic and hepatic testing. An increased incidence of malignancy can be demonstrated only by meta analysis or very long follow-up of large numbers of patients. The risks are very small and probably are offset by benefits in terms of the control of synovitis and the possibility of decreasing concomitant use of corticosteroids.

In the past decade, low-dose methotrexate treatment of RA has become widespread despite substantial uncertainty regarding its mechanism of action, long-term efficacy, and toxicity (Furst and Kremer, 1988). Patient acceptance is high, and side effects are manageable. Fully 60–70% of patients remain on the drug for periods as long as 5 to 7 years (compared to 10% for injectable gold) with a good clinical response (Tugwell *et al.*, 1990). Controversy exists over whether methotrexate's action is immunosuppressive or anti-inflammatory. In small doses used in RA (i.e., 7.5–15 mg orally once a week), there is little effect on a variety of *in vivo* immunologic parameters. Those who favor inhibition of inflammation as a mechanism of action cite a relatively rapid onset of beneficial effects (usually in 3 to 6 weeks), a failure to halt the development of articular erosions on radiographic study, and a rapid recurrence of the joint disease when the drug is stopped. Side effects usually consist of stomatitis and gastrointestinal disturbance; cytopenias are uncommon. The development of hepatotoxicity with chronic administration (as seen in patients treated for psoriasis) has seldom been observed in RA. Occasional fatty infiltration and mild fibrosis is a rare finding on a liver biopsy, but significant hepatic fibrosis or cirrhosis is only rarely encountered. Pulmonary hypersensitivity is rare, although it can be fatal. Despite these concerns, methotrexate alone or in combination with other second-line agents is perhaps the most effective and widely used treatment for severe active RA.

The overall poor response to treatment and the shortened life expectancy in patients with advanced (stage IV) RA have encouraged trials of novel therapies and modalities. Cyclosporine has some benefit when compared to placebo, but only low doses can be used because of nephrotoxicity (Shand and Richardson, 1988). Total nodal irradiation probably provides some relief but the high rate of life-threatening infections has limited its utility (Soden *et al.*, 1989). Products of recombinant technology are currently under study. Gamma interferon has been used in several large multiclinic trials with only modest benefits in RA. Small numbers of patients are being treated with monoclonal antibodies to CD4 or CD5. The results are awaited with interest. Dietary manipulation, particularly of eicosapentaneoics, through the ingestion of fish oils, also provides some benefit in some RA patients (Pike, 1989). Of interest, the effects on cell function and leukotriene B4 release is more impressive than the modest clinical response. Undoubtedly as understanding of the specific factors involved in the perpetuation of rheumatoid synovitis increases, the therapies available will become more specific and effective. It is no longer wishful to believe that control of this devastating disease will come soon.

EDITORS' NOTE:

This chapter on rheumatoid arthritis (RA) collects and organizes much immunologic information on this enigmatic disease. Although the concluding lines are that "it is no longer wishful to believe that control of this devastating disease will come soon," the Editors are not so sanguine. An understanding of the deranged immunology is still insufficiently advanced and, indeed, is progressing rather slowly, looking back on the 1985 account of RA by Morris Ziff in *The Autoimmune Diseases I*. The major advances, to which Firestein and Zvaifler have been substantial contributors, relate to the role of intrasynovial cytokines, which represents an impressive segment of this chapter.

The fact that we remain so much in the dark on the actual cause of RA is illustrated by the three different models cited to explain the immunopathology of the disease, and the authors deal rather even-handedly with each. These are (1) T cells driven by a cryptic antigen; (2) T cells driven by an autologous component, i.e., a DR molecule (as in an AMLR), or an autoantigen (IgGFc, collagen type II or other); or (3) a paracrine–autocrine effect in which the synovium suffers from an extravagant local overproduction (cause unknown) of cytokines secreted by nonlymphoid synovial cells, rather than lymphoid cells.

The interesting point is made by the authors that, in RA, "most synovial lymphocytes are small and quiescent in appearance," although elsewhere the T cells are stated to bear activation markers. However, since circumstantial evidence points to an antigen-driven and T cell-dependent process, this "seems the best site to drill the wells."

The authors touch on collagen type II as a possible autoantigen. The evidence for collagen immunity in RA remains insufficient, but collagen-induced arthritis (CIA) as an experimental model is persuasive, and seems at least as valid a model as EAE for multiple sclerosis; further study of CIA could illuminate the pathogenesis of RA. Heat-shock protein is "all the rage" as a possible autoantigen in RA and other diseases, with mimicries obvious with bacterial proteins; however, the early promise of this lead is not being entirely fulfilled.

The mature or memory class of helper T cells is clearly over-represented and naive T cells under-represented in rheumatoid arthritis, in blood and synovial fluid, shown using the monoclonal antibodies 2H4 and 4B4 (Emery *et al.*, *Arthritis Rheum.* **30,** 849–856, 1987). This leads us to comment that one major feature of autoimmune immune inflammation in general is the enrichment for memory T cells (CD45RO) that express activation markers and adhesion molecules; the latter allow these cells to engage ligands on venules that facilitate their egress into the inflammatory site. The authors, in mentioning the scarcity of naive (CD45RA) cells, make a one-line reference to these as a suppressor–

inducer subset, the only reference to suppressor cells in the chapter: are these "on the way out"? We think not (see Chapter 1), and could note that all considerations of biotherapy for autoimmune disease direct attention to *T-cell vaccination* (see Chapter 16 of this volume) in which immunization with attenuated T cells is thought to be effective by raising a subset of suppressor cells with antiidiotypic responsiveness to pathogenic T cells.

REFERENCES

Alvaro-Gracia, J. M., Zvaifler, N. J., and Firestein, G. S. (1989). *J. Exp. Med.* **170,** 865–876.

Barnes, P. F., Fong, S. J., Brennan, P. J., Twomey, P. E., Mazumder, A., and Modlin, R. L. (1990). *J. Immunol.* **145,** 149–154.

Brennan, F. M., Allard, S., Londei, M., Savill, C., Boylston, A., Carrel, S., Maini, R. N., and Feldmann, M. (1988). *Clin. Exp. Immunol.* **73,** 417–423.

Bull, B. S., Westengard, J. C., Farr, M., Bacon, P. A., Meyer, P. J., and Stuart, J. (1989). *Lancet* **ii**(8669), 965–967.

Burmester, G. R., Jahn, B., Gramatzki, M., Zacher, J., and Kalden, J. R. (1984). *J. Immunol.* **133,** 1230–1234.

Carson, D. (1990). *In* "Internal Medicine" (J. Stein, ed.), pp. 1680–1684. Little, Brown, Boston, Massachusetts.

Cavender, D., Haskard, D., Yu, C.-L., Iguchi, T., Miossec, P., Oppenheimer-Marks, N., and Ziff, M. (1987). *Fed. Proc.* **46,** 113–117.

Cohen, I. R., Holoshitz, J., van Eden, W., and Frenkel, A. (1985). *Arthritis Rheum.* **28,** 841.

Courtenay, J. S., Dillman, M. J., Dayan, A. D., Martin, A., and Mosedale, B. (1980). *Nature* **283,** 666.

Cush, J. J., and Lipsky, P. E. (1987). *Clin. Aspects Autoimmunity* **1,** 2–13.

Cush, J. J., Lipsky, P. E., Postlethwaite, A. E., Schrohenloher, R. E., Saway, A., and Koopman, W. J. (1990). *Arthritis Rheum.* **33,** 19–28.

Dayer, J.-M., Beutler, B., and Cerami, A. (1985). *J. Exp. Med.* **162,** 2163–2168.

Dayer, J.-M., de Rochemonteix, B., Burrus, B., Demczuk, S., and Dinarello, C. A. (1986). *J. Clin. Invest.* **77,** 645–648.

Drug Evaluation Committee of the Japan Rheumatism Foundation. (1988). Long-term comparative studies on gold vs. D-penicillamine and NSAIDs for treatment of early rheumatoid arthritis. I. Evaluation of one year's treatment. *Ryumachi* **1,** 305–318.

Duby, A. D., Sinclair, A. K., Osborne-Lawrence, S. L., Zeldes, W., Kan, L., and Fox, D. A. (1989). *Proc. Natl. Acad. Sci. U.S.A.* **86,** 6206–6210.

Feigenbaum, S. L., Masi, A. T., and Kaplan, S. B. (1979). *Am. J. Med.* **66,** 377–384.

Feldmann, M. (1987). *In* "Autoimmunity and Autoimmune Disease." (Ciba Foundation Sym.) Vol. 129, pp. 88–108. Wiley, Chichester, New York.

Firestein, G. S., Tsai, V., and Zvaifler, N. J. (1987a). *Rheum. Dis. Clin. North Am.* **13,** 191–213.

Firestein, G. S., and Zvaifler, N. J. (1987b). *Arthritis Rheum.* **30,** 864–871.

Firestein, G. S., and Zvaifler, N. J. (1990a). *Arthritis Rheum.* **33,** 768–773.

Firestein, G. S., Alvaro-Garcia, J. M., and Maki, R. (1990b). *J. Immunol.* **144,** 3347–3353.

Firestein, G. S., Xu, W. D., Townsend, K., Broide, D., Alvaro-Gracia, J., Glasebrook, A., and Zvaifler, N. J. (1988). *J. Exp. Med.* **168,** 1573–1586.

Firestein, G. S., *et al., Arthritis Rheum.,* in press.

Fontana, A., Hengartner, H., Weber, E., Fehr, K., Grob, P. J., and Cohen, G. (1982). *Rheumatol. Int.* **2,** 49–53.

Forre, O., Thoen, J., Lea, T., Dobloug, J. H., Mellbye, O. J., Natvig, J. B., Pahle, J., and Solheim, B. G. (1982). *Scand. J. Immunol.* **16,** 315–319.

Franklin, E. C., Holman, H. R., Muller-Eberhardt, H. G., and Kunkel, H. G. (1957). *J. Exp. Med.* **105,** 425–438.
Furst, D. E., and Kremer, J. M. (1988). *Arthritis Rheum.* **31,** 305–314.
Garrod, A. D. (1892). *Lancet* **ii,** 1003–1037.
Gaston, J. S., Life, P. F., Bailey, L. C., and Bacon, P. A. (1989). *J. Immunol.* **143,** 2494.
Gay, S., O'Sullivan, F. X., Gay, R. E., and Koopman, W. J. (1987). *Clin. Immunol. Immunopathol.* **45,** 63–69.
Goto, M., and Zvaifler, N. J. (1983). *J. Exp. Med.* **157,** 1309–1323.
Goto, M., and Zvaifler, N. J. (1985). *J. Immunol.* **134,** 1483–1486.
Gregerson, P. K., Silver, J., and Winchester, R. J., (1989). *Arthritis Rheum.* **30,** 1205–1213.
Guerne, P.-A., Zuraw, B. L., Vaughan, J. H., Carson, D. A., and Lotz, M. (1989). *J. Clin. Invest.* **83,** 585–592.
Hale, L. P., Martin, M. E., McCollum, D. E., Nunley, J. A., Springer, T. A., Singer, K. H., and Haynes, B. F. (1989). *Arthritis Rheum.* **32,** 22–30.
Harrison, R. W., III, and Lippman, S. S. (1989). *Hosp. Pract.* **24,** 63–68, 70–71, 75–76.
Hasler, F., Bluestein, H. G., Zvaifler, N. J., and Epstein, L. B. (1983). *J. Exp. Med.* **157,** 173.
Helfgott, S. M., Dynesius-Trentham, R. E., Brahn, E., and Trentham, D. E. (1985). *J. Exp. Med.* **162,** 1531.
Hirano, T., Matsuda, T., Turner, M. Miyasaka, N., Buchan, G., Tang, B., Sato, K., Shimizu, M., Maini, R., Feldmann, M., and Kishimoto, T. (1988). *Eur. J. Immunol.* **18,** 1797–1801.
Hochberg, M. C. (1989). *Hosp. Pract.* **24,** 185–190.
Holmdahl, R., Klareskog, L., Andersson, M., and Hansen, C. (1986). *Immunogenetics* **24,** 84.
Holoshitz, J., Klajman, A., Druker, I., Lapidot, Z., Yaretzky, A., Frenkel, A., van Eden W., and Cohen, I. R. (1986). *Lancet* **2,** 305–309.
Holoshitz, J., Matitiau, A., and Cohen, I. R. (1984). *J. Clin. Invest.* **73,** 211.
Janossy, G., Duke, O., and Poulter, L. W. (1981). *Lancet* **2,** 839–842.
Kaplan, R. A., Curd, J. G., Deheer, D. H., Carson, D. A., Pangburn, M. K., Muller-Eberhard, H. J., and Vaughan, J. H. (1980). *Arthritis Rheum.* **23,** 911–920.
Kaushansky, K., Lin, N., and Adamson, J. W. (1988). *J. Clin. Invest.* **81,** 92–97.
Keystone, E. C., Minden, M., Klock, R., Poplonski, L., Zalcberg, J., Takadera, T., and Mak, T. W. (1988). *Arthritis Rheum.* **31,** 1555–1557.
Kidd, B. L., Moore, K., Walters, M. T., Smith, J. L., Cawley, M. I. (1989). *Ann. Rheum. Dis.* **48,** 92–98.
Klareskog, L., Forsum, U., Wigren, A., and Wigzell, H. (1982). *Scand. J. Immunol.* **15,** 501–507.
Klareskog, L., Forsum, U., Wigren, A., and Wigzell, H. (1982). *Scand. J. Immunol.* **15,** 501–507.
Konttinen, Y. T., Reitamo, S., Ranki, A., Hayry, P., Kankaanapaa, U., and Wegelius, O. (1981). *Arthritis Rheum.* **24,** 71–79.
Konttinen, Y. T., Nykanen, P., Nordstrom, D., Saari, H., Sandelin, J., Santavirta, S., and Kouri, T. (1989). *J. Rheumatol.* **16,** 339–345.
Krause, A., Protz, H., and Goebel, K. M. (1989). *Ann. Rheum. Dis.* **48,** 636–640.
Kunkel, H. G., Franklin, E. C., and Muller-Eberhard, H. G. (1959). *J. Clin. Invest.* **38,** 424–436.
Kunkel, H. G., Muller-Eberhardt, H. G., Fudenberg, H. H., and Tomasi, T. B. (1961). *J. Clin. Invest.* **40,** 117–129.
Laffon, A., Sanchez-Madrid, F., Ortiz de Landazuri, M., Jimenez Cuesta, A., Ariza, A., Ossorio, C., and Sabando, P. (1989). *Arthritis Rheum.* **32,** 386–392.
Lalor, P. A., Mapp, P. I., Hall, P. A., and Revell, P. A. (1987). *Rheumatol. Int.* **7,** 183–186.
Lindblad, S., Klareskog, L., Hedfors, E., Forsum, U., and Sundstrom, C. (1983). *Arthritis Rheum.* **26,** 1321–1332.
Lotz, M., Tsoukas, C. D., Robinson, C. A., Dinarello, C. A., Carson, D. A., and Vaughan, J. H. (1986). *J. Clin. Invest.* **78,** 713–721.

Malone, D. G., Wahl, S. M., Tsokos, M., Cattell, H., Decker, J. L., and Wilder, R. L. (1984). *J. Clin. Invest.* **74,** 1173–1185.

Miossec, P., Dinarello, C. A., and Ziff, M. (1986). *Arthritis Rheum.* **29,** 461–470.

Miossec, P., Naviliat, M., Dupuy d'Angeac, A., Sany, J., and Banchereau, J. (1990). *Arthritis Rheum.* **33,** 1180–1187.

Mitchell, D. M., Spitz, P. W., Young, D. Y., Bloch, D. A., McShane, D. J., and Fries, J. F. (1986). *Arthritis Rheum.* **29,** 706–714.

Morrissey, P. J., Bressler, L., Park, L. S., Alpert, A., and Gillis, S. (1987). *J. Immunol.* **139,** 1113–1119.

Munthe, E., and Natvig, J. B. (1972). *Clin. Exp. Immunol.* **12,** 55–62.

Nouri, A. M. E., Panayi, G. S., and Goodman, S. M. (1984). *Clin. Exp. Immunol.* **55,** 295–302.

Nykanen, P., Bergroth, V., Raunio, P., Nordstrom, D., and Konttinen, Y. T. (1986). *Rheumatol. Int.* **6,** 269–271.

Paulus, H. E. (1990a). *In* "Internal Medicine" 3rd Ed. (J. Stein, ed.), pp. 1789–1795. Little, Brown, Boston, Massachusetts.

Paulus, H. E. (1990b). *Arthritis Rheum.* **33,** 113–120.

Pearson, C. M. (1964). *Arthritis Rheum.* **7,** 80.

Pekin, T., and Zvaifler, N. J. (1964). *J. Clin. Invest.* **43,** 1372–1382.

Petersen, J., Heilmann, C., Bjerrum, O. J., Ingemann-Hansen, T., and Halkjaer-Kristensen, J. (1983). *Scand. J. Immunol.* **17,** 471–478.

Pike, M. C. (1989). *J. Rheumatol.* **16,** 718–720.

Pope, R. M., Teller, D. C., and Mannik, M. (1974). *Proc. Natl. Acad. Sci. U.S.A.* **71,** 517–521.

Preble, O. T., Black, R. J., and Friedman, R. M. (1982). *Science* **216,** 429–431.

Ranges, G. E., Sriram, S., and Cooper, S. M. (1985). *J. Exp. Med.* **162,** 1105.

Ratcliffe, A., Doherty, M., Maini, R. N., and Hardingham, T. E. (1988). *Ann. Rheum. Dis.* **47,** 826–832.

Rose, H. M., Ragan, C., Pearce, E., and Lipman, M. O. (1948). *Proc. Soc. Exp. Biol. Med.* **68,** 1–6.

Rothschild, B. M. (1989). *In* "Arthritis and Allied Conditions: A Textbook of Rheumatology" (D. J. McCarty, ed.), pp. 3–7. Saunders, Philadelphia, Pennsylvania.

Roudier, J., Rhodes, G., Petersen, J., Vaughan, J. H., and Carson, D. A. (1988). *Scand. J. Immunol.* **27,** 367–371.

Roudier, J., Petersen, J., Rhodes, G. H., Luka, J., and Carson, D. A. (1989). *Proc. Natl. Acad. Sci. U.S.A.* **86,** 5104–5108.

Sakkas, L. I., Demaine, A. G., Welsh, K. I., and Panayi, G. S. (1987). *Arthritis Rheum.* **30,** 231–232.

Sanders, M. E., Makgoba, M. W., and Shaw, S. (1988). *Immunol. Today* **9,** 195–199.

Sansom, D. M., Amin, S. N., Bidwell, J. L., Klouda, P. T., Bradley, B. A., Evison, G., Goudling, N. J., Hall, N. D., and Maddison, P. J. (1989). *Br. J. Rheumatol.* **28,** 374–378.

Sargent, C. A., Dunham, I., Trowsdale, J., and Campbell, R. D. (1989). *Proc. Natl. Acad. Sci. U.S.A.* **86,** 1968–1972.

Saxne, T., Palladino, M. A., Jr., Heinegard, D., Talal, N., and Wollheim, F. A. (1988). *Arthritis Rheum.* **31,** 1041–1045.

Saxne, T., Palladino, M. A., Jr., Heinegard, D., Talal, N., and Wollheim, F. A. (1988). *Arthritis Rheum.* **31,** 1041–1045.

Savill, C. M., Delves, P. J., Kioussis, D., Walker, P., Lydyard, P. M., Colaco, B., Shipley, M., and Roitt, I. M. (1987). *Scand. J. Immunol.* **25,** 629–635.

Scott, D. L., Spector, T. D., and Pawlotski, Y. (1989). *Lancet* **ii**(8678), 1531–1533.

Shand, N., and Richardson, B. (1988). *Scand. J. Rheumatol.* **76,** 265–278.

Sharp, J. T. (1989). *Arthritis Rheum.* **32,** 221–229.

Short, C. L. (1968). *Med. Clin. North Am.* **52,** 549–557.
Short, C. L. (1974). *Arthritis Rheum.* **17,** 193–205.
Slaughter, L., Carson, D. A., Jensen, F. C., Holbrook, T. L., and Vaughan, J. H. (1978). *J. Exp. Med.* **148,** 1429–1434.
Soden, M., Hassan, J., Scott, D. L., Hanly, J. G., Moriarty, M., Whelan, A., Feighery, C., and Bresnihan, B. (1989). *Arthritis Rheum.* **32,** 523–530.
Stamenkovic, I., Stegagno, M., Wright, K. A., Krane, S. M., Amento, E. P., Colvin, R. B., Duquesnoy, R. J., and Kurnick, J. T. (1988). *Proc. Natl. Acad. Sci. U.S.A.* **85,** 1179–1183.
Steere, A. C., Duray, P. H., and Butcher, E. C. (1988). *Arthritis Rheum.* **31,** 487–495.
Sternberg, E. M., Hill, J. M., Chrousos, G. P., Kamilaris, T., Listwak, S. J., Gold, P. W., and Wilder, R. L. (1989). *Proc. Natl. Acad. Sci. U.S.A.* **86,** 2374–2378.
Streeter, P. R., Berg, E. L., Rouse, B. T., Bargatze, R. F., and Butcher, E. C. (1988). *Nature* **331,** 41–46.
Stuart, J. M., and Dixon, F. J. (1983). *J. Exp. Med.* **158,** 378.
Suzuki, R., Suzuki, S., Takahashi, T., and Kumagai, K. (1986). *J. Exp. Med.* **164,** 1682–1699.
Tarkowski, A., Klareskog, L., Carlsten, H., Herberts, P., Koopman, W. J. (1989). *Arthritis Rheum.* **32,** 1087.
Tugwell, P., Bombardier, C., Buchanan, W. W., Goldsmith, C., Grace, E., Bennett, K. J., Williams, H. J., Egger, M., Alarcon, G. S., and Guttadauria, M. (1990). *Arch. Intern. Med.* **150,** 59–62.
van Eden, W., Holoshitz, J., Nevo, Z., Frenkel, A., Klajman, A., and Cohen, I. R. (1985). *Proc. Natl. Acad. Sci. U.S.A.* **82,** 5117–5120.
van Eden, W., Thole, J. E. R., van der Zee, R., Noordzij, A., van Embden, J. D. A., Hensen, E. J., and Cohen, I. R. (1988). *Nature* **331,** 171.
Waaler, E. (1940). *Acta Pathol. Microbiol. Immunol. Scand.* **17,** 172–188.
Ward, P. A., and Zvaifler, N. J. (1971). *J. Clin. Invest.* **50,** 606–616.
Weisman, M. H. (1990). *Curr. Opin. Rheumatol.* **2,** 458–462.
Weiss, M. M. (1989). *Arthritis Rheum.* **19,** 9–21.
Wood, D. D., Ihrie, J., Dinarello, C. A., and Cohen, P. L. (1983). *Arthritis Rheum.* **26,** 975–983.
Wood, N. C., Symons, J. A., and Duff, G. W. (1988). *J. Autoimmun.* **1,** 353–361.
Wooley, P. H., Luthra, H. S., Stuart, J. M., and David, C. S. (1981). *J. Exp. Med.* **154,** 688.
Woodsworth, P. (1990). *Cur. Opin. Rheumatol.* **2,** 423–429.
Xu, W. D., Firestein, G. S., Taetle, R., Kaushansky, K., and Zvaifler, N. J. (1989). *J. Clin. Invest.* **83,** 876–882.
Young, C. L., Adamson, T. C., Vaughan, J. H., and Fox, R. I. (1984). *Arthritis Rheum.* **27,** 32–39.
Young, D. B., Ivanyi, J., Cox, J. H., and Lamb, J. R. (1987). *Immunol. Today* **8,** 215–219.
Zvaifler, N. J., Steinman, J., Kaplan, G., Lau, L. L., and Rivelis, M. (1985). *J. Clin. Invest.* **76,** 789–800.
Zvaifler, N. J. (1990). *In* "Internal Medicine" 3rd Ed., (J. Stein, ed.), pp. 1724–1734. Little Brown, Boston, Massachusetts.

CHAPTER **16**

Principles of Therapeutic Approaches to Autoimmunity

HARTMUT WEKERLE
REINHARD HOHLFELD
Department of Neuroimmunology
Max-Planck-Institute for Psychiatry
Planegg-Martinsried
Germany

I. INTRODUCTION

Autoimmune diseases are caused by pathogenic reactions of immune cells against the body's own constituents. This may sound commonplace, but it is not. Among the many autoimmune phenomena demonstrable in clinical and experimental immunology, only a minority seem to actually lead to disturbance or destruction of tissues. Take as an example the formation of humoral autoantibodies. These immunoglobulins by definition have the capacity of binding to determinants of self-tissues. They include a large proportion of IgM antibodies produced by $CD5^+$ B lymphocytes, which possess a broad spectrum of binding specificity, reacting with determinants on foreign antigens, but also with autoantigens (Casali and Notkins, 1989). These antibodies are truly "natural," preformed antibodies, produced independent of help by T cells, without somatic mutation and class switch (Rajewsky *et al.*, 1987). However, only few of these IgM *autoantibodies,* if any, are indeed pathogenic, i.e., they may be closely associated with particular syndromes (Shoenfeld and Schwartz, 1984), but would not mediate disease even if transferred in large quantities to appropriate recipients. In fact, only very few human or experimental diseases are definitely and solely caused by humoral autoantibodies. One of these is myasthenia gravis, which is based on deficits of the neuromuscular transmission due to autoantibodies binding to the postsynaptic nicotinic acetylcholine receptor (AChR) (Lindstrom, 1985). But even in myasthenia gravis, only some among the anti-receptor autoantibodies seem to be actually pathogenic. There is a poor correlation between the total titer of anti-AChR autoantibodies and disease severity, and within experimentally induced/selected monoclonal anti-AChR hybridoma autoantibodies, only a minority are able to passively transfer experimental myasthenia gravis to naive recipients (Tzartos and Lindstrom, 1980). In other diseases, which have autoantibodies as essential features, the role of the autoreactive immunoglobulins in pathogenesis is even less certain. As mentioned before, in systemic lupus erythematosus, and in its animal models, autoantibodies against nuclear components are regularly produced. Yet, apart from potential roles in idiotypic networks and immunocomplex formation (Mendlovic *et al.*, 1988), no direct pathogenic effect has been documented (Tan, 1989).

Therapies of autoimmune disease have to focus on the elimination of *pathogenic* immune effector molecules or cells. Obviously, the therapeutic measures must be optimally efficient while keeping potential side effects at a minimum. In the first part of this chapter, novel, more or less specific therapeutic strategies will be discussed, as they emerge from our increasing insights into the cellular and molecular mechanisms of immunological autoaggression. Most of these therapies have been successful in special experimental model situations. As will be made clear, some may be applicable to treatment of human disease within a relatively short period, whereas others may still require a much more detailed elaboration and adaptation before clinical use. The second part of this text will be devoted to the therapeutical approaches commonly used in clinical immunology at present. Here, the narrow rim between beneficial immunosuppression and induction of deleterious immunodeficiency will be the focus of the discussion.

II. T CELLS AS TARGETS OF THERAPY

Since 1980, it has become apparent that T cells have an essential role in many, if not most autoimmune diseases. It has been known for a long time that autoimmune T lymphocytes are the effectors in most experimentally inducible, organ-specific diseases including experimental autoimmune encephalomyelitis (Ben-Nun *et al.*, 1981b), neuritis (Linington *et al.*, 1984), uveitis (Caspi *et al.*, 1986), orchitis (Wekerle and Begemann, 1976), thyroiditis (Maron *et al.*, 1983) and adjuvant arthritis (Holoshitz, 1984). In addition, T cells may act as helpers required for the production of high-affinity pathogenic IgG autoantibodies, as shown in (experimental) myasthenia gravis (Hohlfeld *et al.*, 1982; Hohlfeld *et al.*, 1988). T helper cells most probably have a similar role in other antibody-dependent diseases as well, like pemphigus vulgaris and bullous pemphigoid (Stanley, 1989). Furthermore, T lymphocytes have a (hitherto undefined) func-

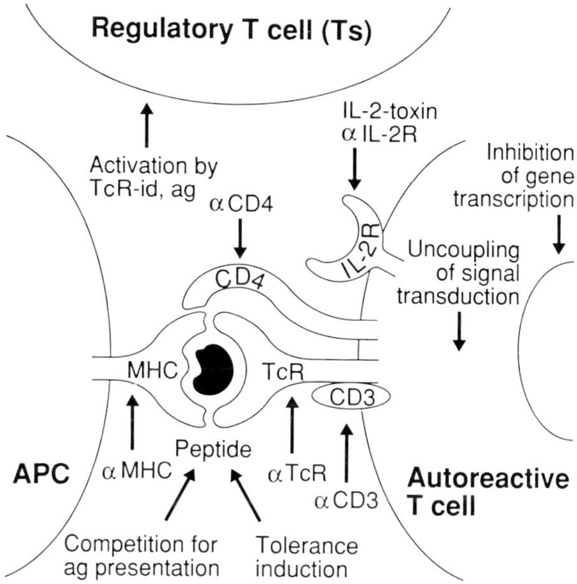

FIG. 1 Possible strategies and sites for (semi-) specific immunointervention. Effective treatment may be achieved by interfering with specific mechanisms as indicated by arrows, or by a synergistic combination of approaches. Ag, antigen; APC, antigen-presenting cell; CD3, complex of surface molecules coupled to the TcR and involved in signal transduction; CD4, surface molecule expressed mainly on helper cells and binding to a nonpolymorphic part of class II MHC molecules; IL-2, interleukin-2; IL-2R, interleukin-2 receptor; MHC, surface molecule encoded by the major histocompatibility complex (the figure refers to a class II MHC molecule, i.e., I-A and I-E in mice and HLA-DR, -DP, and -DQ in humans); TcR, T-cell receptor for antigen; Ts, suppressor T cell; TcR-id, idiotype of the TcR. From Adorini *et al.* (1990). *Immunol. Today* **11,** 384, by permission.

tion in the pathogenesis of lupuslike diseases, as in NZB mice. Their help may be required for isotype class switch and somatic mutation of some of the autoantibodies seen there (Shlomchik *et al.,* 1990).

Since in many human diseases autoimmune T lymphocytes can be expected to act as the key pathogenic agent, determining onset, course, and localization of the disease, these cells should be a most rewarding target for specific therapeutic strategies (Hohlfeld, 1989; Wraith *et al.,* 1989; Adorini *et al.,* 1990). In fact, extrapolating from the natural history of classic T cell-mediated autoimmune disorders, autoimmune T cells could be therapeutically affected by a number of different agents at different stages of their pathogenic careers (Fig. 1).

There is good evidence that, at least in the case of certain organ-specific autoantigens, potentially autoaggressive T cells are normal components of the healthy immune system (Burns *et al.,* 1983; Schluesener and Wekerle, 1985). Under normal circumstances, however, these clones will never be activated, and will never cause *spontaneous* tissue destruction. Hence, the potentially autoaggressive T-lymphocyte clones must be under reliable, safe control by counterregulatory mechanisms, presumably including networklike lymphocytic suppressor circuits (Lider *et al.*, 1988; Sun *et al.*, 1988b). It is conceivable that the potential autoimmune effector or helper T cells may escape their control only under special conditions. Such a situation might be created as a sequela of infectious diseases, as a result of several complementing factors. According to concepts of *molecular mimicry,* for example, an infectious agent may possess a structural protein component with a circumscript peptide sequence that is wrongly recognized by a potentially autoaggressive, organ-specific, self-reactive T-cell clone (Fujinami and Oldstone, 1985; Oldstone, 1987; Singh *et al.*, 1989). The prevalence of the particular self-reactive T-lymphocyte clone in the host immune repertoire is not only codetermined by genetic factors (HLA genes, and T cell-receptor variable-region genes), but also by epigenetic processes leading to the selection of immunocompetent mature T lymphocytes within the thymus (Marrack, 1987; Davis and Bjorkman, 1988; Strominger, 1989).

Cross-recognition of microbial protein epitopes and autoantigenic sequences of self-structures may, however, not suffice to launch the full program of cellular autoaggression. The particular microenvironment created by the infection (and its evoked immune response) may be an additional factor to help autoimmune T-cell clones to overcome their physiological suppression (Botazzo *et al.*, 1985; Kirchner *et al.*, 1988). In a second act of the autoimmune scenario, the activated autoimmune T cells are released into the blood circulation, which provides them with an opportunity to roam through all tissues after having passed through endothelial vessel walls. In their putative target organ, but not in other tissues, these T cells will find their specific *real* antigenic epitope, often after having induced local expression of the relevant major histocompatibility complex (MHC) product required for proper presentation of the processed autoantigen. The actual effector phase of the autoimmune attack may now follow, either as a direct cytotoxic attack against the local antigen-presenting tissue cells (Sun and Wekerle, 1986; Sarvetnick *et al.*, 1990), or indirectly, after recruitment of *unspecific* mononuclear cells for delayed hypersensitivity reactions, or B lymphocytes for antibody-mediated reactions.

The most specific way to neutralize the autoaggressive T lymphocytes would be the best therapy for autoimmune disease. Implicitly, the process of autoantigen recognition by the autoimmune T lymphocytes appears as the most promising target for specific immunotherapy. Any one of the three principal molecule classes involved in (auto-) antigen recognition would be a potential aim for treatment (Fig. 1): the autoantigen, and its critical peptide epitope, the MHC product binding and presenting the epitope, and the variable region of the complementary T cell-receptor α and β chains (not ignoring γ and δ chains as well), which mediate antigen recognition by the pathogenic T lymphocytes. Other molecules involved in T-mediated autoimmune responses, e.g., activation markers distinguishing activated pathogenic T lymphocytes from resting innocent lymphocytes, or adhesion molecules permitting entry of circulating T cells into the tissues, or effector molecules mediating the target-tissue lysis, should, however, by no means be disregarded as targets of therapy.

A. T-Cell Vaccination

The term T-cell vaccination was coined by I. R. Cohen in 1981 (Ben-Nun *et al.*, 1981a). The underlying concept considered cloned organ-specific, autoaggressive T lymphocytes as the pathogenic agents of autoimmune disease very much as pathogenic microbial agents have been shown to be the mediators of infectious diseases. In fact, the mere application of Koch's postulates to define autoimmune disease was not new; this was done before by Witebsky to define truly pathogenic autoantibodies (Milgrom and Witebsky, 1962). The novelty of Cohen's concept resides in the consideration that, as in microbiology, autoaggressive T cells can be attenuated to eliminate their pathogenic potential, while conserving their capacity to elicit counterregulatory control circuits. This concept rests, quite obviously, on two pillars. First, the immune repertoire must contain potentially self-reactive, autoaggressive (T)-lymphocyte clones in its healthy state, and these clones must be normally suppressed by counterregulatory mechanisms. Second, in autoimmune disease, the equilibrium between autoaggressive T cells and their suppressors is lost, but can be reestablished by appropriate stimulation of the suppressor cells. As pointed out, both predictions of the vaccination concept have been confirmed in a number of models of autoimmunity.

Vaccination against autoimmune disease has been carried out successfully in several variations. Originally, an encephalitogenic T-cell line was shown to lose its pathogenic potential on irradiation. Yet, transfer of these *attenuated* T cells rendered the recipients resistant to subsequent active autosensitization with myelin basic protein (MBP) in Freund's complete adjuvant (Ben-Nun *et al.*, 1981a; Ben-Nun and Cohen, 1981). Attenuation of pathogenic T cells can be reached by other procedures as well, including exposure to hyperbaric pressures and fixation by crosslinking agents such as glutaraldehyde (Lider *et al.*, 1987; Sun *et al.*, 1988a).

More recently, vaccination protocols have been developed to induce specific resistance against passively transferred T-line cells. Transfers of sublethal doses of untreated or attenuated activated T-line cells lead to the expansion of recipient T cells specifically reacting against the originally transferred T line, but fail to respond to the tissue-specific autoantigen. Most, but possibly not all, of the induced T cells express the CD8 membrane phenotype and recognize their target epitope in the context of MHC class I products (Sun *et al.*, 1988a,b; Lider *et al.*,

1987). Furthermore, the $CD8^+$ T cells are specifically cytotoxic against the relevant autoaggressive $CD4^+$ T line, ignoring, however, other syngeneic T lines with different or even similar specificities. Finally, in combined transfers, these $CD8^+$ T cells specifically suppress the encephalitogenic activity of their complementary $CD4^+$ target cell line (Sun *et al.*, 1988b).

A third, less specific variant of T-cell vaccination was described as *ergotypic network* interactions. Activated $CD4^+$ T-line cells are able to recruit certain lymphocytes from unselected populations and to push them into proliferation. This recruitment process critically depends on the state of activation of the T-line cells (hence the term *ergo*typic). Although not T-line specific, these cells are able to decrease the pathogenic potential of encephalitogenic or arthritogenic $CD4^+$ T-line cells in transfer assays (Lohse *et al.*, 1989).

B. Immunization Against T-Cell Receptor V Region Determinants

The most specific treatment of T cell-dependent autoimmune diseases would aim at the specific elimination of the pathogenic lymphocyte clones from the affected organism. Clonal identity of (autoimmune) T-cell clones is determined by the T cell-receptor (TcR) variable (V) regions, which thus, at least theoretically, would qualify as ideal targets of specific treatments. Considering the millions of diverse TcR V regions, is receptor-directed therapy realistic? Two recent observations have been encouraging. First, as described, in rodent experimental autoimmune encephalomyelitis (EAE) it became clear that transferred encephalitogenic T-cell lines are able to activate and expand clonotypically specific counterregulatory, cytotoxic $CD8^+$ T clones within the recipient's immune system (Sun *et al.*, 1988b). Although the target antigen involved in this T–T interaction remains to be formally identified, there is evidence in favor of an idiotypic interaction (Lider *et al.*, 1987). Second, quite surprisingly, in several rodent models of autoimmunity, the pathogenic T lymphocytes use a greatly reduced number of available variable-region elements for their antigen receptor. In the PL/J mouse (Acha-Orbea *et al.*, 1988; Urban *et al.*, 1988), for instance, as well as in the Lewis rat (Chluba et al., 1989; Burns *et al.*, 1989), almost all *encephalitogenic* T clones use the Vβ8.2 element. This is especially stunning, since the mouse and rat clones recognize completely distinct peptide epitopes on the MBP molecule: PL/J T cells are specific for sequence Ac-1-9 (Acha-Orbea *et al.*, 1989; Kumar *et al.*, 1989), whereas their Lewis correlates recognize peptide 68–88 (Kibler *et al.*, 1977).

These observations led to two partly interdependent therapeutic strategies. First, it was shown that monoclonal antibodies (MAb) against V-region determinants involved in the autoimmune response can profoundly interfere with inducibility and even progress of organ-specific autoimmune disease (Zamvil *et al.*,

1988). This strategy is not ultimately specific, as it presumably affects any T-cellular response using the V element recognized by the MAb, and, dependent on the individual's genotype, the isotype may be used by a considerable proportion of all clones in the repertoire (Barth *et al.*, 1985; Pullen *et al.*, 1990).

The second, related anti-TcR strategy relies on active immunization of the recipient against critical peptide sequences peculiar to the pathogenic TcR. Immunization of rats against a synthetic peptide representing either the VDJ region (Howell *et al.*, 1989) or a Vβ epitope (Vandenbark *et al.*, 1989) of encephalitogenic T cells was reported to successfully prevent active inducibility of EAE in the recipients, and even to shorten ongoing disease. At present the mechanism of EAE resistance induced by TcR V-peptide immunization remains to be elucidated. Humoral antibodies as well as receptor-specific T lymphocytes may be involved in the process.

C. Blocking the MHC Product/Peptide Epitope Formation

Since T lymphocytes do not recognize protein (auto) antigens in their soluble or native state, but require the presentation of critical peptide epitopes in the molecular context of a suitable MHC product, interference with formation or persistence of the MHC–peptide complex lends itself as a promising target of specific immunotherapy (see Fig. 1; Todd *et al.*, 1988; Adorini *et al.*, 1990).

First attempts to block autoantigen presentation on the presentation side relied on MAbs binding to the MHC products involved in the presentation of autoantigens. That MHC-specific antibodies are most efficient in blocking presentation/recognition of protein antigens has been known for a decade. In treatment of T cell-mediated autoimmune diseases, this approach was further favored by the very unequal autoimmune reactivity of T cells from different MHC haplotypes. Since the proportion of T-lymphocyte clones responding to an (auto)immune epitope is strictly dictated by the individual MHC [in most models by MHC class II products (Kimoto *et al.*, 1981)], blocking of the relevant MHC product of *one* haplotype in heterozygote recipients (Shevach *et al.*, 1972; Schwartz *et al.*, 1976) would confer full resistance to disease induction. This therapeutic strategy was borne out in rodent models of EAE (Steinman *et al.*, 1981; Sriram *et al.*, 1987). Since the rest of the nonbound products of this haplotype, along with *all* products of the *second* haplotype remain undisturbed in binding and presenting antigenic epitopes, a severe suppression of general immune reactivity is not expected, and indeed was not noted in experimental investigations. Unfortunately, antibody blocking of MHC determinants was less successful in primates than in rodents. In particular, in subhuman primates, expression of MHC class II determinants on vascular surfaces led to coagulation incidents that may prevent direct application of these therapies to human disease.

MHC–epitope complex-directed treatment strategies gained new attraction, however, following reports on the relatively strict epitope dominance in T-cell recognition of MBP. It has been known for years that in the Lewis rat, the encephalitogenic T-cell response is almost exclusively focused on epitope(s) located within peptide sequence 68–88 (Kibler *et al.*, 1977). Additional MBP epitopes may be recognized by some Lewis T-cell clones, but it appears that the majority of these are not encephalitogenic (Vandenbark *et al.*, 1985). A similar situation was described for encephalitogenic T-cell clones of mice. In PL/J and B10.PL mice (both with H-2^u) amino acid sequence Ac1-11 (acetylation of the N-terminal Ala is essential for recognition) harbors at least two distinguishable encephalitogenic T-cell epitopes, and incidentally, both epitopes are almost exclusively recognized by T cells using the preponderant Vβ8.2 element (Acha-Orbea *et al.*, 1989; Kumar *et al.*, 1989). Another, minor encephalitogenic epitope for H-2^u-restricted T cells is located between amino acid positions 35 and 47 (Sakai *et al.*, 1988). In the SJL/J mouse (H-s^s), an accumulation of encephalitogenic epitopes was located between amino acid positions 89 and 101 (Acha-Orbea *et al.*, 1989).

Considering the striking epitope dominance in the encephalitogenic T-cell response in three different animal strains, what would be a more straightforward strategy than trying to design a peptide variant that (1) prevents or reverses binding of the encephalitogenic peptide to the salient MHC product, but (2) is not immunogenic by itself? It may not be surprising that indeed several groups reported successful application of this strategy to murine EAE. Variation of the sequence motif of the PL/J-specific encephalitogenic epitope resulted in a peptide that indeed had beneficial effects on EAE when transferred to recipient mice (Wraith *et al.*, 1989; Urban *et al.*, 1989; Kumar *et al.*, 1990). Similar strategies were recently reported using myelin proteolipid protein (PLP) as encephalitogen for SJL/J mice (Lamont *et al.*, 1990). Unwanted, *allergic* T-cell responses against these blocking peptides were apparently not recorded, but further studies will have to establish how reliable this non-immunogenicity remains, longitudinally within one individual, and within a collective.

D. Oral Tolerization

Very recently, a seemingly traditional approach of tolerance induction has gained broad attention: induction of oral (self) tolerance to autoantigens. Following the finding that intragastric instillation of collagen type II into the stomach of rodent recipients could reduce development of autoimmune arthritis following appropriate immunization (Nagler-Anderson *et al.*, 1986), two groups reported that oral administration of MBP (Bitar and Whitacre, 1988; Higgins and Weiner, 1988) could prevent induction of EAE in rats. The mechanism of this oral tolerization is unclear. The sequence of the peptide does not appear to be critical: encephalitogenic and nonencephalitogenic peptides protect equally well (Higgins and Weiner, 1988). As a mechanism of protection, induction of specific $CD8^+$ suppressor T cells and production of antibodies (Fuller *et al.*, 1990) have been proposed (Lider *et al.*, 1989).

III. CONVENTIONAL THERAPIES

A. Corticosteroids

The corticosteroid hormones react with receptor proteins in the cytoplasm of steroid-sensitive cells to form a steroid–receptor complex. This complex moves into the cell nucleus, binds to chromatin, and activates transcription of specific mRNAs. Because different proteins are ultimately synthesized under the influence of steroids in various target cells, the overall effects of steroids in physiologic systems are highly complex and extremely diverse. This holds true, in particular, for the effects of steroids on the immune system (reviewed by Fauci *et al.*, 1976; Cupps and Fauci, 1982).

The antiinflammatory and immunosuppressive properties of corticosteroids are related to at least four major effects. First, steroids have a profound influence on the distribution (*compartmentalization*) and trafficking of leukocytes. This differs among the various white cell populations. A few hours after administration of steroids, there is a significant peripheral blood neutrophilia. This results from an increased release from the bone marrow and an increase in circulatory half-life of neutrophils incapable of normally exiting to inflammatory sites. By contrast, other peripheral blood cells (in particular T cells, monocytes, and eosinophils) are depleted under the influence of steroids. In humans, this effect derives from the temporary redistribution of these cells to extravascular sites. B cells and natural killer (NK) cells are relatively resistant to the lymphodepletive effect of corticosteroids.

Second, steroids alter the functional properties of individual cells of the immune system. Even physiologic concentrations of corticosteroids inhibit T-cell proliferation *in vitro*. *In vivo,* delayed-type hypersensitivity skin reactions are suppressed after a few weeks of steroid therapy. Likewise, the bactericidal activity and chemotaxis of monocytes is extremely sensitive to corticosteroids. By contrast, neutrophils, B cells, and NK cells are relatively resistant.

Third, steroids affect the synthesis and secretion of soluble mediators that serve as signals between immune cells. For example, the production of interleukin-1, interleukin-2, and prostaglandins is inhibited by corticosteroids.

Fourth, steroids have an effect on microvascular permeability and may thus reduce formation of vasogenic edema. The effect on vascular permeability may contribute to the effects on leukocyte migration.

In most (but not all) autoimmune diseases, corticosteroids have remained an important therapeutic principle, although the precise indications and doses vary. For example, corticosteroids are the drug of first choice for the treatment of inflammatory muscle disorders such as *idiopathic* polymyositis and dermatomyositis (Engel and Emslie-Smith, 1989). Treatment may have to be continued for several years in some patients, but eventually the majority of patients can discontinue therapy. By contrast, multiple sclerosis (MS) provides an example that long-term therapy with steroids may not be beneficial. In MS, steroid use is limited to the treatment of acute exacerbations (Weiner and Hafler, 1988).

The continued administration of steroids carries the risk of side effects for which patients must be closely monitored. These include weight gain, exacerbation or precipitation of a diabetic state or hypertension, upper gastrointestinal distress or bleeding from a peptic ulcer, hypokalemia, aseptic necrosis of the femoral head, atrophy of the skin, increased susceptibility to infection, and cataract formation. Therefore the patient's blood pressure, weight, serum electrolytes, and glucose level should be closely followed during treatment. Regular slit-lamp examinations (every 6 months) help to prevent cataracts. Use of regular antacids with meals or histamine-receptor antagonists (cimetidine or ranitidine) protect the upper gastrointestinal mucosa from ulceration and bleeding. Supplementation with calcium and vitamin D minimizes osteoporosis. Potassium replacement may be necessary in patients taking high-dose steroids. The use of antihypertensive therapy is required in some patients.

B. Cyclophosphamide

Cyclophosphamide is the most widely used alkylating agent (reviewed by Calabresi and Parks, 1985). The drug has to be activated by the hepatic cytochrome P-450 system to generate metabolically active metabolites. Hepatic damage is apparently minimized by intrahepatic secondary oxidation reactions, whereas significant amounts of the active metabolites reach the target sites by the circulation. It is not known which of the active metabolites (e.g., phosphoramide mustard, 4-hydroxycyclophosphamide, or nor-nitrogen mustard) plays the key role in the therapeutic and toxic actions of cyclophosphamide. The primary target of the activated metabolites is the DNA molecule. Alkylation of DNA may result in false base pairing, excision of purine residues, and crosslinking of DNA strands. The actions of cyclophosphamide are not strictly cell-cycle specific, but the toxicity is usually expressed in the premitotic phase, and the cycle is blocked at the G_2 phase.

The immunosuppressive actions of the alkylating reagents are secondary to their cytotoxic effects on the various cells of the hematopoietic system, particularly lymphocytes. Early in the course of therapy, the effect of cyclophosphamide is greater on B cells than on T cells (Turk and Parker, 1982). Cyclophosphamide inhibits many of the inflammatory and immune activities of monocytes and macrophages. In experimental models the overall effect of cyclophosphamide on a given immune reaction depends critically on the time point at which cyclophosphamide is administered. The explanation for this is that cyclophosphamide has its greatest effect on rapidly dividing cells. If these happen to be the precursors of immunoregulatory cells, cyclophosphamide may show a paradoxical, partially enhancing effect (Turk and Parker, 1982).

Because of its potentially serious side effects, cyclophosphamide is considered an immunosuppressant of second choice for the treatment of those autoimmune diseases that can be effectively treated with other, less-toxic drugs (e.g., treatment of myasthenia gravis with azathioprine). The main indications for cyclophosphamide in such cases is treatment failure of other drugs or the need to achieve maximal immunosuppression rapidly when the action of other agents would be too slow. In other autoimmune diseases, cyclophosphamide is widely used as a first-line immunosuppressive agent (e.g., Wegener's granulomatosis, systemic necrotizing vasculitis; Haynes *et al.*, 1986).

Cyclophosphamide has serious side effects (reviewed by Calabresi and Parks, 1985). The major and often limiting side effect is bone marrow suppression, which affects leukocytes more than erythrocytes and platelets. The active metabolites are concentrated in the urine, resulting in damage to the epithelium of the bladder (hemorrhagic cystitis, malignant transformation). This toxicity can be reduced by appropriate fluid supply and by the simultaneous application of an uroprotective agent. During prolonged therapy, permanent infertility may develop both in male and in female patients. Of particular concern is the potential for the development of leukemia or lymphoma. Like other cytotoxic agents, cyclophosphamide is potentially teratogenic. Alopecia may develop with chronic therapy but is mild and reversible after treatment is stopped. Additional rarer side effects include myocardial damage and pulmonary fibrosis.

C. Methotrexate

Methotrexate is the prototype of the folic acid antagonists (reviewed by Calabresi and Parks, 1985). Members of this class of cytotoxic drugs are strictly cell-cycle specific. They act by competitively binding dihydrofolate reductase, resulting in decreased thymidine and purine nucleotide synthesis during the S phase of DNA synthesis. Part of the systemic toxicity can be circumvented by folinic acid (leucovorin), which acts as methyl donor and can bypass the need for dihydrofolate reductase.

The immunosuppressive effects of methotrexate are part of the general cytotoxic action on proliferating cells. There is no evidence of a selective action on particular elements of the immune system.

Because of its toxicity, methotrexate has only a limited place in the treatment of autoimmune diseases. For example, methotrexate has been found effective in the treatment of certain collagen–vascular diseases including dermatomyositis, when other forms of immunosuppressive therapy have failed (Engel and Emslie-Smith, 1989). The utility of methotrexate in rheumatoid arthritis is described in Chapter 15. The major toxicities of methotrexate include bone marrow suppression (especially leukopenia and thrombocytopenia), gastrointestinal complications (ulcerative stomatitis, diarrhea, hemorrhagic enteritis), alopecia, dermatitis, interstitial pneumonitis, neurotoxicity, nephrotoxicity, teratogenesis, and severe hepatotoxicity with fibrosis and cirrhosis (Schein and Winokur, 1975).

D. Azathioprine

Azathioprine acts as a purine analog (reviewed by Elion and Hitchings, 1975; McCormack and Johns, 1982). Its active metabolite is 6-mercaptopurine, which is phosphorylated intracellularly to thioinosine monophosphate (T-IMP) by hypoxanthine-guanine phosphoribosyltransferase (HGPRT). T-IMP inhibits several crucial steps in the conversion of inosine monophosphate to adenine and guanine nucleotides. Furthermore, accumulating T-IMP can cause feedback inhibition of the first step in purine biosynthesis. Additional complex biochemical actions may contribute to the cytoxic effects of the antipurine agents.

Azathioprine acts primarily on proliferating lymphocytes. The drug induces B- and T-cell lymphocytopenia of comparable degree. Antigen- and mitogen-induced *in vitro* proliferation of T cells is less inhibited in azathioprine-treated patients than in cyclophosphamide-treated patients. Azathioprine has antiinflammatory properties that are probably associated with the inhibition of promonocyte cell division.

Azathioprine has been used increasingly for the long-term immunosuppressive treatment of autoimmune diseases, particularly in combination with prednisolone. The overall experience has been favorable. Azathioprine has proven effective in a number of autoimmune disorders with an acceptably low incidence of serious side effects. A good example is myasthenia gravis. The prognosis of myasthenia has drastically improved since azathioprine has been used for the management of severe forms of the disease. The most frequent side effects encountered during long-term treatment in 104 patients with severe generalized myasthenia gravis were, in decreasing order of frequency, reversible marrow depression with leukopenia, gastrointestinal complications, infections, and transient elevation of liver enzymes (Hohlfeld *et al.*, 1988). The most serious possible complication was a renal lymphoma after 6 years of treatment with azathioprine.

E. Cyclosporine

Cyclosporine is a lipophilic undecapeptide (molecular weight, approximately 1200; reviewed by Kahan, 1989). The main action of cyclosporine is inhibition of lymphokine production by T cells, particularly synthesis of interleukin-2 (IL-2) and interferon-gamma. The precise mechanism of the inhibition is presently unknown, but there are three major possibilities. First, cyclosporine, which has structural features allowing its binding to calmodulin, could act on calcium-related cytoplasmic processes. However, this does not explain the T-cell selectivity of cyclosporine. Second, cyclosporine could inhibit the generation of cytoplasmic activation proteins that mediate signal transduction from the cytoplasm to the nucleus. The cyclosporine-binding protein called cyclophilin seems to represent one possible target of the cyclosporine effect. Cyclophilin has prolyl-peptidyl *cis-trans* isomerase (PPIase) activity (Fischer *et al.*, 1989; Takahasi *et al.*, 1989). The role of PPIases in T-cell activation is still unknown. The differences among the numerous cyclophilin-containing target tissues in their susceptibility to cyclosporine might be related to the presence of different isoforms of cyclophilin.

Third, cyclosporine could have a direct intranuclear effect. There is evidence indicating that cyclosporine can bind to nuclear transcriptional enhancers that normally regulate the production of lymphokines and cytotoxic enzymes. Specifically, cyclosporine A was found to inhibit the DNA binding of NF-AT (nuclear factor of activated T cells), which binds to the IL-2 enhancer, and AP-3 (activator protein-3), which binds to the IL-2 or IL-2 receptor promoter (Emmel *et al.*, 1989).

Cyclosporine has no effect on events that occur after gene activation. It does not inhibit the constitutive production of lymphokines by T cells, the stability or translation of lymphokine mRNA in the cytoplasm, or the export of protein products.

The effects of cyclosporine apparently spare B cells and macrophages; the only appreciable effect of cyclosporine on accessory cells seems to be disruption of lymphokine-dependent T-lymphocyte–macrophage interactions. The induction of T-suppressor circuits may even be promoted under the influence of cyclosporine.

Cyclosporine has revolutionized the field of organ transplantation and is increasingly being used for the treatment of autoimmune diseases. Cyclosporine has been shown to be effective under appropriate conditions in various autoimmune diseases including uveitis, psoriasis, type I diabetes mellitus, rheumatoid arthritis, myasthenia gravis, and multiple sclerosis. Further indications are currently being investigated in ongoing clinical trials.

Cyclosporine has a number of well-established toxic side effects that may be severe enough to prevent its use or to necessitate discontinuation. Nephrotoxicity is perhaps the most important side effect. Its pathogenesis is not exactly understood. One possibility is that cyclosporine alters the balance of the vasodilator prostacyclin and its vasoconstrictor antagonist thromboxane A_2, leading to renal vasoconstriction.

F. FK 506

FK 506 is a potentially promising new immunosuppressive agent. The mode of action of FK 506 is very similar to that of cyclosporine (Freedman, 1989), although FK 506 has the structure of a macrolide antibiotic, whereas cyclosporine is a polypeptide. Like cyclosporine, FK 506 prevents the synthesis of IL-2 and other lymphokines important in lymphocyte growth and function. Like cyclosporine, FK 506 binds to a cytosolic PPIase (although the FK 506-binding protein is different from the cyclosporine-binding cyclophilin; Freedman, 1989). The sequence of the cDNA of the human FK 506-binding protein is known (Standaert *et al.*, 1990). FK 506 is being evaluated in clinical trials (Thomson, 1990).

G. Apheresis

Plasmapheresis is a procedure in which plasma is removed from the circulation and replaced with colloidal substances such as albumin solution. Leukapheresis is a technique whereby leukocytes or lymphocytes are removed from the circulation without replacement. With both techniques, access is only to the peripheral blood compartment. For the effective removal of circulating factors by plasmapheresis, it is necessary to allow reequilibration between the extra- and intravascular compartments after each plasma exchange. For the removal of relevant cells by leukapheresis, similar *equilibration* between the intravascular compartment and the sites of inflammation would be desirable, but this is limited by the migratory and homing patterns of immune cells.

Of the two apheresis procedures, only plasmapheresis is being used widely in clinical practice. There are two major techniques of plasmapheresis, centrifugal plasma separation and membrane plasma separation (Rock, 1983; Malchesky *et al.*, 1983). In the therapy of autoimmune diseases, the goal of plasmapheresis is to remove circulating autoantibodies and/or inflammatory mediators. The basis for plasmapheresis is most solid in those autoimmune diseases in which autoantibodies have proven pathogenetic significance. The prototypic example of such a disease, myasthenia gravis, may serve to illustrate a number of principles that also pertain to other autoimmune diseases (Toyka, 1990). In myasthenia gravis, the removal of circulating antiacetylcholine receptor (anti-AChR) antibodies results in temporary improvement of neuromuscular transmission. Early clinical effects of plasmapheresis are sometimes observed within hours. Such immediate improvement is probably owing to the removal of autoantibodies that have a direct functional effect on the target antigen (i.e., anti-AChR antibodies that block AChR function, like curare). More delayed effects of plasmapheresis may become obvious only after one or more days. Such delayed improvement is usually attributable to the removal of antibodies that act indirectly, for example, by down-regulating the expression of the autoantigen target. Additional examples of antibody-mediated autoimmune diseases in which plasmapheresis may be clinically useful include the Lambert–Eaton myasthenic syndrome, pemphigus vulgaris, Goodpasture's syndrome, and autoimmune thrombocytopenic purpura.

In diseases in which no pathogenic autoantibodies can be demonstrated, the basis of plasmapheresis is purely empirical. Examples of suspected autoimmune diseases in which plasmapheresis was shown to be useful include the acute and chronic inflammatory polyradiculopathies (Dyck *et al.*, 1986; McKhann *et al.*, 1988). In these disorders the beneficial effect of plasma exchange may be related to the removal of polypeptide cytokines or other inflammatory mediators.

Plasmapheresis protocols usually employ plasma exchanges two to three times weekly for 2 to 6 weeks. At the time of each procedure, approximately 40 ml plasma per kg body weight is removed. In the absence of adjunct immunosuppressive therapy, there is often a *rebound* of autoantibody production after cessation of plasmatherapy. In experienced hands, plasmapheresis is a reasonably safe procedure, but serious complications such as allergic and cardiovascular systemic reactions and electrolyte disturbances can occur.

H. Symptomatic Treatment of Autoimmune Diseases (Target Therapies)

In some autoimmune diseases, functional impairment of the autoimmune target can be partially reversed by agents that specifically act on the target. Two examples may serve to illustrate this therapeutic approach. Anticholinesterase agents represent an extremely effective symptomatic treatment for myasthenia gravis. These drugs, which have few side effects, act by increasing the concentration of acetylcholine in the synaptic cleft of the neuromuscular junction (Hobbiger, 1976). This helps to compensate the loss of AChRs induced by anti-AChR antibodies. The second example of a *target therapy* is 3,4 diaminopyridine. This agent enhances the release of acetylcholine by blocking presynaptic potassium channels, thereby depolarizing the nerve terminal and prolonging the activation of voltage-gated calcium channels. 3,4-Diaminopyridine serves as an effective symptomatic therapy for the Lambert–Eaton myasthenic syndrome (LEMS; McEvoy *et al.*, 1989), the symptoms of which are caused by autoantibodies to presynaptic voltage-gated calcium channels (Vincent *et al.*, 1989). 3,4-Diaminopyridine has also been used to improve impulse conduction across demyelinated nerve segments in multiple sclerosis (Bever *et al.*, 1990).

IV. SEMISPECIFIC IMMUNOTHERAPIES

A. MONOCLONAL ANTIBODIES AGAINST LYMPHOCYTE DIFFERENTIATION ANTIGENS

Monoclonal antibodies (MAbs) against surface antigens expressed on subsets of lymphocytes can be used to deplete or modulate lymphocytes in a semispecific way (Fig. 1). This treatment has been used successfully in one of the best-understood experimental autoimmune diseases, experimental autoimmune encephalomyelitis (EAE), as well as in other experimental autoimmune diseases (reviewed by Hohlfeld and Toyka, 1985; Wraith *et al.*, 1989). The first MAb to be used for the treatment of patients, anti-CD3 (licensed as OKT3), has been very effective in the reversal of transplant rejections (Cosimi *et al.*, 1981). On an experimental basis, the antibody has also been used in autoimmune diseases. Although OKT3 acts only on T cells, it must be considered as a general immunosuppressant. One further disadvantage is that OKT3 has the capacity to activate T cells. This effect contributes to the sometimes severe febrile and circulatory reactions that are often observed during the first days of treatment.

For more selective targeting, MAbs that recognize subsets of T cells have been under investigation (Fig. 1). For example, MAb to the IL-2 receptor bind only to T lymphocytes activated recently, sparing the cells not involved in an immune reaction during the time of MAb treatment. Again, this approach has already been used successfully for the prevention of transplant rejection (Soulillou *et al.*, 1990). Anti-IL-2 MAb may also be useful for the treatment of (early?) stages of some autoimmune diseases. The combined and appropriately timed application of combinations of different MAbs against lymphocyte surface antigens may induce long-lasting tolerance (Mathieson *et al.*, 1990).

The therapeutic use of MAbs has so far been hampered by the fact that only murine MAbs are available. Not surprisingly, such antibodies induce vigorous human immune responses that severely limit the time during which the MAbs can be administered. The problem can be partially overcome by using *humanized* MAbs in which much of the murine sequence has been replaced by human sequence. The most recent of these genetically engineered chimeric antibodies contains only the antigen-binding site of the mouse antibody, rather than the entire variable domain (Riechmann *et al.*, 1988). The remainder of the chimeric protein is a human antibody, which can be selected for its intended function (e.g., complement fixation, activation of human effector cells, or facilitation of attachment of toxic compounds).

Another type of antibody construct has been used to direct human cytotoxic T lymphocytes against a variety of target cells including other lymphocytes. Lanzavecchia and Scheidegger (1987) designed hybrid MAbs with dual specificity against CD3 and either HLA antigens, human Ig, or other antigens. These bifunctional antibodies were able to bridge human cytotoxic T cells to target cells and trigger cytotoxic function via binding to CD3 on the effector cell. It may be possible to develop such hybrid antibodies into useful therapeutic tools. The generation of genetically engineered designer antibodies has been reviewed by Mayforth and Quintans (1990).

B. Monoclonal Antibodies against Adhesion Molecules and Immunomediators

A thus far largely theoretical possibility is to manipulate the immune response with MAbs against accessory (adhesion) molecules such as ICAM-1 and LFA-3. MAbs against cytokines and cytokine receptors may also be candidates for therapeutic use (Ruddle *et al.*, 1990). However, recent progress in the field of cytokine biology indicates that there exist endogenous cytokine receptor antagonists that might serve as more convenient therapeutic agents than antibodies. For example, the primary structure of a human IL-1 receptor antagonist secreted by monocytes has recently been established (Eisenberg *et al.*, 1990). Examples of other down-regulatory mediators include products of the cyclooxygenase or lipooxygenase pathways such as prostaglandin E_2.

C. Immunotoxins

Immunotoxins are conjugates of enzymatically active toxins with antibodies against surface antigens (reviewed by Pastan *et al.*, 1986; Vitetta *et al.*, 1987; Olsnes *et al.*, 1989). The directed toxin (e.g., ricin toxin, diptheria toxin) enters the cytosol of the target cells and inactivates components of the protein-synthesis machinery. Because of the high enzymatic activity of the toxins, the entry of a single molecule into the cytosol may be sufficient to kill a cell. Immunotoxins have been used clinically for the depletion of T cells *in vitro* before transplantation of human bone marrow. However, in spite of a few possible exceptions, systemic treatment with immunotoxins has been disappointing thus far (Olsnes *et al.*, 1989). Full assessment of the role of immunotoxins in immunotherapy will have to await future developments, such as genetically engineered immunotoxins (Vitetta *et al.*, 1987).

EDITORS' NOTE

Wekerle and Hohlfeld expertly scan therapies for autoimmune disease, from futuristic "Star Wars" approaches to the conventional treatments that are used today. They capture the "wave of hope" for interventional biotherapies based on encouraging findings in experimental models and reviewed recently in the context of rheumatoid arthritis.[1]

One might take slight issue with the authors' remark that "only very few human or experimental diseases are definitely and solely caused by humoral autoantibodies." We can cite myasthenia gravis, Lambert–Eaton syndrome, thyrotoxicosis, hemolytic anemia, thrombocytopenic purpura, congenital heart block, (anti-Ro), and the pemphigus diseases. Be this as it may, we agree that the logical targets for biotherapy are the molecular structures associated with the CD4 T cell, as discussed and illustrated in this chapter.

The authors refer to *vaccination* against autoimmune disease. In the autoimmune setting, the term has two connotations. One is the *negative vaccine* idea, in which an autoantigenic molecule is so injected to evoke suppression or *protection,* e.g., as in various of the experimentally induced autoimmune diseases (see Chapter 3); it is presumed that the injected autoantigen will, under particular conditions, elicit tolerance rather than immunity, either by inducing T-cell anergy, or raising a suppressor-cell response. The other sense in which vaccination against autoimmunity is used is by injection of cloned antigen-specific T lymphocytes, which the authors liken to "pathogenic microbial agents"; the obvious explanation is that the vaccination raises an antiidiotypic response, which counteracts the effect of pathogenic T cells. This concept has been further developed by immunizing with peptides derived from the T-cell receptor. However, the actual immunology of T-cell vaccination is far from clear. Presumably the counteracting CD4 helper T cell must recognize the T cell (or receptor peptide) in the context of MHC, and the antiidiotypic (?CD8) effector T cell should attack (in MHC-restricted manner?) the pathogenic receptor-bearing T cell.

Current therapy for autoimmune disease is well covered. We note the increasing use of cyclophosphamide in SLE and vasculitic diseases; the authors do not refer to *pulse* therapy, which has supporters. Methotrexate is used in poly- and dermatomyositis (Chapter 13) and in rheumatoid arthritis (Chapter 15). There are many trials of cyclosporine in autoimmune disease in progress, including those noted by the authors, and in other diseases including primary biliary cirrhosis; at present, the benefits: side-effects ratio seems finely balanced. Plasmapheresis is discussed, but not the related modality of intravenous immunoglobulin that may act by providing a donor source of anti-idiotypic antibody. (Mackay, I. R., Rowley, M. J. and Bernard, C. C. A. (1991). Biological therapies in rheumatoid arthritis: Concepts from considerations on pathogeneis. *In* "Monoclonal Antibodies and Immunotherapy in Arthritis: Clinical and Experimental Aspects" (T. Kresina, ed.), Marcel Dekker Inc., New York.)

Replacement (target) therapies are cited by the authors, referring to myasthenic conditions. These would include also replacements such as vitamin B_{12}, thyroxine, and insulin. On an optimistic note, adequately supplemented patients with autoimmune gastritis or thyroiditis appear to have a normal longevity, so that autoimmunity per se is not necessarily prejudicial to survival.

REFERENCES

Acha-Orbea, H., Mitchell, D. J., Timmermann, L., Wraith, D. C., Tausch, G. S., Waldor, M. K., Zamvil, S. S., McDevitt, H. O., and Steinman, L. (1988). *Cell* **54,** 263–273.

Acha-Orbea, H., Steinman, L., and McDevitt, H. O. (1989). *Annu. Rev. Immunol.* **7,** 371–406.

Adorini, L., and Nagy, Z. A. (1990). *Immunol. Today* **11,** 21–24.

Adorini, L., Barnaba, V., Bona, C., Celada, F., Lanzavecchia, A., Sercarz, E., Suciu-Foca, N., and Wekerle, H. (1990). *Immunol. Today* **11,** 383–386.

Barth, R. K., Kim, B. S., Lan, N. C., Hunkapiller, T., Sobieck, N., Winoto, A., Gershenfeld, H., Okada, C., Hansburg, D., Weissman, I. L., and Hood, L. (1985). *Nature* **316,** 517–523.

Behlke, M. A., Spinella, D. G., Chou, H. S., Sha, W., Hartl, D. L., and Loh, D. Y. (1985). *Science* **229,** 566–569.

Ben-Nun, A., and Cohen, I. R. (1981). *Eur. J. Immunol.* **11,** 949–952.

Ben-Nun, A., Wekerle, H., and Cohen, I. R. (1981a). *Nature* **292,** 60–61.

Ben-Nun, A., Wekerle, H., and Cohen, I. R. (1981b). *Eur. J. Immunol.* **11,** 195–199.

Bever, C. T., Leslie, J., Camenga, D. L., Panitch, H. S., and Johnson, K. P. (1990). *Ann. Neurol.* **27,** 421–427.

Bitar, D., and Whitacre, C. C. (1988). *Cell. Immunol.* **112,** 364–370.

Botazzo, G. F., Dean, B. M., McNeally, J. M., MacKay, E. H., Swift, P. G. F., and Gamble, D. R. (1985). *N. Engl. J. Med.* **313,** 353–360.

Burns, F. R., Li, X., Offner, H., Chou, Y. K., Vandenbark, A. A., and Heber-Katz, E. (1989). *J. Exp. Med.* **169,** 27–40.

Burns, J., Rosenzweig, A., Zweiman, B., and Lisak, R. P. (1983). *Cell. Immunol.* **81,** 435–440.

Calabresi, P., and Parks, R. E. (1985). *In* "The Pharmacological Basis of Therapeutics" (A. Goodman Gilman, L. S. Goodman, T. W. Rall and F. Murad, eds.), pp. 1247–1306. Macmillan, New York.

Casali, P., and Notkins, A. (1989). *Annu. Rev. Immunol.* **7,** 513–535.

Caspi, R., Roberge, F. G., McAllister, C. G., El-Sayed, M., Kuwabara, T., Gery, I., Hanna, E., and Nussenblatt, R. B. (1986). *J. Immunol.* **136,** 928–933.

Chluba, J., Steeg, C., Becker, A., Wekerle, H., and Epplen, J. C. (1989). *Eur. J. Immunol.* **19,** 279–184.

Cosimi, A. B., Colvin, R. B., Burton, R. C., et al. (1981). *N. Engl. J. Med.* **305,** 308–314.

Cotran, R. S. (1987). *Am. J. Pathol.* **129,** 407–413.

Cupps, T. R., and Fauci, A. S. (1982). *Immunol. Rev.* **65,** 133–154.

Davis, M. M., and Bjorkman, P. J. (1988). *Nature* **334,** 395–402.

Dyck, P. J., Daube, J., O'Brien, P., Pineda, A., Low, P. A., Windebank, A. J., and Swansson, C. (1986). *N. Engl. J. Med.* **314,** 461–465.

Eisenberg, S. P., Evans, R. J., Arend, W. P., Verderber, E., Brewer, M. T., Hannum, C. H., and Thompson, R. C. (1990). *Nature* **343,** 341–346.

Elion, G. B., and Hitchings, G. H. (1975). *In* "Handbook of Experimental Pharmacology" (Eichler, O., Farah, A., Herken, H., and Welch, A. D., eds.), pp. 404–425. Springer, Berlin, Germany.

Emmel, E. A., Verweij, C. L., Durand, D. B., Higgins, K. M., Lacy, E., and Crabtree, G. R. (1989). *Science* **246,** 1617–1620.

Engel, A. G., and Emslie-Smith, A. M. (1989). *Curr. Opin. Neurol. Neurosurg.* **2,** 695–700.

Fauci, A. S., Dale, D. C., and Balow, J. E. (1976). *Ann. Int. Med.* **84,** 304–314.

Fischer, G., Wittmann-Liebold, B., Lang, K., Kiefhaber, T., and Schmid, F. X. (1989). *Nature* **337,** 476–478.

Freedman, R. B. (1989). *Nature* **341,** 692.

Fujinami, R. S., and Oldstone, M. B. A. (1985). *Science* **230,** 1043–1046.

Fuller, K. A., Pearl, D., and Whitacre, C. C. (1990). *J. Neuroimmunol.* **28,** 15–26.

Haynes, B. F., Allen, N. B., and Fauci, A. S. (1986). *Med. Clin. North Am.* **70,** 355–375.

Higgins, P. J., and Weiner, H. L. (1988). *J. Immunol.* **140,** 440–445.

Hobbiger, F. (1976). *In* "Handbuch der Experimentellen Pharmakologie" (E. Zaimis, ed.), Vol. 42, pp. 487–581. Springer, Berlin.

Hohlfeld, R. (1989). *Ann. Neurol.* **25,** 531–538.

Hohlfeld, R., and Toyka, K. V. (1985). *J. Neuroimmunol.* **9,** 193–204.

Hohlfeld, R., Kalies, I., Ernst, M., Ketelsen, U.-P. and Wekerle, H. (1982). *J. Neurol. Sci.* **57,** 265–280.

Hohlfeld, R., Michels, M., Heininger, K., Besinger, U., and Toyka, K. V. (1988). *Neurology* **38,** 258–261.

Holoshitz, J., Matitiau, A., and Cohen, I. R. (1984). *J. Clin. Invest.* **73,** 211–215.
Howell, M. D., Winters, S. T., Olee, T., Powell, H. C., Carlo, D. J., and Brostoff, S. W. (1989). *Science* **246,** 668–671.
Kahan, B. D. (1989). *N. Engl. J. Med.* **321,** 1725–1738.
Kibler, R. F., Fritz, R. B., Chou, F. C.-H., Chou, C.-H. J., Peacocke, N. Y., Brown, N. M., and McFarlin, D. E. (1977). *J. Exp. Med.* **146,** 1323–1331.
Killen, J. A., and Swanborg, R. H. (1982). *J. Neuroimmunol.* **2,** 159–166.
Kimoto, M., Krenz, T. J., and Fathman, C. G. (1981). *J. Exp. Med.* **154,** 883–891.
Kirchner, T., Tzartos, S., Hoppe, F., Schalke, B. C. G., Wekerle, H. and Müller-Hermelink, H. K. (1988). *Am. J. Pathol.* **130,** 268–280.
Kumar, V., Kono, D. H., Urban, J. L., and Hood, L. (1989). *Annu. Rev. Immunol.* **7,** 657–682.
Kumar, V., Urban, J. L., Horvath, S. J., and Hood, L. (1990). *Proc. Natl. Acad. Sci. U.S.A.* **87,** 1337–1341.
Lamont, A. G., Sette, A., Fujinami, R. S., Colon, S. M., Miles, C., and Grey, H. M. (1990). *J. Immunol.* **145,** 1687–1683.
Lanzavecchia, A., and Scheidegger, D. (1987). *Eur. J. Immunol.* **17,** 105–111.
Lider, O., Karin, N., Shinitzky, M., and Cohen, I. R. (1987). *Proc. Natl. Acad. Sci. U.S.A.* **84,** 4577–4580.
Lider, O., Reshef, T., Béraud, E., Ben-Nun, A., and Cohen, I. R. (1988). *Science* **239,** 181–183.
Lider, O., Santos, L. M. B., Lee, C. S. Y., Higgins, P. J., and Weiner, H. L. (1989). *J. Immunol.* **142,** 748–752.
Lindstrom, J. (1985). *Annu. Rev. Immunol.* **3,** 109–131.
Linington, C., Izumo, S., Suzuki, M., Uyemura, K., Meyermann, R., and Wekerle, H. (1984). *J. Immunol.* **133,** 1946–1950.
Lohse, A. W., Mor, F., Karin, N., and Cohen, I. R. (1989). *Science* **244,** 820–822.
Malchesky, P. S., Sueoka, A., Matsubara, S., Wojcicki, J., and Nose, Y. (1983). *In* "Plasmapheresis" (Y. Nose, P. S. Malchesky, J. W. Smith, and R. S. Krakauer, eds.), pp. 75–79. Raven Press, New York.
Maron, R., Zerubavel, R., Friedman, A., and Cohen, I. R. (1983). *J. Immunol.* **131,** 2316–2322.
Marrack, P. (1987). *Science* **235,** 1311–1314.
Mathieson, P. W., Cobbold, S. P., Hale, G., Clark, M. R., Oliviera, D. B. G., Lockwood, C. M., and Waldmann, H. (1990). *N. Engl. J. Med.* **323,** 250–254.
Mayforth, R. D., and Quintans, J. (1990). *N. Engl. J. Med.* **323,** 173–178.
McCormack, J. J., and Johns, D. G. (1982). *In* "Pharmacologic Principles of Cancer Treatment" (B. A. Chabner, ed.), pp. 3213–3228. W. B. Saunders, Philadelphia, Pennsylvania.
McEvoy, K. M., Windebank, A. J., Daube, J. R., and Low, P. A. (1989). *N. Engl. J. Med.* **321,** 1567–1571.
McKhann, G. M., Griffin, J. W., Cornblath, D. R., Mellits, E. D., Fisher, R. S., Quaskey, S. A., and The Guillain-Barré Syndrome Study Group. (1988). *Ann. Neurol.* **23,** 347–353.
Mendlovic, S., Brocke, S., Shoenfeld, Y., Ben-Bassat, M., Meshorer, A., Bakimer, R., and Mozes, E. (1988). *Proc. Natl. Acad. Sci. U.S.A.* **85,** 2260–2274.
Milgrom, F., and Witebsky, E. (1962). *J.A.M.A.* **181,** 707–716.
Nagler-Anderson, C., Bober, L. A., Robinson, M. E., Siskind, G. W., and Thorbecke, G. J. (1986). *Proc. Natl. Acad. Sci. U.S.A.* **86,** 7443–7446.
Nussenblatt, R. B., Caspi, R. R., Mahdi, R., Chan, C.-C. Robergé, F., Lider, O., and Weiner, H. L. (1990). *J. Immunol.* **144,** 1689–1695.
Oldstone, M. B. A. (1987). *Cell* **50,** 819–820.
Olsnes, S., Sandvig, K., Petersen, O. W., and vanDeurs, B. (1989). *Immunol. Today* **10,** 291–295.
Osborn, L. (1990). *Cell* **62,** 2–6.
Owhashi, M., and Heber-Katz, E. (1988). *J. Exp. Med.* **168,** 2153–2164.

Pastan, I., Willingham, M. C., and FitzGerald, D. J. P. (1986). *Cell* **47,** 641–648.
Pullen, A. M., Potts, W., Wakeland, E. K., Kappler, J., and Marrack, P. (1990). *J. Exp. Med.* **171,** 49–62.
Rajewsky, K., Förster, I., and Cumano, A. (1987). *Science* **238,** 1088–1094.
Riechmann, L., Clark, M., Waldmann, H., and Winter, G. (1988). *Nature* **332,** 323–327.
Rock, G. (1983). *In* "Plasmapheresis" (Y. Nose, P. S. Malchesky, J. W. Smith, and R. S. Krakauer, eds.), pp. 75–79. Raven Press, New York.
Ruddle, N. H., Bergman, C. M., McGrath, K. M., Lingenheld, E. G., Grunnet, M. L., Padula, S. J., and Clark, R. B. (1990). *J. Exp. Med.* **172,** 1193–1200.
Sakai, K., Sinha, A. A., Mitchell, D. J., Zamvil, S. S., Rothbard, J. B., and McDevitt, H. O. (1988). *Proc. Natl. Acad. Sci. U.S.A.* **85,** 8608–8612.
Sakai, K., Zamvil, S. S., Mitchell, D. J., Hodgkinson, S., Rothbard, J. B., and Steinman, L. (1989). *Proc. Natl. Acad. Sci. U.S.A.* **86,** 9470–9474.
Sarvetnick, N., Shizuru, J., Liggitt, D., Martin, L., McIntyre, B., Gregory, A., Parslow, T., and Stewart, T. (1990). *Nature* **346,** 844–847.
Schein, P. S., and Winokur, S. H. (1975). *Ann. Intern. Med.* **82,** 84–95.
Schluesener, H. J., and Wekerle, H. (1985). *J. Immunol.* **135,** 3128–3133.
Schwartz, R. H., David, C. S., Sachs, D. H., and Paul, W. E. (1976). *J. Immunol.* **117,** 531–540.
Shevach, E. M., Paul, W. E., and Green, I. (1972). *J. Exp. Med.* **136,** 1207–1221.
Schlomchik, M., Macelli, M., Shan, H., Radic, M. Z., Pisetsky, D., Marshak-Rothstein, A., and Weigert, M. (1990). *J. Exp. Med.* **171,** 265–298.
Shoenfeld, Y., and Schwartz, R. T. (1984). *N. Engl. J. Med.* **311,** 1019–1029.
Singh, V. K., Yamaki, K., Donoso, L. A., and Shinohara, T. (1989). *J. Immunol.* **142,** 1512–1516.
Soulillou, J.-P., Cantarovich, D., LeMauff, B., *et al.* (1990). *N. Engl. J. Med.* **322,** 1175–1182.
Sriram, S., Topham, D. J., and Carroll, L. (1987). *J. Immunol.* **139,** 1485–1489.
Standaert, R. F., Galat, A., Verdine, G. L., and Schreiber, S. L. (1990). *Nature* **346,** 671–673.
Stanley, J. R. (1989). *J. Clin. Invest.* **83,** 1443–1448.
Steinman, L., Rosenbaum, J. T., Sriram, S., and McDevitt, H. O. (1981). *Proc. Natl. Acad. Sci. U.S.A.* **78,** 7111–7114.
Strominger, J. L. (1989). *Science* **244,** 943–950.
Sun, D., and Wekerle, H. (1986). *Nature* **320,** 70–72.
Sun, D., Ben-Nun, A., and Wekerle, H. (1988a). *Eur. J. Immunol.* **18,** 1993–2000.
Sun, D., Qin, Y., Chluba, J., Epplen, J. T., and Wekerle, H. (1988b). *Nature* **332,** 843–845.
Takahashi, N., Hayano, T., and Suzuki, M. (1989). *Nature* **337,** 473–475.
Tan, E. M. (1989). *J. Clin. Invest.* **84,** 1–6.
Thomson, A. W. (1990). *Immunol. Today* **11,** 35–36.
Todd, J. A., Acha-Orbea, H., Bell, J. I., Chao, N., Fronek, Z., Jacob, C. O., McDermott, M., Shinha, A. A., Timmerman, L., Steinman, L., and McDevitt, H. O. (188). *Science* **240,** 1003–1009.
Toyka, K. V. (1990). *In* "Current Therapy in Neurologic Disease" (R. T. Johnson, ed.), pp. 385–391. B. C. Decker, Philadelphia, Pennsylvania.
Turk, J. L., and Parker, D. (1982). *Immunol. Rev.* **65,** 99–113.
Tzartos, S. J., and Lindstrom, J. (1980). *Proc. Natl. Acad. Sci. U.S.A.* **77,** 755–759.
Urban, J. L., Horvath, S., and Hood, L. (1989). *Cell* **59,** 257–271.
Urban, J. L., Kumar, V., Kono, D. H., Gomez, C., Horvath, S. J., Clayton, J., Ando, D. G., Sercarz, E. E., and Hood, L. (1988). *Cell* **54,** 577–592.
Vandenbark, A. A., Hashim, G., and Offner, H. (1989). *Nature* **341,** 541–544.
Vandenbark, A. A., Offner, H., Reshef, T., Fritz, R., Chou, C. H. J., and Cohen, I. R. (1985). *J. Immunol.* **135,** 229–233.
Vincent, A., Lang, B., and Newsom-Davis, J. (1989). *Trends Neurosci.* **12,** 496–502.

Vitetta, E. S., Fulton, R. J., May, R. D., Till, M., and Uhr, J. W. (1987). *Science* **238,** 1098–1104.
Weiner, H. L., and Hafler, D. A. (1988). *Ann. Neurol.* **23,** 211–222.
Wekerle, H., and Begemann, M. (1976). *J. Immunol.* **116,** 159–161.
Wekerle, H., Linington, C., Lassmann, H., and Meyermann, R. (1986). *Trends Neurosci.* **9,** 271–277.
Wraith, D. C., McDevitt, H. O., Steinman, L., and Acha-Orbea, H. (1989). *Cell* **57,** 709–715.
Zaller, D. M., Osman, G., Kanagawa, O., and Hood, L. (1990). *J. Exp. Med.* **171,** 1943–1956.
Zamvil, S. S., Mitchell, D. J., Lee, N. E., Moore, A. C., Waldor, M. K., Sakai, K., Rothbard, J. B., McDevitt, H. O., Steinman, L., and Acha-Orbea, H. (1988). *J. Exp. Med.* **167,** 1586–1596.

CHAPTER **17**

Autoimmunity: Horizons

IAN R. MACKAY
Centre for Molecular Biology and Medicine
Monash University
Clayton, Victoria, Australia

NOEL R. ROSE
Department of Immunology and Infectious Diseases
The Johns Hopkins University
School of Hygiene and Public Health
Baltimore, Maryland

I. AUTOIMMUNE DISEASES: IDENTIFICATION AND CLASSIFICATION

The year of preparation of *The Autoimmune Diseases II* (1991) is the 40th anniversary of the first cited adjectival description of "autoimmune," in reference to hemolytic anemia (Young *et al.*, 1951). The prescience of this coinage was shortly fulfilled by the recognition of autoimmune processes in various human diseases of hitherto unknown cause. These included thyroiditis according to experimental and clinical observations (Rose, 1991a), systemic lupus erythematosus, thanks to the discovery of the lupus erythematosus cell by Hargraves *et al.* (1948), and thrombocytopenia purpura consequent to Harrington's self-infusion of disease sera (Harrington *et al.*, 1956). Yet, even after these 40 years, there is still "a pale cast of thought" by those who regard autoimmune phenomena as mostly secondary to an unknown primary etiologic agent or process. Moreover, autoimmunity still creates confusion among clinicians who seek criteria that qualify a disease as "autoimmune," and among basic laboratory scientists who require a better understanding of mechanisms that permit autoimmunity to occur.

Various authors have addressed the uncertainty over the degree to which autoimmunity can be attributed to a provocative primary event, infectious, toxic or other, rather than an occurrence *de novo*. This is a troubling question; autoimmune diseases in some few instances are clearly attributable to an extrinsic cause but mostly occur unheralded, apart from a genetic predisposition. Of equal concern, to those of a catalog persuasion, are the several candidate diseases with marginal qualifications for autoimmunity, e.g., ankylosing spondylitis, ulcerative colitis, and multiple sclerosis. And there are still other diseases for which autoimmunity has been an accepted pathogenesis, e.g., rheumatoid arthritis, but for which an infectious cause still cannot be rejected.

Traditionally, the autoimmune diseases were classified into organ-specific and systemic, but such was the apparent overlap that a "spectrum" was proposed (Roitt, 1984). A classification into the following groupings is suggested:

1. *Organ-specific autoimmune diseases* in which the disease is focused primarily on a single organ, and corresponding organ-specific autoantibodies (or T cells) are demonstrable. In each instance, multiple organ-specific autoantibodies are present. Examples include thyroiditis, gastritis, adrenalitis, and pancreatic insulitis.
2. *Cell-specific autoimmune diseases* in which the disease is focused primarily on a discrete cellular element or product which, although dispersed throughout the body, contains a cell-specific or receptor-specific antigen to which there is a well-defined autoantibody. Examples include hemolytic anemias (antibody to surface antigens of the red blood cell), myasthenia gravis (acetylcholine receptor antibody), and Goodpasture's nephropathy (antibody to the globular domain of Type IV collagen).
3. *"Paradoxical" organ-specific autoimmune diseases* in which there is systemically distributed autoantigen, but the disease is localized mainly to particular tissues or organs, and the demonstrable "marker" autoantibody has no evident relationship to actual pathogenesis. Examples include autoimmune exocrinopathy of Sjögren's syndrome type (antibodies to the nuclear antigens, Ro/SS-A, La/SS-B), polymyositis (antibodies to the Jo1 antigen and others), primarily biliary cirrhosis (antibodies to mitochondrial enzymes), and vasculitis (antibodies to neutrophil cytoplasmic enzymes). The significance of these associations is a major unsolved problem for autoimmunity.
4. *Multisystem autoimmune diseases* with multiple antibodies to widely distributed cell-surface or intracellular antigens, and where pathogenic consequences are attributed for the most part to systemically deposited immune complexes, and also possibly to antibodies to surface antigens of blood and vascular endothelial cells: Prime examples are systemic lupus erythematosus in humans and in the murine models, progressive systemic sclerosis and mixed connective tissue disease.

Autoimmune diseases vary widely in their expression, mediation and outcome, yet are all linked by some common threads of pathogenesis. We can note that specialists in widely different organ–disease systems, e.g., rheumatologists, neuropathologists, endocrinologists, propose strikingly similar formulations for diseases within their own particular specialty, such as rheumatoid arthritis, multiple sclerosis, or autoimmune Type 1 diabetes, respectively. This is illustrated in Figure 1, based on a diagram we have previously presented (Rose, 1991b), which is congruent with concepts of pathogenesis proposed for rheumatoid arthritis by Kingsley *et al.* (1991) and for diabetes mellitus by Nerup and colleagues (1987). We suggest that all autoimmune diseases should fit into this general type of schema, allowing of course for various of the details to be filled in. Among these would be the nature of the antigen, migration patterns of leukocytes, the regulatory mechanisms and, among different autoimmune diseases, the differing utilization of effector mechanisms, including cytokines, antibodies, or cytotoxic T cells.

The diagram allows also for "antigen" to be something other than a self component, i.e., a persisting constituent of a microorganism such as *Borrelia* (Krause *et al.*, 1991), against which the ongoing host response would simulate an autoimmune process. The diagram similarly covers situations in transplantation that resemble autoimmunity, i.e., host-versus-graft and graft-versus-host disease. In host-versus-graft disease, the antigen is from the graft, and the antigen-presenting cell and the T cell are from the host; in graft-versus-host disease, the antigen is from the host, and the antigen-presenting cell and the T cell are from the donor.

> Our prediction is that, within the next five years, knowledge on the basic processes that determine autoimmunity will have advanced sufficiently for the following to be fulfilled. Diseases will be confidently classified as "autoimmune" on the basis that defined reactions with self-antigens are the *major* components in a multifactorial causation, and that a rational classification will exist based on a fully comprehended pathogenesis.

II. AUTOANTIGENS AND COGNATE IMMUNE RESPONSES

The common characteristics of autoantigens have intrigued immunologists for many years, including one of our "forebears," Ernest Witebsky (1929). Clinical immunologists use autoantigens in their diagnostic assays and generally describe reactions in terms of multimolecular organelles, antinuclear, antimitochondrial, or antimicrosomal. Fortunately, new techniques in analytical biochemistry and molecular biology are helping to dissect from these organelles the autoantigenic polypeptides and actual peptide epitopes.

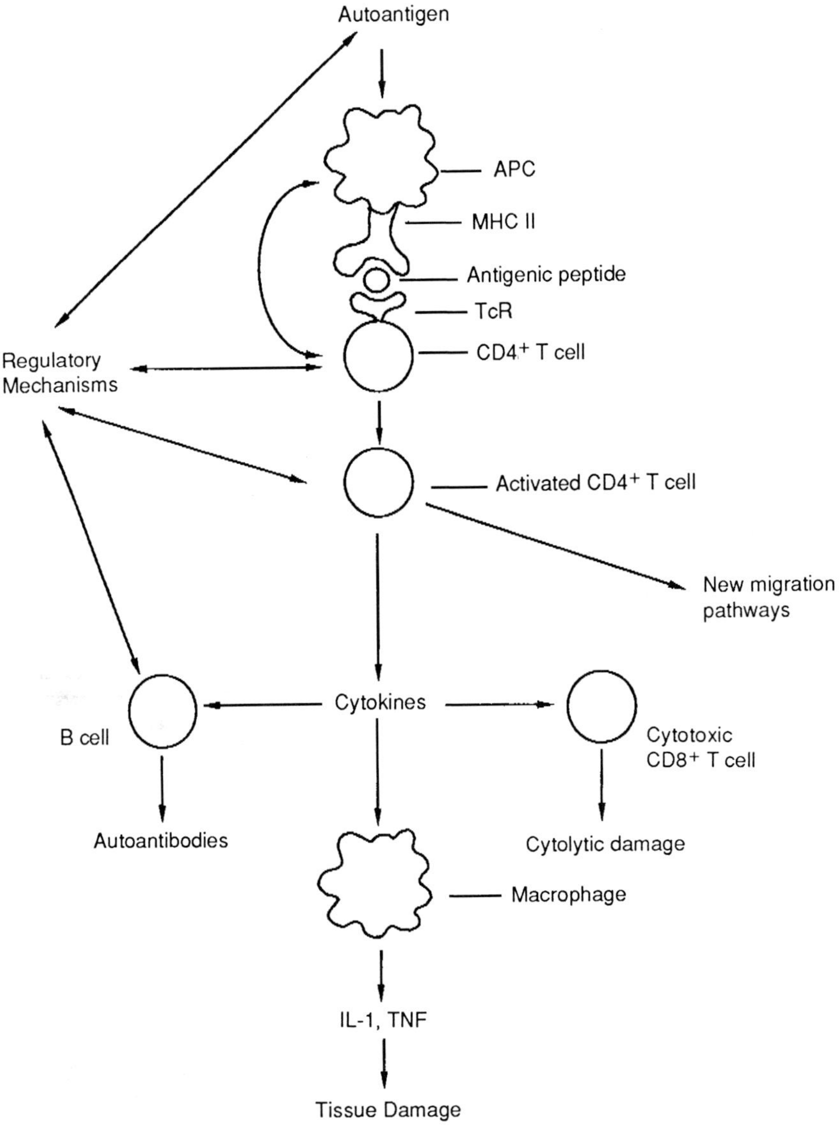

FIG. 1 General scheme for the autoimmune response.

Under appropriate circumstances, practically all constituents of the body could behave as autoantigens, provided the constituent is administered with appropriate adjuvants. Thus, tolerance to self is seldom absolute. On the other hand, there is an undoubted preference for particular constituents of tissues and cells to function as autoantigens. It is being increasingly noted that enzyme molecules are targeted as autoantigens (Banga and McGregor, 1991), and the autoepitopes, when defined, represent important functional sites of the enzyme molecule.

Nearly all of the work so far on "epitope-mapping" has been done for antibodies, i.e., B-cell epitopes, whereas delineating T-cell epitopes on autoantigens have proved more difficult (*vide infra*). Initially, it seemed from studies by immunoblotting that B-cell epitopes may be defined as linear sequences of amino acids. However, autoantibodies, like most conventional antibodies (Benjamin *et al.*, 1984; Laver *et al.*, 1990), appear to react with a large conformational determinant on the antigenic molecule that encompasses discontinuous sequences (Horsfall *et al.*, 1991). As particular examples we can cite the La/SS-B polypeptide (McNeilage *et al.*, 1990) and the Ro/SS-A polypeptide (Boire *et al.*, 1991) that are reactants in Sjögren's syndrome and a subset of systemic lupus erythematosus; the pyruvate dehydrogenase complex that is a reactant in primary biliary cirrhosis (Rowley *et al.*, 1991); the proliferating cell nuclear antigen that is a reactant, occasionally, in cases of systemic lupus erythematosus (Huff *et al.*, 1990); and the 70 kDa constituent of the U_1 RNP complex that is a reactant in mixed connective tissue disease (Cram *et al.*, 1990). As mentioned elsewhere in this volume, this has substantial implications, at least at the B-cell level, for the concept of molecular mimicry as the initiating process for autoimmunity.

Another feature to emerge from recent studies on antigens and autoantibodies is the differing antigenic specificity of natural disease-associated autoantibodies and those induced by deliberate immunization of laboratory animals. This was first shown for the La/SS-B autoantigen by Chan and Tan (1987). As further examples, there are striking differences in natural antibodies to the enzyme pyruvate dehydrogenase complex in primary biliary cirrhosis and those raised by immunizing animals with pyruvate dehydrogenase complex or component subunits (Rowley *et al.*, 1992), and by antibodies to histidyl transfer synthetase (Jo1) in polymyositis and those raised by immunizing mice with histidyl transfer synthetase (Miller *et al.*, 1990); these differences were shown by different patterns of epitope selection on peptide mapping and the exclusive capacity of the natural autoantibodies to inhibit the catalytic activity of enzyme autoantigens. Now that the enzyme glutamate decarboxylase has been unequivocally identified as a major pancreatic islet cell autoantigen in Type I diabetes mellitus, it will be interesting to establish whether there will be differences in natural and experimentally induced antibodies to this molecule.

The isotype (IgM, IgG, IgA) and IgG subclass (IgG1-IgG4) distribution of autoantibodies has received relatively little attention. During maturation, the pre-B cell undergoes genomic switching events under the influence of lymphokines from T cells. Variable immunoglobulin region gene products are linked to constant region products in the following sequence in humans (Flanagan and Rabbitts, 1982):

$$\text{IgM} \rightarrow \text{IgD} \rightarrow \text{IgG3} \rightarrow \text{IgG1} \rightarrow \text{IgA1} \rightarrow \text{IgG2} \rightarrow \text{IgG4} \rightarrow \text{IgE} \rightarrow \text{IgA2}.$$

Primary responses are predominantly of the IgM isotype, secondary responses in bacterial and viral infections are predominantly of the IgG1–IgG3 subclasses, and parasite and reaginic responses IgG4 and IgE. Earlier data for autoimmune disease are reviewed by Yount *et al.*, (1988). The IgG1 subclass usually predominates, exemplified by anti-Sm, anti-RNP and anti-La/SS-B; since the IgG1 subclass is proportionally greater than other isotypes, an increase in such autoantibody is reflected by hypergammaglobulinemia. Other autoantibodies have a more dispersed isotype and subclass distribution (IgM, IgA, IgG1, IgG3), including anti-DNA and rheumatoid factor (Yount *et al.*, 1988). The M2 autoantibodies in primary biliary cirrhosis differ in that IgM and the IgG3 subclasses predominate (Surh *et al.*, 1988). Autoantibodies seem seldom represented among the reaginic IgE isotype and IgG4 subclass; IgE-type antibody to profilin that is cross-reactive with birch pollen profilin could be a possible example (Valenta *et al.*, 1991).

Improvements in methods for studying subclass distribution of autoantibodies (Outschoorn *et al.*, 1992) may clarify the determinants of persisting autoimmune serologic responses. These include the influence of T cells on class-switching events (Schultz and Coffmann, 1991), and the likely resistance to tolerance of B cells that have entered the switch pathway. We can refer here to experiments using nonautoimmune Balb C mice rendered transgenic for genes that encode antibody to DNA. When the heavy chain of the anti-DNA was $C\mu$, the transgenic Balb C mice had many B cells that expressed surface anti-ss DNA of IgM isotype, but no anti-DNA in their serum (Erikson *et al.*, 1991). Schwartz (1991) has commented that when the transgenic construct encodes anti-DNA of IgG2a subclass, transgenic mice mated to Balb C produced progeny with high serum levels of IgG2a anti-ds DNA. Thus the class-switched anti-DNA was resistant to regulation. Along somewhat similar lines, non-autoimmune mice transgenic for the BCL2 gene, under the control of an Ig heavy chain enhancer, had augmented B-cell survival and exhibited features of anti-nuclear autoimmunity (Strasser *et al.*, 1991).

Our prediction is that, within the next five years, the explanation for the particular, indeed in some cases peculiar, epitope selectivity of certain disease-associated autoantibodies will be accommodated by a more satisfying understanding of the escape of B cells from tolerogenesis than we have at present.

III. THE IMMUNE REPERTOIRE

The immune system usually provides a surprisingly effective compromise between the needs for a comprehensive coverage against threats of nonself from the exterior and tolerance of self. Self-tolerance is said by some to entail the creation of "holes" in the immune repertoire. Mitchison (1991) draws a quaint analogy with cheeses, i.e., tiny "Tilsit-cheese"-type holes and large "Emmenthal-cheese"-type holes. The tiny holes are created by a lethal exposure of thymocytes to individual major histocompatibility complex (MHC)-associated self-antigens, and the large holes (at least in mice) are created by exposure of thymocytes to "superantigens" (e.g., bacterial toxins, endogenous tumor viruses), that can delete all reactivities that depend on products of genes for the variable portion of the β chain, Vβ, of the T-cell receptor. The unfavorable evolutionary consequences of such large repertoire deletions created by superantigens suggest that this mechanism must be used very sparingly.

Burnet's early postulate on intrathymic deletion of potentially self-reactive T cells (Burnet, 1962) has now been well validated experimentally in mice for an MHC class II molecule, I-E (Kappler *et al.*, 1987), and this can be taken as a model for intrathymic deletion of T cells with reactivity against any accessible self-structure plus MHC. This process creates a stable "purged" T-cell repertoire which, according to Zinkernagel *et al.* (1991), will remain devoid of any T cells capable of reactivity with what he terms "immunological self"; it was, therefore, claimed that truly autoimmune T cells, i.e., T cells reactive to tolerogenic and immunogenic self, do not (and cannot) exist. This is certainly in accord with the general difficulty in demonstrating clear T-cell reactivity to self-proteins, but we see the distinction between what can, and cannot, be deleted in the thymus as less than clear cut.

Superantigens require some comment since a role is attributed for them in autoimmune disease (*vide infra*). However, superantigens have been identified so far only in mice and may even be unique for that species. The first superantigens to be recognized wore the lymphocyte-stimulatory products of the Mls locus in mice described by Festenstein (1973); responsiveness was later linked to the interaction of these products with TcR Vβ gene products. Subsequently, various microbial superantigens were identified that could bind with high affinity to MHC class II molecules and thereby trigger massive proliferation of T cells expressing TcR Vβ gene products. A further development of interest is the recognition that certain endogenous murine superantigens in fact represent molecules encoded by resident retroviruses (Choi *et al.*, 1991). Returning to autoimmunity, the possibility arises that microbial superantigens could interact with T cells to generate potent helper signals for B cell activation, akin to graft-versus-host disease.

The precise details of intrathymic deletional processes are still to be established other than the occurrence in the thymic medulla by a lethal interaction, visualized as apoptosis, between immature, self-reactive thymocytes and dendritic cells of bone marrow origin that co-express a "thymus-accessible" self-antigen with an MHC molecule. We emphasize that the MHC molecule could make a critical contribution to the configuration of the intrathymic "deletogen" and, if so, to a propensity to autoimmune disease in later life. Perhaps of relevance here is the I-E molecule in autoimmune NOD mice and the prevention of autoimmune disease in such mice by transgenic replacement of I-E (see chapter 3). Finally, it is likely that different deletional conditions will apply for CD4 and CD8 T cells, given the different manner in which antigen is presented to these cell types.

In brief, the eventual "shape" of the T-cell repertoire is created by (1) the large (yet not infinite) and random series of productive rearrangements of Vα and Vβ receptor proteins, (2) high proliferative pressures created within the thymic cortical microenvironment, and (3) the deletional purging that operates on receptor-bearing self-reactive thymocytes before they exit from the medulla; and (4) possible extrathymic pathways of T-cell development. The actual efficiency of purging of T cells with self-reactive potential could be subject to the following influences: (1) the composition of the intrathymic library represented by tissues actually present in the thymus (mesenchyme, lymphoid tissue, squamous epithelium, muscle), and whether these release intracellular molecules; (2) entry into the thymus of circulating blood cells and proteins, and breakdown products of peripheral tissues that gain entry via the blood to the thymic milieu; (3) the efficiency with which these potential autoantigens can bind to and be presented by MHC molecules in the thymic medulla; and (4) the stage during ontogeny at which particular self-molecules are first synthesized. For example, neural myelin, which is a prototype autoantigen, exemplifies a molecule synthesized late in ontogeny.

We can note that T cells continue to be synthesized in postnatal life, and so the question arises whether postnatal deletional tolerance is as efficient as in embryonic life. Another question is the significance of reentry into the thymus of peripheral T cells. In mice, it appears that there is substantial homing to the thymus of peripheral T cells which are exclusively of activated type (Agus *et al.*, 1991). If the immigrants were to include self-reactive cells, these could be subject to deletion, or could act as deletogens by carrying MHC-self-antigen complexes, or might even stimulate antiidiotypic T cells with regulatory functions (Agus *et al.*, 1991).

There was formerly some interest in the treatment of autoimmune disease by thymectomy, with the goal of removing a potential source of forbidden clones. Other than in some cases of myasthenia gravis, it proved ineffective. In fact, there are reported examples in humans of thymectomy for one autoimmune disease being followed by the expression of another (Grinlinton *et al.*, 1991). There is also the challenging observation that certain autoimmune diseases are inducible experimentally by thymectomy (see chapter 3). In the case of experimental gastritis thus induced in mice, transfer of the disease can be achieved by injecting splenic T cells into athymic hosts but not by injection into thymus-intact hosts (Gleeson and Toh, 1991); thus thymic deprivation not only impedes deletion of self-reactive T cells during their genesis, but also abrogates later inactivation of self-reactive T cells.

The entire T-cell "response capacity" must be generated in the thymus since, unlike B cells, T-cell receptors do not undergo post-thymic diversifications. However, the developed peripheral repertoire cannot be created intrathymically, because all of the deletional requirements could not be met, particularly for CD8 T cells that respond essentially to molecules generated intracellularly and presented with MHC class I. Whether peripheral self-reactive CD8 T cells have any significance could depend on the degree of help necessary for CD8 T cells from activated CD4 cells; coincidental up-regulation of MHC class I molecules; the degree of release of intracellular antigen after tissue damage; and other factors. In any event, the peripheral T-cell repertoire requires some degree of modification by extrathymic influences.

Knowledge of peripheral tolerance of T cells has been greatly advanced by transgenic mouse models wherein the transgene linked to an appropriate promoter allows expression of the product to a given tissue or cell type. Transgenic MHC class I or class I molecules, for example, have been expressed extrathymically, e.g. in β-islet cells by the insulin promoter or in liver cells by the β-metallothionine promoter (reviewed by Miller and Morahan, 1992). The transgenic models indicate that a molecule that could not have had thymic representation can indeed induce a general T-cell tolerance, even when that molecule is expressed only in a limited site in the body. The postulated mechanism is cellular anergy, associated with down-regulation of TcR and co-receptor molecules, such as the IL-2 receptor.

Von Boehmer (1989) constructed transgenic mice that expressed a T-cell receptor for the male-associated antigen, H-Y, in the context of syngeneic class I MHC antigens. T cells expressing the transgenic receptor were rescued from apoptosis by the MHC antigens in female mice, but in male transgenics immature ($CD4^+8^+$) T cells were negatively selected, i.e., deleted. Transgene-expressing T cells with a high density of CD8 were absent from the periphery and the remaining T cells could not be readily activated by H-Y stimulator cells because they expressed only low levels of CD8 molecules. Thus autospecific T cells of the $CD4^-CD8^+$ (low) phenotype were spared the deletional processes, remaining as quiescent (anergic) T cells in the periphery.

Transgenic models have acquired further sophistication by mice being rendered doubly transgenic, by mating mice carrying a transgene for an antigenic molecule with mice carrying a transgene for rearranged T-cell receptors specifically reactive with that antigenic molecule, e.g., a foreign class I MHC molecule K^b (Miller and Morahan, 1992). In these experiments, thymic T cells developed that were capable of reacting with the foreign K^b molecule but, in the periphery, contact with the transgene product K^b resulted in reduction of clonotype $CD8^+$ T cells in spleen and lymph nodes. Tolerance *in vivo* was demonstrable since there was failure to reject K^b-bearing tumor cells. However, the anergic T cells could be "awakened" *in vitro* by culture with K^b-expressing spleen cells. The relevance of these experiments for self-tolerance and autoimmunity is that a nondeletional mechanism(s) operates to maintain post-thymic tolerance to some self molecules, and an override of this may result in autoimmune expression.

> Our prediction is that the next five years will see the emergence of the thymus as the real master-mind of the immune system, dictating the specificities to which there will, or will not, be an immune response, conceivably with immunotherapy of the future directed at the thymus itself, postnatally. Peripherally induced T-cell tolerance, including suppression, will be seen as a back-up for the primary thymus-based processes.

IV. T CELLS AND AUTOIMMUNE DISEASE

We must accept that autoantigenicity should be considered, as for a conventional response, in terms of T- and B-cell collaboration, with differing epitopes relevant to these two cell types. T-cell epitopes as short peptides have been clearly defined for those autoimmune diseases that can be established by experimental immunization of laboratory animals, e.g., encephalomyelitis, myasthenia gravis, and collagen arthritis. The effector phase of these diseases is T cell-dependent and antibody appears irrelevant. However, for most human autoimmune diseases, neither the epitope(s) that engages the afferent CD4 helper T cell, nor that which serves as a target for effector CD4 or CD8 T cells, has yet been identified. Indeed it is uncertain whether the same or a different epitope of an autoantigen is required for recruitment of CD4 and CD8 T cells.

An autoantigen that could be engaged by $CD8^+$ effector T cells has not been clearly implicated in any type of autoimmune tissue damage. However, since this possibility exists, reference can be made to the comparable system of minor histocompatibility molecules (also known as minor histocompatibility antigens). The major histocompatibility complex molecules, which in humans are encoded by a discrete region of chromosome 6, influence presentation to T cells, and allograft rejection. Individuals, humans or mice, can be identical at MHC loci, yet develop host-versus-graft or graft-versus-host reactions, attributable to responses to an allelic form of a *minor* transplantation molecule. If this is presented as a complex with an MHC molecule to T cells of an animal lacking that allele (and therefore nontolerant), an immune response is induced (Loveland and

Fischer Lindahl, 1991). The male antigen referred to previously, H-Y, elicits a response in histocompatible females and is probably the best known minor histocompatibility molecule.

There are in mice some 50 minor histocompatibility loci, encoded by chromosomal and even mitochondrial DNA (Fischer Lindahl, 1991a). Their existence, and their products, are demonstrable by the techniques of transplantation immunology, such as skin graft exchange or immunization for a cytotoxic T lymphocyte response, with the latter implying that the products are expressed at the cell surface. An interesting example is produced by the four alleles of the mitochondrially encoded peptide maternally transmitted factor (MTF) which is presented with a (nonclassical) MHC class I molecule (Loveland *et al.*, 1990). Informative data on minor histocompatibility loci have come from Boon and colleagues, who have defined novel antigenic epitopes that are created in mutant tumor cell lines and that evoke cytotoxic T-lymphocyte responses; in their studies, it appeared that an antigen could be derived from transfected DNA without a normal gene structure, leading to the proposal that short subgenic fragments, peptons, would be translated to generate novel antigens for cytotoxic T-lymphocyte responses (Boon and Van Pel, 1989). A speculative application of this idea to autoimmunity was that a mutant subgenic DNA sequence could encode a peptide that could act like a minor histocompatibility antigen in the autologous setting, and so provoke an autoimmune response (Mackay *et al.*, 1990). This is a difficult proposition to test. It also requires the assumption that any accompanying "marker" autoantibodies are consequential to the initial attack on the mutant sequence. Further comment on the pepton hypothesis is made by Fischer Lindahl (1991b).

The meager information on the responsiveness of T cells to autoantigens contrasts with the panoply of humoral autoantibodies. We will comment here on (1) the demonstrability of T-cell reactivity to autoantigens and definition of epitopes; (2) the debate on restricted heterogeneity of TcRs in experimental and naturally occurring autoimmune diseases; and (3) the possibility that surrogate antigens or superantigens provide help for self-reactive B cells.

Attempts in the past to define T-cell reactivity to autoantigens were by indirect cytokine assays based on inhibition of migration of leukocytes or macrophages in the presence of test lymphocytes and an antigen preparation, derived, for example, from thyroid gland (Burek and Rose, 1986), stomach (Whittingham *et al.*, 1975), and liver (Meyer zum Büschenfelde *et al.*, 1974). However, these lapsed because of technical difficulties. The mitogenic response of blood lymphocytes exposed to autoantigen was also used, but the stimulation indices reported were low or borderline ($\sim$ 2–3), perhaps reflecting the scarcity of antigen-reactive T cells in blood. In contrast, T-cell responsiveness to purified autoantigens in experimental autoimmune diseases, such as thyroiditis and encephalomyelitis, is readily demonstrable.

More recently, T cells capable of responding to autoantigens in affected tissues have been identified as judged by the derivation of T-cell lines or clones from blood or tissue homogenates, under the stimulus of IL-2 and the putative autoantigen. As particular examples, we can cite responsive T cells to Type 2 collagen, from blood or rheumatoid synovial lymphocytes (Londei *et al.*, 1989; Lacour *et al.*, 1990); basic protein of myelin, from blood or cerebrospinal fluid lymphocytes in multiple sclerosis (Ben-Nun *et al.*, 1991; Liblau *et al.*, 1991; Wucherpfennig *et al.*, 1991); components of the α subunit of the acetylcholine receptor, from blood lymphocytes in myasthenia gravis (Protti *et al.*, 1990; Link *et al.*, 1990); liver membrane, from liver lymphocytes in autoimmune hepatitis (Franco *et al.*, 1990); 2-oxoacid dehydrogenase enzyme antigens from liver lymphocytes in primary biliary cirrhosis (Van de Water *et al.*, 1991); and thyroid antigens including synthetic peptides by lymphocytes from thyroid infiltrates or blood in autoimmune thyroid disease (Dayan *et al.*, 1991; Tandon *et al.*, 1991). In most of these examples, a T-cell epitope has not been identified, except possibly for myasthenia gravis for which synthetic peptides from the α chain of the acetylcholine receptor were used in stimulation assays (Oshima *et al.*, 1990). These successes stand in contrast to the failure in most of the multisystem autoimmune diseases to identify a source of T-cell stimulation for autoreactive B cells except for the 70-kDa component of U_1-RNP (O'Brien *et al.*, 1990). In various of the examples cited above, we can note that antigen-responsive T cells could also be derived from the blood of healthy controls as well as from disease subjects, albeit less readily.

Another aspect of interest is the variability, or restriction, of T-cell receptors (T-cell receptor V-gene use) in autoimmune responses. The relevance here is that, if the T-cell receptor were to have limited variability, reflecting oligoclonality of the T cell response, the prospects for receptor-directed immunotherapy would be much brighter. The earliest data come from studies in the experimental autoimmune diseases, particularly encephalomyelitis (see chapters 3 and 16), in which T cells reactive with myelin basic protein predominantly used the TcR Vβ gene 8.2 (Acha-Orbea *et al.*, 1989). Curiously, Vβ8.2 was used also in the rat response to myelin basic protein despite differences in the sequence of the T-cell autoepitope and the MHC molecule (Heber-Katz *et al.*, 1989). However, in encephalomyelitis of longer duration, this restriction becomes less evident, and T-cell receptor usage diversifies (Vainiene *et al.*, 1991). Coming to other models, there is a claimed restriction of expression of TcR genes in collagen-induced arthritis, although this is contested (reviewed by Cooke, 1991). A T-cell antigen has not yet been characterized in the autoimmune NOD mouse, but transfer of disease can be effected by T-cell clones derived from pancreatic islets. These T cells were reported to use predominantly Vβ5 (Reich *et al.*, 1989), but it was subsequently reported that islet-specific $CD4^+$ T-cell clones were unrestricted (Candéias *et al.*, 1991).

In human disease, considerable attention has been given to receptor usage by T cells in multiple sclerosis (Wucherpfennig *et al.*, 1991). T-cell clones responsive to epitopes of the neural autoantigen MBP can be derived from blood in subjects with multiple sclerosis, but also from normal subjects. Various autoepitopes could be identified on myelin basic protein (MBP), although sequence 84-102 was a particularly immunodominant peptide. However, it appears that the MHC class II DR2, that is usually present in multiple sclerosis, can present a variety of peptides of myelin basic protein to T cells; thus, cells responding to each of these peptides clearly have escaped intrathymic deletion. The existence of a candidate autoantigen myelin basic protein, and the intractability of multiple sclerosis to conventional therapies, have largely been a stimulus for defining the T-cell contribution to this disease as a forerunner to specific immunotherapy. Further information has come from the use of autopsy brain tissue in multiple sclerosis from which V and C sequences of the TcR were amplified by the polymerase chain reaction (Oksenberg *et al.*, 1990). In such studies, TcR transcripts were detected (as expected) only in multiple sclerosis and not in normal brain; there was a restriction of the Vα gene families used, and Vα10 transcripts were demonstrable in every case studied. Similarly, in autoimmune thyroid disease, there was evidence for limited variability of TcR Vα genes among intrathyroidal T cells (Davies *et al.*, 1991).

In two autoimmune diseases, Sjögren's syndrome and rheumatoid arthritis, an interesting restriction of TcR Vβ expression has been reported. In primary Sjögren's syndrome, in blood and salivary tissue, there was a significant depletion of Vβ6.7a T cells versus controls, including HLA-matched controls. Explanations suggested were a genetic lack of expression of Vβ6.7a, a deletion of cells bearing the "a" allele of the Vβ6.7 gene, or a preferential usage of cells bearing "b" alleles (or alleles other than "a"). Knowledge of the reactant for T cells in Sjögren's syndrome would help in the interpretation of this observation.

In rheumatoid arthritis, synovial fluid cells were used for preparation of RNA and amplification by polymerase chain reaction of TcR transcripts (Sottini *et al.*, 1991). There was a marked depletion in synovial fluid, but not in blood, in the number of Vβ transcripts, suggesting that a "major" antigen associated with the pathogenesis of rheumatoid arthritis had interacted selectively with the Vβ component of the TcR. This major antigen could be acting as a superantigen and was perhaps of endogenous origin, e.g., collagen. Paliard *et al.* (1991) also found a marked limitation, compared with blood, of heterogeneity of TcR β transcripts in rheumatoid synovium in which TcR Vβ14 predominated. The idea proposed was that triggering by a superantigen activated many T cells and, from amongst these, T cells with reactivity with a unique rheumatoid antigen would undergo further stimulation. This idea could have broad application to autoimmunity in general.

We predict that during the next five years there will be a much greater level of understanding of the role of T cells in human autoimmune disease. Enquiry will be directed particularly toward (1) breadth of usage of TcR among lymphocytes responding to autoantigens, with reasonable prospects for immunotherapy directed toward the TcR; (2) effector processes including the possible participation of CD8 T cells; and (3) whether a massive triggering event, such as that initiated by a superantigen, is what sets an autoimmune process in motion.

V. LYMPHOCYTE SURFACE MOLECULES: ADHESION, TRAFFIC, MEMORY

The lymphocyte has a chameleonlike capacity to alter its surface structure according to its stage of differentiation or activation. These surface structures, identified by the raising of monoclonal antibodies in other species, control functions essential to the wandering cells of the lymphoid system, i.e., cellular adhesion, pathways of recirculation, and memory responses. We can note the dependence of expression of adhesion molecules on cytokines, and that properties subserved by adhesion molecules are relevant to the physiologic functions of the immune system, to pathologic responses as in autoimmune disease, and to therapies whereby unwanted interactions between cells or between cells and vascular endothelium can be blocked. Knowledge on lymphocyte membrane molecules has accumulated very rapidly, as is evident from recent reviews (Michl *et al.*, 1991; Patarroyo, 1991).

There is obvious relevance of surface adhesion molecules on lymphocytes and vascular endothelium to autoimmune reactions, which could be itemized as follows. First, contiguitive localization of antigen-presenting cells (APCs) (dendritic cells) and CD4 T cells, noted particularly in the rheumatoid synovium (Janossy *et al.*, 1981), and essential for immune induction in general, depends on expression of adhesion molecules. Second, the type of T cell that will be represented in autoimmune tissue lesions will be of the activated memory type illustrated, in rheumatoid arthritis, by the predominance among synovial T cells of those of the CD45RO phenotype (Emery *et al.*, 1987). Third, the capacity of various cytokines to up-regulate adhesion molecules on lymphocytes and vascular endothelium underscores the importance of cytokine production for the progression of autoimmune damage. Fourth, the feature of formation of new endothelial channels in rheumatoid lesions, and their capacity to attract activated T cells, is relevant to synovial inflammation (Manolios *et al.*, 1991). The functional adhesion-type molecules on the lymphocyte membrane are grouped, according to structural homologies, into three families: integrins, the immunoglobulin superfamily, and selectins. Members of one or another of these families interact specifically with each other, with one or another molecule being cited, according to conventional nomenclature, as "receptor" and "ligand," although which is which seems a matter of choice.

The *integrins* are transmembrane heterodimers among which there are three subfamilies, each defined by a β subunit, β_2, β_1 and β_3. The β_2 integrins (Leu CAMs) include CD11a/CD18 (LFA-1) for which the ligand is ICAM-1 and

CD11b/CD18 (MAC1); the β_2 integrins are the VLA 1–6 proteins, CD49/CD29; and the β_3 integrins include cytoadhesion molecules of which the platelet gp IIb/IIIa is a familiar example. The integrin molecules can be expressed on most hemic cells and facilitate cell–cell adhesion, including T-cell interactions with other lymphocytes, and attachment of lymphocytes to endothelial cells (see below).

The *immunoglobulin superfamily* adhesion molecules (Ig SAM) are so named because they share immunoglobulinlike domains of some 90–100 residues. The major member is CD54 (ICAM-1), the ligand for the integrin CD11a/CD18. CD54 is present on germinal center B cells, dendritic cells, macrophages, and vascular endothelium. The interaction of CD11a/CD18 and CD54 is relevant to the pathology of autoimmune disease, with rheumatoid arthritis as a particular example. The enhanced expression of integrins on T cells facilitates their entry and localization into rheumatoid synovium by reason of upregulated expression of the ligand, CD54, on all components of the synovial microenvironment, notably synovial lining (Type A) cells and vascular endothelium. Another adhesion pathway for T cells mediated by Ig SAMs, depends on CD2, the sheep erythrocyte receptor and CD58 (LFA-3).

Selectins, a third family of adhesion molecules, facilitate adhesion between leukocytes and endothelial cells. The selectins comprise a membrane protein, endothelial leukocyte adhesion molecule (ELAM), expressed on vascular endothelial cells in peripheral lymph nodes and up-regulated by IL-1 and other inflammatory mediators, and the partner on leukocytes (MEL-14, LAM-1 and Leu-8), now known as leukocyte endothelial cell adhesion molecule, LECAM-1. The LECAM selectins have a characteristic structure, comprising an N terminal lectin domain, an epidermal growth factor-like domain, and complement-binding protein-like domains. The neutrophil binds to ELAM-1 by a sialyl-Lewis X determinant, but the binding molecule on T cells has not yet been identified.

A molecule of much relevance to T-cell function is the "leukocyte common antigen," now known as CD45. This is expressed as two isoforms (RA, RO) that distinguish recent emigrant T cells from the thymus; these are naive T cells (CD45RA, 205-240 kDa isoform), and T cells that have been activated by antigen and subserve memory (CD45RO, 180 kDa isoform). The naive T cell carries low levels of activation markers but expresses LECAM-1, whereas activated CD4 memory T cells, which would be the type present in autoimmune lesions, express high levels of various adhesion molecules CD2, CD11a, the CD49/CD29 proteins (VLA 1-6), and CD44.

Surface adhesion molecules dictate different pathways of recirculation for T cells that carry the naive or memory phenotype (Mackay, 1991). Naive T cells are directed by LECAM-1 to traffic from blood through lymph nodes in which new antigens in low concentrations are most likely to be encountered, and to exit via efferent lymph to blood. Activated memory T cells are directed alternatively through capillary endothelium into tissues, and thence drain to lymph nodes via afferent lymphatics. Whether "activated" T cells, which are replicating and short-lived, are wholly equivalent to memory T cells is uncertain. Certainly, activated T cells respond to recall antigens and express memory after adoptive transfer. However, those reluctant to discard the traditional concept of a long-lived memory T cell would visualize that an antigen-experienced T cell might lose activation markers and revert to the CD45RA phenotype, yet retain some capacity for an accelerated (memory) response to antigen (Beverley, 1991).

In addition to this selective traffic of activated/memory CD4 T cells, there is evidence that such cells may have tissue tropisms and undergo preferential recirculation to the site of their original antigen exposure, e.g., the skin or gut. This tissue tropism may depend on particular lymphocyte surface molecules, exemplified by the "skin-homing" cutaneous lymphocyte-associated antigen (CLA) molecule, a presumed ligand on T cells for ELAM-1 (Picker *et al.*, 1991). There is also a "gut-homing" pathway of migration among activated/memory CD4 lymphocytes, as judged by trafficking studies in sheep (Mackay *et al.*, 1992).

> It is our prediction that the wave of interest in adhesion molecules on lymphocytes and vascular endothelium will extend our understanding of autoimmunity. T cells that participate in autoimmune lesions will be exclusively of the activated/memory phenotype and will be refractory to tolerogenesis and will have preferential entry via their surface molecules into autoimmune lesions. Such entry should be susceptible to blockage by monoclonal immunotherapy which even now is an appealing prospect.

VI. EXTRINSIC PROVOCATION OF AUTOIMMUNE DISEASE: VIRUSES, DRUGS, CHEMICALS, ENVIRONMENT

Some autoimmune diseases are clearly related to an antecedent or concurrent infection, and numerous microorganisms have been implicated in etiology. As mentioned earlier, autoimmune diseases mostly occur unheralded and attempts to substantiate an initiating or persisting infection by identifying a particular organism have yielded equivocal results; however, cogent reasons can be given for the absence of consistent identification of infection in autoimmune disease (Sinha *et al.*, 1990). As further points, the conformational nature of autoimmune epitopes casts doubt on the molecular mimicry concept; finally, when a particular tissue susceptible to autoimmune damage, e.g., gastric mucosa, is colonized and damaged by a known organism (*Helicobacter pylori*) with a tropism for that tissue, autoantibodies are conspicuously absent, yet present in the absence of discernible gastric infection.

How and why, then, does autoimmune disease begin? The best supposition would seem to be that infectious, toxic, or environmental damage is merely a nonspecific trigger causing release of sequestered or intracellular autoantigens for which deletional tolerance has not been established; an immune response to such autoantigens is poorly regulated, and so activates cytokine-dependent inflammatory cascades and further tissue damage. On the other hand, the possible environmental initiation of autoimmunity requires close scrutiny of the known examples, because of the important connotations of this issue for, notably, theories of autoimmunity, preventive medicine, immunization practices, and even medico-legal matters. The question covers a very wide range, from ubiquitous virus infection such as Epstein-Barr virus to effects of mercury in amalgam fillings in teeth.

Bacteria that are implicated in autoimmune reactions (although not necessarily in autoimmune disease) include spirochetes, notably, *Treponema pallidum,* group A streptococci (see chapter 12), mycobacteria, and *Yersinia.* Mycobacteria are of interest by reason of the model of adjuvant arthritis in which the mycobacterial arthritogenic antigen is the 65 kDa-heat-shock protein (hsp) 60. This has led to a belief that bacterial hsp induce reactions against conserved regions of host hsp, and ensuing autoimmunity. However, there has been no demonstration of T- or B- cell reactivity to human-specific epitopes of hsp in any disease, including, in particular, rheumatoid arthritis. *Klebsiella pneumoniae* and *Yersinia* species have been implicated in spondylitis and reactive arthritis, although these are not usually claimed as autoimmune diseases. The spondylitic diseases are associated with HLA B27, and there are sequence homologies between the above organisms and the B27 molecule. The two possibilities are that the microbe induces an immune response against host B27, or that there is a "cross-tolerance" induced by the B27 molecule which dampens the host resistance to infection with these microbes.

Viruses have frequently come under suspicion in autoimmune disease. Experimentally, Coxsackie B virus infection is followed by autoimmune myocarditis in mice, but data for myocarditis in man are not yet clear (see chapter 12). There are three human virus infections of particular current interest for autoimmunity: Epstein-Barr virus (EBV), hepatitis C virus and human immunodeficiency virus (HIV).

EBV has been linked over the years to rheumatoid arthritis, but there has been no convincing demonstration of the virus in joint tissues. Recently, the disease most discussed is primary Sjögren's syndrome. In particular, cases have been recorded of Sjögren's syndrome closely succeeding EBV infection; the EBV genome has been identified in affected tissue, the salivary glands; and there is co-identity of the human encoded and EBV-encoded RNAs that associate with the La polypeptide. However, EBV is resident in the salivary glands of most healthy adults, yet Sjögren's syndrome is infrequent. Individuals who develop Sjögren's syndrome probably have a genetic predisposition in that the HLA B8.DR3 alleles are overrepresented, and there is a marked (and presumably constitutional) reduction in T cells with a particular allele "a" of the β chain of the T-cell receptor, Vβ6.7 (Kay *et al.*, 1991). Whether subjects who are B8,DR3$^+$, and deficient in Vβ6.7a, have an anomalous response to persisting EBV infection, or are constitutionally predisposed to autoimmunity by some other mechanism, is uncertain.

A viral infection that is linked to autoimmunity is hepatitis, due to the hepatitis C virus, a parenterally transmitted RNA virus. Reports from Europe initially cited high frequencies of anti-hepatitis C virus by ELISA assays in cases of chronic autoimmune hepatitis, and particularly in that subgroup in which there is an autoantibody to a microsomal cytochrome P450 autoantigen (see chapter 9). Subsequently, tests for anti-hepatitis C virus in chronic autoimmune hepatitis came to be regarded as "false" positive, attributable to hypergammaglobulinemia and reactivity to the fusion proteins associated with recombinant viral proteins used in the immunoassay kits. A further report, based on second generation assay kits, indicated that autoantibodies to cytochrome P450 (LKM antibody) occurred frequently among Italians with chronic autoimmune hepatitis due to hepatitis C virus but not among English cases (Lenzi *et al.*, 1991). Studies in which infection with hepatitis C virus can be demonstrated by the polymerase chain reaction in "hepatitis C virus-associated" chronic autoimmune hepatitis are awaited.

There has been continuing interest in infection with human immunodeficiency virus and autoimmunity. First, there are clinical expressions of HIV infection that simulate autoimmune disease, notably thrombocytopenia, arthritis, and parotid gland enlargement that resembles Sjögren's syndrome. Second, HIV infection is associated with a high frequency of certain autoantibodies, particularly anticardiolipin. Third, there have been speculations over the years that the primary event, the destruction of the CD4 T cell, is not attributable to retroviral damage directly, but to another process, perhaps autoimmune in nature.

Clinical aspects of autoimmunity and HIV infection were discussed in the setting of reports on five cases with some resemblances to systemic lupus erythematosus, and positive tests for nuclear antibodies (Kopelman and Zoller-Pazner, 1988). These cases and the associated literature provide no conviction that HIV provoked multisystem autoimmunity of lupus type; in particular, tests for anti-dsDNA are negative. There is, however, another possibility to consider, i.e., depletion of CD4 T cells in the acquired immune deficiency syndrome (AIDS) is caused (in part, at least) by a highly focused autoimmune response against CD4 T cells. This could be generated by foreign (allogeneic) cells if the idiotype of an anti-MHC class II molecule were to produce an antiidiotypic response that reacted damagingly with structures on the T-cell surface (Kion and Hoffman, 1991). This exemplifies the "surrogate" autoantigen concept referred to in Chapter I.

Autoimmunity can be induced by certain drugs and chemicals, although there is no reason to believe that this is a usual occurrence. Some characteristic examples include induction of erythrocyte antibodies by α methyldopa (see chapter 1), nuclear (histone) antibodies by hydralazine or procainamide (see chapter 7), acetylcholine receptor antibodies (with myasthenia), by d-penicillamine (see chapter 13), and liver and kidney microsomal antibodies by tienilic acid (see chapter 9). In general, in these conditions, the appearance of autoantibody precedes the disease or may be the only expression; symptoms develop slowly; the autoimmune state is drug-dependent in that it recedes when the drug is withdrawn; the autoantibody, compared with spontaneous autoantibodies, may have a more restricted expression as in drug-induced lupus, or may be identical; animal models rarely exist; and, most significantly, the elicited autoantibody has no immunochemical relationship to the configuration of the drug. The T-cell component in drug-induced autoimmune disease is unclear.

In view of the diversity and frequency of drug-induced autoimmune syndromes, it is curious that no satisfying explanation has become available. The drugs may interfere with the function of regulatory T cells or, in the process of catalysis by an enzyme, form a complex that provokes a response to the native molecule.

We believe that insights should come from one of the few model systems in which animals do respond to a chemical by the expression of multisystem autoimmunity. These models include disease induced in rats, mice, and rabbits by heavy metals, such as mercury or gold (Druet *et al.*, 1989). For example, in the mercuric chloride ($HgCl_2$) model in the brown Norway rat, repeated injection of $HgCl_2$ causes lymphoproliferation with an increase in CD4 T cells and B cells, high levels of IgG and IgE autoantibodies of various specificities, and an immune complex type of glomerulonephritis (Goldman *et al.*, 1991). In mice, an analogous disease has been elicited by repetitive injections of mercuric chloride or gold salts (Goter Robinson *et al.*, 1986). The autoantibodies in metal-induced autoimmunity are often of antinucleolar type, with specificities that include fibrillarin and laminin. Metal-induced autoimmune disease is genetically controlled by both MHC and non-MHC genes. Among mice, strains of H-2s haplotype tend to be susceptible while H-2d strains are resistant. It is the MHC 1-A locus that dictates susceptibility. Although in humans drug-induced autoimmunity T cells appear silent, they are essential in mercury-induced disease in mice, since this does not occur in T-cell-deprived animals. Evidence that responding autoimmune B cells are activated polyclonally allows us to infer that they are being driven by a disproportionately active Th-2 subset of CD4 cells. Another feature of interest in metal-induced autoimmunity is the spontaneous autoregulation, with the model providing one of the most credible examples of the regulatory activity of suppressor T cells and antiidiotypic antibodies (Druet *et al.*, 1989; Pusey *et al.*, 1990).

It is our final prediction that no *single* extrinsic etiologic process will account for autoimmune disease; rather, the subtle balance between self-reactivity and self-tolerance [a.k.a. clonal balance (Rose *et al.*, 1981)] will be open to various types of perturbation, as illustrated by the above-cited examples, and by many of the diseases discussed in this volume. Over ninety years have passed since Metchnikoff in 1901 remarked: "Do diseases come from without, or do their causes arise within the organism is a pressing question long discussed by pathologists." For autoimmunity the question still applies, noting that intrinsic genetic susceptibility (lupus mice) and varied extrinsic provocations (microorganisms, chemicals, etc.) might have differing etiologic potencies in different situations. As a final reflection, the undeniable random "bad luck" component to autoimmunity could be determined environmentally, or be due to stochastic somatic genetic errors that accrue during cycles of replication and renewal of lymphoid cells.

REFERENCES

Acha-Orbea, H., Steinman, L., and McDevitt, H. O. (1989). *Ann. Rev. Immunol.* **7,** 371–405.

Agus, D. B., Surh, C. D., and Sprent, J. (1991). *J. Exp. Med.* **173,** 1039–1046.

Banga, J. P., and McGregor, A. M. (1991). *Autoimmunity* **9,** 177.

Benjamin, D. C., Berzofsky, J. A., East, I. J., *et al.* (1984). *Ann. Rev. Immunol.* **2,** 67.

Ben-Nun, A., Liblau, R. S., Cohen, L., Lehmann, D., Tournier-Lasserve, E., Rosenzweig, A., Zhang, J.-W., Raus, J. C. M., and Bach, M. A. (1991). *Proc. Natl. Acad. Sci. U.S.A.* **88,** 2466–2470.

Beverley, P. (1991). *Curr. Biol.* **3,** 355–360.

Boire, G., Lopez-Longo, F.-J., Lapointe, S., and Menard, H.-A. (1991). *Arthritis Rheum.* **34,** 722.

Boon, T., and Van Pel, A. (1989). *Immunogenetics* **29,** 75–79.

Burek, C. L., and Rose, N. R. (1986). *Human Pathol.* **17,** 246–253.

Burnet, F. M. (1962). *Australas. Ann. Med.* **11,** 79.

Candéias, S., Katz, J., Benoist, C., Mathis, D., and Haskins, K. (1991). *Proc. Natl. Acad. Sci. U.S.A.* **88,** 6167–6170.

Chan, E. K. L., and Tan, E. (1987). *J. Exp. Med.* **166,** 1627–1640.

Choi, Y., Kappler, J. W., and Marrack, P. (1991). *Nature* **350,** 203–207.

Cooke, A. (1991). *Clin. Exp. Immunol.* **83,** 345 346.

Cram, D. S., Fisicaro, N., Coppel, R. L., Whittingham, S., and Harrison, L. C. (1990). *J. Immunol.* **145,** 630–635.

Davies, T. F., Martin, A., Concepcion, E. S., Graves, P., Cohen, L., and Ben-Nun, A. (1991). *N. Engl. J. Med.* **325,** 238–244.

Dayan, C. M., Londei, M., Corcoran, A. E., Grubeck-Loebenstein, B., James, R. F. L., Rapoport, B., and Feldmann, M. (1991). *Proc. Natl. Acad. Sci. U.S.A.* **88,** 7415–7419.

Druet, P., Pelletier, L., Rossort, J., Druet, E., Hirsch, R., and Sapin, C. (1989). *In* "Autoimmunity and Toxicology; Immune Dysregulation Induced by Drugs and Chemicals," (M. E. Kammuller, N. Bloksma, and W. Seinen, eds.), 347–366. Elsevier, Amsterdam.

Emery, P., Gentry, K. C., Mackay, I. R., Muirden, K. D., and Rowley, M. (1987). *Arthritis Rheum.* **30,** 849–855.

Erikson, J., Radic, M. Z., Camper, S. A., Hardy, R. E., Carmack, C., and Weigert, M. (1991). *Nature* **349,** 331–334.

Festenstein, H. (1973). *Transplant. Rev.* **15,** 62–68.

Fischer Lindahl, K. (1991a). *Trends in Genetics* **7,** 219–224.

Fischer Lindahl, K. (1991b). *Immunogenetics* **34,** 1–4.

Flanagan, J. G. and Rabbitts, T. (1982). *Nature.* **300,** 709.
Franco, A., Barnaba, V., Kuberti, G., Venvenuto, R., Balsano, C., Musca, A. (1990). *Clin. Immunol. Immunopathol.* **54,** 382–394.
Friedman, S. M., Posnett, D. N., Tumang, J. R., Cole, B. C., and Crow, M. K. (1991). *Arthritis Rheum.* **34,** 468.
Gleeson, P. A., and Toh, B.-H. (1991). *Immunology Today* **12,** 233–238.
Goldman, M., Druet, P., and Gleichmann, E. (1991). *Immunology Today* **12,** 223–227.
Goter Robinson, C. J., Balazs, T., and Egorov, I. K. (1986). *Toxicol. Appl. Pharmacol.* **86,** 159–169.
Grinlinton, F. M., Lynch, N. M., and Hart, H. H. (1991). *Arthritis Rheum.* **34,** 916–919.
Hargraves, M. M., Richmond, H., and Morton, R. (1948). *Proc. Mayo Clinic* **23,** 25–28.
Harrington, W. J., Minnich, V., and Arimura, G. (1956). *Progress in Hematology, Vol. 1.*
(L. M. Tocantins, ed.). Grune and Stratton, New York, p. 156.
Heber-Katz, E., and Acha-Orbea, H. (1989). *Immunology Today* **10,** 164–169.
Horsfall, A. C., Hay, F. C., Soltys, A. J., and Jones, M. G. (1991). *Immunology Today* **12,** 211–213.
Huff, J. P., Roos, G., Peebles, C. L., Houghten, R., Sullivan, K. F., and Tan, E. (1990). *J. Exp. Med.* **172,** 419–429.
Janossiy, G., Panayi, G., Duke, O., Bofill, M., Poulter, L. W., and Goldstein, G. (1981). *Lancet* **ii,** 839–841.
Kappler, J. W., Roehm, N., and Marrack, P. (1987). *Cell* **49,** 273–280.
Kay, R. A., Hay, E. M., Dyer, P. A., Dennett, C., Green, L. M., Bernstein, R. M., Holt, P. J. L., Pumphrey, R. S. H., Boylston, R. W., and Ollier, W. E. R. (1991). *Clin. Exp. Immunol.* **85,** 262–264.
Kingsley, G., Panayi, G., and Lauchbury, J. (1991). *Immunology Today* **12,** 177–179.
Kion, T. A., and Hoffman, G. W. (1991). *Science* **253,** 1138–1140.
Kopelman, R. G., and Zoller-Pazner, S. (1988). *Am. J. Med.* **84,** 82–88.
Krause, A., Brade, V., Schoerner, C., Solbach, W., Kalden, J. R., and Burmester, G. (1991). *Arthritis Rheum.* **34,** 393.
Lacour, M., Rudolphi, U., Schlesier, M., and Peter, H. H. (1990). *Eur. J. Immunol.* **20,** 931.
Laver, W. G., Air, G. M., Webster, R. G., and Smith-Gill, S. J. (1990). *Cell* **61,** 553–556.
Lenzi, M., Johnson, P. J., McFarlane, I. G., *et al.* (1991). *Lancet* **338,** 277–280.
Liblau, R., Tournier-Lasserve, E., Maccazek, J., Dumas, G., Siffert, O., Hashem, G., and Bach, M. A. (1991). *Eur. J. Immunol.* **21,** 1391–1395.
Link, H., Olsson, O., Sun, J., Wang, W.-Z., Andersson, G., Ekre, H.-P. (1990). *J. Clin. Invest.,* **87,** 2191–2196.
Londei, M., Savill, C. M., Verhoef, A., Brennan, F., Leech, Z. A., Duance, V., Maini, R. N., and Feldmann, M. (1989). *Proc. Natl. Acad. Sci. USA,* **86,** 636–640.
Loveland, B. E., and Fischer Lindahl, K. (1991). *In* "Antigen Processing and Recognition" (J. McCluskey, ed.), 172–187. Academic Press, Boca Raton, FL.
Loveland, B. E., Wang, C. R., Yonekawa, H., Hermel, E., and Fischer Lindahl, K. (1990). *Cell* **60,** 971–980.
Mackay, C. R. (1991). *Immunology Today* **12,** 189–192.
Mackay, C. R., Marston, W. L., Dudler, L., Spertini, O., Tedder, T. F., and Hein, W. R. (1992). *Eur. J. Immunol.* In press.
Mackay, I. R., Rowley, M., Loveland, B., and Marzuki, S. (1990). *Immunogenetics* **31,** 61–62.
Manolios, N., Geczy, C., and Schreiber, L. (1991). *Sem. Arthritis Rheum.* **20,** 339–352.
McNeilage, L. J., Macmillan, E. M., and Whittingham, S. F. (1990). *J. Immunol.* **145,** 3829–3835.
Meyer zum Büschenfelde, K.-H., Knolle, J., and Berger, J. (1974). *Klin. Wochenschr.* **52,** 246–248.
Michl, J., Qui, Q.-Y., and Kuerer, H. M. (1991). *Curr. Biol.* **3,** 373–382.

Miller, J. F. A. P., and Morahan, G. (1992). *Ann. Rev. Immunol.* **10,** (in press).

Mitchison. N. A. (1991). *Curr. Biol.* **1,** 87–88.

Nerup, J., Mandrup-Poulsen, T., and Molvig, J. (1987). *Diabetes/Metabolism Rev.* **3,** 779–802.

O'Brien, R. M., Cram, D. S., Coppel, R. L., and Harrison, L. C. (1990). *J. Autoimmunity* **3,** 747–757.

Oksenberg, J. R., Stuart, S., Begovich, A. B., Bell, R. B., Erlich, H. A., Steinman, L., and Bernard, C. C. A. (1990). *Nature* **345,** 344.

Oshima, M., Ashizawa, T., Pollack, M. S., and Atassi, M. Z. (1990). *Eur. J. Immunol.* **20,** 2563–2569.

Outschoorn, I., Rowley, M. J., Cooke, A. D., and Mackay, I. R. (Submitted).

Patarroyo, M. (1991). *Clin. Immunol. Immunopathol.* **60,** 333–348.

Paliard, X., West, S. G., Lafferty, J. A., Clements, J. R., Kappler, J. W., Marrack, P., and Kotzin, B. L. (1991). *Science* **253,** 325–329.

Picker, L. J., Kishimoto, T. K., Smith, C. W., Warnock, R. A., and Butcher, E. C. (1991). *Nature* **349,** 796–799.

Protti, M. P., Manfredi, A. A., Straub, C., Wu, X.-D., Howard, J. F., Jr., and Conti-Tronconi, B. M. (1990). *J. Immunol.* **144,** 1711–1720.

Pusey, C. D., Bowman, C., Morgan, A., Weetman, A. P., Hartley, B., and Lockwood, C. M. (1990). *Clin. Exp. Immunol.* **81,** 76–82.

Reich, E. P., Sherwin, R. S., Kanagawa, O., and Janeway, C. A., Jr. (1989). *Nature* **341,** 326.

Roitt, I. M. (1984). *Triangle* **23,** 67–76.

Rose, N. R. (1991a). *Immunology Today* **12,** 167–168.

Rose, N. R. (1991b). *J. Immunol. Res.* **3,** 37–42.

Rose, N. R., Kong, Y. M., Okayasu, I., Giraldo, A. A., Beisel, K., and Sundick, R. S. (1981). *Immunol. Rev.* **55,** 299–314.

Rowley, M. J., Maeda, T., Mackay, I. R., Loveland, B. E., McMullen, G. L., Tribbick, G., and Bernard, C. C. A. (Submitted).

Rowley, M. J., McNeilage, L. J., Armstrong, J. McD., and Mackay, I. R. (1991). *Clin. Immunol. Immunopathol.* **60,** 356–370.

Schultz, C. L., and Coffmann, R. L. (1991). *Curr. Opinion in Immunol.* **3,** 350–354.

Schwartz, R. S. (1991). *Curr. Biol.,* **1,** 180–181.

Sinha, A. A., Lopez, M. T., And McDevitt, H. O. (1990). *Science* **248,** 1380–1384.

Sottini, A., Imberti, L., Gorla, R., Cattaneo, R., and Primi, D. (1991). *Eur. J. Immunol.* **21,** 461–466.

Strasser, A., Whittingham, S., Vaux, D. L., Bath, M. L., Adams, J. M., Cory, S., and Harris, A. W. (1991). *Proc. Natl. Acad. Sci. USA* **88,** 8661–8665.

Surh, C. D., Cooper, A. E., Coppel, R. L., Leung, P., Ahmed, A., Dickson, R., and Gershwin, M. E. (1988). *Hepatology* **8,** 290–295.

Tandon, N., Freeman, M., and Weetman, A. P. (1991). *Clin. Exp. Immunol.* **86,** 56–60.

Vainiene, M., Offner, H., Morrison, W. J., Wilkinson, M., and Vandenbark, A. A. (1991). *J. Neuroimmunol.* **33,** 207–216.

Valenta, R., Duchêne, M., Pettenburger, K., *et al.* (1991). *Science* **253,** 557–559.

Van de Water, J., Ansari, A. A., Surh, C. D., Coppel, R., Roche, T., Bonkovsky, H., Kaplan, M., and Gershwin, M. E. (1991). *J. Immunol.* **146,** 89–94.

Von Boehmer, H. (1989). *Immunology Today* **10,** 57–61.

Whittingham, S., Youngchaiyud, U., Mackay, I. R., Buckley, J. D., and Morris, P. J. (1975). *Clin. Exp. Immunol.* **19,** 289–299.

Witebsky, E. (1929). *Naturwissenschaften* **17,** 771.

Wucherpfennig, K. W., Weiner, H. L., and Hafler, D. A. (1991). *Immunology Today* **12,** 277–282.

Young, L. E., Miller, G., and Christian, R. M. (1951). *Ann. Intern. Med.* **35,** 507.

Yount, W. J., Cohen, P., and Eisenberg, R. A. (1988). *Monogr. Allergy* **23,** 41–56.

Zinkernagel, R. M., Pircher, H. P., Ohashi, P., Oehen, S., Odermatt, B., Mak, T., Arnheiter, H., Bürki, K., and Hengartner, H. (1991). *Immunol. Rev.* **122,** 133–171.

Index

B

J

K

L

M

N

U